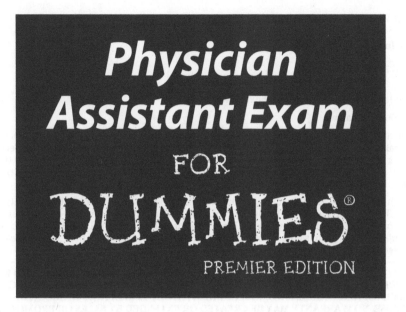

Physician Assistant Exam

FOR

DUMMIES®

PREMIER EDITION

by Dr. Rich Snyder, DO, and Barry Schoenborn

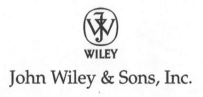

WILEY

John Wiley & Sons, Inc.

Physician Assistant Exam For Dummies® Premier Edition

Published by
John Wiley & Sons, Inc.
111 River St.
Hoboken, NJ 07030-5774
www.wiley.com

About the Authors

Dr. Rich Snyder, DO, is an osteopathic physician who resides in Easton, Pennsylvania. He's a kidney specialist, board-certified in both internal medicine and nephrology. He did his internal medicine residency at Abington Memorial Hospital and completed both clinical and research fellowships in nephrology at the Hospital of the University of Pennsylvania. He also has experience in graduate medical education. As a former associate program director and osteopathic program director at Easton Hospital, he was responsible for both the administration and education of medical residents and medical students.

In addition to maintaining a full-time clinical practice at Lehigh Valley Nephrology Associates, he has authored and co-authored several articles in peer-reviewed journals, including the *American Journal of Kidney Disease* and *Kidney International.* He has also presented at national meetings, including the National Kidney Foundation's Annual Meeting. In addition to being a coauthor of *Medical Dosage Calculations For Dummies,* he has written the books *What You Must Know about Kidney Disease: A Practical Guide to Using Conventional and Complementary Treatments* and *What You Must Know about Dialysis: Ten Secrets to Surviving and Thriving on Dialysis.*

He's also been interviewed regionally and nationally on radio and television about integrative medicine and kidney disease. He can be heard weekly on his show, *Improve Your Kidney Health,* on VoiceAmerica Radio Health & Wellness channel.

Barry Schoenborn lives in Nevada City, California. He's a longtime technical and science writer with more than 35 years of experience. He's written hundreds of user manuals. In the past, Barry's technical writing company worked with the State of California agency CalRecycle to teach scientists and administrators how to write clearly.

Barry's the co-author of *Technical Math For Dummies, Medical Dosage Calculations For Dummies,* and *Storage Area Networks: Designing and Implementing a Mass Storage System.*

He was a movie reviewer for the Los Angeles *Herald-Dispatch* newspaper and wrote a monthly political newspaper column for *The Union* newspaper of Grass Valley, California, for seven years. Barry's publishing company, Willow Valley Press, published *Dandelion Through the Crack: The Sato Family Quest for the American Dream,* which won the 2008 William Saroyan International Prize for Writing.

Dedications

Rich Snyder: This book I dedicate to my mother, Nancy Snyder, a registered nurse and constant source of inspiration and encouragement.

I also dedicate this book to Patty Paul, RN. I speak for everyone at Lehigh Valley Nephrology Associates when I say that you live on in our hearts and minds. Your daughter-in-law, Donielle Paul, PA-C, embodies those same important qualities: kindness, compassion, and a commitment to medical excellence. We are lucky to have her with us in LVNA.

I finally dedicate this book to physician assistants everywhere. Thank you for your decision to work in the medical profession. It is a noble profession, and we thank you.

Barry Schoenborn: I dedicate this book to Frances H. Kakugawa, perhaps the most inspiring person I've ever met. She's the author of ten books, three of which (*Breaking the Silence: A Caregiver's Voice, Mosaic Moon: Caregiving Through Poetry,* and *Wordsworth Dances the Waltz*) have helped hundreds of Alzheimer's caregivers find courage and strength.

This excellent author-poet conducts classes in poetry and journaling for caregivers. In her unique way, she has improved the quality of care for countless Alzheimer's sufferers.

Authors' Acknowledgments

Rich Snyder: I would not have been able to write this book without the heroic efforts of Barry Schoenborn. He is a gifted writer, and his brilliance is outshined only by his great sense of humor. I want to thank Vicki Adang for her help and guidance as well as all of the great editors we had the privilege of working with. I also want to thank Matt Wagner of Fresh Books for being in our corner.

Finally, I would like to thank everyone at Lehigh Valley Nephrology Associates for being the great people they are to work with. Many happy years to come!

Barry Schoenborn: This book wouldn't have been possible without the Herculean efforts of co-author Rich Snyder. It's amazing how much he knows! We were supported by a great team at John Wiley & Sons (Vicki Adang, Danielle Voirol, Jessica Smith, and Tracy Boggier) who worked hard to make this book a reality. They're very talented and also happen to be the nicest people you'll ever meet! Many thanks to our technical editors, Antoinette Polito and Jennifer Snyder. A big thanks, too, to Matt Wagner of Fresh Books Literary Agency, who presented us to Wiley.

Rich and I also are grateful to Intermountain Healthcare and Frank G. Yanowitz, MD, professor of medicine, University of Utah School of Medicine, and medical director, ECG Department, LDS Hospital, Salt Lake City, Utah, for their generosity and permission to use the electrocardiogram materials.

Publisher's Acknowledgments

We're proud of this book; please send us your comments at http://dummies.custhelp.com. For other comments, please contact our Customer Care Department within the U.S. at 877-762-2974, outside the U.S. at 317-572-3993, or fax 317-572-4002.

Some of the people who helped bring this book to market include the following:

Acquisitions, Editorial, and Vertical Websites

Senior Project Editor: Victoria M. Adang

Acquisitions Editor: Tracy Boggier

Senior Copy Editor: Danielle Voirol

Copy Editor: Jessica Smith

Assistant Editor: David Lutton

Editorial Program Coordinator: Joe Niesen

Technical Editors: Antoinette M. Polito, MHS, PA-C; Jennifer A. Snyder, PA-C, DFAAPA

Vertical Websites: Laura Moss-Hollister, Rich Graves, Shawn Patrick

Editorial Manager: Michelle Hacker

Editorial Assistants: Rachelle Amick, Alexa Koschier

Art Coordinator: Alicia B. South

Cover Photo: © iStockphoto.com/Maksim Belyy; © iStockphoto.com/rzdeb

Cartoons: Rich Tennant (www.the5thwave.com)

Composition Services

Project Coordinator: Bill Ramsey

Layout and Graphics: Carl Byers, Carrie A. Cesavice

Proofreaders: Rebecca Denoncour, Lauren Mandelbaum

Indexer: Potomac Indexing, LLC

Publishing and Editorial for Consumer Dummies

   Kathleen Nebenhaus, Vice President and Executive Publisher

   David Palmer, Associate Publisher

   Kristin Ferguson-Wagstaffe, Product Development Director

Publishing for Technology Dummies

   Andy Cummings, Vice President and Publisher

Composition Services

   Debbie Stailey, Director of Composition Services

Contents at a Glance

Table of Contents

Introduction

*Y*ou couldn't ask for a better career than that of a physician assistant (PA). The PA's importance has increased and will continue to increase as healthcare expands. This is especially true in the United States, where people express great concern about providing affordable healthcare for everyone. The doctors can't get there without physician assistants.

To become a physician assistant, you have to pass the Physician Assistant National Certifying Examination (the PANCE). Established PAs must periodically take the Physician Assistant National Recertifying Examination (the PANRE). That's why we wrote this book.

The vast majority of medical diagnostic and treatment scenarios are simple when you're in command of the facts, but you see a lot of overlap in symptoms and alternate choices in treatment. And in the practice of medicine, there's a lot to watch out for. For example, even the noblest treatment may produce electrolyte imbalances or other unforeseen conditions. Even the most effective medications may have unwanted side effects.

Our goal is to give you the best collection of review and test-preparation information you need to pass the PANCE or PANRE without excessive stress and strain. A valuable bonus is that we've included lots of excellent information you can use in your everyday practice.

About This Book

Physician Assistant Exam For Dummies, Premier Edition, puts out a lot of medical information in just a few chapters and in very compact form. This book is a reference, so you can jump in anywhere you like. It's also a repair manual, because it can fill voids you may have in your scholastic background. You can find some unique features here:

- ✔ **This book uses language you'll understand.** When Dr. Rich Snyder says, "This is a bad thing," you immediately get the message. Many medical terms come with brief definitions. Those terms include symptoms, conditions, bacteria and viruses, generic and brand-name medication names, technical words, slang, and abbreviations.

- ✔ **We cover symptoms, diagnosis, testing, and dosing in the context of *both* test preparation and clinical practice.** The emphasis is on test prep, but we wouldn't be doing our job if we didn't talk about real life. We cover countless useful techniques, such as ordering that additional *definitive* test, ordering the best imaging, knowing first-line and second-line treatments, and following a patient's progress on various meds. The scenarios we describe are based on classic presentations and are likely to appear on the PANCE or PANRE. Many examples are based on real-life experiences.

   Nonetheless, this book is a *test-preparation book*. We've put in huge amounts of information applicable to daily clinical practice, but in the main, we've focused on your managing the PANCE or PANRE. You'll see numerous conditions in clinical practice over the years, but if they aren't likely to appear on the test, we've had to omit them.

- ✔ **We include practice questions to test your knowledge in nearly every chapter.** After answering a question, make sure to read the answer explanation, even if you chose the correct answer, because this book educates through wrong answers as well as correct ones. We've put in abundant information about why the wrong answers are wrong.

✔ **We give you one complete practice exam in the book and four additional digital full-length tests.** These tests, which are available on the CD accompanying this book or via download (if you're using a digital version of this book), provide you with even more practice so you're ready to go on test day.

✔ **You see an insight or two from a doctor, who (sadly) treats patients with advanced conditions.** Many of these patients are older, with multiple afflictions. Barry will be the first to tell you that he wouldn't trade places with Rich for the proverbial million bucks.

✔ **This book isn't dull (we hope), as other test prep books tend to be.** Because it's a *For Dummies* book, you can be sure that it's relatively lively and easy to read. The only reason this book doesn't have a lot of light moments is that so much in medicine isn't funny. When people may die, we don't make jokes.

Conventions Used in This Book

We designed this book to be user-friendly, maybe even user-affectionate. The subject matter is quite challenging, so we don't think you need a book that's hard to read. We use the following conventions:

✔ When talking about exam topics, we often use *PANCE* as shorthand to refer to both the PANCE and the PANRE. Reading "PANCE or PANRE" all the time gets a little tedious.

✔ *Italic type* highlights new terms, bacteria names, and virus names. Once in a great while, we use italics for emphasis.

✔ Whenever possible, we provide alternate names for disease conditions, signs, or tests. For example, *otitis externa* is also known as *external otitis* and *swimmer's ear*.

✔ Each drug name appears first with its generic name and then with a commercial brand name in parentheses. For example, we say "hydrocodone (Vicodin)" to show you both the generic name and the brand name. In some cases, only the generic form is available. However, when you take the PANCE or PANRE, the questions include only the generic drug name, so make sure you know generic names as well as you know your own.

✔ We usually write numbers as numerals, not words. For example, the text says "vaccinate at ages 3 months and 6 months," not "vaccinate at ages three months and six months." The same idea applies to units. We write "g," not "gram." We write "dL," not "deciliter," wherever possible. And we also include the greater-than and less-than symbols in text. Why? Because we want to give you the numbers and units as you'll see them every day in your career.

✔ Web addresses are in `monofont`. If the address breaks across two lines of text, no extra characters indicate the break. Just type what you see into your browser.

What You're Not to Read

We'd love you to read all the words in this book in the order in which they appear, but life is short. You don't have to read chapters that don't interest you. This book is a reference book, and it's designed to let you read only the parts you need.

Sidebars (that's what they're called in publishing) are the blocks of text that have a gray background. They're interesting and highly useful in your understanding of the main text, but they contain info that isn't essential to the topic at hand. You're under no obligation to read them.

Foolish Assumptions

In writing this book, we had to make a few assumptions about you:

✔ **You're getting ready to take the PANCE or PANRE.** You're nearing completion of a two-year or three-year PA program, and all indications are that you'll successfully complete your coursework and are ready to sit for the PANCE. Or if you're already working as a PA, we assume that it's time for you to take the PANRE.

✔ **You got a full exposure to medical concepts via your textbooks, your lectures, and your rotations.** If you're prepping for the PANCE, we assume you've had a quality education. If you're going to take the PANRE, we assume you've been in the trenches for several years.

✔ **You have access to detailed medical texts.** Remember, this book is largely a review. We can't stuff all things medicine into one volume, so consult your texts when you need to.

✔ **You want to take some practice exams.** We include a printed exam in the book and four addition digital exams on the companion CD or via download (if you have a digital version of this book).

How This Book Is Organized

This book has seven parts. After the introductory chapters, we concentrate on all major body organ systems. Some chapters are longer than others because the PANCE and PANRE devote more questions to them.

Part 1: Scratching the Surface of the PANCE and PANRE

Part I gives you an overview of the PA exams. It deals with test-taking procedures and strategies you can use to ensure success. We describe the importance of the tests and what you need to do after the test to become a fully certified and licensed PA. Then we offer tips for preparing for the test and tell you what to expect on test day. We also give you some insights into the test — the breakdown of the questions, how the test is scored, that kind of stuff.

Part II: Getting to the Heart of the Test: Four Foundational Systems

Four topics — cardio, pulmonary, the gastrointestinal system, and bones and joints — make up approximately half the questions on the PANCE, so we devote Part II to these vital organ systems.

Part III: Reviewing Surgical Topics and Other Organ Systems

Part III contains chapters about surgery; the genitourinary system; the eyes, ears, nose, and throat; and reproductive medicine. These topics yield a fair number of questions on the test, though not quite as many as the topics in Part II.

Part IV: Pursuing Primary Care, Pharmacology, and Behavioral Health

Part IV addresses special medical topics: pediatrics, health maintenance and medical ethics, behavioral health and psychiatry, and pharmacology and toxicology. You'll likely encounter a couple of questions on each of these topics on the test.

Part V: The Brain, Blood, Bugs, Skin, and Glands

Part V provides a review of the endocrine system, hematology and oncology, neurology, dermatology, and infectious diseases. These topics won't constitute a big portion of the exam, but they'll be represented.

Part VI: Tackling a PANCE Practice Test

When you're ready to tackle PANCE questions, flip to Part VI. You find a complete 300-question PANCE practice examination in Chapter 20. Chapter 21 explains the correct answers and why the other answer choices are incorrect.

Part VII: The Part of Tens

The three chapters in the Part of Tens are filled with useful information in compact form. We cover medical triads, common medical abbreviations, and mistakes that test-takers make.

CD-ROM

The companion CD contains four practice tests: three PANCEs and one PANRE. You can take timed versions of all four tests to simulate the real testing experience, or you can take untimed versions of two of the PANCE practice tests for extra practice and review of the material. We've also included more than 300 flashcards that cover facts related to each of the 13 categories tested on the PANCE. Finally, you can find a slideshow of dermatologic conditions that you should be able to identify on sight. We give you more detailed information about the CD in the appendix. *Note:* If you're using a digital version of this book, please go to http://booksupport.wiley.com for access to the additional content.

Icons Used in This Book

Icons are the drawings in the margins of this book, and we use several icons to call out special kinds of information.

Examples are sample test questions that appear at the ends of sections and that highlight particular conditions or diseases. We provide an answer and explanation immediately after the question. (And there's more — at the end of a chapter, you usually find six numbered sample questions, which we don't mark with the icon because they're in their own practice-questions section.)

The Remember icon points out something you should keep in mind, whether you're taking the exam or examining and treating a patient.

A Tip is a suggestion that usually points out a trick for remembering information for the test or a quick and easy way to get things done.

The Warning icon flags a serious situation where you should exercise care and perhaps seek additional advice. Numerous diagnostic situations can be critical to the well-being of the patient, and you need to be aware of them.

Where to Go from Here

You can go to any chapter from here. The book isn't linear, so you can start anywhere. First, check the table of contents for the names of the parts and the chapters. Then pick any chapter you're interested in. If you can't decide, begin with Chapter 1 — it includes broad concepts about the PANCE and PANRE and becoming a PA, and you'll probably need to read it at some point. If you have a particular body organ system you want to concentrate on, such as the cardiovascular system (Chapter 3) or the genitourinary system (Chapter 10), go straight to it. We give you an index, too, at the back of the book. Or, if you'd like, you can take one of the tests to see how well you do and figure out what you need to brush up on.

Part I

Scratching the Surface of the PANCE and PANRE

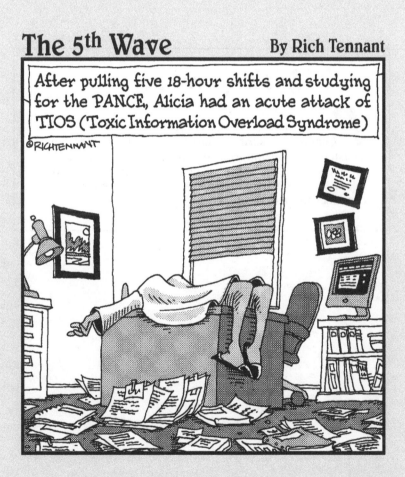

The 5th Wave   By Rich Tennant

After pulling five 18-hour shifts and studying for the PANCE, Alicia had an acute attack of TIOS (Toxic Information Overload Syndrome)

In this part . . .

Part I is an overview of the PANCE and PANRE. Chapter 1 describes steps to becoming a physician assistant and the importance of the exams. Chapter 2 gives you details about the process of preparing for and taking the test. It includes the basic techniques for succeeding with test questions.

Chapter 1

Becoming a Physician Assistant

In This Chapter

▶ Going from student to physician assistant

▶ Preparing for the PANCE or PANRE

*P*hysician assistants have been around since the 1960s. Dr. Charles Hudson suggested the idea to the American Medical Association in 1961. Then Dr. Eugene Stead Jr. of the Duke University Medical Center assembled a class made up of U.S. Navy hospital corpsmen and applied techniques he had learned about fast-tracking doctors in World War II. The first class graduated in 1967.

To become a physician assistant today, you have to take and pass the Physician Assistant National Certifying Examination (PANCE). And to continue working in the field, you have to be recertified every 6 years by taking and passing the Physician Assistant National Recertifying Examination (PANRE). (Starting in 2014, recertification will be required every 10 years.) These tests are tough — they're lengthy and have challenging questions. But if you prepare well, you'll have a surprisingly easy time, and we're confident that you'll rise to the challenge.

This chapter gives you a quick overview of what a physician assistant does. It also outlines the PANCE and PANRE.

Knowing What to Expect as a PA

A *physician assistant* (PA) is a well-educated healthcare professional who is nationally certified and licensed by the state in which he or she practices. The PA practices medicine under the supervision of a physician. A physician assistant can have a large degree of autonomy, depending on his or her experience and the doctor's willingness to delegate.

PAs prevent, diagnose, and treat illness and injury by providing many healthcare services, including the following:

✔ Conducting physical exams

✔ Ordering and interpreting tests

✔ Counseling people on preventive healthcare

✔ Assisting in surgery

✔ Writing prescriptions

If you see the letters PA after a person's name, that means *physician assistant*.

In this section, we discuss PA education programs, steps to take after you receive your certification, and your job prospects as a PA.

Training to become a PA

To become a PA, you must pass the PANCE. But first, you need to get an education through an accredited PA program. Currently, the United States has more than 160 such programs. The program at Duke University in North Carolina is probably best known because the nation's first PAs were trained at and graduated from Duke.

PA training at the graduate level takes 2 to 3 years and involves a combination of classroom studies and clinical rotations. Admissions departments are selective, and for many programs, your GRE score must be relatively high. So why do we say this? It's a confidence builder. If you survived PA education and training, you're more than capable of acing the PANCE!

What you do when you're a PA

After you're certified as a physician assistant, you have to fulfill some legal requirements, keep up with medical developments, and celebrate your profession, all the while treating patients. Here's a quick list of things to do:

- ✔ Get a license.
- ✔ Get a job as a physician assistant and put all your training to good use caring for patients.
- ✔ Get professional liability insurance.
- ✔ Register with the Drug Enforcement Administration (DEA), as needed.
- ✔ If you're in the United States, join the American Academy of Physician Assistants (www.aapa.org).
- ✔ Earn and report 100 hours of continuing medical education (CME) hours every 2 years. You can obtain CME hours by attending seminars, journal reading, and online study. Many PAs choose to attend a conference to obtain most or all of their CME credits.
- ✔ Celebrate National Physician Assistant Week on October 6 through October 12. October 6 is the day the first PA class graduated at Duke University and just happens to be the birthday of Dr. Eugene Stead, creator of the PA program.
- ✔ Reregister your certificate with NCCPA (National Commission on Certification of Physician Assistants) every 2 years.
- ✔ Take the PANRE after 6 years (or 10 years starting in 2014).

Employers often pay for the PA's professional liability insurance, registration fees with the DEA, state licensing fees, and credentialing fees.

Sizing up your prospects

So after you've gone through years of training and hours of testing, will you be able to find a job? Yes, most likely. Will it pay well? Yes, relatively so. Given that most PA programs in colleges and universities charge pretty high tuition, you'll need a good job.

In its 2010 census report, the American Academy of Physician Assistants reported that the median income for PAs ranged from $85,000 to $101,000. Income varies depending on experience, specialty, practice setting, and location.

The U.S. Bureau of Labor Statistics (www.bls.gov) indicates the following:

✔ Employment of PAs is expected to grow by 39 percent from 2008 to 2018, much faster than the average for all occupations.

✔ More PAs will provide primary care and assist with medical and surgical procedures because PAs are "cost-effective and productive members of the healthcare team." Cost containment is likely to be a factor. States will continue to expand the PA's scope of practice by allowing them to perform more procedures.

✔ Besides working in traditional office-based settings, PAs should find a growing number of jobs in hospitals, academic medical centers, public clinics, and prisons. Job opportunities should also be good in rural and inner-city healthcare facilities.

These days, a physician in private practice can't function without a PA or a nurse practitioner (NP), and the ever-increasing healthcare demands of public institutions, hospitals, and clinics should ensure job security.

Introducing the Tests

The National Commission on Certification of Physician Assistants administers the two tests that are required of PAs: the PANCE, which certifies you to work as a PA, and the PANRE, which you take every 6 years (or 10 years starting in 2014) for recertification. In this section, we provide a quick overview of each test. We give you more details about applying for and taking the tests, as well as their content, in Chapter 2.

Getting your PANCE on

The PANCE is the essential exam for certification, and certification is essential for licensure. This exam has 300 questions and takes 5 hours to complete, not including breaks.

The PANCE is a testimonial to your knowledge. Doctors and nurses take qualifying examinations, so for a PA, certification is expected, too. This tells the world you're ready to do the work.

A few simple — but not easy — steps are involved in preparing for the PANCE. You've already accomplished the first few items:

✔ Enter a PA program at an accredited school.

✔ Take the classes and do the clinical rotations.

✔ Buy an excellent test preparation book. Why, that's what's in your hands!

✔ Begin a concerted program of test preparation based on the medical facts and the sample questions in this book. This book is as much about strategies for approaching test questions as it is about medical topics.

What's your specialty? Earning a CAQ

A practicing PA can earn a Certificate of Added Qualification, or CAQ. This certificate recognizes the PA for advanced knowledge and a skill set in a particular specialty. Current CAQ specialties include nephrology, orthopedic surgery, cardiothoracic surgery, emergency medicine, and psychiatry. Here are the requirements for the CAQ:

✔ Having worked the equivalent of 2 years full time as a PA with at least 50 percent of that time spent in that particular specialty

✔ Obtaining continuing medical education (CME) hours that are specific to the specialty

✔ Having a supervising physician write a letter of support stating a high level of performance

✔ Taking a multiple-choice examination of 120 questions in that specialty area

Reviewing for the PANRE

The Physician Assistant National Recertifying Examination (PANRE) is just what it says — a periodic recertifying examination that ensures that your knowledge is up to date. Every 6 years, a PA must successfully complete the PANRE. This test has 240 questions (instead of the PANCE's 300), and there are four test blocks instead of five. You still average, however, about a minute per question (60 questions in 60 minutes).

The PANRE offers you content options. About 60 percent is the same generalist exam as the PANCE, but you choose the emphasis of the other 40 percent. Here are your three options:

✔ Adult medicine

✔ Surgery

✔ Primary care

A recertifying PA may want to choose adult medicine or surgery if that's where he or she works. If you choose primary care, then the PANRE content won't be at all different from the PANCE. And even if you choose the surgery or the adult medicine option, a large portion of the examination will still contain general medicine questions.

Chapter 2

Presenting the PANCE and PANRE

* *

* *

The logistics of the PANCE and PANRE are well-documented, and so are the test structures and the question structures. Take a careful look at the logistics and structures, because knowledge of both is essential to doing your best on the tests. *Logistics* comprises all the administrative details before, during, and after the test. *Structure* is all about the mix of questions and the rather predictable structure of the questions. By studying structure, you acquire two valuable skills: the ability to balance your preparation to take advantage of the question mix and the ability to quickly identify and process different question structures during the test.

You don't want to mess up the test because of a misunderstanding about administrative details, and of course there's no reason to go into the test without fully understanding how the questions work. We cover both logistics and structure in this chapter.

Beyond Studying: Preparing to Take the PANCE or PANRE

In most cases, the logistics of applying for the tests are straightforward. If your situation is different — for example, if you're not a recent graduate from a PA program — consult the PANCE pages on the website for the National Commission on Certification of Physician Assistants (www.nccpa.net/Pance.aspx).

Applying to take the test

Before you can take the PANCE, you need to graduate from an accredited PA program. About 3 months before you graduate, go online and apply to take the test. Visit https://www.nccpa.net/PA/LoginNew.aspx to create an online account. Then follow the directions for registering and pay the $475 fee.

Your school's PA program confirms your eligibility. After NCCPA gets your application and your money, you receive an acknowledgment in about 3 to 5 business days. That acknowledgment includes instructions for scheduling your test at a Pearson VUE test center (www.vue.com/nccpa/). You choose the test date and the location. You can first take the test as soon as 7 days after you graduate or up to 6 months later.

If you're already a physician assistant, you need to take and pass the PANRE before your 6-year (or 10-year) PA certification expires. You can take the test in year 5 or 6. You have four chances to pass — two per year. The process is the same as for the PANCE — apply online to take the test and pay the $350 fee. Soon after, you can choose a test date and test center location.

If you're a recertifying PA, don't wait too long in your 6th year to apply. If you apply less than 45 days before your certification expires, you'll have to do extra work, such as submitting the application manually and getting a waiver (written permission) from NCCPA.

Locating the test center

You take the PANCE or PANRE at a Pearson VUE testing center. Pearson VUE has about 200 test centers in the United States, so make sure you know where your test center is. For example, co-author Barry lives in Nevada City, California, which is 65 miles northeast of Sacramento. Sacramento has *two* Pearson testing centers, and one of them is called a "Sacramento" center even though it's in Roseville, California. It would be best if Barry located the test center exactly, or he'd risk doing something really dumb, like going to the wrong one. Co-author Rich lives in Easton, Pennsylvania. He'd have to drive down to Allentown, a good 25 miles away, if he were taking one of the tests.

Drive to the test center some days before the test, and when you do, consider the traffic patterns for the morning you'll be traveling to the test center.

Chillaxing before the test

You worked your gluteus maximus off to prepare, and you did all the administrative steps correctly. So on the day before the test, you might as well relax. Here are some tips to help you stay cool:

- ✔ Make sure you have plenty of gasoline in the car.
- ✔ Avoid foods that will mess up your GI tract the following morning. You don't want a case of the dire rear (diarrhea).
- ✔ Meditate, don't medicate. Take deep, cleansing breaths. This isn't a good time to booze it up.
- ✔ Set your alarm clock.
- ✔ Get a good night's sleep.

If you feel you must study, look at common medical triads, common abbreviations, and common test-taker mistakes. We give you this info in Chapters 22, 23, and 24. And if you feel the need to get in a last-minute review, then use the handy-dandy digital flashcards that came with this book.

Making It through Test Day

When the day you're scheduled to take the PANCE or PANRE arrives, stay calm. Eat a good breakfast. Take a deep breath every so often. Then head out the door knowing you've done everything you can to ace the exam. Here's what you can expect after you leave the house.

Planning for a timely arrival

On the day of the test, give yourself plenty of time to get to the test center. You never know what sort of traffic jams, detours, or acts of God you may face during your drive. Make sure you know where you're going, what time you need to arrive, and how long getting there takes. Plan to arrive at the test center about 30 minutes before the scheduled testing time.

The testers won't accept "the freeway ate my drive time" as an excuse. Don't be late to your test, and above all, don't go to the wrong test center. There's a cutoff time for checking in, and if you arrive too late, you won't be admitted. You'll forfeit your fee and you'll have to reapply — and pay for the exam again!

Oh, and please don't go there on the *wrong day*. Such things have happened before.

Getting in the door

Checking in to take the PANCE or PANRE is roughly equivalent to boarding a commercial airline flight, except you don't have to submit to a random search. When you arrive at the test center, you must show two forms of valid, current identification. One ID must have a "permanently affixed photo with your printed name and signature," and the second ID must have your printed name and signature. The first amounts to a driver's license, a passport, or a military ID. The second one can be just about anything.

You won't get in if the names on your IDs don't match or if they're different from your name as listed in NCCPA's record. These are not trusting people, folks — they fear that you'll send in a ringer to take the test for you. You should expect to be subjected to a digital fingerprint or palm scan and to be photographed.

Knowing what's allowed in the testing room

The list of things that the test administrators *do* and *don't* allow is unfortunately long. Get ready. The NCCPA website informs you about these restrictions numerous times.

Items that are disallowed

You can't take paper, pens, pencils, calculators, watches, cell phones, and other gadgets into the test room. Bring nothing personal into the test room except essential medical aids and the clothes on your back.

You receive a locker outside of the test room to store your personal items. Although snacks aren't allowed in the test room, bring along some fruit, nuts, or whatever munchies you need to make it through a long day, and store them in your locker. You'll be at the test center for at least 5 or 6 hours and will need to maintain your energy. You can access your locker during breaks in the test.

Items that are allowed

You can bring in some medical aids without applying for a special dispensation. Just as when you travel by air, pack your small items in a plastic bag no bigger than quart size. Acceptable items that need to go in a bag include the following:

- Tissues
- Cough drops or pills (must be unwrapped and not in a bottle/container)
- Eye drops

✔ Hearing aids

✔ Earplugs (or the proctor can provide you with a set of disposable earplugs)

✔ Eyeglasses (without the case)

✔ An inhaler

✔ A paper face mask

✔ A glucose meter

Here are some allowable items that don't need to be in the bag:

✔ A pillow for supporting your neck, back, or an injured limb

✔ Braces (for your wrist, leg, neck, and so on) and neck collars (for neck injuries)

✔ Bandages or casts, including eye patches, slings for broken or sprained arms, and other injury-related items that can't be removed

✔ Crutches, canes, walkers, or other medical walking aids

✔ A wheelchair or motorized chair or scooter

✔ An insulin pump or other medical device attached to the body

Knowing what to expect before and during the test

After you're shown to the testing room, you get an orientation to the computer and a chance to take a brief tutorial. This gives you an idea of how the testing software works. (If you're gonna screw up, do it now, not when it counts during the official test. Ask your questions about answering the questions or how the program works. When it's finally time to take the test, you should have nothing to do but read and evaluate questions.)

Expect that an audio and/or video tape is being made of the testing process.

The center staff gives you an erasable marker and a white board, which is very handy for writing down the numbers of questions you want to revisit.

The test is divided into 60-question blocks. Each block is 1 hour in duration, although you can finish early. After you finish the questions in your block, a "scheduled break" message appears on the screen. You have a total of 45 minutes of scheduled break time between blocks, and you can use this time any way you want, including going to your locker. If you like, you can take a short break between the first two blocks and a longer one later — the breaks just can't add up to more than 45 minutes, or you'll lose testing time.

Arranging for special accommodations

If you have a chronic health problem, an injury from an accident, or a disability — which may be a physical, hearing, visual, or learning disability — you can apply to NCCPA for a special accommodation. Here are some typical accommodations:

✔ Extended testing time (50 percent or 100 percent more time to complete the test) with no additional break time

✔ Frequent breaks and/or additional break time

✔ An individual testing room for people whose disability necessitates separation from all other examinees

✔ A reader, which means you'll be taking the test in a separate room

When applying for the test, you fill out a Special Testing Accommodations form and send it to NCCPA. If NCCPA approves your request, they forward the information to the Pearson VUE testing center.

Try to avoid unscheduled breaks in the middle of a block. Such breaks reduce the time available for the block — the clock doesn't stop. Also, you can't access personal items, and you'll be delayed by a security check on your return.

Looking at what happens after the test

After the test, you wait, but don't be on (surgical) pins and (hypodermic) needles — everything will be fine. NCCPA gets the test results about 2 weeks after the test date. Then they notify you by e-mail that they've posted your results. Go to the NCCPA website and look at your personal certification record. Congratulations! You passed! We knew you would.

And if you don't pass? Wait 90 days. You can take the test again. You have up to six tries in a 6-year period to pass the test if you don't pass it the first time.

Now take the next steps to becoming a licensed, practicing physician assistant. See Chapter 1 for more info on PAs.

Understanding How the Exam Is Scored

You're likely concerned with your total test score and whether it's high enough to pass. Each question can yield either a 1 (correct) or a 0 (wrong) — you get 1 point for each correct answer and nothing for wrong or unanswered questions, so there's no penalty for guessing. A raw score of 300 on the PANCE or 240 on the PANRE is a perfect score.

However, you'll never see the count of questions you got right or wrong. The test-makers have a complex system of weighting the questions based on difficulty to produce a scaled score. For test-takers, there's no way to correlate the raw score to the scaled score.

Your scaled score will be somewhere between 200 and 800, and NCCPA will tell you whether your score is high enough to pass. The details, if any, will be available to you when you see your exam results.

Some sources suggest that you need at least 60 percent correct answers, and we speculate that 62.5 percent is a good figure. However, analyze the math here. If you don't know which questions have less weight and which ones have more weight, the percentage of correct answers doesn't mean much. We can say the following about your score:

- ✔ A good performance on "easy" questions can increase your number and percentage of correct answers, but you don't know which ones NCCPA considers to be easy.

- ✔ A good performance on "hard" questions can increase your scaled score. Again, you don't know which questions NCCPA considers to be hard.

- ✔ A good performance in one subject area can offset a poor performance in another area. You can move faster and more confidently through subject areas you know very well, leaving you more time to ponder items you don't know as well.

- ✔ Although all subject areas are important, the topics in Chapters 3 to 6 of this book (heart, 16 percent; lungs, 12 percent; bones and joints, 10 percent; and gastrointestinal, 10 percent) account for almost half of the test questions. See the later section "Checking out question topics" for details on subject areas.

Your goal isn't to slide by, so don't worry about any minimum passing score. Your goal should be to answer *all* the questions you can correctly.

Familiarizing Yourself with the Test Format

Acquaint yourself with the broad organization of the test. The test format has two organizational components: the percentage distribution of question types and the structure of the questions themselves.

Test-makers have made careers thinking up this stuff. Just as you and your peers expect to be outstanding PAs, these folks expect themselves to be fine test-makers. They aren't in business to cut you any slack.

Although there's dignity in all work and the test-makers probably mean you no harm, we're sorry to report that you must consider the test-makers to be your adversaries. We've done the reconnaissance for you, and in this section, we tell you what you're up against.

Understanding the test organization

The PANCE is 5 hours long and contains 300 multiple-choice questions, and the PANRE is 4 hours long and contains 240 multiple-choice questions. In both tests, 60 questions are in a block, and you have 60 minutes to complete each block.

You can answer the questions in a block in any order, and you can review and change your choices. Use the time well; after the block is closed, you can't go back.

On both tests, the questions are organized in a random manner. Questions on any topic may appear in any block.

Scheduled breaks occur between blocks. You have a total of 45 minutes of scheduled break time, so that basically gives you about 11.25 minutes between PANCE blocks or 15 minutes between PANRE blocks if you divide the break time evenly. In that time, you can answer nature's calls, go to your locker, or do (almost) whatever you like.

Checking out question topics

PANCE questions cover about 18 topics, depending on how you classify them. In this book, we use body organ systems as the basis for the topic categories.

The approximate mix of questions on the test is well-documented. Some subject areas require more preparation because the test includes more questions about them. You need understanding and knowledge in these two broad categories:

- **Body organ systems:** Know the disorders of the major organ systems, including causative factors, significant labs, and treatment.
- **Task areas:** Know the general tasks common in working with all body organ systems, including history, examination, and best imaging.

Table 2-1 summarizes the percentage and number of questions per body organ system on the PANCE. Although the PANRE is still a general test covering the same 18 topics, PANRE questions are a little different in that the mix of topics varies, depending on which content concentration you chose: adult medicine, surgery, or primary care.

Table 2-1	Percentage and Number of Questions per Body Organ System	
Body Organ System	*Percentage of Questions*	*Approximate Number of PANCE Questions*
Cardiology	16	48
Pulmonary	12	36
Musculoskeletal	10	30
Gastrointestinal (GI)	10	30
Eyes, ears, nose, throat	9	27
Reproductive*	8	24
Endocrine	6	18
Genitourinary (GU)	6	18
Psychology/Behavioral	6	18
Neurology	6	18
Dermatology	5	15
Hematology	3	9
Infectious diseases (ID)	3	9

Reproductive encompasses all women's health issues.

Table 2-2 summarizes the percentage of questions within each body organ system asked about each task area.

Table 2-2	Percentage of Questions per Task Area
Task Area	*Percentage of Questions*
Formulating the most likely diagnosis	18
Pharmaceutical treatments	18
Health history and performing physical examinations	16
Clinical intervention	14
Employing laboratory and diagnostic information	14
Health maintenance	10
Applying basic science concepts	10

Examining the question structures

Every question on the PANCE and PANRE is a multiple-choice question with five answer choices. Only one answer choice is correct for each question. However, the questions may be presented in one of two structures.

"You know it or you don't" questions are often only one line long. They're often concerned with a symptom or a drug therapy. Here's an example:

Which of the following medications works by increasing the pancreatic secretion of insulin?

(A) Metformin (Glucophage)

(B) Acarbose (Precose)

(C) Glucagon

(D) Glimepiride (Amaryl)

(E) Cosyntropin (ACTH)

The "I've got to study this" questions use a multiple-line setup and usually have to do with how a patient presents. Here's an example:

You are evaluating a 25-year-old woman who has been transferred to the ICU secondary to profound hypotension. Her blood pressure is 75/40 mmHg with a pulse of 120 beats per minute. Her monitor shows she is in a normal sinus rhythm. Despite intravenous fluids and pressor medications, her blood pressure remains low. You suspect adrenal insufficiency. What would be your next step?

(A) Check a stat random cortisol level.

(B) Do a 24-hour urinary free cortisol.

(C) Do an ACTH stimulation test.

(D) Do a low dose dexamethasone suppression test.

(E) Give hydrocortisone 100 mg intravenously stat.

The test has no negative questions. A question won't ask "All of the following are true *except.*" Also, the test has no *K questions.* That is, no answer choices will say, for example, "A and C only" or "B, D, and E."

Knowing conventions

Knowing how the PANCE presents information in a question can give you insight into how to study. Here are a few notes on how info will appear on the test:

- ✔ The test always gives the generic name of a drug and provides the trade name only when necessary, so make sure you know generic names.

- ✔ Temperatures are given in both Fahrenheit and Celsius.

- ✔ While taking the test, you can click on "Lab Values" to find out normal lab values for healthy adults.

- ✔ Although acronyms are common in clinical practice, the test questions use few acronyms, so be familiar with spelled-out names.

For techniques to help you correctly answer test questions, flip to Chapter 24.

Part II

Getting to the Heart of the Test: Four Foundational Systems

The 5th Wave   By Rich Tennant

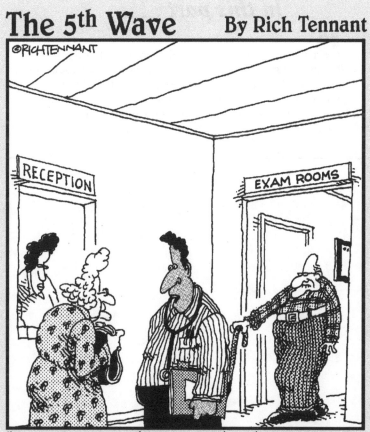

"Sometimes a tightness in the chest can be a sign of high blood pressure. In your husband's case, however, I just loosened his belt a little."

In this part . . .

Part II has chapters devoted to four vital body organ systems. The topics in this part constitute about 50 percent of the questions you'll see on the test. Look at Chapter 3 for cardio, Chapter 4 for pulmonary, Chapter 5 for the gastrointestinal system, and Chapter 6 for bones and joints.

Chapter 3

Tending to the Heart and the Great Vessels

*W*ithout a doubt, the heart is the most important organ of the body. Co-author Rich is a kidney specialist, and he definitely concurs. The creators of the PANCE and PANRE also agree, because a whopping 16 percent of the test comprises heart-related topics. The importance of the heart makes this chapter one of the most important ones in the book.

In this chapter, you read about all kinds of great and terrible stuff — cardiomyopathies, angina, congestive heart failure, congenital heart disease. As in the other body organ system chapters in this book, we've interspersed practice questions to keep you on your toes, with more at the end of the chapter to help you review and make you heart smart.

Keeping Blood Pressure in Line

You know that abnormal blood pressure is a component of many disease conditions. Blood pressure is useful for assessing health, too. That's why along with temperature, heart rate, and respiratory rate, blood pressure is called a *vital sign*.

Hypertension is the term for high blood pressure, and it's an epidemic in the United States. It's called the "silent killer" because it's a significant risk factor for coronary artery disease (CAD) and stroke, and it's also the second leading cause of kidney disease, right behind diabetes mellitus. In fact, CAD and diabetes often coexist.

This section covers both hypertension and hypotension.

Defining hypertension

The Joint National Committee on Prevention, Detection, Evaluation, and Treatment of High Blood Pressure (JNC) cites four blood pressure categories. Table 3-1 shows the numbers from the JNC's seventh report. If you haven't memorized these before, now is a good time.

The blood pressure categories list *or* numbers, not *and* numbers. If the systolic and dia-stolic blood pressure are in different ranges, the patient goes in the higher range. For exam-ple, if someone has a blood pressure of 130/98 mmHg, he or she has Stage 1 hypertension, even though the systolic blood pressure is in the range of prehypertension. The elevated diastolic blood pressure marks it as Stage 1 hypertension.

Table 3-1	JNC 7 Blood Pressure Categories for Adults	
Category	Systolic (mmHg)	Diastolic (mmHg)
Normal (desirable)	90–119	60–79
Prehypertension	120–139	80–89
Stage 1 hypertension	140–159	90–99
Stage 2 hypertension	160 or greater	100 or greater

You need a minimum of three elevated readings to establish a diagnosis of hypertension. You may get these readings from several office visits; however, many people also measure their blood pressure at home. The gold standard for diagnosis is actually ambulatory blood pressure monitoring — it should be used way more than it's prescribed.

You're evaluating a 65-year-old man at his annual physical. On examination, you get a blood pressure reading of 158/90 mmHg. Blood pressure measurements similar to this have been obtained on prior office visits and at his home. Which of the following would you prescribe?

(A) Lisinopril (Zestril)

(B) Metoprolol (Lopressor)

(C) Hydrochlorothiazide (HCTZ)

(D) Clonidine (Catapres)

(E) Terazosin (Hytrin)

The correct answer is Choice (A). This question asks what you'd pick first-line for someone coming into your office for hypertension. When Rich was in medical school, the first-line medications were lisinopril or hydrochlorothiazide. Choice (A), lisinopril, is first-line, because ACE inhibitors like lisinopril do so much above and beyond lowering blood pres-sure. They're heart protective. They help improve mortality in the setting of congestive heart failure, and they help lower proteinuria in someone with diabetic nephropathy. They do a lot of good stuff.

What's a second-line med? Well, based on the ON-TARGET trial, it's amlodipine (Norvasc), which is more of a vasodilator. Third-line is Choice (C), hydrochlorothiazide (HCTZ). Choices (B) and (D) are used later on and in specific instances. Choice (B), metroprolol, is used with someone after a myocardial infarction when the person has an indication of heart failure in the treatment. Choice (D), clonidine, is used when other medications don't work. Side effects of clonidine include dry mouth, lethargy, and hypotension. Choice (E), terazo-sin, is used in someone who has both benign prostatic hyperplasia (BPH) and problems with high blood pressure.

Handling essential and resistant hypertension

Hypertension comes in two types. The first is the *essential,* or run-of-the-mill, hypertension. Experts feel the cause of essential hypertension is a combination of a genetic predisposition and environmental influences, including a high-sodium diet, obesity, a sedentary lifestyle, tobacco abuse, alcohol abuse, and metabolic syndrome, to name a few. Usually, essential hypertension can be partially controlled by diet and exercise and additionally controlled by a blood pressure medication.

The second type of hypertension is *resistant hypertension,* which refers to high blood pressure that's resistant to treatment using environmental and lifestyle measures. On the PANCE or in clinical practice, the following case scenarios should be a tipoff that someone has resistant hypertension:

- ✔ Anyone less than 18 or more than 65 years of age who develops acute uncontrolled blood pressure when it was previously controlled or wasn't even an issue
- ✔ Anyone (of any age) whose blood pressure is still difficult to control, despite being on three or more optimally dosed, antihypertensive medications, usually including a diuretic

The PANCE may ask you to identify the causes of resistant hypertension. You should be familiar with several causes in terms of identification, evaluation, and management. We cover them next.

Chronic kidney disease (CKD)

The most common cause of resistant hypertension is chronic kidney disease (CKD). You read about chronic kidney disease in Chapter 10, but recognize that it affects more than 30 million people. Hypertension and diabetes mellitus are the two leading causes of chronic kidney disease. Clinically, in someone with resistant hypertension, you should check a blood urea nitrogen (BUN) and serum creatinine level to look for evidence of intrinsic renal parenchymal disease.

Renal artery stenosis (RAS)

Renovascular disease, especially renal artery stenosis (RAS), is a common cause of resistant hypertension. The most common cause of renal artery stenosis is atherosclerosis at the proximal ostium of the renal artery — right where it branches off of the big trunk known as the *aorta.* The renal artery becomes narrow enough to cause high blood pressure.

There's a distinct difference between renovascular disease and renal artery stenosis. Renal artery stenosis is a significant narrowing, significant enough to cause symptoms of resistant high blood pressure. Many people can have narrowing of the renal artery; however, the artery is not narrow enough to cause sky-high blood pressure. That being said, renovascular disease can still raise blood pressure.

Here are three key points about identifying renal artery stenosis:

- ✔ On physical examination, you may hear an audible flank or abdominal bruit, usually with the bell of the stethoscope.
- ✔ With an initial presentation of renal artery stenosis, you may see flash pulmonary edema, with normal heart function and patent coronary arteries.
- ✔ Acute renal failure, hypotension, and/or hyperkalemia after the use of an ACE inhibitor is a tipoff that renal artery stenosis is likely present. When the artery is really narrow, it becomes dependent on the blood pressure hormone angiotensin for renal perfusion. Block this hormone in someone with renal artery stenosis, and the person can get acute renal failure and hyperkalemia.

The gold standard for diagnosis of renal artery stenosis is the angiogram. A Doppler ultrasound isn't a bad initial test; however, the results are often operator-dependent and can be less reliable in someone with a large body habitus. A captopril renal scan may pop up on the PANCE as an initial screening test, but it isn't used much clinically anymore.

Treatment for renal artery stenosis is somewhat controversial. Certainly angioplasty and stent placement together is one recommended treatment. Studies show that angioplasty with or without stenting is safe and effective, but a number of trials don't demonstrate improvement in blood or renal function. Just the same, on the PANCE, recognize angioplasty with or without stenting as a treatment option.

 Another form of renal artery stenosis is called *fibromuscular hyperplasia.* This is stenosis of the *distal* part of the renal artery. Unlike atherosclerosis, the narrowing is caused by hyperplasia of one of the layers of the blood vessel, the tunica media. You commonly see fibromuscular hyperplasia as new onset high blood pressure in a young woman in her late teens to even twenties or thirties. The diagnosis is made by angiogram, and the treatment is angioplasty. On an angiogram, the typical appearance of the artery is a "string of beads."

Hyperaldosteronism

You see *hyperaldosteronism* with new onset hypertension and low potassium. The potassium stays low despite replacement, and the high blood pressure is resistant to treatment. The initial screening for hyperaldosteronism involves obtaining two blood tests, namely an aldosterone level and a renin level (the plasma renin activity to be exact). The aldosterone/renin ratio confirms the diagnosis. For hyperaldosteronism, the aldosterone level is usually greater than 16, and the renin level is suppressed, usually unmeasurable.

If those blood tests suggest that hyperaldosteronism may be present, the next step is to order a CT scan of the abdomen and pelvis to look at the adrenal glands. The most common cause of hyperaldosteronism is adrenal adenoma, and the second most common cause is bilateral adrenal hyperplasia. The treatment for adenoma may be surgical removal, depending on the size of the adenoma. The treatment for bilateral adrenal hyperplasia is to block aldosterone secretion using an aldosterone blocker like spironolactone (Aldactone). Remember that a major side effect of spironolactone is hyperkalemia.

Pheochromocytoma

Pheochromocytoma is usually an adrenal-producing tumor that can cause refractory labile hypertension. The blood pressure can be refractory to treatment, or it can be very labile, either super high or super low, bouncing up and down like a yo-yo (typically described as *paroxysmal*). The initial screening is biochemical, comprising urinalysis and blood testing. Here are some high-yield points about pheochromocytoma:

- The screening tests include a plasma metanephrines and/or a 24-hour urinary collection for vanillylmandelic acid (VMA) and urinary metanephrines. The metanephrines test is the more sensitive test.

- If the metanephrines are elevated, then obtain a CT scan to look at the adrenal glands for an adrenal adenoma. A more sensitive study may be needed to help establish the diagnosis.

- Remember the 10 percent rule: The pheochromocytma is familial 10 percent of the time, extra-adrenal 10 percent of the time, malignant 10 percent of the time, and present in both adrenal glands 10 percent of the time. If an adenoma is present, the treatment is usually surgical removal.

Coarctation of the aorta

Coarctation of the aorta is a common congenital pediatric cause of hypertension. With this condition, narrowing of the aorta causes a difference in the blood pressures between the upper and lower extremities. The area affected is the ductus arteriosus.

A classic physical exam finding is *radial-femoral delay,* meaning that there's a significant delay between the radial and the femoral pulses. In someone with coarctation, the upper torso is highly vascularized, and the legs can be small and spindly. Depending on the degree of narrowing, the lower-extremity pulses may not be palpable at all.

Here are some other key points concerning coarctation of the aorta:

✔ Initial presentation can include claudication-type symptoms, similar to what you see in older adults with really bad peripheral vascular disease (PVD)

✔ Upper-extremity hypertension and lower-extremity hypotension with decreased palpable pulses is typical for this condition.

✔ Depending on clinical presentation, treatment can be conservative or involve surgery of the stenosed area.

✔ A figure-three sign and scalloped ribs are classic signs on radiograph.

Other causes of resistant hypertension include Cushing's syndrome (see Chapter 15), carcinoid syndrome (see Chapter 4), obesity, and obstructive sleep apnea (which can be present in someone who is obese).

Which of the following is the most common cause of secondary (or resistant) hypertension?

(A) Carcinoid syndrome

(B) Renal artery stenosis

(C) Chronic kidney disease (CKD)

(D) Hyperaldosteronism

(E) Obstructive sleep apnea

The correct answer is Choice (C). The most common cause of resistant hypertension is actually intrinsic renal parenchymal disease. The second most common cause is Choice (B), renal artery stenosis. Choice (E), obstructive sleep apnea, is probably the least-recognized cause of refractory hypertension. Carcinoid syndrome, Choice (A), can be a cause of refractory hypertension where the carcinoid tumor secretes serotonin. You can read more about this in Chapter 4. Choice (D), hyperaldosteronism, is a cause of refractory hypertension and hypokalemia but isn't the most common cause of resistant hypertension.

Helping extremely high pressure

On the PANCE, expect to see common clinical scenarios involving very high blood pressure (and very low blood pressure, too, which we cover in the next section). Be aware of two basic scenarios concerning high blood pressure: hypertensive urgencies and hypertensive emergencies.

Hypertensive urgency concerns someone who presents with really high blood pressure: a systolic blood pressure ≥ 180 mmHg or a diastolic blood pressure ≥ 110 mmHg. The affected person is relatively asymptomatic and has no signs of end-organ damage on exam — no dizziness, no chest pain, no blurry vision, no nothing. He or she doesn't usually require inpatient hospitalization but does require aggressive blood pressure management and follow-up.

Hypertensive emergency concerns someone who presents with blood pressure readings ≥ 180 mmHg systolic or ≥ 120 mmHg diastolic with symptoms and signs of end-organ damage. He or she may have a change in mental status, chest pain, kidney failure, or pulmonary edema, possibly in combination. The affected person can have damaged organs, and that may not be reversible, depending on the intensity of the initial symptoms.

A person in hypertensive emergency needs to be hospitalized, usually in an intensive care unit, with gradual blood-pressure lowering over the first 24 to 48 hours. Cerebral perfusion, especially cerebral autoregulation of blood pressure, can get all messed up when the systolic blood pressure is too high. The general rule of thumb is to lower the blood pressure by no more than 20 percent of the mean arterial pressure (MAP) daily for the first couple of days. In other words, lower the blood pressure very slowly when you're treating a hypertensive emergency.

Be aware of commonly used medications to treat hypertensive emergency and their precautions and side effects. Many times, a continuous intravenous infusion is needed to tightly regulate the blood pressure. A healthcare provider often begins with one medication and adds another if needed to help bring the blood pressure under control. Consider the following meds:

- ✔ Nitroprusside (Nipride) is a potent vasodilator. A person on this medication needs to be in the ICU and should have an arterial line placed (usually in the radial artery) to measure blood pressure changes minute by minute. Side effects include cyanide toxicity, so thiocyanate and cyanide levels need to be monitored. Also, be careful giving this med to people with kidney disease or who are on dialysis.

- ✔ Labetalol (Trandate) can be given as a continuous infusion. Rich likes using this first-line. Remember that this medication is both an alpha blocker and a beta blocker. It can bring down the blood pressure nicely.

- ✔ Nicardipine (Cardene) is an intravenous calcium channel blocker. It also lowers blood pressure nicely.

Raising low blood pressure

Hypotension has many causes, including infection, volume depletion, adrenal insufficiency, anemia, blood pressure medications, and so forth. Because of the depth of this topic, your focus for test purposes should be on the main causes of low blood pressure, which we bring up here. (*Note:* Cardiac tamponade is a medical emergency that can cause hypotension. You can read about cardiac tamponade in the later section "Probing the Pericardium.")

Cardiogenic shock

Cardiogenic shock occurs when the systolic function of the heart goes kaput. Often, this occurs as a consequence of a myocardial infarction (MI), especially an ST elevation myocardial infarction (STEMI) affecting the anterior wall. The person in cardiogenic shock usually has some history of underlying coronary artery disease (CAD). On examination, the person is hypotensive, with significant jugular venous distention (JVD). Rales are present, as is a significant hypoxemia. Edema may be present as well. The person may be intubated because the hypoxemia is so bad as a result of the increased work of breathing.

Here are some key points concerning cardiogenic shock:

- ✔ Because there are different types of shock, part of the identification depends on using invasive monitoring (a Swan-Ganz catheter, for example). In cardiogenic shock, you expect the following hemodynamic pattern: elevated systemic vascular resistance, low cardiac output (low cardiac index), elevated pulmonary capillary wedge pressure, elevated central venous pressure, and elevated pulmonary artery diastolic pressure. Simply put, *everything* is elevated except the cardiac output, which is low because the systolic function of the heart sucks big time, as we medical professionals say.

- ✔ The mainstay of treatment involves using ionotropes and/or diuretics if the blood pressure allows. Examples of ionotropes are dopamine, dobutamine (Dobutrex), and milrinone (Primacor). Furosemide (Lasix) in high doses is also used.

- ✔ When the systolic function is really bad, an intra-aortic balloon pump (IABP) can be inserted. Sometimes, especially in the setting of a really bad myocardial infarction, emergent cardiac surgery may be required.

Orthostatic hypotension

Orthostatic hypotension means that the blood pressure is okay when the patient is in one position, but if he or she stands or sits up, the blood pressure drops. Orthostatic hypotension is established by one of the following criteria:

- ✔ **Systolic change:** The person has a drop of 20 mmHg in his or her systolic blood pressure when switching from one position to another, usually when assuming a standing position.

- ✔ **Diastolic change:** The person has a drop of 10 mmHg in his or her diastolic blood pressure when switching from one position to another, again usually when assuming a standing position.

Causes of orthostatic hypotension include blood pressure medications, volume depletion, adrenal insufficiency, aortic stenosis, cardiomyopathy, and anemia, among others. Other causes include amyloidosis and autonomic neuropathy that can be associated with variations of Parkinson's syndrome (also known as *multiple-system atrophy*). The most common cause of autonomic neuropathy is diabetes mellitus.

Here's a big testing-taking tip: The difference between orthostatic hypotension due to volume depletion and anemia versus autonomic neuropathy has to do with the pulse. In autonomic neuropathy, the heart rate doesn't increase when the patient stands up. You'd expect an increase in the heart rate (not necessarily a tachycardia) when the blood pressure drops.

The treatment for orthostatic hypotension depends on what's causing it — a blood pressure medication, anemia, volume depletion, and so forth. When the hypotension is due to autonomic neuropathy, be aware of a couple of meds used for treatment:

- ✔ Midodrine (ProAmatine) is an alpha agonist that raises blood pressure. It's short-acting and can be given 2 to 3 times a day. A major side effect is supine hypertension.

- ✔ Fludrocortisone (Florinef) is a synthetic aldosterone that raises blood pressure. Side effects can be hypertension, edema, volume overload, and hypokalemia. Fludrocortisone can also be used in the treatment of primary adrenal insufficiency, because it's a replacement for missing aldosterone.

Analyzing Acute Coronary Syndrome

Chest pain (angina pectoris) and congestive heart failure are two of the biggest reasons people are admitted to the hospital. In this section, you read about the various components of acute coronary syndrome (ACS), which is due to coronary artery disease (CAD). Acute coronary syndrome encompasses many of the reasons that someone comes to the hospital: stable angina, unstable angina, and the infamous myocardial infarction (heart attack). In this section, you also read about variant angina.

Some risk factors for CAD are modifiable; some are not. The modifiable risk factors for CAD include hypertension, diabetes, smoking, hyperlipidemia, a sedentary lifestyle, obesity, overuse of alcohol, and a chronic inflammatory state. Inflammation is a big risk for CAD. Nonmodifiable risk factors for CAD include age, gender, and family history.

Sorting out stable versus unstable angina

With *stable* angina, the patient never had any chest pressure at rest; chest pressure occurred only with activity. Chronic stable angina often occurs predictably, usually after physical activity or as a result of a significant emotional stressor. One of the classic scenarios of stable angina is the obese middle-aged man who hasn't engaged much in any sort of physical activity. He watches the news and finds out that he is going to be the recipient of a few inches of snow. The next day, he goes out and tries to shovel the snow and ends up getting chest pressure similar to what he felt the other few times he engaged in physical activity. His wife calls 911, and he's admitted to the hospital with acute coronary syndrome. Other similar examples include the weekend warriors — out-of-shape older "athletes," more commonly men, who do strenuous physical activity once a week.

By contrast, unstable angina occurs in the gentleman sitting at home watching the news and getting chest pressure while *thinking* about shoveling snow. *Unstable angina* occurs at rest.

Here are two key points concerning chest pain:

- ✔ Men tend to have the classic pain patterns, with chest pressure and radiation to the left arm. It's often described as more of a pressure than a sharp pain. In addition, nausea and/or diaphoresis can be present. Sometimes, especially in the setting of an acute myocardial infarction, there can be a "sense of doom" as well.

- ✔ The patient may have symptoms typified as *angina equivalents,* which refers to symptoms that you can miss because they mimic the symptoms of something else. For example, some people may express cardiac chest pain through right upper-quadrant pain, midepigastric pain, or even a toothache.

Women differ from men, especially in the way they experience chest pain. Women may not experience the classic chest pressure with radiation to the left arm. They may "not feel well," or they may have more nausea or abdominal symptoms. These symptoms cannot be discounted, and the clinician needs to look for more angina equivalents.

You're evaluating a 67-year-old man who was admitted for a non-ST-elevation myocardial infarction (NSTEMI). He underwent a cardiac catheterization and was told that aggressive medical management was needed. Despite beta blockers, nitropaste, and aspirin, he's still having bouts of angina. Which of the following medications could you add to his regimen at this time?

(A) Atorvastatin (Lipitor)

(B) Furosemide (Lasix)

(C) Lisinopril (Zestril)

(D) Ranolazine (Ranexa)

(E) Indomethacin (Indocin)

The correct answer is Choice (D), ranolazine. Many cardiologists prescribe this medication to provide additional help with angina symptoms for someone on maximal medical therapy. Choice (A), atorvastatin, decreases the cholesterol level and has an anti-inflammatory effect but doesn't treat symptomatic angina. Choice (B), furosemide, is used to treat congestive heart failure (CHF). Choice (C), lisinopril, is used for both acute coronary syndrome and congestive heart failure but again doesn't help with symptomatic angina. Choice (E), indomethacin, is used for musculoskeletal pain and is first-line for treating pericarditis.

Reviewing basic criteria for myocardial infarction

You should be familiar with the nuts and bolts of myocardial infarction (MI for short). A person is said to be having an MI if there's a positive enzyme leak in the blood and accompanying ECG changes. The clinical presentation may not always be reliable. For example, you may miss an MI in a person with diabetes and bad neuropathy.

Although we review ECG changes in the next section, you should also be aware of some of the labs used in evaluating an MI. Here are a couple of points:

✔ The troponin I rises within the first few hours of an MI and can stay elevated for at least a week, if not more.

✔ The creatine phosphokinase (CPK) and the CK-MB fraction especially start rising in the first few hours but peak in around a day, only to return to baseline in about 2 to 3 days.

The thrombolysis in myocardial infarction (TIMI) score is a great scoring system that any clinician can use during the history and physical. This scoring system is based on cardiac risk factors as well as known coronary artery disease. You can use the TIMI score to risk-stratify patients being admitted to the hospital.

Knowing the NSTEMI and STEMI

There are two types of myocardial infarctions, depending on how much of the myocardium is affected. NSTEMI stands for *non-ST-elevation myocardial infarction*. This MI doesn't involve the entire myocardium. It's not a transmural MI. A diagnosis of NSTEMI is made by positive cardiac enzymes, and you'll likely see ST depression or T-wave inversion on the ECG, indicating that ischemia is going on.

STEMI stands for *ST-elevation myocardial infarction*. This is the biggie, reflecting an infarct that affects the whole wall of the myocardium. Classic ECG patterns include hyperacute ST segment elevation with (later on) the formation of a Q wave when the infarct is complete. Here are some specific patterns to be aware of concerning STEMI as seen on the ECG:

✔ **Anterior wall myocardial infarction:** This causes ST elevation in leads V1 through V3, and it can also affect V4. The coronary artery affected is the left anterior descending (LAD), which supplies the left ventricle. Common clinical presentations of an acute anterior wall myocardial infarction can include acute pulmonary edema and cardiogenic shock, which you read about earlier in "Raising low blood pressure."

✔ **Inferior wall myocardial infarction:** This MI causes an ST elevation in leads II, III, and aVF on an ECG. In addition to common clinical presentations of chest pain, someone with an inferior wall MI can present with nausea, vomiting, and GI upset. Why? Remember that the inferior wall sits near the vagus nerve; consequently, an MI in this area can mimic GI symptoms via vagal nerve stimulation. The artery affected by an inferior wall MI is the right coronary artery (RCA). Here are some other key points concerning an inferior wall MI:

  • If you see a test question in which a person with an inferior wall MI presents with hypotension, there may be extension of the inferior wall MI to affect the right ventricle. In another scenario, a person with an inferior wall MI is given nitroglycerin to help with the chest pain and all of a sudden experiences a drop in blood pressure. There's extension to involve the right ventricle and hypokinesis of that right ventricle. The treatment is fluids, fluids, fluids, with isotonic saline to increase preload.

  • Another complication of an inferior wall MI is a ventricular septal defect. We mention this because it's also a cause of congenital heart disease that you read about later in "Viewing ventricular septal defect."

✔ **Lateral wall MI:** There's a high lateral wall MI and a low lateral wall MI. You see ST segment elevation in leads I and aVL for an MI in the high lateral wall, and you see ST segment elevation in leads V5 and V6 for an MI in the low lateral wall. A STEMI of the high lateral wall can affect the circumflex artery. There are usually no significant hemodynamic complications associated with this.

✔ **Posterior wall MI:** This MI can be a tricky one to determine. The clinical presentation can be similar to an inferior wall MI (that is, GI symptoms can predominate). On an ECG, you see ST depression in the anterior leads (V1 and V2 big time). You need to use the mirror trick: Flip the ECG over to see the ST elevation.

Just because someone comes into the hospital on warfarin (Coumadin) doesn't mean that he or she can't have an MI. Warfarin isn't an antiplatelet drug; it works on the extrinsic clotting pathway. Warfarin doesn't inhibit platelet aggregation/clumping. That's why aspirin and clopidrogel (Plavix) are used in treating acute coronary syndrome.

You need to be aware of several important points concerning ECG interpretation of a STEMI:

✔ During an acute MI, there's initially T wave elevation that converts to hyperacute ST segment elevation. You often see ST segment elevation in two contiguous leads in the setting of a STEMI.

✔ Within a few hours, you can begin to see negative T waves or T wave inversion as the MI evolves. The T wave inversion can persist for months after the MI.

✔ A Q wave can take hours to days to develop (depending on the MI) and means that the damage done to that particular area is irreversible. Look at Figure 3-1. Q waves are in the inferior leads, meaning that in a recently completed MI, either the MI has run its course or it's an old inferior wall MI.

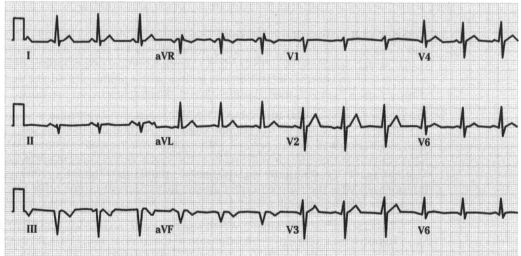

Figure 3-1:
A STEMI rhythm strip with Q waves.

Treating ACS

Many of the PANCE questions concerning acute coronary syndrome involve evaluation, treatment, or both. Because the treatment of acute coronary syndrome overlaps so much with so many conditions, much of the focus is on recognizing clinical presentation and ECG changes. Here are some key points for treating different aspects of acute coronary syndrome:

- The standard of care treatment for a STEMI is a trip to the cardiac catheterization lab for an emergent cardiac catheterization, with angioplasty and possible stent. If you're practicing in an area where a cardiac catheterization lab isn't readily available, then the second-line treatment is thrombolysis with a medication like tPA.

- Statin therapy is usually administered in the setting of an MI. A lipid profile is usually ordered if the patient has been fasting or within 24 hours of admission when someone presents with acute coronary syndrome. If the LDL-C is ≥ 100 mg/dL, a statin should be prescribed on hospital discharge.

- Clopidogrel (Plavix) is an antiplatelet agent that's routinely given, along with aspirin, in the treatment of a STEMI. Clopidogrel can be maintained for a while, especially to reduce clotting off of a cardiac stent if a stent has been placed. An uncommon side effect of clopidogrel is thrombotic thrombocytopenic purpura (TTP) — rare but possible. You can find info on TTP in Chapter 18.

Reviewing variant angina

In *variant angina,* or *Prinzmetal's angina,* a person comes in with crushing chest pressure. ECG changes indicate an acute coronary syndrome, and there may be an enzyme leak (that is, positive troponins and CK-MB fraction).

POW! BAM! Holy infarction, Batman!

For unstable angina and an NSTEMI, you see some overlap in treatment. One of the great acronyms for recalling the treatments of both is the mnemonic OH, BATMAN:

O = Oxygen: Ischemia implies oxygen deprivation, which leads to increased myocardial oxygen demand and increased myocardial work. The goal of treatment is to reduce the workload of the heart. Every person admitted to the hospital with acute coronary syndrome (ACS) is given oxygen via nasal cannula.

H = Heparin: This blood thinner works by potentiating antithrombin III. It's used to prevent clotting and to thin the blood during an ACS. Heparin can be given for unstable angina, but it's almost always given to a person with an NSTEMI.

B = Beta blocker: This is a standard of care for anyone with ACS, particularly an NSTEMI or a STEMI. It decreases the workload of the heart and should improve morbidity and mortality in someone with ACS. It's also used in treating congestive heart failure (CHF). The most common beta blockers used are metoprolol (Lopressor) and atenolol (Tenormin).

A = Aspirin: Anyone with an MI needs to chew an aspirin right away. Aspirin is an antiplatelet agent that has saved countless lives.

T = Thrombolysis: Thrombolysis is used in the setting of a STEMI if and only if a cardiac catheterization lab isn't available within a few hours of the ischemic event. For a STEMI, time is of the essence.

M = Morphine: Morphine is used in managing pain associated with an MI. Morphine can also be used in treating congestive heart failure/pulmonary edema.

A = ACE inhibitors: ACE inhibitors can help in preserving the myocardium in the setting of an MI. They're usually given in the first 24 hours unless acute kidney failure is present.

N = Nitroglycerin: Nitroglycerin is a coronary artery vasodilator and is used to help in the management of ACS. In the setting of an NSTEMI, it's usually given as a continuous infusion along with heparin. It can also be given as a pill (isosorbide mononitrate [Imdur]) or as a topical nitropaste that can be applied across the chest.

The person with ACS is on multiple therapies at one time. For example, the person with an NSTEMI is on IV heparin and nitroglycerin, on oxygen via nasal cannula, and on oral metoprolol (Lopressor). You've likely ordered many of these medications yourself.

On a cardiac catheterization, the coronary arteries are clean as a whistle — there's no atherosclerosis to be found. What's happening is that the arteries are going into vasospasm, or intense coronary artery vasoconstriction. Here are two key points concerning variant angina:

- ✓ Diagnosis can be made via an ergonovine challenge test. In a controlled situation, this can reproduce the previously mentioned symptoms if variant angina is present.

- ✓ The treatment is the use of vasodilators, such as nitroglycerin, and calcium channel blockers, such as nifedipine (Procardia XL).

The treatment for variant angina (nitroglycerin and calcium channel blockers) is similar to the treatment for two other conditions: esophageal spasm and Raynaud's phenomenon. You read about these conditions in Chapters 5 and 6.

Clarifying Congestive Heart Failure

Congestive heart failure (CHF) is a leading cause of hospital admissions. One of the most frustrating things for both clinician and patient is the high readmission rate for this condition.

You're familiar with many of the common clinical presentations of shortness of breath as it pertains to CHF. These presentations can include orthopnea, paroxysmal nocturnal dyspnea (PND, not to be confused with post-nasal drip), shortness of breath at rest (SOB), and dyspnea on exertion (DOE). Many affected people complain of increased swelling in the legs (edema) or weight gain of several pounds in a period of a few days.

Common clinical findings on physical examination for CHF can include hypoxemia, jugular venous distention (JVD), an S3 gallop (in systolic heart failure), and an S4 (in diastolic dysfunction or diastolic heart failure). Hepatojugular reflux (HJR) may be present. The person may have increased abdominal girth (he or she gains fluid around the belly).

Realize that CHF is a *symptom* that something's wrong with the heart. When you see a PANCE question about CHF, you should be thinking, "Why does the person have CHF?" There are three basic answers to that question:

- ✓ Systolic heart failure
- ✓ Diastolic heart failure
- ✓ Valvular dysfunction

Many people have more than one of these conditions, and some people (more than you'd think) have all three. Although Rich is a kidney doctor, he sees many people with CHF. They can be a challenge to treat.

We discuss systolic and diastolic heart failure in this section. Valvular disorders, such as mitral regurgitation and aortic stenosis, can be common causes of congestive heart failure, especially among older people. Read more about these two conditions later in "Vexing Over Valvular Disorders." Questions about them will be on the PANCE.

Seeing and treating systolic heart failure

Systolic heart failure is a failure of the heart to work well as a pump. On an echocardiogram, you see this failure as a reduced ejection fraction. Assuming that the heart has a normal ejection fraction of 65 percent, anything less than 50 percent is thought to represent some degree of a pump problem. Common causes of systolic heart failure include ischemia due to CAD (that is, an ischemic cardiomyopathy), hypertension, and other causes of cardiomyopathy, especially a dilated cardiomyopathy (which you read about later in "Muscling In on the Cardiomyopathies").

On the PANCE, you'll be asked not only about the medications for treating systolic heart failure but also about key side effects and potential drug-drug interactions. Here's a list of meds typically used in treating systolic heart failure:

- ✔ **Furosemide:** Furosemide (Lasix) is used to help treat the volume overload and pulmonary edema associated with congestive heart failure. It can be given intravenously or orally. Before it does its main job — facilitating a diuresis — it works in the pulmonary circulation to decrease preload. Side effects of this medication and other loop diuretics include hypokalemia, hypomagnesemia, and metabolic alkalosis.

- ✔ **ACE inhibitors and ARBs:** Angiotensin converting enzyme (ACE) inhibitors and angiotensin receptor blockers (ARBs) prolong morbidity and mortality in systolic CHF. The medications can actually cause remodeling of the cells of the left ventricle and decrease left ventricular hypertrophy (LVH). Side effects include a cough (ACE inhibitors only) and hyperkalemia (both ACE inhibitors and ARBs). An uncommon side effect of an ACE inhibitor is angioedema. When you start anyone on one of these classes of medication, you need to check a blood chemistry panel after a week or so for the serum creatinine and potassium levels.

- ✔ **Digoxin:** Digoxin (Lanoxin) improves systolic heart failure symptoms and morbidity, but it doesn't improve mortality. In CHF, digoxin has been shown to help reduce sympathetic tone. This medication is also an atrioventricular nodal blocker that can be used in managing rate control for atrial fibrillation. Digoxin is renally eliminated, so in cases of chronic kidney disease or acute kidney failure, the dosing of this medication needs to be greatly reduced or even held. Clinicians follow blood levels closely when they prescribe digoxin.

Watch for symptoms of digoxin toxicity. When the digoxin level is very high, symptoms of toxicity include nausea, vomiting, dizziness, and palpitations. On an ECG, you can see many types of arrhythmias, including junctional rhythm. The most common arrhythmia you see with digoxin toxicity is paroxysmal atrial tachycardia with block. Note that hypercalcemia can make digoxin toxicity worse, as can hypokalemia. You treat digoxin toxicity by using Fab antibody fragments (Digibind) that bind digoxin. Because digoxin is heavily protein-bound, it can't be removed by hemodialysis.

- ✔ **Beta blockers:** Beta blockers are used in treating chronic systolic heart failure. They improve morbidity and mortality. They can reduce sympathetic tone, as can digoxin. Beta blockers also have a mortality benefit in treating the post-MI patient. Commonly prescribed medications include metoprolol (Lopressor) and carvedilol (Coreg).

- ✔ **Spironolactone:** Spironolactone (Aldactone) is added after a person is on digoxin, an ACE inhibitor, a beta blocker, and a loop diuretic. Spironolactone can help with survival in patients with CHF. It also can help reverse left ventricular hypertrophy, as can an ACE inhibitor.

Spironolactone has to be carefully dosed in patients with a glomerular filtration rate (GFR) < 30 mL/min. It's contraindicated in advanced kidney disease because it can cause hyperkalemia. The kidney function and potassium levels need to be watched, especially if the person is also on an ACE inhibitor.

In general, treating heart failure involves more than just using the meds we describe here. The patient should get daily exercise and adhere to a diet that is low in sodium (1,500–2,000 mg/day limit) and high in fruits and vegetables. Fluid restriction is often recommended. Avoiding medications like NSAIDs is also important, because they can cause high blood pressure and salt and water retention and can blunt the effect of loop diuretics. NSAIDs can also cause hyperkalemia and acute kidney failure.

Diagnosing and treating diastolic heart failure

Systolic heart failure is a problem with the heart's pumping. By contrast, *diastolic heart failure* is a problem with the heart's relaxing. Common causes include ischemia and hypertension. A major cause is obesity. Diastolic dysfunction, especially with the current obesity epidemic in the United States, is more common than systolic dysfunction, although the two can coexist. On an echocardiogram, the cardiologist can diagnose diastolic dysfunction/diastolic heart failure based on the inability of the heart to relax.

Systolic and diastolic heart failure are called *left-sided heart failure,* which is important because problems with the left side of the heart can affect the right. In fact, the most common cause of right-sided heart failure is left-sided heart failure (a mantra).

Treatment for diastolic heart failure is a little different from treatment for systolic heart failure. The mainstay treatment medications for diastolic heart failure are beta blockers and calcium channel blockers. They help the heart relax.

You're evaluating a 77-year-old man who presents to the hospital with shortness of breath. A chest radiograph shows pulmonary edema. His blood pressure is 128/66 mmHg, and his oxygenation level is 96 percent on 6 liters via nasal cannula. You order a BNP level, which is 2,000 pg/mL. The ECG shows normal sinus rhythm at 68 beats per minute and no acute ST-T wave changes. Which of the following combinations of medications would you administer to this person?

(A) Furosemide (Lasix) and heparin

(B) Aspirin and heparin

(C) Furosemide (Lasix) and hydrochlorothiazide

(D) Nitroglycerin and heparin

(E) Nitroglycerin and furosemide (Lasix)

The correct answer is Choice (E), nitroglycerin and furosemide. This man has a chest radiograph that shows pulmonary edema. The treatment for acute pulmonary edema is oxygen, furosemide, nitroglycerin, and maybe morphine. The nitroglycerin is a potent vasodilator and can ease the work of breathing in acute pulmonary edema/decompensated congestive heart failure. Choices (B) and (D) would be used in the treatment of acute coronary syndrome. The meds in Choice (C) aren't really given together. Furosemide and heparin, Choice (A), would be given together if the person had CHF in the setting of acute coronary syndrome (an NSTEMI, for example). Clinically, in the setting of CHF due to acute coronary syndrome, other medications would be given, including aspirin and nitroglycerin.

Note the inclusion of the brain (B-type) natriuretic peptide (BNP) in the question. It's secreted by the ventricles and can be elevated chronically in states of ventricular stretch, such as chronic CHF or a cardiomyopathy. In acute decompensated CHF, these levels can be elevated from baseline. Clinicians can trend these over time.

Muscling In on the Cardiomyopathies

A *cardiomyopathy* is an abnormality of heart function secondary to changes in the structure of the heart muscle. The most common cause of congestive heart failure is an ischemic cardiomyopathy, which we mention in the earlier section "Seeing and treating systolic heart failure." In this section, you read about the other types of cardiomyopathies that you may see on the PANCE.

Note that in many if not all cases, you can make the diagnosis by an echocardiogram interpretation (in addition to a history and physical). Often, a cardiac catheterization has to be done to rule out coronary artery disease (CAD) as a cause of the cardiomyopathy.

The three classifications of cardiomyopathy you need to be familiar with are dilated, restrictive, and hypertrophic.

Dealing with dilated cardiomyopathy

If you look at a *dilated cardiomyopathy* (DCM) on an echocardiogram, you'll likely see dilatation of both atria and both ventricles. Basically, the heart becomes weakened and enlarged and can't pump blood very well. The common causes of dilated cardiomyopathy include long-term alcohol consumption, viruses, and certain medications. For example, the antineoplastic agent doxorubicin (Doxorubicin) and the monoclonal antibody trastuzumab (Herceptin) can be causes of a dilated cardiomyopathy.

The most common initial presenting symptoms are those of CHF, and dilated cardiomyopathy is diagnosed by echocardiogram. The mainstay of treatment is removing the offending agent (for example, stopping drinking) and using ACE inhibitors and beta blockers together.

Recognizing restrictive cardiomyopathy

Restrictive cardiomyopathy (RCM) refers to a condition in which the heart's walls are rigid, limiting the heart's stretching and filling with blood. The most common causes of restrictive cardiomyopathy are the infiltrative conditions, and examples of common infiltrative conditions include amyloidosis and sarcoidosis. You can read about these conditions in other chapters — Chapter 18 for amyloidosis and Chapter 4 for sarcoidosis.

Handling hypertrophic cardiomyopathy

Hypertrophic cardiomyopathy (HCM) commonly occurs in young people. The typical scenario is the young person who has a syncopal episode during an athletic event. This condition can cause death.

Hypertrophic cardiomyopathy can be genetically inherited, usually in an autosomal dominant manner. The diagnosis is made by the history and physical exam findings and is confirmed by echocardiogram. Here are some key points concerning a hypertrophic cardiomyopathy:

- ✔ On physical examination, the murmur increases with the Valsalva maneuver, because you're decreasing the amount of blood going into the left ventricle.

  On the PANCE, a physical examination question may want you to differentiate between the murmur accompanying a hypertrophic cardiomyopathy and the murmur accompanying aortic stenosis (AS). In aortic stenosis, the murmur decreases with the Valsalva; this is the direct opposite of hypertrophic cardiomyopathy. However, both conditions have a midsystolic ejection murmur.

- ✔ The medical treatment for hypertrophic cardiomyopathy can include the use of beta blockers and calcium channel blockers to relax the left ventricle.

- ✔ Surgical treatment can include a surgical myomectomy in which part of the interventricular septum is shaved. Alcohol septal ablation has also been used in the treatment of this condition.

- ✔ Because hypertrophic cardiomyopathy carries with it an increased risk of sudden death, it's recommended that an implantable cardioverter defibrillator (ICD) be placed in someone with this condition, especially if he or she has a strong family history of sudden death.

Vexing Over Valvular Disorders

The most common valvular issues you'll likely be tested on are problems with the mitral and aortic valves. The other valves (the pulmonic and tricuspid valves) are important as well, but the good stuff occurs with the first two valves. Not only should you be familiar with the clinical presentations and causes of some of these valvular problems, but you also need to know the pertinent clinical exam findings for each of them.

Meeting the mitral valve

The *mitral valve* is located in between the left atrium and the left ventricle. You need to be familiar with three murmurs concerning the mitral valve: mitral stenosis, mitral valve prolapse, and mitral regurgitation.

Mitral stenosis

Mitral stenosis is a failure of the mitral valve to fully open over time. The most common cause of this condition is rheumatic fever. Your physical examination findings can vary, depending on whether you're talking about early mitral stenosis or late mitral stenosis. Early on, you may hear a very loud S1 and an opening snap after the S2. As the stenosis progresses, the S1 is very decreased or absent. On an echocardiogram, you may see an enlarged left atrium.

Mitral valve prolapse

Mitral valve prolapse (MVP) is a common murmur in young people, particularly women. You'll likely see a test question in which MVP is linked to anxiety and panic disorder.

Here are two key physical examination points concerning MVP:

- ✔ On cardiac auscultation, you hear a midsystolic click followed by a late systolic murmur, which is best heard at the heart apex.
- ✔ The intensity of MVP is increased by the Valsalva maneuver and by the handgrip maneuver.

For test-taking purposes, the two cardiac conditions in which the intensity of the murmur increases with Valsalva are MVP and hypertrophic cardiomyopathy. The Valsalva decreases the volume of fluid going into the left ventricle, so it accentuates these murmurs.

Mitral regurgitation

Mitral regurgitation refers to an incompetent mitral valve. The mitral valve doesn't close properly when the heart pumps out blood, so blood leaks from the left ventricle through the mitral valve into the left atrium. It's a common valvular problem in older people and can be a cause of congestive heart failure. On physical examination, you can hear a holosystolic murmur, usually heard best at the left sternal base. The severity of the murmur may vary, with mild, moderate, and severe degrees.

Assessing the aortic valve

The *aortic valve* is located between the left ventricle and the aorta. The two major disorders you can see with the aortic valve are aortic stenosis and aortic regurgitation.

Aortic stenosis

Aortic stenosis (AS) refers to a narrowing of the aortic valve area. Over time, this trileaflet valve becomes calcified. The more severe the narrowing of the valve, the more significant the left ventricular hypertrophy (LVH) that can develop over time.

On physical examination, you can hear a midsystolic murmur as well as a decreased S2, which is best heard at the second right intercostal space. Recall that the *S2* refers to a closure of the aortic and pulmonic valves. With aortic stenosis, the A2 part can be diminished or even absent if the aortic stenosis is severe.

Other physical exam findings include *pulsas parvus et tardus* (weak and late pulse) as well as a narrow pulse pressure. This is the opposite of aortic regurgitation, which has a widened pulse pressure. Aortic stenosis decreases with the Valsalva maneuver.

In terms of the three different (but sometimes overlapping) clinical presentations of aortic stenosis, remember the mnemonic SAD: S = syncope, A = angina, and D = dyspnea. The presenting symptoms in someone with aortic stenosis can actually can help predict, to a degree, his or her life span without intervention:

Clinical Presentation	Average Life Span
AS and dyspnea	2 more years
AS and syncope	3 more years
AS and chest pressure/angina	5 more years

Here's a key point about aortic stenosis: Cardiac chamber catheterization provides a definitive diagnosis. It can directly measure the pressure on both sides of the aortic valve. The pressure gradient may be used as a decision point for treatment. It's useful in symptomatic patients before a cardiac intervention is planned.

Aortic stenosis can be classified as mild, moderate, or severe. The valve area is normally 1.5–2 cm². A valve area of about 1 cm² is classified as moderate aortic stenosis. If it's < 0.8 cm², it's classified as severe aortic stenosis. The narrower the valve area is as measured by echocardiogram, the more severe the presenting symptoms.

You're evaluating a 65-year-old man who complains of shortness of breath. On physical examination, he has a midsystolic murmur and decreased S2. You also note diminished carotid upstroke bilaterally. Which one of the following is true?

(A) He likely needs a mitral valve replacement.

(B) This murmur would decrease with a Valsalva maneuver.

(C) He would be expected to have a widened pulse pressure.

(D) The cause of the murmur is likely rheumatic fever.

(E) His life span without surgical intervention is at least five years.

The correct answer is Choice (B). This man has aortic stenosis. He would likely need an *aortic* valve replacement rather than a mitral valve replacement, Choice (A). Regarding Choice (C), he would have a narrow pulse pressure; you'd see a widened pulse pressure with aortic regurgitation. Rheumatic fever, Choice (D), is a cause of mitral and tricuspid stenosis, and this guy has aortic stenosis with shortness of breath. Regarding Choice (E), his life span without surgical intervention is unfortunately about 2 years.

Aortic regurgitation

Aortic regurgitation (AR) is a common murmur. The aortic valve is leaking, and blood flows in the reverse (wrong) direction from the aorta into the left ventricle. The first clue to the presence of aortic regurgitation (also called *aortic insufficiency,* or AI) is a widened pulse pressure. Recall that *pulse pressure* is simply the difference between the systolic and diastolic blood pressures. The wider the pulse pressure, the more significant the aortic regurgitation. You may see a blood pressure like 150/45 mmHg. You can see a widened pulse pressure in isolated systolic hypertension as well. Here are three key points about aortic regurgitation:

✔ In addition to a widened pulse pressure, aortic regurgitation can cause a diastolic murmur (a diastolic rumble).

✔ Causes of aortic regurgitation include endocarditis, acute aortic dissection, syphilis, and the seronegative spondyloarthropathies, including ankylosing spondylitis and reactive arthritis.

✔ With symptomatic aortic regurgitation, surgical intervention — aortic valve replacement (a valve job but with no oil change) — is often warranted. With asymptomatic aortic regurgitation, surgery is indicated only if the ejection fraction is ≤ 50 percent.

Testing the tricuspid valve

The *tricuspid valve* is located between the right atrium and the right ventricle. Tricuspid valve problems aren't as common as mitral and aortic valve problems. The two main valvular conditions concerning the tricuspid valve are tricuspid regurgitation and tricuspid stenosis.

Tricuspid regurgitation questions on the PANCE may concern two different scenarios:

✔ You're evaluating someone with moderate to severe pulmonary hypertension and a harsh murmur at the right sternal base. Because of the increased right-sided heart pressures, you may see tricuspid regurgitation. In addition, you may see elevated jugular venous pressure (JVD) and/or lower-extremity edema.

✔ You see an infection of the tricuspid valve. The most common clinical scenario is right-sided endocarditis caused by *Staphylococcus aureus,* which you usually see with intravenous drug abuse (IVDA).

On physical examination of someone with tricuspid regurgitation, you hear a holosystolic murmur best at the left sternal border.

Tricuspid stenosis, in which blood has difficulty getting through the valve, isn't commonly seen clinically. Remember that rheumatic fever is almost always the cause. As with mitral stenosis, you can hear an opening snap that occurs after the S2.

Pushing the pulmonary valve

The *pulmonary valve* is located between the right ventricle and the pulmonary trunk. The two main valve problems are pulmonic stenosis and pulmonic regurgitation.

You commonly see *pulmonic stenosis* as one aspect of congenital heart disease (which you read about in the next section). Pulmonic stenosis is diagnosed by an echocardiogram. When severe, it can cause significant right ventricular hypertrophy (RVH). On physical examination, it can cause a wide-split S2.

Pulmonic regurgitation is usually somewhat physiologic in everyone. When pulmonic regurgitation is present, the clinician needs to look for causes of pulmonary hypertension, including rheumatic fever and rheumatologic conditions, drugs and toxins, connective tissue disorders, and most commonly "idiopathic" pulmonary hypertension. On physical examination, you may find a right ventricular heave and an early diastolic murmur. The treatment is personalized, based on the underlying cause and the other comorbid conditions.

Diagnosing Congenital Heart Disease

Many types of congenital heart disease exist. This section covers the conditions you're likely to see on the PANCE. Many of the congenital heart diseases you read about here are detected at birth and have telltale signs and features that you need to know.

Analyzing atrial septal defect

In *atrial septal defect* (ASD), someone has a defect or opening in the atrial septum between the right and left atria. Over time, this causes blood from the left atrium to enter the right atrium. Atrial septal defect increases the volume of fluid and blood over what the right-sided circulation would normally handle. Initially, the left-sided pressures are higher than the right-sided pressures.

If the flow of blood from the left atrium to the right atrium continues, a kind of reversal happens. Increased pressure develops on the right side. The patient then develops a right-to-left shunt, which is called *Eisenmenger's syndrome.* You can see this shunt in any type of cyanotic congenital heart disease, but it's most likely to come up in reference to atrial septal defect.

Here are some key points about atrial septal defect:

- ✓ You can hear a midsystolic murmur with an increased P2 component of the S2.
- ✓ The most common type of atrial septal defect is ostium secundum.
- ✓ There's a fixed splitting of the S2, which is a common giveaway on medical exams.
- ✓ A good imaging procedure to see whether a shunt is present is a specific kind of echocardiographic study called a *bubble study* (a transcranial Doppler with bubble contrast).
- ✓ The treatment is surgical intervention. The outcome is better if persistent pulmonary hypertension hasn't yet developed.

Persistent patent ductus arteriosus

The *patent ductus arteriosus* (PDA) is a link between the pulmonary artery and the arch of the aorta that's supposed to close during the first month or so after birth. In a patient with patent ductus arteriosus, this connection stays intact, which is not a good thing. Blood from the aorta flows backward into the pulmonary circulation and the lungs, which can cause all kinds of problems, including pulmonary edema and congestive heart failure.

With untreated patent ductus arteriosus (just as with an untreated atrial septal defect), the affected person can develop Eisenmenger's syndrome (a right-to-left shunt). The treatment is usually surgical.

Note that NSAIDs can be used to help close the patent ductus arteriosus, because prostaglandins can help keep this shunt open. That being said, surgical intervention can be curative.

Viewing ventricular septal defect

Ventricular septal defect is a congenital tear in the ventricular septum. It causes a left-to-right shunt. Unlike atrial septal defect and patent ductus arteriosus, the ventricular septal defect isn't a form a cyanotic congenital heart disease. Here are a few key points concerning ventricular septal defect:

- It's the most common cause of congenital heart disease in newborns.
- It doesn't cause Eisenmenger's syndrome (a right-to-left shunt).
- It's one of the big four heart defects in tetralogy of Fallot.
- On physical examination, you hear a holosystolic murmur. For PANCE purposes, recall that the two other causes of holosystolic murmurs are mitral regurgitation and tricuspid regurgitation.
- Although ventricular septal defect can sometimes be treated by just following it closely, it usually requires surgical intervention.

The telling tetralogy of Fallot

Tetralogy of Fallot (TOF) is a congenital heart defect, the most common cyanotic heart defect, and the most common cause of blue baby syndrome. In terms of PANCE questions, you just need to know the parts of the syndrome. Here are four aspects of tetralogy of Fallot:

- Ventricular septal defect (VSD)
- Right ventricular hypertrophy
- Pulmonic stenosis
- Overriding aorta

Because tetralogy of Fallot is a form of cyanotic congenital heart disease, manifestations include cyanosis. The cyanosis is a cause of the secondary polycythemia that you see in cyanotic congenital heart disease. The treatment for this condition is primarily surgical.

Going Ga-Ga Over Conduction Disorders

Rich has been around awhile and has taught both medical residents and physician assistants. Before that, he was a med student. Rich knows that when it comes to cardiology, two of the biggest causes of consternation, angst, and pain are answering physical-exam questions and identifying heart rhythms. During an in-training exam in cardiology, he once saw one of his colleagues abruptly drop to the floor, assume the fetal position, and start sucking his thumb. Another person stood up and began screaming in an unintelligible language. This is complicated stuff, and we know it.

We don't want you to go crazy. Just read this section carefully, and you'll increase your mastery of conduction-system disorders.

Sometimes you'll be the only person on the cardiology service with normal sinus rhythm (NSR). (Well, hopefully the cardiologist's will be normal, too.) Check out Figure 3-2 for a refresher on what a normal sinus rhythm looks like. Flip back here as often as you'd like to see how ECGs of the conditions we describe in this section differ from the norm.

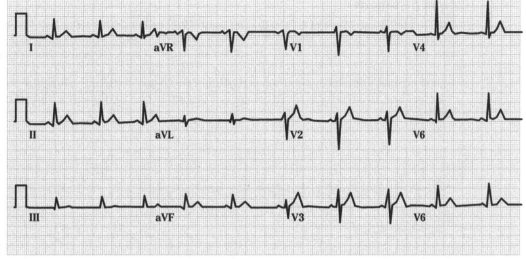

Figure 3-2:
An ECG
of a nor-
mal sinus
rhythm.

Annihilating atrial flutter and atrial fibrillation

Atrial flutter and atrial fibrillation are probably the two most common arrhythmias you'll deal with during your clinical career.

Atrial flutter

Atrial flutter is recognizable on an ECG or rhythm strip because of its saw-tooth appearance. Look at Figure 3-3 to see what we mean.

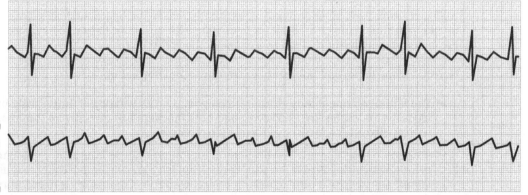

Figure 3-3:
An ECG of
atrial flutter.

Here are two important points about atrial flutter:

- ✔ Beta blockers and calcium channel blockers can be used for rate control, as can digoxin (Lanoxin), which also functions as an AV nodal blocker.

- ✔ On physical examination, the rhythm can be irregular or regular, depending on the atrial flutter. For example, a 2:1 atrial flutter can sound very regular, whereas a 3:1 atrial flutter sounds very irregular.

Atrial fibrillation

Atrial fibrillation involves an atrium that is "fibrillating" rather than conducting. Imagine all sorts of atrial impulses being thrown at the AV node. In this situation, you're called to see a patient with a tachycardia and you're trying to figure out what's causing the abnormal rhythm.

A-fib is probably the most common arrhythmia you'll deal with in the hospital setting, even more so than atrial flutter. Figure 3-4 gives an example of a rhythm strip showing atrial fibrillation.

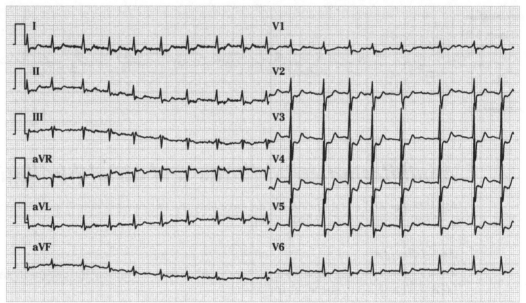

Figure 3-4:
An ECG
of atrial
fibrillation.

A-fib can result from an underlying illness that stresses the heart, such as sepsis or pneumonia. You should check a TSH level in anyone with atrial fibrillation to evaluate for possible underlying hyperthyroidism as a cause of the arrhythmia.

Here are some important points about treating atrial fibrillation:

- The initial treatment focuses on rate control. Just as with atrial flutter, calcium channel blockers like diltiazem (Cardizem) and beta blockers like metoprolol (Lopressor) as well as digoxin (Lanoxin) can be used for rate control.

- If a person has been in atrial fibrillation for longer than 48 hours, or if you encounter a person with atrial fibrillation and its duration isn't known, empiric anticoagulation with intravenous heparin with transition to oral warfarin (Coumadin) is mandatory to decrease the risk of embolic stroke.

- A person with acute congestive heart failure and atrial fibrillation can be very hard to treat, because he or she has lost the 20 percent "atrial kick" to the left ventricle.

You can convert someone from atrial fibrillation to normal sinus rhythm (NSR) in a few different ways. In many cases, just slowing down the ventricular rate with the medications we've mentioned is enough. Other medications that are used to try to convert A-fib to normal sinus rhythm include amiodarone (Cordarone), sotalol (Betapace), and procainamide (Procan-SR).

Electrical cardioversion can also be done, although this requires the person to be anticoagulated for several weeks prior, and a transesophageal echocardiogram is usually done to make sure that there isn't a clot in the area of the atrium known as the *left atrial appendage*.

Reviewing some conduction system blocks

Many different kinds of blocks can occur along the cardiac conduction system, from the sinus node to the AV node to the bundle of Purkinje fibers. Here you read about the different blocks of the conduction system and how to evaluate them. (Other kinds of blocks are mental. Rich, for example, had a severe case of writer's block when initially writing this chapter.)

First-degree AV block

First-degree AV block is fairly simple. The normal PR interval is ≤ 200 milliseconds (0.2 seconds). In a *first-degree AV block,* the PR interval is longer than that. It's fixed; it doesn't vary or change. Causes can include medications like beta blockers or medical conditions that can affect conduction of the sinus node, such as an aortic valve abscess. Figure 3-5 gives you a look at a strip showing a first-degree AV block.

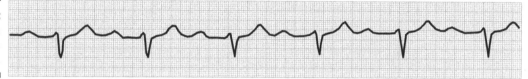

Figure 3-5: An ECG of a first-degree AV block.

Type I and Type II second-degree AV blocks

You can divide the second-degree AV block into two types — Type I and Type II. With this block, the focus is again on the PR interval. Figure 3-6 shows an example of a Type I second-degree AV block.

Think of Type I (also called *Wenckebach*) as a PR interval that's like Pinocchio's nose: With each beat, the PR interval gets longer and longer, before you lose a QRS complex. Then the cycle repeats itself. Type I has a pretty benign prognosis, and it's usually just watched closely.

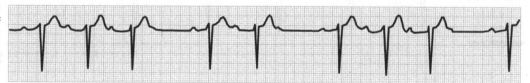

Figure 3-6: An ECG of a Type I second-degree AV block.

The Type II second-degree AV block (Mobitz Type II) is a baddie. It has some serious implications. Figure 3-7 shows an example of a Mobitz Type II AV block.

With Mobitz Type II, the PR interval is fixed, but not all the P waves conduct to the ventricle. Thus, you can see some dropped QRS complexes. The atrial conduction is okay, so your P-to-P intervals are fine. If the atria aren't able to conduct to the ventricle, you get a P wave but not a corresponding QRS complex.

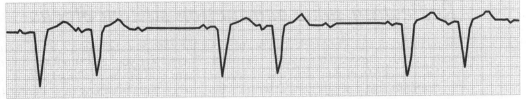

Figure 3-7:
An ECG of a
Mobitz Type
II AV block.

A big point about this conduction disturbance is that it can be a warning sign of impending transition to third-degree (complete) heart block and so is an indication for a pacemaker, especially if a lot of QRS complexes are being dropped.

Third-degree AV block

With a third-degree AV block, the P wave isn't being conducted to the QRS. The atria and the ventricles are kind of doing their own thing. This is an indication for a pacemaker. Figure 3-8 shows an example of a third-degree AV block.

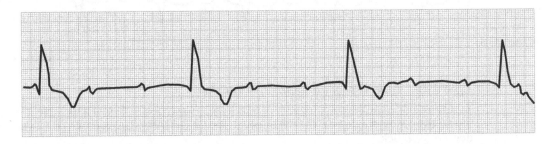

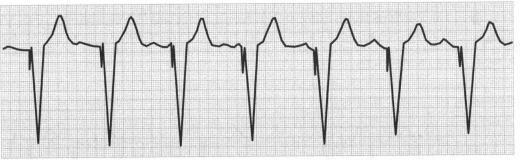

Figure 3-8:
An ECG of a
third-degree
AV block
and an ECG
of a paced
rhythm.

Sinus bradycardia and sick sinus syndrome

Sinus bradycardia can be symptomatic or asymptomatic. For example, some athletes can have resting pulses in the high 50 BPM range to the low 40 BPM range, and that's symptomatic of nothing except being in great shape. But in many people, the bradycardia is symptomatic. Common causes of sinus bradycardia include medications like beta blockers and calcium channel blockers. Causes can also include electrolyte abnormalities, including hyperkalemia, and ischemia to the area. The affected person can feel dizzy, weak, or lightheaded, or even experience a syncopal or near-syncopal episode. Treatments can involve evaluating and treating the abnormal electrolytes and discontinuing the offending medications. In some cases, a pacemaker may be needed.

Sick sinus syndrome (where do we get these terms?) can cause long symptomatic sinus bradycardia and can cause long sinus pauses. It can also be part of a condition called tachy-brady syndrome. Sick sinus syndrome can be an indication for a pacemaker.

Battling bundle branch blocks

For the PANCE, know your right and left bundle branch blocks. Be able to diagnose them and be aware of the important causes of each one.

Right bundle branch blocks

You can see *right bundle branch blocks* (RBBBs) when you look at leads V1 to V4 on an ECG. You see a big-time R wave in these leads, as compared to an S wave. You can also see what looks like rabbit ears in the leads (see Figure 3-9). In addition, you see widening of the QRS wave, and the T wave is in the opposite deflection to the R wave. This means if the R wave is up, the T is down.

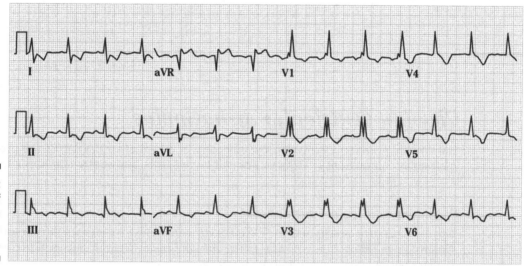

Figure 3-9: An ECG of right bundle branch block.

Common causes of right bundle branch blocks include a pulmonary embolus or pulmonary hypertension. Most of the time, there's no treatment for a right bundle branch block except evaluating and treating the underlying cause.

Left bundle branch blocks

Left bundle branch blocks (LBBB) can be old or new. If you see a new left bundle branch block, you need to worry that an ischemic event (STEMI) affecting the left ventricle has occurred. A cardiac catherization may need to be done to evaluate the coronary artery anatomy. Figure 3-10 shows an example of a left bundle branch block.

On an ECG, you focus primarily on leads V5 and V6. You see a broad notched or slurred R wave in leads I, aVL, V5, and V6 and a widened QRS greater than three blocks.

Patients with a left bundle branch block require complete cardiac evaluation, and those with a left bundle branch block and syncope or near-syncope may require a pacemaker. Some patients with a left bundle branch block, a markedly prolonged QRS, and congestive heart failure may benefit from a pacemaker, which provides rapid left ventricular contractions.

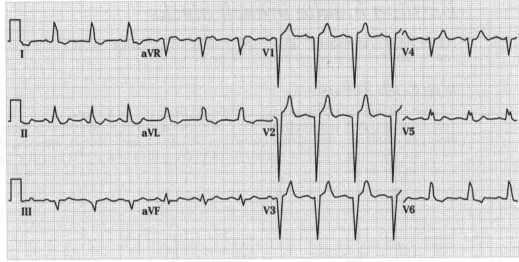

Figure 3-10: An ECG of left bundle branch block.

Viewing ventricular arrhythmias

The three big ventricular problems you need to be aware of for the PANCE are premature ventricular contractions (PVCs), ventricular tachycardia, and ventricular fibrillation. The latter two are life-threatening.

Premature ventricular contractions

Premature ventricular contractions (PVCs) occur commonly. Sometimes the person can feel a "skipped beat." Many times, an ECG picks this up. Concerning the causes of premature ventricular contractions, think about the three *i*'s:

- **Irritability:** The causes of myocardial irritability are hypoxemia and electrolyte abnormalities, including hypokalemia and hypomagnesemia. Correcting these conditions can really help treat myocardial irritability.

- **Infection:** Infection can be a big-time cause of premature ventricular contractions, especially in the hospital setting. Infection increases the metabolic demand of the body, and the heart has to work faster.

- **Ischemia:** Ischemia can also be a cause of premature ventricular contractions and requires further investigation.

Sometimes a person has premature ventricular contractions but no organic cause can be found. This is part of what makes medicine fascinating (or extremely frustrating).

Ventricular tachycardia

Ventricular tachycardia (V-tach) comes in two flavors (see Figure 3-11):

- *Non-sustained V-tach,* which is a string of PVCs together, usually for 8 beats or less

- *Sustained V-tach,* a life-threatening arrhythmia that can become ventricular fibrillation

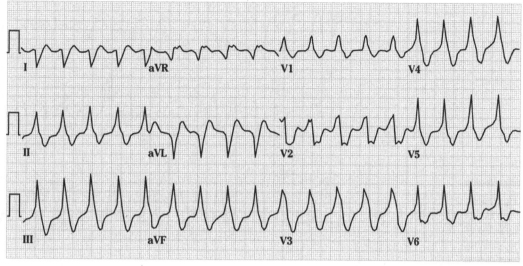

Figure 3-11:
An ECG of
V-tach.

V-tach can occur in the setting of myocardial infarction, particularly in the first 24 hours after an anterior wall myocardial infarction, although it can occur after any type of STEMI. (See the earlier section "Knowing the NSTEMI and STEMI.")

Look at electrolytes as possible causes or contributing factors of V-tach (for example, low potassium and magnesium levels). Also, look at medications and conditions that can prolong the QT interval as predisposing factors. Be aware that there are also hereditary causes of long QT intervals, including congenital long QT syndrome (LQTS). Acquired causes can be secondary to the use of certain medications, including some psychotrophic drugs. Many antiarrythmic medications can also prolong the QT interval.

The treatment depends on whether the person has a blood pressure and a pulse:

- **The person doesn't have a blood pressure or doesn't have a pulse:** First do an electrical cardioversion.

- **The person has both a blood pressure and a pulse:** Several medications, including lidocaine (Xylocaine) and amiodarone (Cordarone), can help stabilize the situation.

Be aware of the side effects of the antiarrythmics. Lidocaine can cause neurotoxicity, so follow blood levels to minimize the risk. Amiodarone has many possible side effects, including pulmonary fibrosis, hypothyroidism and hyperthyroidism, increased liver function levels, and blue-gray sclera.

Torsades de pointes ("twisting of the points," from ballet) is a distinct form of V-tach that requires magnesium sulfate to be given as an intravenous push as part of the initial treatment. In addition to magnesium replacement, temporary cardiac pacing is also recommended. Cardioversion may or may not be needed, depending on how the individual responds to therapy.

Torsades has a characteristic look you should be familiar with. Figure 3-12 should just scream "torsades de pointes" at you.

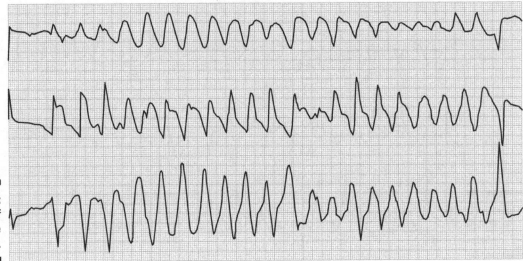

Figure 3-12:
An ECG of
torsades de
pointes.

Ventricular fibrillation

Ventricular fibrillation (also known as V-fib) is a life-threatening emergency. V-fib requires emergent electrical cardioversion, because it's associated with sudden cardiac death. Figure 3-13 shows an example of V-fib.

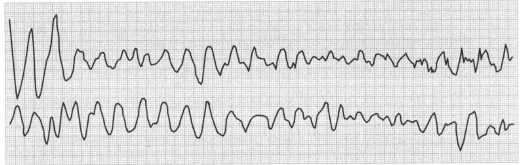

Figure 3-13:
An ECG
showing
ventricular
fibrillation.

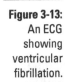

Which of the following is an adverse effect of procainamide (Procan-SR)?

(A) Teratogenesis

(B) Pulmonary fibrosis

(C) Neurotoxicity

(D) Drug-induced lupus syndrome

(E) Hyperkalemia

The correct answer is Choice (D). Procainamide, an antiarrythmic medication used in the treatment of ventricular tachycardia, can cause a drug-induced lupus. Choice (A), teratogenesis, is due to ACE inhibitors and statin therapy. Choice (B), pulmonary fibrosis, is due to amiodarone (Cordarone). Choice (C), neurotoxicity, can be associated with lidocaine (Xylocaine). Choice (E), hyperkalemia, is a side effect of ACE inhibitors, ARBs, and spironolactone (Aldactone).

Probing the Pericardium

The pericardium, the outer covering of the heart, can get inflamed and irritated from a variety of conditions. For PANCE purposes, be familiar with pericarditis, pericardial effusion, and cardiac tamponade.

Linking pericarditis to multiple causes

Pericarditis is simply an inflammation of the pericardium. Causes of pericarditis may be viral (think Coxsackie B virus), autoimmune (think lupus), medication-induced (think cyclosporine, warfarin, and heparin), or malignant (think Kaposi's sarcoma or metastatic disease from another solid tumor malignancy, most commonly lung carcinoma). *Uremic pericarditis* is an effect of untreated, advanced kidney disease. And don't forget about tuberculosis as a cause of pericarditis — tuberculosis, as you read about in Chapter 4, can do just about anything. In case the list isn't long enough, other possible causes of pericarditis are bacterial, fungal, radiation-induced, and that famous catch-all *idiopathic* (meaning "we don't have a clue").

Here are some key points concerning pericarditis:

- The classic pain pattern of pericarditis is often pleuritic. The patient feels relief when sitting up and forward.
- You can best hear an audible pericardial friction rub (think of Velcro) with the person sitting up and forward. The sound is often triphasic.
- The treatment for pericarditis is initially indomethacin (Indocin), but prednisone and colchicine (Colcrys) can also be used if the condition is refractory to NSAIDs.
- The typical ECG findings for acute pericarditis include diffuse ST elevation and PR segment depression.

Building up to pericardial effusion

Pericardial effusion is a buildup of fluid in the pericardial space. If it occurs gradually, there may not be any hemodynamic compromise. It comes in four flavors: transudative, exudative, hemorrhagic, and malignant. The big causes of a pericardial effusion, which are similar to the causes of pericarditis, are connective tissue disorders, malignancies, infections, and medications. Don't forget tuberculosis as another cause of a pericardial effusion.

Look for chest pain, pressure symptoms, and on radiography, the so-called "water-bottle heart." Look for Ewart's sign (dullness to percussion). To make you crazy, we'll also say that a small effusion may have no symptoms.

Here's a possible PANCE subtlety: pericardial effusion is also present after a repair of atrial septal defect secundum (ASD).

Acting swiftly to relieve cardiac tamponade

Cardiac tamponade occurs when a pericardial effusion gets really big really, really quickly and in effect cuts off the left ventricle and blocks inflow. Picture the pericardium rapidly filling with fluid. Cardiac tamponade can be a cause of hypotension. Here are some key points about cardiac tamponade:

✔ On physical examination, jugular venous distention (JVD), Kussmaul's sign, and pulsus paradoxus can be present. Be familiar with these signs. (And please don't confuse Kussmaul's sign with Kussmaul respirations. *Kussmaul's respirations* are tachypnea seen in the setting of a metabolic acidosis. *Kussmaul's sign* is an increase in JVD on inspiration due to the pericardial effusion.) There are also diminished heart sounds.

✔ The ECG shows decreased amplitude and poor R wave progression. Electrical alternans can also be present.

✔ If a person has a Swan-Ganz catheter, you see equalization of pressures in someone with cardiac tamponade. The heart is literally getting squeezed in there. You see the pulmonary artery diastolic (PAD) pressure (an example of right-sided pressures) equal the pulmonary capillary wedge pressure (PCWP) (which is the awesomest way to measure left-sided pressures).

In contrast, in cardiogenic shock, the person usually has a PCWP that's greater than the PAD pressure (reflecting a left-sided or systolic problem — a pumping problem), although both can be elevated.

✔ You can confirm the diagnosis of cardiac tamponade by bedside echocardiogram. It shows collapse of the right atrium and ventricle. There can also be obstruction of the flow of blood from the left ventricle as the buildup of fluid causes shifting of the interventricular septum to the left. This is not good.

✔ The treatment is a pericardiocentesis using the xiphoid process of the sternum as a guide.

Evaluating Endocarditis

Endocarditis is an inflammation of the heart valve, and for the PANCE, you should know the different flavors: infective endocarditis and subacute bacterial endocarditis.

The staph: Looking for vegetation with infective endocarditis

Infective endocarditis (IE) is a baddie. It commonly affects the mitral valve, although IV drug users may have right-sided endocarditis causing tricuspid regurgitation (see the earlier section "Testing the tricuspid valve" for details on that condition). The most common cause of infective endocarditis is *Staphylococcus aureus*.

The diagnosis of infective endocarditis is made by at least two sets of blood cultures being positive (where *S. aureus* is concerned) and the presence of vegetation on a cardiac valve. This requires a transesophageal echocardiogram (TEE) to diagnose; it may be missed on a transthoracic echocardiogram (TTE).

The PANCE may ask you about a plethora of signs concerning infective endocarditis on physical examination. Sometimes the initial cause is intermittent and relapsing fevers. Cyanosis may or may not be present (note that there are many causes of cyanosis outside of pulmonary disorders).

Other big physical exam findings include Roth spots, Janeway lesions, and/or Osler's nodes. *Roth spots* are retinal, flame-shaped hemorrhages in the eye that you can see on fundoscopic examination. *Janeway lesions* are splinter hemorrhages that you see on the fingernails. *Osler's nodes* are papular, erythematous lesions found on the palms and soles.

The treatment for infective endocarditis is 6 weeks of intravenous antibiotics, usually a beta-lactam agent such as penicillin or the antibiotic vancomycin (Vancocin), and an amino-glycoside antibiotic such as gentamicin (Garamycin) for the first week or two. Any more than this, and the person is at risk of developing aminoglycoside ototoxicity.

Depending on the extent of the vegetation, a cardiothoracic surgeon is often consulted to see whether intervention is warranted.

The strep: Searching for structural issues with subacute endocarditis

Subacute endocarditis (SBE) is primarily caused by *Streptococcus viridans*. Less-common causes include other *Streptococcus* species and *Enterococcus*. Here are three key points about subacute endocarditis:

- It's less acute than infective endocarditis in its presentation.

- When you find subacute endocarditis, order a transesophageal echocardiogram (TEE) not only to look for vegetation but also to look for evidence of a structural heart problem (an incompetent valve).

- Subacute endocarditis requires at least 4 to 6 weeks of antibiotics to treat. The standard treatment is a minimum of 4 weeks of high-dose intravenous penicillin with an aminoglycoside such as gentamicin (Garamycin).

Worrying about the Vascular System

Cardiovascular doesn't refer to just the heart; it also refers to the blood vessels. Guess what! For the PANCE, you have to worry about the arteries and veins as well as the heart. Before you read this section, make sure your distal pulses are strong and palpable.

Dissecting the aorta, so to speak

One scenario you never want to miss is the person with a history of uncontrolled hypertension who presents to the emergency room with acute chest pain radiating to the back or with acute abdominal pain radiating to the back. With this scenario, think about *acute thoracic dissection* and *abdominal dissection,* respectively. These are tears in the inner wall of the aorta.

Here are some key points about aortic dissection:

- On physical examination, if you find a difference in the blood pressure between the arms, think about a thoracic dissection. Also check the pulses in both feet, because these can be affected if someone has an abdominal dissection.

- The diagnosis is best confirmed by a CT scan of the thorax or abdomen with IV contrast. If dye can't be given, then the next best test is a transesophageal echocardiogram (TEE). A plain chest radiograph isn't specific enough.

- Treatment depends on whether you're dealing with a Type A or Type B dissection. The *Type A dissection* indicates a more proximal tear and is treated with surgery. The *Type B dissection* (anatomically occurring distal to the left subclavian artery) is treated medically.

✔ The medical treatment for acute aortic dissection is the abrupt lowering of blood pressure to 120–130 mmHg systolic. This involves the combination of a potent vasodilator, such as an intravenous calcium channel blocker like nicardipine (Cardene), along with a beta blocker to prevent reflex tachycardia that can make the symptoms worse.

Acute aortic dissection is treated differently from an acute stroke. An acute aortic dissection involves an abrupt lowering of blood pressure. With an acute stroke, you lower blood pressure gradually in order to maintain cerebral perfusion.

It's recommended that men 65 to 75 years of age who have smoked be screened once for an abdominal aortic aneurysm (AAA) by an abdominal ultrasound.

Establishing arterial patency

For the PANCE, you should be familiar with three arterial medical conditions: temporal (giant cell) arteritis, peripheral arterial disease (PAD), and acute arterial occlusion. In each of these conditions, you're dealing with a problem of arterial patency.

Temporal arteritis

Temporal arteritis (TA) is a rheumatologic condition, an inflammation of the temporal artery. The classic presenting symptoms are a headache and an acute loss of vision. Other associated symptoms can include jaw claudication. Here are three points about temporal arteritis:

✔ Part of the diagnostic workup includes obtaining a sed rate, which is elevated in temporal arteritis.

✔ The diagnosis is confirmed by a temporal artery biopsy. However, because of sampling error (the chance of missing the inflamed area), even if the biopsy is negative, the person gets treated if the symptoms are present.

✔ The treatment is steroids.

A condition that's closely associated with temporal arteritis is *polymyalgia rheumatica* (PMR), which is associated with proximal muscle weakness and pain. We talk about PMR in Chapter 6.

Peripheral arterial disease

Peripheral arterial disease (PAD) is very common in the United States. Here we talk about it as it affects the arteries of the lower extremities. A classic presenting symptom is *claudication,* pain in the legs that occurs with walking and is relieved by rest. For PANCE purposes, know how to evaluate peripheral arterial disease and the options for managing it. Here are some key points:

✔ Risk factors for peripheral arterial disease include diabetes mellitus, hypertension, hyperhomocysteinemia, and high levels of inflammation in the body (an elevated C-reactive protein level). If you find peripheral arterial disease, look for other potential concomitant medical conditions.

✔ The initial finding on physical examination is diminished distal pulses. A good test in a physical examination is the ankle brachial index (ABI). An ABI score of < 0.8 is suggestive of peripheral arterial disease.

✔ An initial screening test for peripheral arterial disease is a Doppler arterial ultrasound of the lower extremity.

✔ The gold standard for the diagnosis of peripheral arterial disease is a contrast arteriogram to evaluate the location and severity of the blockage.

Acute arterial occlusion

An *acute arterial occlusion* is a surgical emergency. The most common scenario is the acute loss of a pulse in one of the extremities, indicating that something is seriously wrong. This can happen as a result of a vascular event (such as an abdominal aortic dissection) or a hypercoagulable state that can cause an arterial thrombosis (such as antiphospholipid antibody syndrome and/or factor V Leiden mutation that's homozygous).

As we said, acute arterial occlusion is a surgical emergency. The patient must go to the operating room for an emergent thrombectomy or embolectomy.

Evaluating the venous system

The veins are a little easier to deal with than the arteries. For the PANCE, be familar with four venous system conditions: superficial venous thrombophlebitis, varicose veins, venous insufficiency, and deep venous thrombosis.

Superficial venous thrombophlebitis

Superficial venous thrombophlebitis is an infection of a superficial vein. The initial presentation can be redness, warmth, and pain over the vein. The treatment involves oral antibiotics and anti-inflammatories like ibuprofen (Motrin).

Varicose veins

Varicose veins are dilated superficial veins that can occur on the legs. Risk factors include obesity and occupations that involve standing for a long time. Over time, varicose veins can become painful. The affected person can also experience leg cramps.

Treatment can include venous stripping. A nonsurgical approach is the use of sclerosing agents. Anti-inflammatories also have a role in initially decreasing the inflammation.

Venous insufficiency

Venous insufficiency is usually due to an incompetent valve in the veins. Recall that the venous system includes one-way valves. As a valve works less efficiently, the person can have edema, and venous stasis can develop as a result. Risk factors include obesity. The treatment is compression stockings and weight loss.

Deep venous thrombosis

Deep venous thrombosis (DVT) commonly presents as acute swelling of an affected extremity, usually a lower extremity, although it can affect the upper extremities as well. The key to diagnosis is having a high clinical suspicion that a deep venous thrombosis may be present as well as making an appraisal of risk factors. Here are some key points concerning deep venous thrombosis:

- Risk factors include Virchow's triad — stasis, hypercoagulable state, and injury to the endothelium — see Chapter 22. Additional risk factors include obesity, malignancy, and taking oral contraceptive pills. Causes include a long plane ride or car trip. The keys to answering PANCE questions likely lie in the patient's history.

- Physical exam findings suggestive of a lower-extremity deep venous thrombosis are a Moses' sign (also known as Bancroft's sign) and a Homans' sign. Note that these signs are only 50 percent predictive for a deep venous thrombosis.

- The diagnosis of a distal deep venous thrombosis can be made with a lower-extremity Doppler venous ultrasound. It may miss more proximal deep venous thromboses (for example, in the ileofemoral area).

> ✔ The D-dimer can help in the initial triage of a deep venous thrombosis. If the D-dimer is negative, it's less likely that any type of deep venous thrombosis is present.
>
> ✔ People who have deep venous thrombosis are at risk of pulmonary embolism. The more proximal the deep venous thrombosis, the higher the risk.

The treatment for deep venous thrombosis is heparin and warfarin (Coumadin). For an initial deep venous thrombosis, the time to be on warfarin is 3 to 6 months, depending on comorbid conditions and risk factors.

Practice Cardiovascular System Questions

These practice questions are similar to the PANCE cardiology and vascular system questions.

1. You're evaluating a 78-year-old man who presents to the emergency room with a heart rate of about 140–150 beats per minute. On the monitor, you see a narrow-complex tachycardia, but it's impossible to determine the underlying rhythm. You apply carotid massage, and the patient breaks into a normal sinus rhythm. What's the likely original rhythm?

   (A) Atrial fibrillation

   (B) Atrial flutter

   (C) Sinus tachycardia

   (D) Supraventricular tachycardia

   (E) Ventricular tachycardia

2. You're evaluating a 40-year-old man who presents with chest pressure with pain radiating down his left arm. His ECG is shown here:

   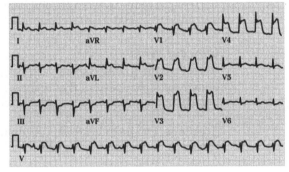

   After reading this ECG, which one of the following would you do next?

   (A) Start indomethacin (Indocin).

   (B) Start aspirin, intravenous heparin, and nitroglycerin.

   (C) Take the patient emergently to the cardiac catheterization lab.

   (D) Give aspirin and a beta blocker. Then give IV heparin and nitroglycerin.

   (E) Start intravenous dobutamine (Dobutrex).

3. You're evaluating a 35-year-old man who presents to your office with a headache. On physical examination, his blood pressure is 240/120 mmHg. On fundoscopic examination, you note the presence of papilledema. What's this person's underlying diagnosis?

    (A) Hypertensive emergency

    (B) Hypertensive urgency

    (C) Stage I hypertension

    (D) Stage III hypertension

    (E) Prehypertension

4. Which class of medications would you recommend for a young man with a history of high blood pressure who also has significant anxiety and panic disorder?

    (A) ACE inhibitors

    (B) Beta blockers

    (C) Alpha blockers

    (D) Hydrochlorothiazide

    (E) Calcium channel blockers

5. You're evaluating a 25-year-old woman who presents with palpitations. On examination, you hear a midsystolic click. Which one of the following would you recommend concerning evaluation of her heart condition?

    (A) She should be screened for major depressive disorder.

    (B) She should be screened for a bleeding diathesis.

    (C) She should be screened for rheumatic fever.

    (D) Her murmur would decrease with a Valsalva maneuver.

    (E) She may need a beta blocker if the palpitations continue.

6. Which one of the following would be used in the treatment of peripheral arterial disease (PAD)?

    (A) Indomethacin (Indocin)

    (B) Pentoxifylline (Trental)

    (C) Ranolazine (Ranexa)

    (D) Warfarin (Coumadin)

    (E) Dabigatran (Pradaxa)

Answers and Explanations

Use this answer key to score the practice cardiovascular questions from the preceding section. The answer explanations give you insight into why the correct answer is better than the other choices.

1. **D.** You can use carotid massage or Valsalva maneuvers to evaluate tachycardia. This intervention can either slow the rate down enough to identify the underlying rhythm or stop the rhythm in its path. Supraventricular tachycardia (SVT) — most commonly paroxysmal supraventricular tachycardia (PSVT) — breaks with a Valsalva maneuver or with adenosine. With Choices (A), (B), and (C) — atrial fibrillation, atrial flutter, and sinus tachycardia — these rhythms slow down, but they usually don't break. For Choice (E), ventricular tachycardia, the initial treatment is lidocaine.

2. **C.** This person is having an acute STEMI (ST elevation myocardial infarction) involving the anterior wall. You can see the fireman's hats on the ECG. This man needs to be taken to the cardiac catheterization lab pronto. Choice (E), dobutamine, isn't applicable here because you have no indication that he's in cardiogenic shock. Choices (A), (B), and (D) — starting indomethacin; starting aspirin, intravenous heparin, and nitroglycerin; and giving aspirin and a beta blocker followed by IV heparin and nitroglycerin — aren't necessarily wrong, but none of them is the best answer.

3. **A.** This person has a headache and papilledema, which is a sign of damage due to hypertension. This is called *hypertensive emergency*. A blood pressure ≥ 180 mmHg systolic with no symptoms is an example of a hypertensive *urgency,* Choice (B). Recall that Stage I hypertension, Choice (C), is a systolic blood pressure of 140–159 mmHg and/or a diastolic blood pressure of 90–99 mmHg. With the new criteria from the Joint National Committee on Prevention, Detection, Evaluation, and Treatment of High Blood Pressure (JNC), there's no Stage III hypertension, Choice (D), only Stages I and II.

4. **B.** In someone who has hypertension and panic disorder, beta blockers, Choice (B), are a good choice because the side effects include calming the person down. Alpha blockers, Choice (C), could be used in an older man with benign prostatic hyperplasia. ACE inhibitors, Choice (A), should be given first-line to anyone with hypertension, but you try to personalize your therapy as much as possible. Hydrochlorothiazide (Microzide), Choice (D), is used in the treatment of hypertension, as are calcium channel blockers, Choice (E).

5. **E.** This person has mitral valve prolapse, as seen with a midsystolic click. It's associated with panic disorder, not depression, Choice (A). If palpitations occur with mitral valve prolapse, a beta blocker, Choice (E), first-line wouldn't be unreasonable. Choice (B), bleeding diathesis, concerns the association between aortic stenosis and gastrointestinal bleeding secondary to arteriovenous malformation (AVM), which is termed *acquired von Willebrand's disease*. Regarding Choice (C), you can see mitral stenosis and tricuspid stenosis with rheumatic fever. Mitral valve prolapse would increase in the setting of a Valsalva maneuver, Choice (D).

6. **B.** Choice (B), pentoxifylline, is an older medication used in treating peripheral arterial disease. Choice (A), indomethacin, is used to treat varicose veins and phlebitis by decreasing the inflammation. Choice (C), ranolazine, is an antianginal medication used in treating coronary artery disease for someone on maximal medical therapy; the ranolazine helps with symptoms. Choice (D), warfarin, is used in anticoagulation therapy for atrial fibrillation as well as for the treatment of a deep venous thrombosis. Choice (E), dabigatran, is a new medication used in treating atrial fibrillation.

Chapter 4

Taking a Deep Breath: The Lungs

. . . .

In This Chapter

▶ Evaluating obstructive and restrictive lung disease

▶ Considering the pleura

▶ Looking at infectious processes

▶ Evaluating childhood lung problems

▶ Investigating lung cancer

▶ Exploring the pulmonary vasculature

. . . .

*P*ulmonary topics account for a significant amount of content on the PANCE and PANRE. In this chapter, you review lung-related topics, including asthma, chronic obstructive pulmonary disease, bronchitis, and pleural-based disorders, among others. We also include common pulmonary processes that affect children.

Evaluating Obstructive Lung Disease

This section covers obstructive lung diseases that are diagnosed through a pulmonary function test (PFT). We review evaluating and managing asthma, chronic obstructive pulmonary disease (COPD), bronchiectasis, and cystic fibrosis. If you recall, obstructive lung disease is differentiated from restrictive lung disease based on the findings of the PFT.

With obstructive lung disease, spirometry findings include a reduction in the FEV1 (forced expiratory volume in 1 second) and a reduction in the FEV1/FVC (forced vital capacity) ratio. You read about spirometry findings in the section "Chronic obstruction: Correcting COPD." With this condition, the findings on spirometry actually define how bad someone's COPD is.

Ameliorating asthma

Asthma is a chronic inflammatory process of the airway. An asthma attack can be stimulated by a hyperresponsiveness to environmental exposures or other triggers. Asthma is reversible, and it can resolve either on its own or with treatment. Asthma is very common in the younger population, especially African-Americans. During the teenage years, males are more likely than females to have asthma.

Offering insights on asthma

Triggers for asthma can include seasonal allergies, environmental allergens (mold, dust, and so on), salicylic acid derivatives (see Sampter's triad in Chapter 22), exercise, changes in weather or temperature, and gastroesophageal reflux disease (GERD).

Allergic rhinitis, GERD, and/or cough-variant asthma are the three primary differential diagnoses for chronic cough in the outpatient setting. GERD can sometimes present solely as a cough without any symptoms of heartburn at all, appearing predominantly at night. This is great information for a PANCE question.

Here are key points about asthma:

✔ Clinical presentation includes rapid onset of shortness of breath, tightness in the chest, and/or cough during an acute asthma exacerbation. You may hear an audible wheeze.

✔ Physical examination can demonstrate tachypnea, wheezing, and decreased air movement on lung auscultation. Accessory muscle use is a bad sign — it indicates that the person is tiring and may need to be intubated for airway protection.

✔ Labs can show a CBC demonstrating a mild eosinophilia. Although bronchial thickening, hyperinflation, and focal atelectasis suggest asthma when they're present, the chest radiograph can be normal.

✔ The diagnosis is made by spirometry — an FEV1/FVC < 0.8 is diagnostic. But a more important measurement for asthma is the peak flow. During an asthma exacerbation, the peak flow, as measured by a peak flow meter, is usually substantially reduced from the patient's baseline.

The peak flow is vital both in the early evaluation of an asthma attack and also chronically to assess efficacy of treatment. Different calculations, based on a person's height, weight, and gender, can determine what a normal peak flow should be. Variations from this can determine how reduced the peak flow is from normal during an asthma exacerbation.

If you obtain an ABG that's normal during an acute asthma exacerbation (that is, a normal pH and a normal pCO_2), that's a very bad prognostic sign that the patient is tiring and is having trouble getting rid of the excess carbon dioxide. During an acute asthma episode, you should see a respiratory alkalosis characterized by an elevated pH and low pCO_2. There may or may not be a low P_aO_2 as well.

During an acute asthma exacerbation, treatment includes intravenous steroids and beta-2 agonists (for example, albuterol sulfate). After the acute exacerbation is over, the treatment depends on the type and severity of asthma.

Examining asthma classifications and treatments

Asthma has different classifications. It can be either intermittent or persistent. The only type of intermittent asthma is *mild intermittent asthma*. Here, the asthma exacerbations are infrequent, and they usually resolve through treatment with a short-acting beta-2 agonist such as albuterol.

The three kinds of persistent asthma are mild, moderate, and severe. The differences have to do with the frequency and severity of symptoms:

✔ **Mild persistent asthma:** The person has fewer than two asthma exacerbations in a 7-day period. He or she also never has more than one exacerbation per day. Usually the treatment involves an inhaled corticosteroid.

✔ **Moderate persistent asthma:** The person has daily asthma symptoms and nighttime symptoms more than once per week. The treatment usually involves an inhaled corticosteroid plus a long-acting beta-2 agonist.

✔ **Severe persistent asthma:** The person is exhibiting nearly continuous symptoms with frequent nocturnal exacerbations. Other medications, such as montelukast (Singulair) may be used. Steroids may be needed for an acute exacerbation.

Understand that treating asthma requires a stepwise approach that depends on the frequency and severity of symptoms.

When you're answering test questions about asthma, the classification and treatment are big topics. You repeatedly see questions in which a patient diagnosed with a certain classification of asthma is failing prescribed medical therapy. You may then be asked which classification of asthma he or she has now or how you should change his or her therapy.

You're evaluating a 45-year-old woman with a history of recurrent asthma exacerbations. She's admitted with severe shortness of breath. The patient has limited audible wheezing, is tachypneic, and is using accessory muscles. An ABG is pH 7.18, pCO_2 69, and pO_2 56. What is your next step?

(A) Do bilevel positive airway pressure (BiPAP).

(B) Put the patient on a 100% nonrebreathing mask.

(C) Do emergent intubation.

(D) Give a stat dose of methylprednisolone (Solu-Medrol).

(E) Give a stat nebulizer treatment with albuterol.

The answer is Choice (C), emergent intubation. This patient has *status asthmaticus,* a particularly severe asthmatic attack that doesn't respond adequately to usual therapy. The first thing you assess for any patient (or on any test question) is the ABCs (airway, breathing, and circulation). You need to stabilize the airway. Limited wheezing in this scenario indicates decreased air movement and is also an ominous sign. This patient is getting tired and needs help. BiPAP won't work here because the patient is too fatigued.

Chronic obstruction: Correcting COPD

Chronic obstructive pulmonary disease (COPD) is an inflammatory disease of the lungs caused by one of two medical conditions:

- **Chronic bronchitis:** A productive cough for at least 3 months per year for 2 consecutive years

- **Emphysema:** A lung disease characterized by airway inflammation and loss of elasticity of the alveoli over time, secondary to destruction of the walls of the alveoli; continued smoking makes this process worse

Diagnosing COPD

Here are the key points concerning COPD:

- The biggest risk for developing COPD is cigarette smoking. Environmental exposures, such as long-term exposure to second-hand smoke, are also important predisposing factors. Other risk factors include occupational exposures to chemicals and other pulmonary irritants. Alpha-1 antitrypsin (ATT) deficiency is a genetic cause of emphysema.

- Clinical presentations of an acute COPD exacerbation include shortness of breath and productive cough.

- Physical examination can show tachypnea, a decreased pulse oximetry, and cyanosis if hypoxemia is present.

- COPD isn't diagnosed by chest radiograph findings. However, radiography can be suggestive, especially if you see hyperinflation of both lung fields. Emphysematous bullae may or may not be present on a chest radiograph.

- CT scan findings can show two patterns of emphysemas: centrilobular or panacinar. *Centrilobular emphysema,* which is due to chronic tobacco use, causes changes that predominantly affect the upper lobes as seen on CT scan. *Panacinar emphysema* causes changes in the lower lobes as seen on CT scan and commonly occurs with alpha-1 antitrypsin deficiency.

Alpha-1 antitrypsin deficiency is characterized by elevated liver function tests and worsening emphysema. The condition, which is autosomally inherited, can be either homozygous or heterozygous, and it usually affects people at a very young age. You diagnose it by checking an alpha-1 antitrypsin level. For people with lung involvement, treatment can involve administering alpha-1 antitrypsin protein. This condition can also cause liver failure in a young person, especially if the affected person is homozygous for this condition. In cases of fulminant liver failure, the patient may need a liver transplant.

Physiologic characteristics in a question can help tip you off that COPD is present. For example, the classic description of someone with chronic bronchitis is an obese individual with cyanosis, often termed "the blue bloater." This is also referred to as the Pickwickian syndrome, named after the character Samuel Pickwick, the main character in Charles Dickens's novel *The Pickwick Papers*. Joe, a "fat boy," eats lots of food and constantly falls asleep. Joe and others with chronic bronchitis often have alveolar hypoventilation and suffer from obstructive sleep apnea as well. Indications of *obstructive sleep apnea syndrome* include being overweight and falling asleep at any time of day.

The diagnosis of COPD is confirmed via a pulmonary function test (PFT). Changes from baseline can be followed by spirometry in a pulmonologist's office. To determine the severity of COPD, look at three basic parameters:

- ✓ **FEV1 (forced expiratory volume in 1 second):** The FEV1 is how much air can be forced out in 1 second. You look at the FEV1 level to see how far from the predicted value it lies. For example, if the FEV1 is < 50 percent of what the predicted value should be, then the patient has severe COPD. After establishing the FEV1, see whether the FEV1 improves after administering a bronchodilator.

- ✓ **FVC (forced vital capacity):** The FVC is how much air can be forced out during a forced exhalation, like when doing a PFT.

- ✓ **FEV1/FVC ratio:** A normal value for many people is > 0.7, or 70 percent. If the FEV1/FVC ratio is less than 70 percent, then there's likely some degree of airflow obstruction.

Knowing someone's FEV1 level and FEV1/FVC ratio and how far off they are from their predicted values is important because you may see significant decreases in these levels before a person becomes symptomatic.

Treating COPD

The treatment for an acute COPD exacerbation consists of intravenous steroids and a combination of short-acting beta-2 agonists (albuterol or levalbuterol [Xopenex]) and anticholinergic agents (ipratropium bromide), usually given via a nebulizer. If there's evidence of an acute infection, antibiotics are administered as well.

Other agents used to treat COPD include theophylline, which increases the contractility of the diaphragm. Oxygen is given if hypoxemia is present. The long-term treatment is for the patient to stop smoking. Pulmonary rehabilitation can also be prescribed.

Be aware (and beware) that in an acute exacerbation of COPD, you may see an *acute respiratory acidosis* characterized by a low pH and a very elevated pCO_2. Patients with COPD can be "chronic retainers." A tipoff to this is an elevated carbon dioxide on a CHEM-7 blood test. An ABG here shows a *chronic respiratory acidosis*, with a low pH and a slightly elevated pCO_2.

If you see a question in which a patient has an acute COPD exacerbation with a change in mental status and an acute respiratory acidosis, the treatment is either BiPAP or intubation. A person has to be able to take a deep breath for BiPAP to work, so the treatment depends on how responsive the patient is.

Which one of the following statements concerning the management of COPD is true?

(A) Intravenous steroids and beta-2 agonists are given for an acute exacerbation.

(B) Oxygen administration is avoided because it can elevate CO_2 levels.

(C) Theophylline (Theo-Dur) decreases diaphragmatic contractility.

(D) Common causes of infection include anaerobic organisms.

(E) The influenza vaccine should be given every ten years.

The answer is Choice (A). Choice (A), intravenous steroids and beta-2 agonists, are the standards of treatment for a COPD exacerbation. Oxygen, Choice (B), actually is one of the treatments for COPD, although it's usually titrated slowly to achieve an oxygen saturation of 92 percent. Concerning Choice (C), theophylline actually increases, not decreases, diaphragmatic contractility. It also can function as a bronchodilator. Anaerobic organisms, Choice (D), are common causes of aspiration pneumonia, particularly in someone with very bad oral dentition. *Haemophilus influenzae* and *Branhamella catarrhalis* are common causes of COPD exacerbations. Influenza can also cause a COPD exacerbation. The influenza vaccine, Choice (E), is given annually, not every 10 years. Patients with both COPD and asthma should be vaccinated for influenza yearly.

Dilated air sacs: Beating bronchiectasis

Bronchiectasis is a chronic condition characterized by dilation of the alveolar air sacs. The airways can become huge and dilated, and affected patients can have difficulty clearing mucous.

Bronchiectasis is usually an irreversible condition secondary to long-standing lung inflammation. Often, the inflammation has been occurring for years. Causes include cystic fibrosis (which you read about in the next section), pulmonary infections, and malignancy.

Here are a few clinical points you need to know about bronchiectasis:

- ✔ The person often has a chronic productive cough with significant sputum production.

- ✔ Cyanosis and/or clubbing (the fingernail kind, not the bar-hopping kind) can be present.

- ✔ The imaging test to best help in diagnosing bronchiectasis is the high-resolution CT scan. A pulmonologist may perform a bronchoscopy to make sure a lung malignancy isn't present. In addition, the bronchoscope can be used to "suck out all the junk" — stuff that the affected person is unable to clear.

- ✔ Antibiotics and bronchodilating agents are given for acute exacerbations.

One often-repeated PANCE question involves a person who has long-standing bronchiectasis and develops nephrotic proteinuria with no hematuria. What does this mean? The answer is *secondary amyloidosis* — the protein buildup is due to long-standing inflammation from the bronchiectasis.

You are evaluating a 56-year-old man who presents with clubbing. He denies any fevers or chills. He does not have a smoking history. On physical examination, you note the presence of palmar erythema and telangiectasias. His abdominal examination is positive for the presence of a fluid wave. Which one of the following is a likely cause of his clubbing?

(A) Bronchiectasis

(B) Lung cancer

(C) Endocarditis

(D) Cirrhosis

(E) Kidney disease

The answer is Choice (D), cirrhosis. Clubbing is a nonspecific clinical sign that you can see in a variety of disorders, including Choices (A) through (D) of this question. The lack of fevers and chills is a sign that endocarditis isn't likely to be present. The man has no history of a chronic cough with productive sputum, which would be a tipoff that bronchiectasis isn't present. This person has the findings of cirrhosis, including palmar erythema, telangiectasias, and a fluid wave suggesting the presence of ascites. Clubbing is not typically a sign of kidney disease, Choice (E). Unlisted causes of clubbing include other lung processes as well as inflammatory bowel disease (IBD) and many malabsorption syndromes.

Chasing cystic fibrosis

Cystic fibrosis (CF) is an abnormality of exocrine gland function. In this condition, a disorder of the cystic fibrosis transregulator (CFTR) gene messes up the normal flow of the chloride channel. Because the movement of chloride also affects the cellular movement of water, the person may have a lot of thick mucus production. Here are some key points concerning cystic fibrosis:

- Cystic fibrosis is a genetic condition inherited in an autosomal recessive manner.

- The major body organs affected by cystic fibrosis are the lungs, pancreas, and testes:

    - **Lungs:** Someone with cystic fibrosis can present with productive cough with excessive sputum production. Long-standing cystic fibrosis can be a cause of bronchiectasis (see the preceding section).

    - **Pancreas:** Because cystic fibrosis affects the pancreatic exocrine function, the affected person can present with malabsorption symptoms. He or she can also have pancreatitis and/or pancreatic insufficiency from long-standing cystic fibrosis.

    - **Testes:** A man with cystic fibrosis can present with infertility.

- A person with cystic fibrosis can have cyanosis and/or clubbing.

- A diagnosis of cystic fibrosis is determined by an elevated sweat chloride test. While genetic testing may be done to evaluate for abnormalities in the CFTR gene, an abnormal sweat chloride test alone confirms the diagnosis.

- Treatment includes antibiotics and bronchodilators. Nebulized antibiotic therapy (for example, inhaled tobramycin) has been used. Because of pancreatic insufficiency, the patient may need supplemental enzyme therapy. Extensive chest physiotherapy may also be required.

Reviewing Restrictive Lung Disease

A *restrictive pattern* on a pulmonary function test (PFT) is a reduced diffusion capacity of the lungs for carbon dioxide (D_{LCO}). In this section, you review lung disease caused by occupational exposure, interstitial lung disease (ILD), and granulomatous diseases, including sarcoidosis.

After the dust settles: Exploring occupational exposures

Occupational exposure to the dust of various materials is a significant cause of pulmonary problems. In this section, you review these dust-related lung diseases — which are various types of *pneumoconiosis* — including lung disorders related to exposure to silica, asbestos, and coal.

Silicosis

Silicosis is caused by inhaling dust from silica. People who are exposed to silica, including stoneworkers and sandblasters, are at risk. Here are some key points about silicosis:

- A high-yield chest radiograph finding is eggshell calcifications. This refers to hilar adenopathy, which may be calcified.

- The treatment is generally supportive, including antibiotics when needed and steroids for superimposed inflammation.

- People with silicosis are at greater risk for the development of tuberculosis (so-called silicotuberculosis).

Asbestosis

Asbestosis is caused by inhalation of asbestos dust, which over time causes inflammation and fibrotic changes (scarring) in the lung. Anyone who has been involved in construction work, especially working on older buildings where asbestos was in the walls and part of the insulation, is at risk. Here are the key points about asbestosis:

- Cigarette smoking is really bad if you have asbestosis because asbestosis increases the risk of lung cancer. It can also exponentially increase the damage smoking does to the lungs.

- Asbestosis is associated with the development of malignant melanoma.

- Important chest radiograph findings include increased interstitial lung markings, pleural thickening, and pleural plaques.

Coal worker's pneumoconiosis

Coal worker's pneumoconiosis, as the name suggests, involves coal miners who develop lung problems due to inhalation of coal dust. This causes significant inflammatory and fibrotic changes in the lung. The key point concerning coal worker's pneumoconiosis is that a chest radiograph demonstrates nodules in the upper lung zones.

Caplan's syndrome is a combination of pneumoconiosis and rheumatoid arthritis (RA). The characteristic finding is long nodules on a routine chest radiograph. (For more about evaluating lung nodules, head to the section "Scrutinizing the lung lesion" later in this chapter.)

Investigating interstitial lung disease

Interstitial lung disease (ILD) comes in several types. It's usually of an insidious onset, with progressive shortness of breath and exertional dyspnea. ILD refers to the inflammation of the lung parenchyma, which surrounds the lung alveoli. The cause of ILD isn't known; it's thought that an abnormal immune response in the lungs may play a role. It may be a side effect of medication, including the chemotherapy agent busufan (Myleran) and the antiarrythmic agent amiodarone (Cordarone). You see it in many rheumatologic conditions, including rheumatoid arthritis (RA). Many cases of ILD are termed idiopathic because the underlying cause is unknown.

Here are the key points concerning ILD:

- Many of the subtypes of ILD are defined by the histology that's found on lung biopsy, the gold standard for diagnosing ILD. Common types include *usual interstitial pneumonia* (UIP) and *desquamative interstitial pneumonia* (DIP).

- A chest radiograph shows interstitial infiltrates in a reticulonodular pattern.

✔ The diagnosis can be confirmed with a high-resolution CT scan. With ILD, you can often see a radiologic finding of "honeycombing."

✔ The role of steroids and other immunosuppressive agents in treating ILD isn't yet fully defined. The overall prognosis of ILD is not very good.

Cryptogenic organizing pneumonia (formerly referred to as *Bronchiolitis obliterans with organizing pneumonia* [BOOP]) is an uncommon type of ILD, diagnosed via lung biopsy. It affects the small airways and alveoli. It's been linked to many medical conditions, including infections and connective tissue diseases. BOOP can be very steroid responsive. If you see a PANCE question about BOOP, think "treatment with steroids." It actually responds well to treatment. (Note that BOOP has nothing to do with Betty Boop, the 1930s Hollywood cartoon character.)

Sarcoidosis: Gasping about granulomatous disease

Granulomatous diseases come in many forms, but the one that you see most on the PANCE is sarcoidosis. *Sarcoidosis* is a noncaseating granulomatous disease that can affect multiple organs, including the lungs, liver, eyes, and skin. Here are some key points concerning sarcoidosis:

✔ Clinical presentation consists of shortness of breath (SOB) and cough. Sarcoidosis usually has an insidious onset.

✔ The lungs are the most common site of involvement.

✔ Common lab findings can include an elevated erythrocyte sedimentation rate (ESR), an elevated angiotensin converting enzyme (ACE) level, and hypercalcemia.

✔ You may see kidney stones, an elevated 24-hour urinary calcium excretion, and tubulointerstitial disease.

✔ The classic chest radiograph finding is bilateral hilar lymphadenopathy. Other possible findings include bilateral pulmonary infiltrates.

Besides sarcoidosis, several other conditions can cause bilateral hilar lymphadenopathy on a chest radiograph. They include silicosis, beryliosis, fungal diseases, and lymphoma.

✔ You need a lung biopsy to confirm the diagnosis of sarcoidosis.

✔ The treatment of choice is steroids, and sarcoidosis is very responsive to treatment.

Blanketing the Lungs: The Pleura

You may see questions about conditions that affect the pleura. In this section, you review the evaluation and management of pleural effusions, the pneumothorax, and pleurisy.

Fluid around the lungs: Probing the pleural effusion

Normally, the pleura is an empty space; a *pleural effusion* is simply fluid that occupies that space. Pleural effusions can be unilateral or bilateral.

In evaluating pleural effusions, a thoracentesis helps you determine the etiology. The fluid is sent for LDH, protein, Gram stain and culture, cell count with differential, cytology, glucose, and pH tests. This section helps you interpret the results.

Measuring protein and LDH: Transudative and exudative pleural effusions

Light's criteria say that if an effusion meets any one of three characteristics, then it meets criteria to be an *exudate:*

✔ The ratio of pleural fluid total protein to serum total protein is > 0.5.

✔ The ratio of pleural fluid LDH level to serum LDH level is > 0.6.

✔ The pleural LDH is > ⅔ the value of the total LDH.

An *exudative* pleural effusion (caused by local factors) can be caused by pneumonia, a malignancy, or connective tissue disease, such as rheumatoid arthritis. Rheumatoid arthritis can also cause the pleural fluid glucose to be very low. A pneumonia, empyema (pus in the pleural space), connective tissue diseases, and malignancy can also present with a very low pleural fluid pH (usually less than 7.3).

A *transudative* effusion (caused by systemic factors) is an effusion where the ratio of pleural fluid protein to serum protein level is < 0.5. Common causes include congestive heart failure, kidney disease, and cirrhosis.

A pulmonary embolism can be associated with either a transudative or exudative effusion.

Considering types of fluid in the pleural space

Here are the types of fluid you may find in the pleural space:

✔ A *hemothorax* is blood in the pleural space. This can occur after a trauma or interventional procedure.

✔ A *chylothorax* occurs when lymphatic fluid is in the pleural space. This usually results from a leak in the thoracic duct. Causes include trauma and lymphoma.

✔ An *empyema* is pus in the pleural space. It fits all of Light's criteria (see the preceding section). In addition, the pH may be low. The culture and Gram stain are usually positive as well. Sometimes the fluid is so fibrin-rich that a chest tube — with or without a lysing agent such as streptokinase (SK) — is used to try to make the fluid amenable to drainage. Sometimes surgical intervention, such as a thoracotomy, is needed.

Clearing the air on pneumothorax

A *pneumothorax* is air that occupies the pleural space. You should know about the following types of pneumothoraces:

✔ A *primary spontaneous pneumothorax* happens just like that — spontaneously, not precipitated by a traumatic event. It can occur in the absence of documented lung disease. This type of pneumothorax typically happens to men, usually between their teenage years and their early 30s. These men tend to have tall and thin builds. There's usually no history of underlying lung disease with a primary pneumothorax.

✔ A *secondary spontaneous pneumothorax* usually occurs in people who have a smoking history and documented emphysema. If blebs (large blisters filled with serous fluid) or bullae are present, they can spontaneously rupture.

✔ A *traumatic pneumothorax* means the patient has a hole in his or her chest. Knife wounds and rib fractures are common causes.

✔ In a *tension pneumothorax,* the pneumothorax results in hypoxia and low blood pressure. This is a medical emergency because it can lead to cardiac arrest. Any type of pneumothorax could conceivably develop into a tension pneumothorax, which can be a result of a motor vehicle accident, trauma, or barotrauma.

The tension pneumothorax is potentially fatal if not diagnosed and treated early. In a tension pneumothorax, an air leak continues to put more air in the pleural space. Basically, air is able to get in but can't get out. The trapped air can affect the function of the heart and other organs in the thoracic space as they're in essence squeezed. This can affect venous return, and hypotension can result. Symptoms can include chest pain, shortness of breath, and in a rare few, abdominal pain.

On physical exam, the person with tension pneumothorax can be tachycardic, hypotensive, and/or hypoxemic. On lung examination, you find absent breath sounds over the collapsed lung. In addition, there can be tracheal deviation and a mediastinal shift to the opposite side. Note that tracheal deviation can be an inconsistent finding.

You need to get the air out of the pleural space rapidly. How do you do that? By placing a large-gauge needle in the second intercostal space at the midclavicular line. This is a temporizing measure, but it allows the built-up air to escape.

How can you determine who needs a chest tube? It depends on the size of the pneumothorax. On a normal chest radiograph, the lung markings should extend to the periphery. With a pneumothorax, you can often see where the lung markings are in comparison to a normal chest radiograph. If the pneumothorax is small, you can watch it; if it's a larger pneumothorax, then a chest tube may be needed.

Pleural pain: Not putting up with pleurisy

Pleurisy is pain due to inflammation in the pleural space. Pleurisy is most commonly caused by a viral process. The treatment is supportive, but pain medication may be prescribed. With pleurisy, you need to make sure that the person can take a deep breath; if not, he or she is at increased risk for a superimposed bacterial infection.

Investigating Infectious Processes

You have to know about several lung-related infectious processes for the PANCE. In this section, you review the evaluation and treatment of pneumonias, acute bronchitis, influenza, and tuberculosis.

Knocking out pneumonias

Broadly speaking, *pneumonia* is an inflammation of the lung, the alveoli in particular. It's typically caused by an infection, with bacteria as the most popular players. Although pneumonia is highly treatable, it remains a leading killer of some segments of the population in the Third World.

Pneumonias come in several types, including community-acquired pneumonias, healthcare-associated pneumonias, and pneumonias found in immunocompromised hosts.

When you answer test questions about pneumonia, pay close attention to the key points presented. Is the presentation of the pneumonia abrupt or insidious? Is the person a nursing home resident (think healthcare-associated pneumonia)? Is the person immunocompetent or immunocompromised? What is the nature of the sputum? What was on the sputum Gram stain? Does the patient present with bad dentition? Tooth decay can provide evidence for an anaerobic cause of the person's pneumonia.

Community-acquired pneumonias

Community-acquired pneumonias (CAP) are classified into typical and atypical types. A *typical* pneumonia causes fever, chills, rigors, and the classic toxic look. An atypical pneumonia (walking pneumonia) doesn't present with the features of typical (classic) pneumonia. *Walking pneumonia* gets its name because the person with an atypical form of community-acquired pneumonia can have milder, more subtle symptoms than the classic CAP. However, the person usually still feels horrible.

The bacterial causes of CAP that you need to know for the PANCE include *Streptococcus pneumoniae, Haemophilus influenzae, Moraxella catarrhalis, Legionella pneumophila, Chlamydophila pneumoniae,* and *Mycoplasma pneumoniae.* They sound like the characters in a gladiator movie!

When pneumonia is suspected, broad-spectrum antibiotics are used to cover the typicals and atypicals.

Streptococcal pneumonia

A common cause of CAP is *Streptococcus pneumoniae.* The usual presentation is productive cough with rust-colored sputum, fever, chills, rigors, and a toxic look. Here are the key points about streptococcal pneumonia:

- ✔ Lung examination shows dry rales and increased tactile fremitus along the area.

- ✔ Labs can show an elevated white count +/– a left shift or significant bandemia. *Bandemia* refers to production of immature neutrophils by the bone marrow, usually in response to a significant infection. A sputum Gram stain and culture should be collected if possible. Many times, getting a good sputum sample is impossible. With streptoccocal pneumonia, the Gram stain shows the presence of Gram-positive cocci in pairs and/or chains. Note that hyponatremia, as defined by a low serum sodium, can also be present.

- ✔ A urinary pneumococcal antigen can be ordered. But even if this test is negative, it doesn't rule out the presence of streptococcal pneumonia.

- ✔ A chest radiograph may show a lobar infiltrate.

- ✔ The usual initial antibiotic choices are fluoroquinolones, including levofloxacin (Levaquin), and a third-generation cephalosporin such as ceftriaxone (Rocephin) plus a macrolide antibiotic such as azithromycin (Zithromax).

Hemophilus influenzae and *Moraxella catarrhalis* are two other causes of CAP. They are also two very common pathogens in patients with COPD. The antibiotic coverage is the same as in streptococcal pneumonia.

Legionnaires' disease

Legionnaires' disease (also known as Legionellosis) is generally caused by *Legionella pneumophila,* although there are other serotypes as well. This organism is thought of as an atypical cause of CAP, although patients can be very sick when diagnosed.

For test-taking purposes, know that you can find *Legionella* bacteria wherever water is. Think about air conditioners, water heaters, plumbing, shower stalls — you get the idea. Inhale respiratory droplets that contain the bacteria, and you've been infected.

Concerning labs, a leukocytosis with bandemia may or may not be present. You can check for a urinary *Legionella* antigen as well. Affected patients can present with nausea, vomiting, and/or diarrhea. They can also have a relative bradycardia as well. On lab tests, hyponatremia may be present. (*Note:* Although hyponatremia is nonspecific and can be seen with many pneumonias, it has been reported with *Legionella* pneumonia.)

The treatment is usually a fluoroquinolone such as levofloxacin (Levaquin), although the macrolide class of antibiotics can be prescribed as well.

Mycoplasma pneumonia

Like Legionnaires', mycoplasma pneumonia is an atypical (walking) type of CAP. The bacterium *Mycoplasma pneumoniae* is a common etiology of pneumonia, especially in young people. The chest radiograph findings can be variable, although you can see opacification of certain segments of the lungs' lower lobes. Here are a couple of points about mycoplasma pneumonia:

- ✔ Getting a sputum culture for mycoplasma can be difficult if not impossible. A serologic test for cold agglutinins can be used to diagnose mycoplasma.

- ✔ *Mycoplasma* lacks a cell wall, so you can use the macrolide class of antibiotics or the fluoroquinolones to treat this pneumonia. Tetracycline derivatives, including doxycycline, have also been used.

When you're reviewing for the PANCE, make sure you recognize other associations for a given causative organism. For example, mycoplasma can cause atypical pneumonia, bullous myringitis, and hemolytic anemia.

Chlamydial pneumonia

Chlamydophila pneumoniae (formerly known as *Chlamydia pneumoniae* or TWAR, Taiwan acute respiratory agent) is a common cause of pneumonia in kids and young people. The chest radiograph findings are similar to other atypical CAP. Because this bacterium can be difficult to isolate in sputum (just like mycoplasma), you need blood antibody testing to identify the organism. Both macrolide antibiotics and tetracycline derivatives can be used to treat.

Chlamydophila psittaci is a cause of pneumonia for people who work with sick birds, usually parrots. People working in a vet's office or pet shop are at risk. Patients can be very sick, with high fever and gastrointestinal symptoms. On physical examination, splenomegaly may be present.

Healthcare-associated pneumonias

Healthcare-associated pneumonias (formerly called *hospital-acquired pneumonias*) can affect people living in nursing homes or rehabilitation centers or people who've spent more than a few days in the hospital.

Gram-negative bacteria

The organisms responsible for healthcare-associated pneumonias are different from CAP organisms, tending to be more Gram-negative in scope. Examples include *Pseudomonas aeruginosa* and *Klebsiella pneumoniae.*

Treatment needs to reflect more Gram-negative coverage, including the use of third- or fourth-generation cephalosporins. Fluoroquinolones do have some Gram-negative coverage. If the person has been in the critical care unit for a while, the big Gram-negative guns can be prescribed, including the carbapenem class of beta-lactam antibiotics and monobactam aztreonam (Azactam). An infectious-diseases healthcare provider usually prescribes the stronger antibiotics.

Although the aminoglycoside antibiotics do have good Gram-negative coverage, they have very poor lung penetration. They're great for complicated urinary tract infections or infections of the genitourinary system. Aminoglycosides have also been prescribed for endocarditis. That being said, they aren't great for lung infections.

Staphylococcus aureus

We can't leave a discussion of healthcare-associated pneumonias without talking about *Staphylococcus aureus.* It used to be one of those rare bugs you read about, but now you find it everywhere, even in the community. *Staph aureus* pneumonia can be a superimposed bacterial infection if the person has influenza. You also find it in nursing homes, residential care facilities, and hospitals. If someone has any type of indwelling lines or catheters, he or she is at higher risk of getting a staph infection.

Classically, the pneumonia associated with *Staphylococcus aureus* is a cavitary pneumonia. A chest radiograph can show multiple cavitary lesions called *pneumatoceles.*

The treatment depends on which kind of staph infection you're dealing with. Is it methicillin-sensitive staph aureus (MSSA) or methicillin-resistant staph aureus (MRSA)? For MSSA, penicillin antibiotics like piperacillin-tazobactam (Zosyn) can be used. For MRSA, first-line agents can include vancomycin, although with increasing MRSA resistance, other agents like linezolid (Zyvox) have been used.

Pneumonias in the immunocompromised patient

Many types of pneumonia can affect people who are immunocompromised. One such type of pneumonia (and this is likely to be on the test) is *pneumocystis pneumonia* (PCP). It's also called *pneumocystis jirovecii pneumonia* and was formerly called *pneumocystis carinii pneumonia.* Here are the main points concerning this fungal pneumonia:

- ✔ It tends to occur in immunocompromised hosts, including people with HIV whose CD4 count is < 200 and people receiving chemotherapy.

- ✔ It can be a very destructive pneumonia, actually destroying the parenchyma of the lung. Serum LDH levels can be high, reflecting this destruction.

- ✔ A chest radiograph can show opacification of both lung fields.

- ✔ An arterial blood gas (ABG) has special significance for this pneumonia. If the pO_2 is < 60 mmHg, signifying hypoxemia, then steroids are given in addition to trimethoprim/sulfamethoxazole (Bactrim). Trimethoprim/sulfamethoxazole is often given for 21 days of therapy.

You're admitting a 54-year-old man to the hospital for pneumonia. He was found drunk, passed out in an alley. He has a known history of alcohol abuse. Which of the following is the most likely causative organism of his pneumonia?

(A) *Staphylococcus aureus*

(B) *Pseudomonas aeruginosa*

(C) *Legionella pneumophila*

(D) *Streptococcus pneumoniae*

(E) *Klebsiella pneumoniae*

The correct answer is Choice (E), *Klebsiella pneumoniae.* Certainly, although the gentleman in question may also have streptococcal pneumonia, the keys in the question ("drunk" and "alcohol abuse") point to *Klebsiella* as the answer. By the way, another *Klebsiella* pneumonia reference is the presence of currant jelly sputum.

For each answer choice, you need to make a connection to the question. For Choice (C), Legionnaires', to be right, the question could say something about working as a plumber or with air conditioning and heating. For *Staph aureus,* the question could say something about being hospitalized with a central venous catheter — the bacteria are spread via the blood to the lungs.

Analyzing acute bronchitis

You can breathe easy now — this section should be a piece of cake. The most common etiologies of bronchitis are viral, including the adenovirus (also a common viral cause of pharyngitis), respiratory syncytial virus (or RSV), and rhinovirus (the cause of the common cold).

Acute bronchitis can also have bacterial causes. These causes are basically what you read about earlier in "Knocking out pneumonias." All the causes of the typical CAP can be causes of acute bronchitis.

Whereas *chronic bronchitis* is characterized by a chronic cough, *acute bronchitis* is characterized by an acute airway inflammation. Catchy, huh, how "chronic" matches "chronic" and "acute" matches "acute?" (***Note:*** Chronic bronchitis is associated with COPD — see the earlier section "Chronic obstruction: Correcting COPD" for details.) Anyway, imaging studies such as chest radiographs are nondiagnostic for acute bronchitis. The diagnosis is made on clinical presentation with shortness of breath and wheezing, along with a negative chest radiograph.

Antibiotics are prescribed for people whose symptoms don't resolve, for people with underlying lung disease, for geriatric patients, or for people whose immune status is in question.

Investigating influenza

Influenza (the flu) is an infectious disease caused by viruses of the family *Orthomyxoviridae*. The virus causes outbreaks during late fall and winter. The most common viral types are influenza A and B, with A being more common than B.

Both virus types produce similar symptoms, which can begin 24 to 48 hours after infection. They include cough, fever, rigors, arthralgias, and myalgias. Sometimes you can isolate the virus from the nose or pharynx — that is, a nasal swab can be done.

Several medications have been used in treating influenza:

- Oseltamivir (Tamiflu) can treat both influenza A and B, but it's effective in lessening the duration and intensity of symptoms only if it's given in the first 24 to 48 hours. Zanamivir (Ralenza) is a newer medication that works in a manner similar to oseltamivir.

- Amantadine, the same medication prescribed for Parkinson's disease, is used to treat influenza A, but it isn't effective against influenza B. Again, for this medication to have any effect, it has to be given early. Another medication that sounds like amantadine, rimatadine (Flumadine), works in a similar manner.

Vaccines can effectively prevent influenza virus infection. They're typically administered widely — look for a flu clinic near you. The flu vaccine is reformulated every year and manufactured 6 months before flu season starts so it's ready when people need it.

A common test question asks about the association between children with viral infections (primarily influenza), the use of salicylates, and the development of *Reye's syndrome,* a deadly medical condition that can affect the liver and brain. Bottom line: Don't give salicylate derivatives of any kind to children under the age of 19.

For which of the following people would you most strongly recommend the flu vaccine?

(A) A woman under the age of 65 with no documented health problems

(B) A nurse working the day shift in a hospital

(C) A researcher working in a lab

(D) A 25-year-old librarian

(E) A 55-year-old person diagnosed with acute bronchitis that has resolved

The correct answer is Choice (B). Any person over the age of 65, healthcare professional, or person with a compromised immune system (or suffering from a chronic medical condition) should get the vaccine. Choice (A) is wrong because she isn't over the age of 65. Choice (C) is in the lab; contact with people is minimized, so vaccination is less important. The same concerns Choice (D). Who goes to the library, anyway?

Tuberculosis: Preparing for the TB test

The causative organism of tuberculosis (TB) is *Mycobacterium tuberculosis*. It's transmitted from person to person, usually by respiratory droplets.

Initial symptoms of TB can show a cough that gets progressively worse. There can also be type B constitutional symptoms. Hemoptysis may or may not be present.

Looking at types of TB

There are several types of tuberculosis and several disseminations. The World Health Organization estimates that about a third of the world's population is infected with *M. tuberculosis.*

Primary tuberculosis concerns initial exposure to the mycobacterium, which triggers an inflammatory reaction in the lungs. Chest radiograph findings can show hilar adenopathy and nonspecific infiltrates; however, they don't always show up on a chest radiograph.

A *Ghon nodule* is simply a tuberculous lesion that has healed. It looks small and calcified on a chest radiograph.

For someone who has a problem with the immune system, primary tuberculosis in the lung can spread. In *primary progressive tuberculosis,* the TB can spread via the lymphatics, and the lung disease worsens. It can spread into the pleura and cause a pleural effusion. The mycobacterium can also spread in the blood (through *hematogenous dissemination*) to other body organs, leading to *extrapulmonary TB.*

Tuberculosis can reactivate. Some latent infection is usually somewhere in the body. The most common place for reactivation is in the upper lobes of the lung, specifically the apical and posterior regions. This can be a cavitary pneumonia.

Miliary tuberculosis is tuberculosis that has disseminated throughout the body. It can affect any organ, and it occurs less than 5 percent of the time. Classic chest radiograph findings make it look like someone took a machine gun and shot out the lungs. These bullet-like small nodules appear throughout both lung fields. (No, it's not called "military" tuberculosis.)

TB skin tests

At some point, everyone who has applied for a job in healthcare has undergone skin testing for tuberculosis. What's a positive test? The size of the wheal, not the redness, is what matters. But interpreting whether someone's positive means not only looking at the size of the wheal or induration but also paying attention to the risk factors. Here are key points you need to know:

- ✔ If the wheal is > 5 mm, the following groups are considered to be positive for TB: people with HIV, those who have been in contact with someone who has active TB, and those who are on chronic immunosuppressive therapy, such as prednisone and anti-rejection medications (cyclosporine [Neoral] and tacrolimus [Prograf]).

- ✔ If the wheal is > 10 mm, the following groups are considered to be positive: people who are active drug users (they inject), healthcare personnel, and other employees and residents of high-risk areas, including nursing homes, residential care facilities, and jails. Other significant risks include chronic medical conditions that can render people relatively immunosuppressed, including diabetes, advanced kidney disease (and/or dialysis), and COPD. In addition, people who've emigrated to this country from endemic areas fall into this category.

- ✔ Any individual who has a wheal > 15 mm is considered positive and has risk factors for developing tuberculosis.

Treating TB

Different therapies and drug regimens can be used to treat TB. Many of them can last 6 to 9 months. For PANCE purposes, you should be familiar with side effects of the medications:

- ✔ Isoniazid (INH), which is usually the first-line treatment, can cause a peripheral neuropathy. It may also cause low levels of vitamin B_6, so supplementation with vitamin B_6 is recommended. Because isoniazid carries a risk of hepatitis, liver function tests need to be monitored while the person is on the medication.

- ✔ Rifampin can turn the urine and secretions a funky orange color. Rifampin is a potent enzyme inducer that can affect the metabolism of many drug classes, including HIV meds. It has gastrointestinal effects, can cause thrombocytopenia, and can be toxic to the liver.

- ✔ Pyrazinamide can cause some minor joint pains, but the main effect is liver toxicity. It can raise serum uric acid levels.

- ✔ Ethambutol's significant side effect concerns the eye. It can cause color blindness, and in some studies, it caused optic neuropathy.

Addressing Childhood Lung Conditions

Lung conditions that affect adults are not the same as the ones that affect the pediatric population. Kids have smaller airways, and their respiratory muscle structure is less developed. Pediatric conditions that we cover in this section include croup, epiglottitis, respiratory syncytial virus (RSV), and whooping cough.

A barking cough: Catching up with croup

Most people who have children or have worked with children are aware of the sound of a croup cough. It's a distinct sound, almost like the barking of a seal. Croup can affect the upper airways, especially the larynx and trachea. That's why another term for croup is *laryngotracheobronchitis.*

Croup is common in very young children. You can see it in children as young as 5 to 6 months and as old as 3 to 4 years. The cause of croup is usually viral, and the most common cause is parainfluenza. Note that croup can be caused by other viruses, such as the influenza virus and rhinovirus, the commonest cause of the common cold.

A child can present with typical upper respiratory infection symptoms, but as the inflammation of the upper airway gets worse, you begin to hear *stridor,* a high-pitched wheeze that's worse on inspiration. The child is also likely to have a mild fever. The croup symptoms tend to worsen at night. Other symptoms can include hoarseness and significant accessory muscle use, as well as signs of cyanosis.

Kids like to put anything and everything in their mouths, so make sure you rule out other causes of upper airway obstruction, such as a foreign body or a big epiglottis. Use a radiograph to check the out the lungs and the cervical soft tissues of the neck.

The treatment is paying attention to the ABCs and stabilizing the airway, if needed. The hallmark of treatment is humidified oxygen. In the hospital, so-called croup tents can be used.

Recognizing emergency epiglottitis

Epiglottitis is an inflammation of the epiglottis, causing it to enlarge (swell), which can obstruct the child's small airways. It's usually caused by a bacterial infection, namely *Haemophilus influenzae* type B. Epiglottitis affects younger children, usually between ages 2 and 6, although it may occur in older children. Vaccination has greatly diminished the occurrence of epiglottitis.

Children may present with an upper respiratory infection that quickly worsens, with hypoxemia, tachypnea, and accessory muscle use. Kids with epiglottitis are pretty toxic looking; they can be drooling and sitting upright, often in a "sniffing position," with their head and nose tilted forward and upward as if smelling something. On physical examination, you see an erythematous, edematous, angry-looking epiglottis.

Although epiglottitis and croup can be similar in presentation, there are differences. Epiglottitis can worsen a lot faster than croup. Stridor may be present in epiglottis, but the barking cough of croup is not. A cervical soft tissue radiograph also shows a swollen epiglottis in epiglottitis.

Epiglottitis is an emergency that needs to be recognized swiftly. If the epiglottis gets too swollen, it can completely block the airway, creating a potentially life-threatening situation. So the treatment for epiglottitis is first to stabilize the airway. If intubation is needed, you want to avoid the trauma of repeat intubations and intubation attempts; they can compromise an already swollen airway. Intravenous antibiotics need to be administered as well.

Reacting to respiratory syncytial virus (RSV)

Respiratory syncytial virus (RSV) can cause upper respiratory infection symptoms in very young children. People at high risk for RSV include babies of several months and those who are premature or immunocompromised in some way.

In most cases, RSV will run its course, and supportive measures are needed. Sometimes, however, the virus is bad enough that the child can become symptomatic. RSV is the leading cause of bronchiolitis in children

In certain patients, RSV can affect the lower airways, cause inflammation of the bronchioles, and increase the risk of developing pneumonia.

Sizing Up Lung Malignancy

Lung cancer is a leading cause of morbidity and mortality. For the PANCE, be familiar with the evaluation, characteristics, and management of lung cancer. The two major types of lung cancer you need to know are small-cell lung cancer and non-small-cell lung cancer.

Lung cancer can manifest in various ways. Commonly, the affected person presents with a cough that won't go away despite antibiotics, treatment for GERD, and treatment for asthma. Type B constitutional symptoms, including fevers, chills, and weight loss, may or may not be present. Sometimes an initial manifestation is hemoptysis. When this occurs, the pulmonologist often performs a bronchoscopy to see whether he or she is dealing with an endobronchial lesion.

After diagnosis, staging is important for any type of lung cancer. Common sites of metastasis include the liver, bone, brain, and adrenal glands. CT scans of the thorax, abdomen, and pelvis as well as a bone scan should be a part of the metastasis workup. PET scanning can also be used to determine how active the cancer is.

Of course, what's most important is to know the histologic type of cancer that you're dealing with. Obtaining a biopsy is key.

The saying "An ounce of prevention is worth a pound of cure" has never been more apt than when you're talking about lung cancer. The key is for the patient to stop smoking and avoid exposure to any type of smoke if possible.

In this section, we take a look at primary lung malignancies. We also explain how to evaluate a lung nodule that unexpectedly appears on a chest radiograph.

You can have cancer in the lung that isn't "lung cancer." Many solid organ cancers, including breast cancer and renal cell cancer, can metastasize to the lung.

Focusing on small-cell lung cancer

Small-cell lung cancer is the type of cancer that, when diagnosed, you can assume has already metastasized. It's an aggressive cancer, and it's usually not amenable to any type of surgical intervention. The long-term prognosis isn't good, and the treatment usually involves chemotherapy, although radiation therapy is sometimes indicated.

For PANCE purposes, realize that lung cancer, like many other solid organ cancers, is associated with paraneoplastic phenomenon. Here are some paraneoplastic phenomena associated with lung malignancies:

✔ **Ectopic ACTH secretion:** The affected person can manifest all the symptoms of Cushing's syndrome and can also have hypokalemia and a metabolic alkalosis as well as high blood pressure. (See Chapter 15 for info on Cushing's.)

✔ **Syndrome of inappropriate antidiuretic hormone hypersecretion (SIADH):** SIADH, which manifests as hyponatremia, has many causes. For information on evaluating and managing hyponatremia, refer to Chapter 10.

✔ **Lambert-Eaton syndrome:** This autoimmune phenomenon is characterized by muscular weakness affecting the legs and the arms. For test-taking purposes, be able to differentiate between Lambert-Eaton syndrome and myasthenia gravis. You read about the differences in Chapter 16.

Seeing the bigger picture: Non-small-cell lung cancer

Non-small-cell lung cancer (non-small-cell lung carcinoma, or NSCLC) includes a number of types of cancer:

✔ *Adenocarcinoma* is the most common type of non-small-cell lung cancer. Its location is more peripheral than central. In someone who develops lung cancer but has no smoking history, you're dealing with an adenocarcinoma more often than not.

✔ *Squamous cell cancer* is the second most common type of non-small-cell lung cancer. Squamous cell cancer tends to be more central. A common paraneoplastic syndrome associated with squamous cell carcinoma is hypercalcemia. The primary treatment of squamous cell cancer is surgery, although chemotherapy and/or radiation may be needed, depending on the extent of metastasis at time of presentation.

✔ *Large-cell lung carcinoma* (LCLC) accounts for 5 to 10 percent of all lung cancers. A history of smoking cigarettes increases the risk.

✔ *Bronchoalveolar cancer* (BAC) is another type of non-small-cell lung cancer, but it's a little different from its counterparts. It primarily affects women, and it's the only lung malignancy not associated with tobacco use. Bronchoalveolar cancer isn't felt to be an aggressive cancer, and it has a better survival rate than other forms of lung cancer.

You're evaluating a man who says he has pain in his left arm and hand. He was newly diagnosed with lung cancer and is scheduled to go for a staging workup. Nothing has helped the pain. On exam, you notice that one pupil is smaller than the other and that his eyelid is drooping. What is your next step?

(A) Obtain a stat CT scan of the head.

(B) Obtain a stat CT scan of the chest.

(C) Obtain a neurological consultation.

(D) Order carotid Dopplers.

(E) Obtain an orthopedic consultation.

The answer is Choice (B), get a CT scan of the chest. The patient likely has a Pancoast tumor with accompanying Horner's syndrome. A *Pancoast tumor* is a non-small-cell lung cancer that's found in the apex of the lung. It can compress the brachial plexus and cause pain in the ipsilateral arm and hand. It can also affect sympathetic nerve fibers — if they're inhibited, the triad of Horner's syndrome can result: miosis (constricted pupil), ptosis (sagging eyelid), and anhidrosis (lack of sweating). You'll likely see this question in one form or another on the test.

Scrutinizing the lung lesion

A common scenario you deal with clinically is inadvertently finding a lung lesion on a chest radiograph. You're looking for something, and bam! There it is. What do you do about it? You assess the lesion on the radiograph:

1. **Check the other lung findings to make sure that you're just dealing with a pulmonary nodule.**

   Other lung findings should be normal. Examples of abnormal findings include the presence of atelectasis or a recurrent pneumonia that won't go away despite repeated treatment with antibiotics. The presence of adenopathy, especially hilar adenopathy, should be inspected on the chest radiograph.

2. **Know the size of the lung lesion.**

   The number 3 is the key. If the lung lesion is < 3 cm, you likely have a lung nodule. If it's > 3 cm, you're likely dealing with a lung mass. The larger the lung lesion, the more likely that you're dealing with a malignancy.

3. **Look at the edges of the lesion.**

   A lung malignancy has irregular or spiculated borders. Benign lesions tend to have smooth edges.

4. **See whether the lesion contains calcium.**

   More often than not, calcification suggests a benign lesion. In fact, calcification has many benign causes, including old, healed infections or reaction to a foreign body. Granulomas are a perfect example of a nonmalignant calcified lung lesion. However, if the calcification is irregular or eccentric, there's a higher chance that you're dealing with a malignancy.

5. **If all else fails and you need a better assessment of the solitary nodule, obtain a CT scan.**

6. **After you've looked at the characteristics of the lesion, look at the characteristics of the person.**

   Is he or she old or young? A smoker? An older person who smokes has a higher chance of malignancy. You can watch people who are at lower risk with serial imaging, but for those who are at higher risk, you may need to get a biopsy to find out what you're dealing with.

You're evaluating a 55-year-old man who presents to the ER with hemoptysis. He states that he hasn't been feeling well for a while. He says he has intermittent episodes of dizziness and diarrhea that comes on for no reason. He also feels flushed. This has been occurring for a few weeks. You obtain a chest radiograph, and it shows a tumor located on the right mainstem bronchus. What does this lung mass likely represent?

(A) Small-cell lung cancer

(B) Legionellosis

(C) Tuberculosis

(D) Carcinoid tumor

(E) Pulmonary embolus

The correct answer is Choice (D). *Carcinoid tumor* is a neuroendocrine tumor that, although not aggressive, is treated like a lung mass. Some patients can have the symptoms mentioned in the question, including dizziness, diarrhea, and flushing, because the tumor secretes serotonin. A CT scan is used for staging, because the most common place of spread is to the liver. The treatment is surgery.

Note that a carcinoid tumor can initially present in places other than the lung. Examples include intestinal carcinoid tumors, which are commonly in the appendix, and carcinoids in the breast.

As for the other answer choices, small-cell lung cancer, Choice (A), would be more diffuse on chest radiograph; it wouldn't appear as an isolated mass near the mainstem bronchus. The time course is too long for legionellosis, Choice (B); the symptoms don't fit, and neither does the chest radiograph. This presentation is not typical of TB, Choice (C). Concerning Choice (E), the classic symptoms for a pulmonary embolus include abrupt onset of short-ness of breath and pleuritic chest pain. Hemoptysis isn't felt to be a major symptom, although it sometimes occurs. The chest radiograph is usually normal, and the ECG can show a sinus tachycardia. You wouldn't see a lung mass on the chest radiograph.

Probing the Pulmonary Vasculature

Pulmonary embolism and pulmonary hypertension are two pulmonary circulation condi-tions that are high-yield for the PANCE. And for good reason, too — you see these condi-tions clinically time and time again.

Blood clots: Evaluating the pulmonary embolism

As the name suggests, a *pulmonary embolism* (PE) is an obstruction of the pulmonary artery or one of its many branches due to embolus. A pulmonary embolism is commonly due to a deep venous thrombosis (DVT), which we cover in Chapter 3.

Common presenting symptoms include sudden onset pleuritic chest pain, sweating, and tachycardia. Physical examination can reveal tachycardia, low blood pressure, and/or hypoxemia, depending on the extent of the clot.

ABG can show hypoxemia as well as a respiratory alkalosis secondary to tachypnea. The most common ECG finding is sinus tachycardia. You may also see right axis deviation and T wave inversion in the anterior leads. In addition, there can be poor R wave progression. The S1Q3T3 pattern is present less than 10 percent of the time.

You can order various imaging studies to evaluate for a pulmonary embolism: ECG, chest radiograph, and ventilation/perfusion (V/Q) scan. As with the ECG, the chest radiograph is usually normal. The V/Q scan looks for ventilation/perfusion mismatching. You can inter-pret V/Q scans as low probability, intermediate probability, or high probability. High proba-bility is diagnostic for a pulmonary embolism. However, if a person has underlying lung disease, such as emphysema, the V/Q scan isn't a reliable test.

The gold standard for evaluating the pulmonary vasculature is the angiogram. However, given advances in radiologic imaging, the CT angiogram has become a popular method (and perhaps the preferred choice) for identifying a pulmonary embolism.

Remember that the diagnosis of a pulmonary embolism is based on clinical suspicion. If someone has risk factors that would increase his or her risk of developing deep venous thrombosis and/or pulmonary embolism, then you need to act on it. Even if someone has a low probability V/Q scan, it doesn't completely rule out that a pulmonary embolism is present. Virchow's triad (in Chapter 22) is a nice way of examining for possible risk factors for deep venous thrombosis and/or pulmonary embolism.

If you have a high clinical suspicion that a person has a pulmonary embolism, start anticoagulation therapy with intravenous heparin. Thrombolytics are used for people with major pulmonary embolism such as a saddle embolus, which can be fatal if not treated super aggressively.

Which one of the following is associated with the presence of a pulmonary embolus?

(A) Sinus bradycardia

(B) Right ventricular hypokinesis on echocardiogram

(C) Diffuse ST segment elevation

(D) Kerley B lines

(E) ST elevation in the anterior leads

The correct answer is Choice (B). With a significant pulmonary embolism, you see right ventricular hypokinesis, given the acute high pressures in the pulmonary artery secondary to the pulmonary embolism. Concerning Choice (E), ST elevation in two contiguous leads is the definition of a myocardial infarction. Diffuse ST segment elevation, Choice (C), is associated with acute pericarditis. PR segment depression is also a common ECG finding with pericarditis. You'd expect to see sinus tachycardia, not sinus bradycardia, Choice (A), with pulmonary embolism. An inferior wall myocardial infarction can present with sinus bradycardia. Choice (D) is seen on a radiograph of someone with congestive heart failure.

Taking the pressure off pulmonary hypertension

Pulmonary hypertension is an increase in blood pressure in the pulmonary artery, pulmonary vein, or pulmonary capillaries. A cardiac echocardiogram can suggest elevated pulmonary pressures; however, the definitive test is a right heart catheterization.

Pulmonary hypertension comes in two types, and they have simple names — primary and secondary:

✔ **Primary:** Primary pulmonary hypertension (PPH) is an uncommon form of pulmonary hypertension that mainly affects women in their late 20s and early 30s. Treatment consists of long-term anticoagulation with warfarin (Coumadin) and intravenous prostaglandins like epoprostenol (Flolan). Calcium channel blockers can be used in treating primary pulmonary hypertension, but they need to be instituted in a controlled fashion. Not everyone responds to calcium channel blockers, so pulmonary pressures need to be monitored by pulmonary artery catheterization.

Other medications used in the treatment of primary pulmonary hypertension can include sildenafil (Viagra or Revatio) and bosentan (Tracleer). Sildenafil is an example of a *phosphodiesterase inhibitor,* which helps improve pulmonary blood flow — it's not just for erectile dysfunction! Bosentan is an example of an endotheial receptor antagonist that's used to improve blood flow and vasodilate the pulmonary artery. Endothelin is a potent vasoconstrictor. Side effects of this medication include hypotension and elevated liver function levels.

✔ **Secondary:** Secondary pulmonary hypertension has many etiologies. The most common cause of right heart problems is left heart problems (see Chapter 3 for details). Left ventricular systolic dysfunction, diastolic dysfunction, and valvular problems (for example, mitral regurgitation) can all cause secondary pulmonary hypertension.

Many of the pulmonary problems you read about earlier in this chapter can cause secondary pulmonary hypertension. For example, as COPD advances, it can cause right heart failure, termed *cor pulmonale*. Treatment, which can be difficult, can involve the use of diuretics and management of the underlying condition. Medications to try to lower pulmonary pressures can also be used, depending on the cause of the cor pulmonale (that is, primary versus secondary pulmonary hypertension).

Connective tissue disorders, such as scleroderma and mixed connective tissue disease (MCTD), can cause secondary pulmonary hypertension as well.

Practice Pulmonary Questions

These practice questions are similar to the PANCE questions about pulmonary matters.

1. You're treating a 74-year-old male nursing home resident who was admitted with shortness of breath and fever. His temperature on admission was 38.3°C (101°F). On physical exam, the gentleman is toxic looking and has decreased lung sounds at the right base. The chest radiograph shows an infiltrate at the right lower lobe. What's the most likely causative organism?

    (A) *Streptococcus pneumoniae*

    (B) *Legionella pneumophila*

    (C) Viral pneumonia

    (D) *Klebsiella pneumoniae*

    (E) Anaerobes

2. A 35-year-old man develops worsening dyspnea on exertion, occurring over the last few weeks. He has no cardiac risk factors. A chest radiograph reveals bilateral hilar adenopathy. Labs show an elevated erythrocyte sedimentation rate and an elevated angiotensin converting enzyme (ACE) level. What is this person's likely diagnosis?

    (A) Lymphoma

    (B) Silicosis

    (C) Sarcoidosis

    (D) Tuberculosis

    (E) Caplan's syndrome

3. Which one of the following is a cause of a respiratory alkalosis?

    (A) Neuromuscular disease

    (B) Pulmonary embolism

    (C) Kyphosis

    (D) Diarrhea

    (E) Nasogastric section

4. What is the treatment of choice for mild persistent asthma?

    (A) Inhaled steroids

    (B) Daily albuterol

    (C) Methacholine (Provocholine)

    (D) Daily ipratropium bromide (Atrovent)

    (E) Nebulized albuterol and Atrovent

5. Steroids are used in treating severe asthma and COPD exacerbations. Side effects of long-term steroid use include which of the following?

    (A) Osteoporosis

    (B) Lethargy

    (C) Hypotension

    (D) Adrenal insufficiency

    (E) Weight loss

6. Which one of the following statements about acute respiratory distress syndrome (ARDS) is false?

    (A) A chest radiograph can show bilateral opacification of both lung fields.

    (B) Causes of this acute lung injury can include severe sepsis, trauma, and blood transfusions.

    (C) The role of steroids in the treatment of ARDS is controversial.

    (D) Many patients with ARDS will experience multi-organ dysfunction syndrome (MODS).

    (E) Treatment includes using high tidal volumes to maintain oxygenation.

Answers and Explanations

Use this answer key to score the practice pulmonary questions from the preceding section. The answer explanations give you some insight into why the correct answer is better than the other choices.

1. **D.** A nursing home resident is likely to have a healthcare-associated pneumonia caused by Gram-negative bacteria, such as *Klebsiella pneumoniae*, or by *Staphylococcus aureus*. Choices (A) and (B), *Streptococcus pneumoniae* and *Legionella pneumophila*, represent causes of community-acquired pneumonia (CAP). For the answer to be anaerobes, Choice (E), the question would have to contain clues such as a history of aspiration of food contents or bad dentition (the mouth is dirty).

2. **C.** Although many of the answers could demonstrate bilateral hilar adenopathy on a chest radiograph as well as an elevated sed rate (nonspecific), only sarcoidosis, Choice (C), is associated with an elevated ACE level. Remember that Choice (E), Caplan's syndrome, is a combination of rheumatoid arthritis plus lung nodules.

3. **B.** Pulmonary embolism can cause respiratory alkalosis. We discuss acid-base in detail in Chapter 10, but we'd be remiss if we didn't include at least one question on acid-base in a pulmonary chapter. Choices (A) and (C), neuromuscular disease and kyphosis, are causes of a respiratory acidosis. Diarrhea, with loss of bicarbonate in the stool, is a cause of a metabolic acidosis. Choice (E), nasogastric section, causes a metabolic alkalosis. Other causes of a metabolic alkalosis include vomiting and diuretic use.

4. **A.** Inhaled steroids are the treatment of choice for mild persistent asthma. For intermittent asthma, the use of a short-acting inhaler like albuterol, Choice (B), is okay. But after someone begins to have more frequent asthma exacerbations, using an inhaled steroid is recommended. The key word here is *persistent*. Choice (C), methacholine, can be used to test for asthma, not to treat it. Ipratropium bromide (Atrovent), Choice (D), is used in the treatment of COPD. Nebulized albuterol and Atrovent together, Choice (E), are used in the treatment of advanced COPD — many patients actually have their own nebulizers.

5. **A.** Steroids are a leading cause of osteoporosis, Choice (A). Steroid use can be associated with a steroid psychosis, not lethargy. They can elevate blood pressure, not cause hypotension. Steroid use can cause Cushing's syndrome, and abrupt discontinuation of steroids — not the long-term use of steroids — can precipitate adrenal insufficiency. They're associated with weight gain, not weight loss.

6. **E.** Patients with ARDS can be difficult to oxygenate; the use of low tidal volumes plus the use of positive end expiratory pressure (PEEP) is vital in the management of ARDS. You don't want to use high tidal volumes, because the lungs won't tolerate it.

All the other choices are true statements. Choice (A) is true because a chest radiograph can show bilateral opacification of both lung fields. Differentiating between pulmonary edema and multilobar pneumonia can be difficult.

Choice (B) is true because severe sepsis, trauma, and blood transfusions are the main causes of ARDS. You can think of ARDS as a hyperactive immune system reacting to some inciting event that causes the lung problems. Infections and significant trauma are the leading etiologies. Transfusion-associated acute lung injury (TRALI) is another cause, and as the name suggests, it's associated with blood transfusions.

Choice (C) is true because although steroids have been tried in treating ARDS, they aren't considered a standard of care in ARDS.

Choice (D) is true because ARDS can affect multiple organs, especially the liver and kidney. ARDS has a high fatality rate.

Chapter 5

Hungering for the Digestive System

Although the heart is one of the most important organs in the body, for many people, the key to the heart is through the stomach — the GI tract. There's nothing like a good meal and regularity thereafter to make a person feel positively well. In this chapter, you review many clinical conditions that affect the gastrointestinal tract. From the esophagus to the opposite end, nothing is left untouched as you explore this important body system.

This chapter describes medical conditions affecting the esophagus, the stomach, and the small and large intestines. For good measure, we throw in the liver, pancreas, and gallbladder (we cover more gallbladder pathology in Chapter 7). You also read about vitamin and nutritional deficiencies, many of which can be caused by problems with absorption.

Going Down the Esophagus

For test-taking purposes, you need to be aware of various conditions that affect the esophagus. In particular, you should know esophagitis, bleeding problems, and motility/digestive problems. Before you go on to the rest of this section, review the basic anatomy and histology of the esophagus: The old saying is "Over the teeth, past the gums, look out stomach, here it comes!"

Inviting inflammation: Esophagitis

Esophagitis is inflammation of the esophagus. You need to know various causes in both immunocompetent and immunocompromised patients.

GERD

Gastrosophageal reflux disease (GERD) reflects a problem with the lower esophageal sphincter (LES). Because the LES is "incompetent," the affected person has reflux of gastric contents into the esophagus. The most common clinical complaints include heartburn, an "acid taste" in the mouth, and a nonproductive cough. Other symptoms can include dysphagia and increased salivation.

Be aware of atypical presentations of GERD, such as a chronic cough that occurs at night or laryngitis but no other upper respiratory infection type symptoms.

Left untreated, this regurgitant LES can cause big-time damage, including ulcers, Barrett's esophagitis, and cancer (we cover those conditions later). GERD is also a leading risk factor for the formation of esophageal strictures. Lifestyle modifications to reduce GERD include not eating before bedtime and avoiding foods that reduce LES tone, such as chocolate. Weight loss can also help. In addition, be aware of medications that can reduce LES tone, such as calcium channel blockers and nitrates.

For sleeping, the affected person should keep the head of the bed (HOB) raised at least 30 degrees. Medications used to treat GERD include H2 blockers, proton pump inhibitors, and prokinetic agents such as metoclopramide (Reglan). For those who fail medical management, surgical intervention, namely a Nissen fundoplication, may be required.

Barrett's esophagus

Barrett's esophagus is an inflammation of the distal part of the esophagus. It involves a metaplasia as the epithelium of the esophagus changes from a squamous to a columnar epithelium. The diagnosis is made by an endoscopy with biopsy. In addition, you should know two other key testing points:

- ✔ Risk factors include GERD and tobacco use.

- ✔ Barrett's esophagus increases the risk of developing adenocarcinoma in the distal one-third of the esophagus. This is a very important association. We discuss adenocarcinoma later in "Esophageal cancer."

The treatment of Barrett's esophagus includes treatments to eliminate the reflux. The use of medications, including proton pump inhibitors, is strongly recommended. If symptoms persist, surgical intervention may be needed. Given the increased risk, someone with Barrett's esophagus often requires routine endoscopic surveillance. The clinician looks for abnormal cellular changes. If a high-grade dysplasia is present, an endoscopy with repeat biopsy is done several times per year to follow these changes closely.

Infectious esophagitis

Candida albicans, cytomegalovirus (CMV), and *herpes simplex virus* (HSV) are infectious causes of esophagitis. Although they can occur in individuals with normal immune systems, you see them more often in the elderly and in people with compromised immune systems, such as patients with HIV.

Someone with infectious esophagitis presents with dysphagia and odynophagia. The patient may also present with weight loss because difficult and painful swallowing makes the patient reluctant to eat.

You can identify infectious esophagitis on biopsy. For HSV and CMV, you see vesicular lesions that are typical of those disorders. For *Candida,* you see a whitish plaque that's consistent with *Candida* genus infections.

A person with severe esophagitis many not be able to swallow food, let alone pills. You may need to administer medications intravenously. Here are the medications for treating infectious esophagitis:

- ✔ For esophageal candidiasis, the treatment is fluconazole (Diflucan). Fluconazole can elevate the liver function tests.

- ✔ For HSV, use acyclovir (Zovirax). Acyclovir can cause both neurotoxicity and nephrotoxicity, so a common practice is to have intravenous saline hanging if the acyclovir is given intravenously to reduce the risk.

- ✔ For CMV, use ganciclovir (Cytovene). Gancyclovir can cause neutropenia as a side effect.

Pill-induced esophagitis

Taking a lot of large pills, especially "horse pills," can lead to a pill-induced esophagitis. For example, some forms of oral potassium can be difficult to swallow and can lead to pill-induced esophagitis. Other commonly implicated medications include the bisphosphonate medication alendronate sodium (Fosamax) and nonsteroidals like ibuprofen. The key to treatment is to minimize the number of pills the person has to take. See whether you can substitute a liquid form of the medication and, if appropriate, suggest that the patient take the medication with food.

Narrowing but not swallowing

Some conditions can cause a narrowing of the esophagus, which makes swallowing very difficult. Here are five conditions that you may encounter on the PANCE and in your practice.

Achalasia

Achalasia refers to a failure of the lower esophageal sphincter (LES) to relax and failure of the lower esophagus to have meaningful peristalsis. This can make swallowing and digesting food impossible. The diagnosis is strongly suggested by a barium swallow, which reveals what looks almost like a bird's beak at the distal end of the esophagus — be sure you know this radiographic sign for the test. The diagnosis of achalasia can be confirmed via esophageal manometry.

Treatment for this condition can be medical or surgical. The medical treatment involves using botulinum toxin injections to try to relax the sphincter. Surgical intervention includes a *Heller myotomy,* in which the muscles of the lower esophageal sphincter are cut. It's considered very effective.

Esophageal rings and webs

Esophageal webs and rings are common anatomic abnormalities of the esophagus. They usually cause a narrowing of the esophageal lumen. Here are two conditions to know for the test:

- **Schatzki's ring:** Schatzki's ring is an anatomic narrowing of esophageal mucosa toward the distal end of the esophagus. Presenting symptoms include difficulty swallowing. The diagnosis is made by a barium swallow or esophagogastroduodenoscopy (EGD). (By the way, that's the longest word we use in this book.) Management includes dilating the affected area.
- **Plummer-Vinson syndrome:** This is a triad of dysphagia due to an esophageal web, glossitis (a swollen but very smooth tongue), and iron deficiency anemia. It's very common in people of Scandinavian descent and in postmenopausal women. The treatment often includes iron replacement therapy and balloon dilatation of the esophagus via endoscopy.

Esophageal stricture

Esophageal stricture is a condition caused by a narrowing of the esophagus. Causes include inflammation, motility disorders, and toxic ingestions. (Esophageal stricture is what happens when you drink lye, which is never a good idea.) If esophagitis is the cause of the stricture, then you can administer medications (see the earlier section "Inviting inflammation: Esophagitis"). Also, depending on the severity of the stricture, a balloon dilatation, which can be done via endoscopy, may be needed.

Esophageal spasm

Esophageal spasm, sometimes called *corkscrew esophagus,* is a gastrointestinal cause of chest pain and pressure. It's brought on by eating. The affected person may experience an intense chest pain that can mimic acute coronary syndrome. Esophageal spasm is often a diagnosis of exclusion. The treatment includes nitrates and/or calcium channel blockers. (These meds are also the treatment for coronary artery spasm, or Prinzmetal's angina. Go figure.)

Esophageal cancer

Esophageal cancer can cause weight loss, dysphagia, and odynophagia. Be aware of two types of this cancer for the test. *Adenocarcinoma* is linked with Barrett's esophagitis (see the earlier section "Barrett's esophagitis" for details). The other histologic subtype is *squamous cell carcinoma,* which is related to tobacco and alcohol use.

Esophageal cancer can be diagnosed via an endoscopy as a mass obstructing the esophageal lumen. A barium swallow can demonstrate an *apple-core deformity,* showing a filling defect within the esophageal lumen.

The treatment for esophageal cancer is usually surgical, and it can involve an esophagectomy — a lengthy, complicated, high-mortality procedure. Not that there are any good cancers, but esophageal cancer is a particularly bad one.

Bleeding from the esophagus

For the PANCE, be aware of three types of esophageal bleeding — Mallory-Weiss tears, Boerhaave's syndrome, and esophageal varices.

Mallory-Weiss tears

Mallory-Weiss tears are tears or lacerations in the distal part of the esophagus. The most common test scenario involves a person with a history of recurrent retching or vomiting, perhaps following an alcoholic binge. The key is in the history. In a test question, look for someone with a history of bulimia or alcohol abuse who presents with acute hematemesis.

You diagnose Mallory-Weiss by endoscopy. If the patient has areas of active bleeding, they can be treated with either cautery or a sclerosing agent.

Boerhaave's syndrome

Boerhaave's syndrome is usually a perforation in the distal esophagus. Increases in intra-esophageal and intrathoracic pressure, often secondary to vomiting and retching, frequently precede the perforation. Large meals and alcohol intake are contributing factors. Symptoms include severe chest and abdominal pain and the rapid development of fever, tachypnea, and shock. The treatment is surgical intervention, parenteral feedings, and IV antibiotics.

Esophageal varices

Esophageal varices can present with painless, acute hematemesis, usually in someone with a history of cirrhosis/end-stage liver disease. As a consequence of increased portal venous pressures, these veins rupture, leading to bleeding. Esophageal varices is an emergent condition. For the PANCE, here are the take-home points:

✔ For the management of esophageal varices, familiarize yourself with certain medications. Order an intravenous proton pump inhibitor as well as an intravenous octreotide (Sandostatin) infusion. (This is different from the subcutaneous octreotide you may order in someone with acute kidney failure in the setting of liver disease.) If you're given the option of using intravenous vasopressin (Pitressin), that's a good choice as well.

✔ You want to volume resuscitate these patients, usually with isotonic saline. Check a CBC and PT/INR to make sure that the liver can clot the blood. In an acute bleed and an elevated INR, the person also needs fresh frozen plasma (FFP) — vitamin K is not

> enough to do the trick, because the liver is unable to utilize the vitamin K to synthesize clotting factors because of the cirrhosis.
>
> ✔ The diagnosis and management is done via endoscopy. You may see longitudinal red wale markings. The area is usually sclerosed, or band ligation is done.

Which of the following would be contraindicated in the emergent management of esophageal varices?

(A) Intravenous vasopressin

(B) Fresh frozen plasma

(C) Subcutaneous octreotide

(D) Intravenous normal saline

(E) Intravenous proton pump inhibitor

The correct answer is Choice (C). With acute esophageal varices, you want to use intravenous octreotide as a continuous infusion, not give it subcutaneously. All the other choices are inappropriate in this situation.

Stomaching the Gastric Area

After traveling through the esophagus (and who wouldn't want to do that?), your next destination is the lively gastric area. Containing the cardia, fundus, antrum, and pylorus, this area is just ripe for pathology and future PANCE questions. The stomach is a happening place where much of the digestion takes place. The chief cells make pepsinogen, and the paneth cells make hydrochloric acid (part of gastric acid) to keep gastric pH low. In this section, you read about gastritis, peptic ulcers, and gastric cancer.

Inviting inflammation yet again: Gastritis

Inflammation of the stomach is referred to as *gastritis*. Gastritis can be classified as type A or type B:

> ✔ Type A is *fundal gastritis* (in the fundus of the stomach), and it's felt to be autoimmune in nature. It's associated with inflammatory processes such as pernicious anemia.
>
> ✔ Type B is *antral gastritis* (in the antrum of the stomach). Risk factors and causes include the use of nonsteroidals (NSAIDs), *Helicobacter pylori* infection, alcohol use, and the use of oral steroids.

H. pylori, which is a Gram-negative micro-aerophilic rod- or spiral-shaped bacterium that lives on the surface of the gastric area, is a leading cause of gastritis — you can bet that you'll see questions about this on the test.

How can you search for *H. pylori?* Well, let us count the ways. It can be detected through a urea breath test. Antibodies can be detected in the blood, although the blood test isn't the most reliable. It can be confirmed via biopsy of the affected mucosa via endoscopy. Or it can be detected in the stool via assay, which is often done after treatment to ensure that the bacteria have been eradicated.

Be familiar with the medications used for treating *H. pylori* gastritis. Treatment involves the use of a proton pump inhibitor (PPI) like pantoprazole (Protonix) as well as antibiotics such as amoxicillin (Trimox) and clarithromycin (Biaxin). The duration of treatment is usually 7

to 14 days. Other medications have included metronidazole (Flagyl) and bismuth salicylate (Pepto-Bismol). Be aware that different medication regimens also have different eradication rates. The best eradication is the triple-threat combination of a PPI, clarithromycin, and amoxicillin.

Untreated *H. pylori* infections can increase the risk of developing gastric lymphoma, specifically the development of a MALToma (mucosa-associated lymphoid tissue lymphoma). See the later section "Going after gastric cancer" for info on stomach cancer.

Uncovering the ugly peptic ulcer

Peptic ulcer disease refers to significant inflammation of the lining of the stomach (gastric ulcers) and/or the small intestine (duodenal ulcers). The ulcer forms after the lining of the stomach or duodenum breaks down.

Nothing is uglier than an ulcer, especially a gastric ulcer. The risk factors for gastric ulcers are much the same as for gastritis and can include alcohol, NSAID use, steroids, cigarette smoking, and *Helicobacter pylori* (see the preceding section for info on gastritis and *H. pylori*). Symptoms of a gastric ulcer can include pain induced by eating. If the person is bleeding from a gastric ulcer, you can see dark, tarry (melenic) stools.

In a PANCE question, a gastric ulcer can present with bleeding and pain made worse with eating. A duodenal ulcer can present with pain made better with eating.

The gastric or duodenal ulcer can be diagnosed via an endoscopy. A gastric ulcer is often biopsied to differentiate a malignant gastric ulceration from a benign gastric ulcer.

The treatment for a gastric ulcer is similar to treatment for gastritis. In general, you should be aware of the H2 antagonists, proton pump inhibitors (PPIs), and sucralfate:

- **H2 antagonists:** The commonly used H2 blockers include ranitidine (Zantac) and famotidine (Pepcid). They work by inhibiting H2 secretion from the gastric parietal cells. Although H2 agonists are generally well-tolerated, a possible side effect is increased risk of sedation, especially in older people.

- **Proton pump inhibitors (PPIs):** PPIs are a very commonly prescribed class of medications. Examples include pantoprazole (Protonix) and esomeprazole (Nexium). Note that because they block the secretion of hydrochloric acid from the parietal cells, they can elevate the serum gastrin levels. A common side effect of PPIs is diarrhea. Note that PPIs can also alter the bioavailability of certain supplements and medications that require a more acidic pH for absorption. From a kidney standpoint, they can cause hyponatremia and interstitial nephritis (for info on kidney conditions, see Chapter 10).

  Be aware of the interaction between the PPI pantoprazole and clopidogrel (Plavix). Pantoprazole can decrease the efficacy of clopidogrel.

- **Sucralfate:** Sucralfate (Carafate) works by forming a protective coating over the affected area. It's usually prescribed to be taken 3 to 4 times a day. A common side effect of this medication is hypophosphatemia. It can also interact with the quinolone class of antibiotics, decreasing their absorption.

Going after gastric cancer

Gastric cancer is a nasty, nasty cancer with very poor long-term survival rates. Symptoms that indicate that a malignancy may be present are abdominal fullness (early satiety after eating a little bit), a decreased appetite, and type B constitutional symptoms such as fever, weight loss, and night sweats. Gastric ulcers are often biopsied in order to make sure that malignancy isn't present.

Here are some key test points concerning gastric cancer:

- *Helicobacter pylori* is more than a cause of gastritis and peptic ulcer disease (PUD); it's also a leading cause of gastric cancer, which histologically is an adenocarcinoma. It can form a lymphoma. Additional risk factors for gastric cancer include smoking, drinking alcohol, and eating foods that contain a lot of nitrates.

- Just to make life difficult, there are two types of gastric adenocarcinomas — intestinal type and diffuse type. On a test, if you see linitis plastica, or *leather bottle stomach,* think about the diffuse type of gastric cancer. (At least it's not caused by *H. pylori.*)

- Leser-Trélat syndrome, in which you see a bunch of seborrheic keratoses, is a sign of gastric cancer.

- The diagnosis of gastric cancer is made by endoscopy and biopsy. This is the gold standard.

- Treatment for gastric cancer is usually a partial or subtotal gastrectomy.

A *gastrinoma* is a tumor usually found in the duodenum, though it sometimes occurs in the pancreas. The tumor secretes gastrin; if you were to measure a gastrin level, it would be elevated big time. The triad of Zollenger-Ellison syndrome is the tumor itself, peptic ulcer disease, and high gastrin levels. People with this syndrome present like someone with peptic ulcer disease would, including abdominal pain and/or GI bleeding. The treatments include PPIs. Chemotherapy and surgery may also be needed, depending on the staging of the tumor at the time of diagnosis.

Which of the following statements concerning gastric cancer is correct?

(A) The primary treatment is chemotherapy.

(B) Paraneoplastic phenomena include acanthosis nigricans.

(C) The leading cause of gastric cancer is NSAID use.

(D) It is associated with an increased risk of inflammatory bowel disease (IBD).

(E) This type of malignancy has a low rate of metastatic spread.

The correct answer is Choice (B). Paraneoplastic phenomena associated with gastric cancer include acanthosis nigricans and Leser-Trélat syndrome. Choice (A) is wrong because gastric cancer is usually treated with surgery, primarily a partial or subtotal gastrectomy. The leading cause of gastric malignancy is *H. pylori,* not NSAIDs, so you can eliminate Choice (C). There's no direct association with inflammatory bowel disease, and at the time of diagnosis, the malignancy is usually metastatic, so Choices (D) and (E) are wrong as well.

Can I Buy a Bowel?

A lot of pathology concerns the small and large intestines, and many bowel-related conditions begin with the letter *i.* Here you see conditions such as irritable bowel syndrome (IBS), ischemic bowel, inflammatory bowel disease (IBD), celiac disease, and diverticulitis. Okay, those last two don't begin with an *i,* but we put them here anyway because they contain a lot of *i*'s. Finally, we touch on colon cancer. To read about the infectious causes of diarrhea, go to Chapter 19, where we cover infectious disease.

Identifying irritable bowel syndrome (IBS)

Irritable bowel syndrome (IBS) is a diagnosis of exclusion after other conditions have been ruled out. It's a clinical diagnosis — you can't diagnose this condition with endoscopy and biopsy or barium swallow as you can with many other GI conditions, because the findings are often normal. Common symptoms include constipation, diarrhea, or a combination of both.

A stereotypical candidate for IBS is someone (mostly younger and female) under a great deal of stress who has problems with either diarrhea or constipation during the day, most of the time having the conditions normalize at night during sleep. In a typical PANCE question, you get hints such as "it has been going on for a while," "both endoscopy and colonoscopy are negative," "and stool studies, including those for ova and parasites (O&P), are negative." A very common syndrome associated with IBS is fibromyalgia syndrome (FMS).

The treatment for IBS includes recognizing the triggers, including food, physical stressors, and psychological stressors. Many of the anticholinergic medications, such as dicyclomine (Bentyl), have been tried in treating IBS.

Investigating ischemic bowel

Ischemic bowel, also known as *ischemic colitis,* commonly occurs in older individuals. Risk factors and medical conditions associated with ischemic bowel include atherosclerosis of the intestinal vessels (in the superior mesenteric artery and celiac artery), atrial fibrillation or the presence of a left ventricular mural thrombus (which can increase the risk of an embolic phenomenon to the intestinal vessels), and a hypercoagulable state. Low blood pressure, especially in someone who has significant atherosclerosis of the mesenteric vessels, can precipitate mesenteric ischemia due to hypoperfusion of these vessels.

Here are key points about ischemic bowel:

✔ The classic presentation is pain out of proportion to clinical findings. The person (usually with one of the preceding risk factors) can have diffuse midepigastric pain but also have a benign physical examination.

✔ The pain worsens after eating a meal. Blood flow to the mesenteric area increases after a meal to aid with digestion, and the timing of the abdominal discomfort in relation to eating can point to ischemic bowel.

✔ A person can have *mesenteric angina* or mesenteric ischemia, which is an acute problem. If a large amount of the bowel is affected, expect to see a lactic acidosis and an anion gap on the CHEM-7. If the affected person's abdominal pain is just an episode of angina, you may not see a lactic acidosis.

✔ If findings suggest an acute mesenteric event, the best way to get a look at the intestine is an exploratory laparotomy. A CT scan of the abdomen and pelvis with oral contrast may suggest bowel wall thickening, but this is a nonspecific pattern that you also see with other types of colitis. That being said, the CT scan is probably the best test for looking at the integrity of the bowel wall.

On a CT scan, if you see *thumbprinting* — a radiologic sign suggesting narrowing of the intestinal lumen secondary to bowel wall edema — think about ischemia, especially in the context of a PANCE question. If a bleed is present, magnetic resonance angiography (MRA) is used more often to detect the area of bleeding, especially in the setting of a rapid GI bleed.

Recognizing inflammatory bowel disease (IBD)

Inflammatory bowel disease (IBD) is a comprehensive term covering two different but overlapping conditions: Crohn's disease and ulcerative colitis. Both of these conditions confer an increased risk of colon cancer.

Crohn's disease is an inflammatory condition that can involve any area of the GI tract from the mouth to the anus, although it's usually predominant in the ileum and ileocecal region of the small intestine. When confined to this area, it's called *regional enteritis*. Histologically, Crohn's disease is characterized by noncaseating granulomas on tissue biopsy. The etiology behind the inflammation is unknown. Note that this condition affects all layers of the intestine. When it affects the small intestine, especially the ileum, Crohn's can cause malabsorption of key nutrients, especially the fat-soluble vitamins A, D, E and K. See the later section "Concerning celiac disease and malabsorption" for more information.

Here are the key points about Crohn's disease:

- It usually occurs in younger people, with an initial onset in the teenage years up to the mid-30s.

- It's characterized by the presence of *skip lesions* (areas of inflammation next to areas of normal mucosa) as well as what looks like a cobblestoning mucosa on colonoscopy.

- Crohn's can affect the anus. If on you're asked about the presence of anal fissures on the PANCE, think Crohn's disease.

- Treatment can involve steroids and salicylate derivatives such as mesalamine. Antibiotics such as metronidazole (Flagyl) can be used. In advanced cases that have been refractory to treatment, you can use intravenous infliximab (Remicade).

- Surgery is not curative in Crohn's disease; there can be frequent exacerbations.

Ulcerative colitis (UC) overlaps with Crohn's disease to some extent, but here are some key differences:

- Unlike Crohn's, ulcerative colitis involves only the superficial mucosa, not all layers of the intestine.

- Ulcerative colitis doesn't have these skip lesions; the area of inflammation is continuous.

- Ulcerative colitis is predominantly in the sigmoid-rectal region. In fact, a common presenting symptom of ulcerative colitis is hematochezia and a colonoscopy that demonstrates ulcerative proctitis. Crohn's, on the other hand, is predominantly in the small intestine (ileum), is sometimes in the large intestine, and can affect the anus.

- Crohn's disease has a higher rate of strictures than ulcerative colitis. Both are associated with the possible development of obstruction, abscess formation, perforation, and fistula formation.

- Ulcerative colitis increases the risk of developing sclerosing cholangitis. Remember Charcot's triad of right upper-quadrant (RUQ) pain, fevers, and jaundice for the diagnosis of cholangitis.

- Ulcerative colitis treatment can consist of steroids, although it primarily consists of 5-ASA derivatives. They can be given either orally or rectally.

Both ulcerative colitis and Crohn's disease can be associated with extraintestinal manifestations, which makes sense because both conditions are inflammatory. They can be associated with eye disease (uveitis and iritis) and certain skin lesions, including pyoderma gangrenosum (not a pretty sight) and erythema nodosum. If the PANCE asks you about the lesion of a pyoderma gangrenosum, think ulcerative colitis — necrotic lesions are common with ulcerative colitis. Erythema nodosum can be seen in many conditions; for PANCE purposes, when you see this condition or a picture of this condition, think of either IBD or sarcoidosis.

IBD is also associated with inflammatory arthritis. IBD, psoriatic arthritis, ankylosing spondylitis, and reactive arthritis (previously known as Reiter's syndrome) are examples of the seronegative spondyloarthropathies. All are associated with HLA-B27 expression. The arthritis associated with IBD is thought to affect more of the peripheral joints, especially during an active flare of IBD.

Which of the following conditions can be associated with caseating granulomas?

(A) Crohn's disease

(B) Sarcoidosis

(C) Ulcerative colitis

(D) Tuberculosis

(E) Silicosis

The correct answer is Choice (D). Tuberculosis is associated with caseating granulomas. Choices (A) and (B) are associated with noncaseating granulomas. Although you can see silicosis with tuberculosis, it in and of itself isn't associated with granuloma formation. Ulcerative colitis, Choice (C), is not associated with granuloma formation.

Concerning celiac disease and malabsorption

A *malabsorption syndrome* is an inability to absorb key nutrients in the small intestine. In this section, we cover nutritional deficiencies and celiac disease.

Vitamin deficiencies

Your intestine is responsible for the absorption of many vitamins and nutrients. One main cause of vitamin deficiencies is the lack of absorption in the small intestine due to conditions such as Crohn's disease and the malabsorption syndromes, such as celiac disease. Here's a quick review of some basic aspects of vitamin and nutritional deficiencies:

- Vitamin A is important for maintenance of vision and of the immune system. Symptoms of Vitamin A deficiency include night blindness and increased susceptibility to infections.

- Vitamin C is important for collagen formation. A deficiency of vitamin C is called *scurvy,* which can present as spongy gums, bleeding from mucous membranes, spots on the skin, and lethargy.

- You know there are different kinds of vitamin B. Vitamin B1 is thiamine, and a deficiency causes Wernicke's encephalopathy — the triad of cerebellar ataxia, nystagmus, and confusion, commonly seen in alcoholics. Vitamin B3 is niacin, and a niacin deficiency causes pellagra, with the triad of dementia, diarrhea, and dermatitis. Vitamin B_6 is responsible for helping with nerve health. A deficiency of B_6 or an excess of B_6 can cause a neuropathy.

- A deficiency of Vitamin D causes problems with bone, namely osteomalacia.

- Vitamin E (alpha-tocopherol) is a lipid-soluble antioxidant. A Vitamin E deficiency messes you up, and it may show up as spinocerebellar ataxia and myopathy, various neurological signs, and anemia, to name but a few.

- Vitamin K is important for clotting of the blood, and a deficiency of this vitamin causes excess bleeding problems.

Celiac disease

Celiac disease, which is also known as *gluten-sensitive enteropathy* or *celiac sprue,* is an auto-immune reaction in the small intestine caused by gluten. Gluten can be found in wheat, rye, and barley. Histologically, you can see flattening of the small intestinal villi. Celiac disease is the most common form of malabsorption syndrome, affecting approximately 1 in 100 people.

The affected person can present with bloating, abdominal distention, and altered bowel habits, such as constipation and/or diarrhea. Celiac disease can also cause weight loss. It's an uncommon cause of elevated liver function tests (transaminitis), and it can cause cirrhosis.

Here are several key points concerning celiac disease:

- ✔ You'd order antigliadin antibody and tissue transglutaminase antibody in anyone you suspected has celiac disease.

- ✔ The gold standard test to confirm the diagnosis is an endoscopy with biopsy of the small intestine.

- ✔ The treatment includes the elimination of anything with gluten, which means prescribing a gluten-free diet for your patient. Many grocery stores have special gluten-free aisles.

- ✔ It's important to correct any nutritional deficiencies that may have resulted from celiac disease. This can include iron deficiencies, B_{12} and/or folate deficiencies, other vitamin deficiencies, and low magnesium levels.

 Celiac disease can be associated with other medical conditions. A common one you may see on the PANCE is *dermatitis herpetiformis,* a blistering/bumpy type of rash commonly seen on the extremities, including the knees and elbows. It can also appear on the back. The treatment includes adherence to a gluten-free diet. A medication called dapsone (Aczone) is also used for treating this condition.

Diagnosing diverticulosis and diverticulitis

One of the most common conditions occurring in the older population is *diverticulosis,* which is simply an outpouching or formation of pockets of the colonic mucosa through weaknesses in the intestinal wall. This pouching most commonly occurs in the sigmoid colon. Realize that diverticulosis is a leading cause of hematochezia as well. For the most part, diverticulosis is painless, and the bleeding associated with it is painless bleeding.

For PANCE purposes, be aware of the factors that increase the risk of developing diverticulosis: older age, a Western-based diet (low in fiber content with excessive meat ingestion), and abnormal bowel habits, including straining and constipation.

One complication of diverticulosis is *diverticulitis,* an infection of the diverticula. Here are some key points:

- ✔ Symptoms of diverticulitis include acute left lower-quadrant abdominal pain and fever. Labs can show a leukocytosis. The diagnosis can be confirmed by a CT scan.

- ✔ Mild cases can be managed as an outpatient with a low-residue diet, clear liquids, and an oral antibiotic. Moderate to severe cases are often treated in the hospital. Treatment includes making the patient NPO, giving intravenous fluids, and ordering intravenous antibiotics. The most common antibiotics prescribed are metronidazole (Flagyl) and a fluoroquinolone such as levofloxacin (Levaquin) or ciprofloxacin (Cipro).

- ✔ Complications of diverticulitis can include perforation, abscess, bleeding, obstruction, and/or fistula formation. Again, diagnosis is via CT scan. A localized abscess is often amenable to CT-guided drainage.

✔ With diverticulitis, the third time's the charm. After three attacks, discuss the need for possible surgery with the patient. Surgical options can include a hemicolectomy with reanastomosis or a colostomy initially if significant inflammation is involved.

Conquering colon cancer

Colon cancer is a topic you'll surely be tested on, because colorectal cancer is the third most commonly diagnosed cancer in males and the second in females, especially in developed countries.

Watching for risk factors

Risk factors for colon cancer include a low-fiber Western diet, inflammatory bowel disease (including Crohn's disease and ulcerative colitis), and heredity. A big hereditary condition that you should be aware of is familial adenomatous polyposis (FAP). With this condition, you see many polyps throughout the colon, and the incidence of cancer is very high. Most people with familial adenomatous polyposis will develop colon cancer before age 40. The treatment for FAP is a colectomy.

Looking at the signs, symptoms, and treatment of colon cancer

Signs and symptoms of colon cancer can include bleeding and abnormalities of bowel habits, including constipation and diarrhea. If the tumor is large enough and much of the colonic lumen is obstructed, then symptoms of obstruction, including abdominal pain, distention, nausea, and vomiting, may be present.

On a colonoscopy, you may see a polyp. Different types and different characteristics of polyps can imply a benign or a malignant prognosis. For example, hamartomatous polyps are completely benign. If the polyp is a tubular adenoma, it has a low risk of malignancy, but it still has a malignancy risk. If a villous adenoma is present, it has a very high malignancy potential. Any polyp with a sessile base has a higher risk of developing into cancer.

Here are three essential points about colon cancer:

✔ The most common site of metastasis is the liver.

✔ Therapy can include surgery and chemotherapy. Common chemotherapeutic agents used in the treatment of colon cancer include 5-fluorouracil (5-FU) and certain platinum-based compounds, including oxaliplatin. A main side effect of 5-FU is diarrhea — very significant diarrhea.

✔ After the colon cancer is diagnosed, you use the carcinoembryonic antigen (CEA) level to monitor recurrence and response to therapy.

Screening for colon cancer

The PANCE is likely to ask about when someone should be screened as well as risk factors for colon cancer. This is a big topic, so expect big questions. Someone who has no family history of colon cancer should begin the following screening tests for colon cancer at age 50 (note that the current guidelines talk about screening until age 75):

✔ A colonoscopy every 10 years

✔ A sigmoidoscopy every 5 years (Barry considers this to be "colonoscopy light")

✔ Annual fecal occult blood testing (FOBT)

Evaluating the GI bleed

Upper GI bleeding is bleeding from the esophagus, stomach, and small intestine proximal to the ligament of Treitz. Causes can include esophagitis, Mallory-Weiss tears, Boerhaave's syndrome, esophageal and gastric varices, gastritis, and gastric cancer.

Common causes of bleeding from the lower GI tract include diverticulosis, colon cancer, hemorrhoids, angiodysplasia, and arteriovenous malformations, or (AVMs). Arteriovenous malformations are dilated venous plexi that can be difficult to find on a colonoscopy. In addition to recognizing arteriovenous malformations as a cause of lower GI bleeding, one common condition where you see arteriovenous malformations is

with aortic stenosis (AS). The combination of aortic stenosis and arteriovenous malformations is called *Heyde's syndrome.*

The management of a GI bleed includes adequate intravenous access (two 18-gauge IVs) with volume repletion, and the person is usually NPO. Assessing for any coagulaopathy is important, as is serial hemoglobin and hematocrits (H/H) to assess bleeding loss. A nasogastric tube can be placed to obtain an aspirate if you're worried about an upper GI bleed. It's also used if there's an active bleed to minimize the risk of vomiting and aspirating the blood. For information on managing GI bleeding from a surgical point of view, see Chapter 7.

If someone has a first-degree relative who was diagnosed with colon cancer when younger than 60 years or two relatives diagnosed with colon cancer at any age, the patient should begin screenings at age 40 (not age 50) or 10 years before the age at which the relative was diagnosed, whichever comes first.

For example, if someone has a sister diagnosed with colon cancer at the age of 55, then that person should have his or her first screening done at age 40 rather than age 50. If that same person has a sister diagnosed with colon cancer at age 50 and another diagnosed with colon cancer at age 45, then you'd recommend that your patient have his or her first colonoscopy at age 35. In people with a family history, the follow-up is every 5 years instead of every 10 years.

Here are a few more notes on cancer screening for people with a high risk of colon cancer:

✔ In someone with a history of hereditary nonpolyposis colorectal cancer (NPCC), it's recommended that he or she get an annual colonoscopy after age 20.

✔ Someone with familial adenomatous polyposis (FAP) should get a colonoscopy done annually starting in his or her teenage years. Sadly, colorectal cancer is probably coming; it's just a matter of when.

Putting Up with the Pancreas

The pancreas is an important organ that has many functions in the body, both endocrine and exocrine. Concerning endocrine function, the pancreas produces insulin, glucagon, and somatostatin (or it's supposed to). You read about the abnormalities of some of the endocrine functions of the pancreas in Chapter 15. Concerning exocrine function, the pancreas secretes digestive enzymes such as the proteases, lipase, and amylase. It secretes bicarbonate as well.

Common abnormalities of the pancreas that you'll likely find on the PANCE include acute pancreatitis, chronic pancreatitis, and pancreatic cancer. Be aware that pancreatitis and pancreatic inefficiency can also contribute to malabsorption of certain essential vitamins and nutrients.

Improving acute pancreatitis

Pancreatitis is inflammation of the pancreas. Acute pancreatitis can be a source of increased morbidity and mortality. The two most common causes of acute pancreatitis include gallstones and alcohol abuse. Other causes include high triglycerides (usually greater than 1,000 mg/dL), medications (examples include sulfa-based meds and diuretics), and infections (including mumps).

The clinical presentation of acute pancreatitis is usually left upper-quadrant pain or midepigastric pain with radiation to the back.

Two physical examination signs of acute pancreatitis include Cullen's sign and Grey Turner's sign. *Cullen's sign* refers to periumbilical bruising related to acute pancreatitis. *Grey Turner's sign* refers to bruising and ecchymosis of the flank area, related to hemorrhagic pancreatitis.

The diagnosis of acute pancreatitis is suggested by an elevated amylase and lipase. The lipase, which can be very elevated (sometimes in the thousands), is the most specific test for pancreatitis.

Be aware that medical conditions other than pancreatitis can also cause an elevation in serum amylase and lipase levels. For example, intestinal problems, kidney failure, and certain cancers (lung and pancreatic, among others) can increase serum amylase levels. Concerning lipase levels, medications such as NSAIDs and morphine can elevate these levels, as can obesity and gallbladder problems. But on the PANCE, if you're given a scenario with a significantly elevated lipase level, think acute pancreatitis.

An abdominal plain film may exclude other etiologies. The radiograph may range from unremarkable to a localized ileus of a segment of the small intestine (sentinel loop) or the colon cutoff sign in advanced disease. The pancreas may be calcified on a radiograph, which can be a sign of chronic pancreatitis. The diagnosis of acute pancreatitis is confirmed by a CT scan of the abdomen with IV contrast. On CT, you see significant edema and inflammation of the pancreas. A phlegmon may or may not be present. A *pancreatic pseudocyst,* which is a fluid-filled area around the pancreas, may be present.

Acute pancreatitis increases the body's systemic inflammatory response system. Pancreatitis can have many complications, both local and systemic. Locally, a pseudocyst may form. If the pancreatitis is aggressive, it can transform into a hemorrhagic pancreatitis or a necrotizing pancreatitis — these conditions are really bad. Systemic complications can include multi-organ dysfunction syndrome, including worsening of liver and kidney function. Lung function can deteriorate through the formation of acute respiratory distress syndrome (ARDS).

Various scores have been used to evaluate the acuity of someone with pancreatitis in the ICU. Examples include the SOFA score and the APACHE score. When assessing the severity of pancreatitis, one scoring system that you may be asked about is Ranson criteria. This scoring system, which is based on lab abnormalities, includes looking at certain parameters at the time of admission and 48 hours later. At the time of admission, parameters include a person's age, blood glucose level, WBC count, AST level, and LDH level.

Pancreatitis can cause third spacing of fluid, and the patient can be liters behind in terms of volume requirements. Recall that the *third space* is the area of the body that normally does not collect fluid. The management of acute pancreatitis includes making the patient NPO; aggressive, aggressive hydration with normal saline; and intravenous pain medication. Aggressive volume resuscitation is needed because of the third spacing of fluids. Labs are monitored and a workup is begun, including evaluation of the biliary tract and a fasting lipid profile.

Which of the following medications can be used in the treatment of acute necrotizing pancreatitis?

(A) Amoxicillin (Amoxil)

(B) Imipenem-cilistatin (Primaxin)

(C) Levofloxacin (Levaquin)

(D) Metronidazole (Flagyl)

(E) Doxycycline (Doryx)

The correct answer is Choice (B). In someone with necrotizing pancreatitis, imipenem-cilistatin is the one antibiotic that has been used effectively to treat the infection.

Treating chronic pancreatitis

With chronic pancreatitis, the nature of the pain is the same as with acute pancreatitis — left upper-quadrant pain or midepigastric pain with radiation to the back. However, the labs are a little different. The lipase may be normal to just slightly high. In this case, you're dealing not with acute pancreatitis per se but with an exacerbation of chronic pancreatitis.

For the PANCE, be aware of one telltale sign of chronic pancreatitis: You can see calcification of the pancreas on an abdominal radiograph (KUB). You can also see this calcification on a CT scan.

Two complications deriving from chronic pancreatitis are diabetes (failure of the endocrine pancreatic function) and malabsorption (failure of the exocrine pancreas). In the case of malabsorption, the patient often needs supplemental pancreatic enzymes, which he or she takes with each meal.

Recognizing pancreatic cancer

Pancreatic cancer is a bad cancer with a very high mortality rate. If you see a test question that concerns painless jaundice, think pancreatic cancer until proven otherwise; obstructive jaundice that's usually painless is the most common presentation of pancreatic cancer. The jaundice comes from blockage of the bile duct.

Other signs of pancreatic cancer include weight loss, itching (due to elevated bilirubin levels), and abdominal distention. Sometimes the patient feels pain with radiation to the back. Risk factors for pancreatic cancer include obesity, advanced age, tobacco use, diabetes, diets high in meat and low in fruits and vegetables, and alcoholism.

Here are other key points to be aware of concerning pancreatic cancer:

- ✔ The tumor marker associated with pancreatic cancer is CA 19-9.

- ✔ Diagnostic studies used in evaluating pancreatic cancer include the CT scan and endoscopic ultrasound. The head of the pancreas is the most common site of diagnosis of tumors. Tumors located in the body or tail of the pancreas tend to be more aggressive.

- ✔ Histologically, pancreatic cancer is an adenocarcinoma.

- ✔ Pancreatic cancers do not respond well to chemotherapy, so the main treatment is surgical. A pancreaticoduodenectomy (Whipple procedure) is used to remove the carcinoma when it's at the head of the pancreas. If the body and/or tail is affected, often the treatment is a distal pancreatectomy. With this type of surgery, the spleen is often removed as well. Both procedures are major surgeries, and the prognosis for a person with a pancreatectomy is very poor. There are no good cancers, but pancreatic cancer is one of the worst.

Two signs associated with pancreatic cancer are Trousseau's sign and Courvoisier's sign:

- **Trousseaus' sign of malignancy:** This sign has been described as a migratory thrombophlebitis, where clots can form in the legs or in the portal venous system. This sign makes sense because any type of cancer can make someone hypercoagulable and increase the clotting risk.

- **Courvoisier's sign:** With this sign, you can actually palpate a gallbladder on physical examination because it's so distended. You see Courvoisier's sign with pancreatic cancer and with gallbladder cancer.

Looking at the Liver

The liver does vital things, including controlling the metabolism, processing toxins and medications, manufacturing proteins, clotting blood, and regenerating anions into bicarbonate. Why are these points important to know? Because when the liver doesn't work, you begin to see problems with metabolism, bleeding, and acidosis. The most common forms of liver injury that you see on the PANCE concern hepatitis.

Be aware of the two main forms of liver injury. Hepatitis concerns inflammation of the liver. It's characterized by *transaminitis,* or elevated liver function tests, such as an elevated aspartate aminotransferase (AST) and alanine aminotransferase (ALT). There's also a *cholestatic pattern* of liver injury, which causes elevation of alkaline phosphatase and total bilirubin. Examples include biliary tract obstruction as well as medications, a common example being erythromycin.

Helping people with hepatitis

On the test, you'll likely be asked to discern not only the pattern of liver injury based on the labs and clinical exam but also the cause and prognosis of that cause. This may sound a little complicated, but it's fairly easy. Here are some general points to consider when you're evaluating a question about someone with hepatitis:

- If you see a question in which the AST and ALT are elevated and the AST level is twice the ALT level (a 2:1 ratio), think about alcoholic hepatitis.

- On a test question (or clinically), if you see an AST and ALT level in the thousands with the 2:1 ratio, another inflammatory process other than just alcoholic hepatitis is affecting the liver.

- Viral hepatitis usually causes the ALT level to be greater than the AST level

Many of the causes of hepatitis that you'll see on the test are viral hepatitis: hepatitis A, hepatitis B, hepatitis C, hepatitis D, and hepatitis E. In addition, you may see questions concerning medication-induced hepatitis (think statins) as well as Epstein-Barr virus (EBV) and cytomegalovirus (CMV).

Hepatitis A
Hepatitis A is a viral form of hepatitis that has a fecal-oral route of transmission and is usually spread through eating contaminated food or water. It can also spread if someone comes into direct contact with a person who has hepatitis A. The good news about this form of hepatitis is that it usually gets better on its own and it doesn't turn into a chronic form of

hepatitis. IgM antibodies to hepatitis A indicate an acute infection. Because this condition is self-limiting, no specific treatment is needed, other than avoiding other hepatotoxins.

Hepatitis A usually occurs in younger individuals, most commonly in people who travel to countries where it may be endemic. Here are two key points about hepatitis A:

- ✔ If you're traveling to an area where there's a high prevalence of this condition, then vaccination with a hepatitis A vaccine is recommended.
- ✔ Anyone with any other form of hepatitis (specifically B and/or C) should be immunized to hepatitis A.

Hepatitis B

Hepatitis B is a viral form of hepatitis that's transmitted through body fluids, usually from sexual contact or a blood transfusion. It can also be transmitted through sharing needles.

As with other forms of hepatitis, most people actively infected with hepatitis B just feel bad. They feel tired and weak, like they have the flu. They may have jaundice. Note that hepatitis B can present acutely and resolve. In some people, it develops into a chronic form. In a few people, it can turn into fulminant liver failure.

For the test, be familiar with the antibody and antigen tests for hepatitis B:

- ✔ **Envelopes:** There are two envelope tests: the hepatitis B envelope antigen and the hepatitis B envelope antibody. The hep B envelope *antigen* means that the virus is actively replicating and that the person is highly infective. The hep B envelope *antibody* means that the virus is replicating and the person is infective but to a lesser degree (that is, there's less viral replication).

- ✔ **Surface dudes:** You again have two surface tests: the hepatitis B surface antigen and the hepatitis B surface antibody. The hep B surface *antigen* means that the person is still dealing with an active infection. The hep B surface *antibody* is what you test for (to see whether it's positive) after someone has been immunized against hep B. The surface antibody also means the person has built up antibodies to the hep B virus and is immune to any infection.

  Follow the sequence of events. When someone has a hepatitis B infection, the hep B surface antigen is the usually the first one you see. The hep B envelope antigen appears after the hep B surface antigen. In general, as soon as the person is able to clear the infection, you see the envelope antibody and then the surface antibody. Note that we say *usually* and *in general* because there are exceptions to this rule. For the test, know the general process of things.

- ✔ **Core:** In one special case, the hep B surface antigen isn't the first antigen positive in the setting of an infection. Sometimes the body does such a good job of clearing the virus initially that the only test that's positive is the hep B core antibody. Because the infection is acute, this is an IgM antibody, not an IgG antibody.

In many people, hepatitis B resolves, and they develop antibodies against it. In some cases, someone develops a chronic hepatitis secondary to hep B. If the hepatitis B surface antigen stays elevated for 6 months or longer, that person is said to have a chronic hepatitis. Usually the ALT level stays elevated in that regard. Also, many people are chronic carriers of the hepatitis B infection.

Hep B is a DNA virus, so you can always order a quantitative hepatitis B DNA level to see how much the virus is replicating. Chronic hepatitis B is associated with the development of hepatocellular carcinoma; often you need to order a liver biopsy.

You're evaluating a 45-year-old woman whom you believe has acute hepatitis. You find that she is hepatitis B surface antigen positive and hepatitis B surface antibody negative. What would you tell her about her hepatitis B at this point?

(A) She is no longer infected.

(B) She is still in the infectious stage.

(C) She has hepatitis C.

(D) She has already been vaccinated against the disease.

(E) She needs to be vaccinated against hepatitis B.

The correct answer is Choice (B). She is still infectious and infective and hasn't yet developed antibodies to hepatitis B. For Choice (C) to be correct, you'd expect to see some indication that she had hepatitis C or that the antibody tests were positive for hepatitis C. If she were already vaccinated against the disease, then the hepatitis B surface antibody would be positive and the antigen, negative. She doesn't need to be vaccinated against hepatitis B because she's actively infected.

Hepatitis D

Hepatitis D is next, ahead of hepatitis C. This isn't because we're rebels who want to go out of order (Barry is, Rich isn't) but because hepatitis D is associated with hepatitis B. A person can be infected with both B and D at the same time (co-infection), or hepatitis D can infect someone already diagnosed with hepatitis B (superinfection).

Three things you need to know about hepatitis D:

✔ It can make the hepatitis B much worse.

✔ It's associated with many of the same risk factors as hepatitis B, especially the part about sharing needles.

✔ It's also known as the *delta agent* and can't replicate without hepatitis B.

Hepatitis C

Hepatitis C is like hepatitis B in a couple of ways. First, the route of transmission is the same, and a primary way that hep C spreads is through blood transfusions. Like hep B, hep C can be an acute hepatitis that resolves, develops into a chronic hepatitis, or develops into fulminant liver failure.

Unlike hep B, hep C is an RNA virus, not a DNA virus. And unlike hep B, you don't have six freakin' antibodies to worry about. If a person has hep C, the antibodies to hep C are positive. Note that hepatitis C antibodies don't show up until about 4 months after the initial exposure.

You need to quantitate the hep C RNA to determine the viral load. If the viral load is significant, then the person has an ongoing infection. You can follow the viral load and the ALT levels over time. Sometimes, the liver can clear the viral load with resolution of the infection. Most people, however, develop a chronic infection. Chronic hepatitis C is associated with development of liver cancer.

Always consider treating hepatitis C. A biopsy may be done to see whether fibrosis is present, but ordering a biopsy isn't a hard and fast rule among GI doctors. For PANCE purposes, a biopsy is needed to determine the extent of fibrosis. The genotype of the hepatitis C is also important. The three different genotypes are types 1, 2, and 3. Basically, type 1 is difficult to treat with therapy. The other two genotypes tend to respond better.

The therapy for hep C involves pegylated interferon and ribavirin. Both of these can have serious side effects. The interferon can cause a flu-like illness as well as depression. Ribavirin can wreak havoc on the blood count and cause pancytopenia.

Other types of hepatitis

Epstein-Barr virus causes infectious mononucleosis ("the kissing disease"). It's also associated with hepatitis. Note that liver function tests can be associated with mononucleosis at the time of diagnosis. This virus also causes a hemolytic anemia. The treatment is supportive, the key being to recognize the initial presentation. Remember that with mono, one can have cervical adenopathy, exudative pharyngitis, and splenomegaly.

Cytomegalovirus-induced hepatitis is a rarer sort of infection. Almost everyone already has IgG antibodies to the cytomegalovirus. You see this virus wreaking havoc more commonly in transplant recipients. Cytomegalovirus can cause hepatitis, and it can also cause colitis or retinitis. The treatment is either ganciclovir (Cytovene) and/or valganciclovir (Valcyte). You may see one or the other on a test but not both.

As if there weren't enough causes of hepatitis, many medications and toxins can cause an acute hepatitis. Look at the following practice question.

Which of the following medications can cause an acute transaminitis?

(A) Erythromycin (Ery-Tab)

(B) Simvastatin (Zocor)

(C) Hydralazine (Apresoline)

(D) Hydroxychloroquine (Plaquenil)

(E) Gentamicin (Garamycin)

The correct answer is Choice (B). Many commonly prescribed medications have side effects. Choice (A), erythromycin, can cause elevated liver function tests, but it usually causes a cholestatic-like picture over a transaminitis. Choice (B), simvastatin, is associated with a transaminitis. Statins can also cause muscle damage (rhabdomyolysis is an example) and even memory loss in some people. Choice (C), hydralazine, can cause a drug-induced lupus-like syndrome. Because hydralazine is a vasodilator, it can cause a reflex tachycardia as well. Choice (D), hydroxychloroquine, can cause macular degeneration. Choice (E), gentamicin, is kidney toxic, causing a nephrotoxic acute tubular necrosis (ATN).

Keeping cirrhosis in check

Any hepatic process, especially hepatitis or long-standing alcoholism over time, causes cirrhosis of the liver. Cirrhosis is not reversible. For the PANCE, be familiar with various aspects of cirrhosis.

Because the liver is responsible for regulating metabolism, processing medications, and processing the body's various hormones, many things can change when cirrhosis is present. Men can develop gynecomastia (also known as "man-boobs"). People with cirrhosis feel tired and weak.

From an acid-base perspective, chronic liver cirrhosis can cause a respiratory alkalosis. The liver also regenerates bicarbonate, so at very late stages of liver disease, a metabolic acidosis can be present. (See Chapter 10 for details on acid-base.)

People with cirrhosis can have problems with blood clotting, which is manifested by an elevated PT/INR. If there's significant portal hypertension and splenomegaly, then leukopenia and thrombocytopenia may also be present. Liver disease itself can cause a macrocytic anemia.

As cirrhosis progresses, you see elevation in the portal venous pressures. Ascites occurs when the portal venous pressures are greater than 30 mmHg. For chronic compensated cirrhosis, the treatment is sodium restriction, and if ascites is present, the use of spironolactone (Aldactone) and/or furosemide (Lasix).

It doesn't take much for someone to go from a compensated state of cirrhosis to a decompensated state. GI bleeding, spontaneous bacterial peritonitis (SBP), and bacteremia all can cause the liver to decompensate. In decompensated cirrhosis or end-stage liver disease, you may see some or all of the following:

- **Hepatic encephalopathy, which is due to an elevated NH_3 level (hyperammonemia):** The treatments include lactulose and rifaximin (Xifaxan) second line.

- **Bleeding secondary to hypoprothrombinemia:** Oral and/or subcutaneous therapies are unlikely to be effective with a cirrhotic liver. In this situation, you may need to give fresh frozen plasma. We cover the treatment of coagulopathies in Chapter 18.

- **An increased risk for renal failure:** Examples include prerenal azotemia, acute tubular necrosis (ATN), and the hepatorenal syndrome (HRS).

- **Hypotension:** As the liver fails, the systemic vascular resistance drops, and consequently, so does blood pressure.

Looking at liver cancer

Liver cancer is very bad news. Here are the key points about liver cancer:

- The most common cause of hepatocellular carcinoma (HCC) is hepatitis C.

- Any type of cirrhosis can, over time, lead to an increased risk of cancer. Hepatitis B and certain toxin exposures are also risk factors for the development of liver cancer.

- Hepatocellular carcinoma is associated with the tumor marker alpha-fetoprotein.

- After the diagnosis of cancer, the liver should be biopsied. Therapies can include cryo-ablation (freeze that tumor off!) or radiofrequency ablation (heat that tumor off!), depending on the size of the tumor. Surgical resection may also be indicated. These patients are often poor chemo candidates.

The liver is a common site of metastasis for many cancers, including colon and lung malignancies. Rectal cancers tend to metastasize in the lung first because the inferior rectal vein drains into the inferior vena cava rather than into the portal venous system, as do renal cell cancers.

Fixing a Wrecked Rectum

The rectum and anus can be sources of PANCE questions. Many of these conditions affecting the rectum and anus are also painful, so when someone says something is "a pain in the butt," it's not just an expression.

Helping patients with hemorrhoids

Hemorrhoids may be external or internal. The ones that can hurt — and the ones that you can see on examination — are the external hemorrhoids. They're distal to (below) the pectinate (or dentate) line. Symptoms can include pain with defecation, anal pruritus, and irritation around the affected area. The most common symptom is hematochezia.

Internal hemorrhoids, or hemorrhoids originating above the pectinate (or dentate) line, come in four degrees, depending on how far down the anal canal they go. For example, mild cases (grades 1 and 2) either bleed or descend with bleeding but go back to their original positions after the acute flare is over. The more advanced grades of internal hemorrhoids (grades 3 and 4) may be visible after bowel movements and need to be reduced. A grade 4 hemorrhoid is the worst and may be visible to the naked eye.

Treatment depends on the grade. The lower grades get more conservative treatment, including diet modification and hydration. Higher grades may need topical anesthetic preparations or specialized suppositories. Surgical intervention is an option if other measures are unsuccessful.

Fingering fecal impactions

As a medical professional, Rich has had to do his share of manual disimpactions for fecal impaction. It's not a pretty sight. The stool consists of this hard ball-like material, almost looking clay-like. The goal is not to let the stool get to this state.

Many people will discuss their bowel issues with you, rather openly we may add. Common symptoms of a fecal impaction you may hear about are abdominal pain, distention, and bloating. They may say that they "can't pass gas."

Usually the fecal material is confined to the colon, but an impaction can affect much of the large intestine and, on rare occasions, the small intestine. Left untreated, the person risks colon perforation, necrosis of the rectal tissue, and ulcers of the rectal tissue. Note that a colon fully distended by fecal material can cause urinary symptoms as well.

The treatment usually involves digital disimpaction as well as enemas. Other therapies take longer and aren't valuable when the impaction needs to be removed immediately.

The fecal impaction is often due to constipation that has gotten worse and worse. Remember that *constipation* is usually having 3 or fewer bowel movements per week. In addition, it can be tremendously difficult to move the bowels (leading to straining) and/or there can be a sense of not being fully empty ("I still gotta go").

Common causes of constipation can include opioid pain medications, calcium channel blockers, hypothyroidism, and electrolyte problems such as hypokalemia and hypercalcemia that can slow down bowel motility. Neuropathic disorders like diabetic gastroparesis can also be contributory.

A colonic malignancy can present with constipation and incomplete emptying. When other differential diagnoses are excluded and the constipation persists, you need to think of a colonic malignancy and order a colonoscopy.

The treatment can consist of dietary changes such as increased fiber, stool softeners, and laxative agents that can clean out the stool.

Reaching for rectal cancer

The risk factors for rectal cancer are somewhat similar to the risk factors for colon cancer. These include older age, tobacco use, a diet higher in fat, a family history of cancer, and human papillomavirus (HPV) infection.

Signs and symptoms of colon cancer can include hematochezia and/or blood mixed with the stool. The patient may also have obstructive symptoms, especially if the mass is large enough to obstruct the rectal lumen. Other type B constitutional symptoms, including weight loss, can also occur, depending on the extent and spread of the cancer. Sometimes an initial hint of this condition is the palpation of a mass during a digital rectal examination. The diagnosis is confirmed by a sigmoidoscopy.

The treatment of the rectal cancer often depends on the stage of the cancer. Early-stage cancers are more confined to the rectum and have no lymph node involvement. Early stages can be treated with surgical resection. For Stage II and higher, chemotherapy and radiotherapy may be considered. Common sites of metastasis include the lungs and the liver. Stage IV cancer is consistent with metastasis.

Probing for perirectal abscess

A perirectal abscess can be a painful experience. The person often presents with rectal pain and fever. Another possible symptom is constipation, and sometimes drainage from the abscess is present. Often, you can palpate a mass on examination.

The etiology of the abscess is usually bacterial in nature. Common causative organisms include *Staphylococcus* and *E. coli*. All abscesses require surgical intervention, with an incision and drainage (I&D) recommended. If left unattended, a fistula can form. And that's no fun, either.

Figuring out anal fissures

An *anal fissure* is a small tear in the anal canal. Risk factors include constipation, improper hygiene, and any condition that causes intestinal straining, such as the birth of a child. For test purposes, if you see a question concerning anal fissures, Crohn's disease should be in your differential diagnosis. (We discuss Crohn's earlier in "Recognizing inflammatory bowel disease [IBD].")

The key point to remember with anal fissures is that you need to worry about the anal sphincter as well. If you don't relax the contracted anal sphincter, the fissure may not heal.

Treatment can be medical or surgical. Common conservative therapies include more fiber in the diet and laxatives as needed. In addition, topical vasodilators such as nitro are sometimes enough to help the sphincter relax. If medication treatment fails, a sphincterotomy is often considered.

Practice Questions about the Digestive System

Here are some lively questions about the GI system.

1. Which one of the following statements concerning colon cancer screening is correct??

   (A) After the age of 50, a person should obtain a sigmoidoscopy every 10 years.

   (B) Fecal occult blood testing (FOBT) should be done every year after the age of 35.

   (C) A colonoscopy should be done every 5 years, first starting at age 60.

   (D) If a person's brother has a history of colon cancer, the sibling should obtain a colonoscopy 5 years prior to the age at which her sibling was diagnosed.

   (E) After the age of 50, a colonoscopy should be done every 10 years.

2. Which of the following is an example of a physiologic function of the pancreas?

   (A) Secretion of cholecystokinin

   (B) Secretion of pepsinogen

   (C) Secretion of glucagon

   (D) Absorption of calcium

   (E) Absorption of bicarbonate

3. You're evaluating a 65-year-old man with advanced colon cancer for a possibility of recurrence. Which of the following laboratory studies would you order at this time?

   (A) CEA

   (B) CA 19-9

   (C) CA 125

   (D) Erythrocyte sedimentation rate (ESR)

   (E) Alpha-fetoprotein (AFP)

4. Which of the following medications has been used in the treatment of hepatitis B?

   (A) Ribavirin (Rebetol)

   (B) Interferon alpha (Intron-A)

   (C) Steroids

   (D) Plasmapheresis

   (E) Lamivudine (Epivir)

5. Which of the following tests would you order for someone in whom you suspect celiac disease?

   (A) Carcinoembryonic antigen (CEA)

   (B) Anticentromere antibody

   (C) HLA-B27

   (D) Tissue transglutaminase antibody

   (E) Anti-Smith antibody

6. Which one of the following medications would you give to treat someone with cytomegalovirus esophagitis?

   (A) Acyclovir (Zovirax)

   (B) Ganciclovir (Cytovene)

   (C) Fluconazole (Diflucan)

   (D) Interferon alpha (Intron-A)

   (E) Steroids

Answers and Explanations

Use this answer key to score the practice digestive system questions in the preceding section. The answer explanations give you some insight into why the correct answer is better than the other choices.

1. **E.** For anyone with no significant family history of colon cancer, it's recommended that the person obtain a colonoscopy every 10 years, starting at age 50. A sigmoidoscopy should be done every 5 years after the age of 50, and fecal occult blood testing should be done annually. If the person has a first-degree relative who was diagnosed with colon cancer, the person should have a colonoscopy 10 years before the age at which his or her sibling was diagnosed.

2. **C.** Understanding physiology is just as important as understanding pathology. The pancreas has an endocrine and an exocrine function. The pancreas secretes bicarbonate and glucagon. It does not absorb bicarbonate or calcium, Choices (D) and (E). The absorption of calcium takes place in the small intestine. Pepsinogen, Choice (B), is secreted by the chief cells of the stomach. Cholecystokinin, Choice (A), is secreted by the duodenum.

3. **A.** The CEA is elevated in colon cancer. CA-19-9, Choice (B), is elevated in pancreatic cancer, and CA 125, Choice (C), is a tumor marker elevated in ovarian cancer. The sed rate, Choice (D), is usually elevated in an inflammatory state, so it's nonspecific. Choice (E), alpha-fetoprotein, is elevated in hepatocellular cancer.

4. **E.** Choices (A) and (B), ribavirin and interferon alpha, are used in the treatment of hepatitis C. Choice (C), steroids, is used in the treatment of autoimmune hepatitis, a condition you see predominantly in young women. Choice (D), plasmapheresis, is used to treat thrombotic thrombocytopenic purpura (TTP). Choice (E), lamivudine, has been used in the treatment of hepatitis B, although it's primarily used to treat HIV.

5. **D.** Someone with celiac disease has a sensitivity to the protein gluten. Wheat can stimulate a gluten sensitivity in a susceptible person. The antibody tests used to diagnose celiac disease are an anti-gliadin antibody test and a tissue transglutaminase antibody, Choice (D). Choice (A), carcinoembryonic antigen, is a tumor marker used to monitor potential recurrence of colon cancer. Choice (B), anticentromere antibody, is the antibody for CREST syndrome. Choice (C), HLA-B27, is associated with seronegative spondyloarthtopathies, including inflammatory bowel disease, Reiter's syndrome, and ankylosing spondylitis. Choice (E), anti-Smith antibody, is present in someone who has systemic lupus erythematosus.

6. **B.** Ganciclovir (Cytovene), Choice (B), is used in treating cytomegalovirus (CMV) esophagitis. Acyclovir, Choice (A), is used in treating herpes simplex virus (HSV) esophagitis, and fluconazole, Choice (C), is used in treating *Candida* esophagitis. Interferon alpha, Choice (D), is used in treating hepatitis C, and steroids, Choice (E), are used in treating autoimmune hepatitis.

Chapter 6

Knowing the Hard Facts about Bones and Joints

This chapter covers the myriad medical conditions that deal with the musculoskeletal system. Many of these conditions can be debilitating, whether you're talking about rheumatologic conditions (such as rheumatoid arthritis or gout), orthopedic problems (such as osteoarthritis), or hip or knee pain. Because musculoskeletal conditions affect millions of Americans, you can bet you'll see questions about them on the PANCE or PANRE.

This chapter is a unique mix of medicine, surgery, and the complex interplay between them. You read about a lot of different conditions, and you'll probably get sick of reading about antibody tests and radiologic findings for the different disorders. In this chapter, we start with the rheumatologic conditions you're likely to see on the test.

Reviewing the Rheumatologic Conditions

Make no bones about it: With rheumatology, the clinical presentations of many connective tissue diseases can overlap. A person can also be diagnosed with more than one rheumatologic condition. Your primary goal is to differentiate among similar conditions on the PANCE. This means understanding the radiologic findings of some of the medical conditions, as well as becoming familiar with certain significant antibody tests. Co-author Rich, a kidney doctor, sees many rheumatologic patients because a lot of connective tissue diseases have renal manifestations.

Reading up on rheumatoid arthritis

Rheumatoid arthritis (RA) is an autoimmune, symmetric polyarticular arthritis that can be severely debilitating — it affects similar joints on both sides of the body. Rheumatoid arthritis and osteoarthritis (OA, which we cover in the later section "Paining over osteoarthritis") are both very common causes of arthritis, although rheumatoid arthritis occurs more often in women than men. When teenagers develop rheumatoid arthritis, they're diagnosed with juvenile rheumatoid arthritis (JRA).

Explaining rheumatoid arthritis

For testing-taking purposes, you should know some of the diagnostic criteria for rheumatoid arthritis as well as the options for treatment. Diagnostic criteria include the following:

- Morning stiffness in the joints, lasting for at least an hour. The time course is important.

- The arthritis should be bilateral and symmetrical and affect more than two joints at any one time for more than 6 weeks. Examples can include the metacarpophalangeal joints (MCP) and proximal interphalangeal joints (PIP). The joints are usually swollen and tender.

  The test may ask you to differentiate between rheumatoid arthritis and osteoarthritis. Remember that rheumatoid arthritis affects the MCP and PIP but doesn't usually affect the distal interphalangeal joints (DIP).

- Positive lab tests include the anticyclic citrullinated peptide (anti-CCP), which is specific for rheumatoid arthritis. Note that rheumatoid factor, which is commonly ordered in someone suspected of having rheumatoid arthritis, can be negative more than 50 percent of the time.

- Classic radiographic findings in someone with rheumatoid arthritis show an erosive arthritis, joint space narrowing, and joint destruction, usually in hand and wrist areas.

People with *Caplan's syndrome* have both rheumatoid arthritis and pneumoconiosis (see Chapter 4 for details). In Caplan's syndrome, nodules are in the lung. Patients with rheumatoid arthritis can also have *rheumatoid nodules,* which occur under the skin. Rheumatoid nodules are another diagnostic criterion for rheumatoid arthritis. In addition, boutonniere deformities (flexion of the PIP with DIP hyperextension) as well as swan neck deformities (the complete opposite of the boutonniere deformity, with flexion of the DIP and hyperextension of the PIP) are also found in inflammatory conditions like rheumatoid arthritis.

Treating rheumatoid arthritis involves disease-modifying antirheumatic drugs (DMARDs). Start such medications early, because rheumatoid arthritis is an erosive, inflammatory arthritis that can destroy the joints. Here are the key points about medicines for rheumatoid arthritis:

- Prednisone can be given either orally or directly into the joint space. Be wary of prednisone's numerous major side effects — it has over 25 of them. Big-time side effects include osteoporosis, hyperglycemia, gastritis, psychosis, and avascular necrosis.

- Hydroxychloroquine (Plaquenil) is used in mild cases of rheumatoid arthritis. Anyone taking this med needs to have routine ophthalmologic examinations, because it can cause macular degeneration. This drug can also be used to treat mild forms of lupus.

- Methotrexate (Rheumatrex) is a very commonly prescribed medication for treating rheumatoid arthritis. It's an example of an immunosuppressive medication. Methotrexate can cause anemia and can affect liver and kidney function, so follow patients closely with complete blood count, kidney, and liver function tests.

  Methotrexate can cause folate deficiency, so a patient who's taking methotrexate needs folic acid (also known as vitamin B_9) replacement.

- A class of medications called the *biologics,* including etanercept (Enbrel) and adalimumab (Humira), are used for severe rheumatoid arthritis. Etanercept works by inhibiting tumor necrosis factor, a potent pro-inflammatory cytokine.

Still's disease: Diagnosing juvenile rheumatoid arthritis (JRA)

Juvenile rheumatoid arthritis (JRA, also known as *juvenile idiopathic arthritis,* or JIA) is the same as Still's disease. It's an autoimmune condition that can affect teenagers, with males more affected than females. A quatrad (four things) is associated with Still's disease:

✔ Joint pain and swelling

✔ Fevers

✔ Rash on the chest, abdomen, and both upper and lower extremities

✔ Uveitis

You may also see lymphadenopathy and hepatosplenomegaly on physical examination, in addition to an inflamed and generalized rash.

Labs can demonstrate a positive antinuclear antibody (ANA) and positive rheumatoid factor (RF). The rheumatoid factor may not be positive all the time, so a negative rheumatoid factor doesn't exclude a diagnosis of JRA.

Treatments for juvenile rheumatoid arthritis include steroids, methotrexate (Rheumatrex), and the other disease-modifying antirheumatic drugs. Close follow-up with an eye doctor is also recommended.

Learning about lupus

Systemic lupus erythematosus (SLE), or just plain *lupus,* is a systemic autoimmune disease that can involve multiple organs and body systems, including the joints, heart and pericardium, lungs, brain (in lupus cerebritis), and kidneys. As with rheumatoid arthritis, women are affected more than men. You need to be aware of some criteria in making the diagnosis. *Remember:* You don't need all these criteria to make the diagnosis of systemic lupus erythematosus — four or more will do:

✔ The appearance of a malar (butterfly) rash on the face or a discoid rash

✔ Photosensitivity

✔ Painful and swollen joints

✔ Photophobia

✔ Mouth ulcerations

✔ Evidence of cardiac involvement, including pericarditis; Libman-Sacks endocarditis is a common example

✔ Evidence of kidney disease, including abnormal kidney function, and/or evidence of hematuria and/or proteinuria

✔ Evidence of any neurological involvement

✔ An abnormal complete blood count, including anemia, low platelets, or a low white cell count

✔ Any abnormal antibody testing, including a positive antinuclear antibody (ANA) or low complements, such as a low C3 and C4 (the complements are low because they're consumed by an overstimulated immune system). Other serologies can include a positive anti-double-stranded DNA (anti-dsDNA) antibody and anti-Smith antibody. The anti-dsDNA is thought to correlate well with evidence of kidney involvement — it rises as the degree of kidney involvement increases.

The treatment for systemic lupus erythematosus can range from steroids and hydroxychloroquine (Plaquenil) to stronger immunosuppressive medications such as methotrexate (Rheumatrex), mycophenolate (Cellcept), and/or cyclophosphamide (Cytoxan). If you see active kidney involvement, give medications such as mycophenolate (CellCept), tacrolimus (Prograf), or cyclophosphamide (Cytoxan) in addition to high-dose prednisone.

How many types of lupus are there?

How do I afflict thee? Let me count the ways. In addition to systemic lupus erythematosus (SLE), other types of lupus include discoid lupus erythematosus (DLE) and drug-induced lupus (DIL). Discoid lupus can cause alopecia and scaly, disc-like patches on the skin.

Commonly prescribed medications, including quinidine and hydralazine (Apresoline), can cause drug-induced lupus. You can see an antihistone antibody in the case of drug-induced lupus. In the case of meds like hydralazine, experts think that if a person is a "slow acetylator," the risk of drug-induced lupus increases. *N-acetylation speed* is the rate at which the liver metabolizes the drug.

Scrutinizing scleroderma

Scleroderma, also known as *progressive systemic sclerosis* (PSS), is an autoimmune disease that affects the connective tissues. The skin is predominantly involved, although various organs, including the lungs and kidneys, can be affected as well. The skin actually becomes tight due to collagen buildup.

Scleroderma can cause pulmonary hypertension, and serial cardiac echocardiograms are often ordered to monitor pulmonary arterial pressures. Kidney function and blood pressure need to be monitored as well.

Antibodies associated with scleroderma include the anti-Scl-70 antibodies. Treatment can involve steroids and immunosuppressive medications like mycophenolate (CellCept) and methotrexate (Rheumatrex).

CREST syndrome, which has nothing to do with toothpaste, is closely related to scleroderma. *CREST syndrome* has five components: calcinosis, Raynaud's phenomenon (the digits turn white to blue to red, often in that order, in cold weather), esophageal dysmotility, sclerodactyly (a tightening of the fingers and toes rather than the whole body), and telangiectasias — that's CREST. The treatment is multidisciplinary and can involve pharmacotherapy and surgical intervention. You see Raynaud's phenomenon in many connective tissue diseases and autoimmune conditions like the ones in this chapter.

Which one of the following antibodies is associated with scleroderma?

(A) anti-Scl-70 antibody

(B) anti-SSA antibody

(C) anti-ribonucleoprotein P antibody (anti-RNP)

(D) anti-double-stranded DNA antibody

(E) anticentromere antibody

The answer is Choice (A). Anti-Scl-70 antibodies are positive for scleroderma. Anti-RNP, Choice (C), is diagnostic for mixed connective tissue disease (MCTD), which in rheumatologic terms means "a little bit of everything." MCTD encompasses many connective tissue diseases, and you confirm it with antibody testing. Choice (E) is positive for CREST syndrome, and Choice (B) is positive for Sjögren's syndrome.

We threw this question in because with antibodies and rheumatology, sometimes the questions can get funky, with all kinds of antibodies being offered as answers. For the PANCE, you should be familiar with the various rheumatologic conditions and their respective antibodies.

You're seeing a patient diagnosed with scleroderma in the office, and you notice that his blood pressure is 146/80 mmHg. What would be your next step?

(A) Start hydrochlorothiazide (Microzide).

(B) Start lisinopril (Zestril).

(C) Start amlodipine (Norvasc).

(D) Start metoprolol (Lopressor).

(E) Start terazosin (Hytrin).

The answer is Choice (B), starting lisinopril (Zestril), which is an ACE inhibitor. This patient is experiencing scleroderma renal crisis. Significant inflammatory changes occur in the small arteries of the kidney, mediated in part by the renin-angiotensin-aldosterone system. That's why the use of an ACE inhibitor is so important here: It can help save kidney function. Anyone with scleroderma should have his or her blood pressure on the lower side (SBP in the 120s or 130s). Even if the kidney function gets worse, you increase the ACE inhibitor. This is the one exception to the rule that you should stop ACE inhibitors in the setting of renal failure. The other medications aren't bad blood pressure medications, but in the setting of scleroderma, your first choice is always going to be an ACE inhibitor. Scleroderma is big payoff test topic and an important piece of clinical knowledge; you should especially be aware of scleroderma renal crisis.

If the patient had Raynaud's phenomenon instead of scleroderma, the answer to the example question would've been a calcium channel blocker, such as nifedipine (Procardia XL). Nifedipine works well in Raynaud's phenomenon because it's a vasodilator and can improve blood flow to the extremities. In addition to nifedipine, the use of topical nitroglycerin ointment or paste on the affected digits is also prescribed to treat Raynaud's phenomenon. Nitro is a potent vasodilator.

Dry eyes and mouth: Seeking out Sjögren's syndrome

Sjögren's syndrome (also known as *sicca syndrome*) is an autoimmune condition. It's characterized by dry eyes and dry mouth (sicca symptoms) or just dry mouth (xerostomia). Antibodies actually form against the salivary and lacrimal glands. Sjögren's syndrome can also affect other organs, including the kidneys — it can cause a form of renal tubular acidosis and low potassium levels. Note that Sjögren's syndrome frequently occurs with other autoimmune conditions, including rheumatoid arthritis and systemic lupus erythematosus.

Sjögren's syndrome can be diagnosed labwise by testing for anti-SSA and anti-SSB antibodies. The condition is confirmed by a biopsy, usually on the lip or parotid gland.

You can use *Schirmer's test* to test for dry eyes. A special type of filter paper is placed in each of the bottom eyelids. After several minutes, the paper is removed and the moisture content of the paper is measured.

Treating Sjögren's syndrome includes the use of artificial tears and an eye patch. Many people carry around water bottles to keep their mouths moist. Hydrating gum is available as well. Depending on the extent and severity of the disease, stronger immunosuppressive medication may be needed.

Sjögren's syndrome is not an innocuous disease; it increases the risk of developing malignancies and other lymphoproliferative diseases, such as lymphoma.

Managing monoarticular arthritis: Gout and pseudogout

Talk about pain, and nine times out of ten someone will tell you that three of the most painful things in medicine are childbirth (well, men are just guessing about this), a kidney stone, and an acute gout flare. In this section, you read about two common causes of acute monoarticular arthritis: gout and pseudogout.

Getting a grip on gout

Gout is caused by the deposition of uric acid crystals into a joint space. The most common place is the first metatarsophalangeal (MTP) joint — you can call it the hallux, the big toe, or the great toe. Whatever you call it, gout can hurt like hell. In some stories, gout is so painful that even putting a bedsheet over the affected foot causes the person to scream in pain. Depending on the severity of the gout, it can also present in the knee or other joints. Understand that gout is more than just uric acid crystals in the joint — it's a deforming arthritis.

Gout is more common in men. It's thought that either the body produces too much uric acid or the kidney isn't excreting enough uric acid. Risk factors for the developing gout include alcohol use, increased purine intake (such as from meat), and diuretics that can deplete volume. Any of these factors can cause a gout exacerbation. Recall that one of the side effects of the diuretic hydrochlorothiazide (HCTZ) is hyperuricemia.

On physical examination, if a joint has significant uric acid deposition, you can see tophi around the joint.

The diagnosis of gout (or pseudogout) is obtained by tapping the joint (*needle aspiration,* also called performing an *arthrocentesis*). As with pleural effusion (see Chapter 4), the nature of the synovial fluid tells you what you're dealing with. Tapping the joint is simple, and it provides a big payoff for the PANCE. With gout, you see needle-shaped negatively birefringent crystals. The synovial fluid may show an elevation in the white blood cell count as well.

The serum uric acid level is notoriously unreliable during an acute episode of gout — it can be high, low, or normal. The goal of treatment over time, however, is to reduce the uric acid level to less than 6.5 mg/dL and keep it there. This level minimizes the risk of future attacks.

During an acute flare of gout, treatment options include colchicine, indomethacin (Indocin), and/or steroids. Steroids can be given orally for a steroid taper or injected directly into the joint during an acute flare. Be careful using NSAIDs if the patient has underlying kidney disease.

The treatment for chronic gout is adhering to a low-purine diet and avoiding alcohol. Medications such as allopurinol (Zyloprim) and febuxostat (Uloric) work by inhibiting the formation of xanthine oxidase, an enzyme that breaks down purines.

During an acute gout attack, never give allopurinol as initial therapy. You'll only make a gout flare worse. However, if a person's already on allopurinol, don't stop it. Allopurinol doesn't relieve acute attacks of gout, but you can use it to treat chronic gout.

Detecting the faker, pseudogout

Pseudogout is also known as *calcium pyrophosphate deposition disease* (CPPD). Whereas with gout you have uric acid deposition, pseudogout involves the deposition of crystals of calcium pyrophosphate dihydrate. The initial presentation can be very similar to gout, with incredible pain and swelling in a joint.

With pseudogout, synovial fluid examination reveals positively birefringent crystals that are shaped like rhomboids. In contrast, with gout, you see negatively birefringent crystals under polarized light.

Pseudogout has a classic radiologic appearance: Because of calcium deposition into the joint, you see *chondrocalcinosis*. In English, this means that in a radiograph of someone diagnosed with pseudogout, you'd see what looks like a thick chalk line drawn along the affected joint.

The treatment for pseudogout is supportive, similar to the treatment of acute gout. Treating acute pseudogout can include NSAIDs like indomethacin (Indocin) and/or steroids (either oral or via intra-articular injection). Look for an associated condition, especially hemochromatosis or primary hyperparathyroidism.

You're evaluating a 40-year-old man who presents with a hot, swollen left knee. He doesn't have a history of gout. On exam, the knee is tender and warm to the touch. Flexion and extension is limited due to pain and swelling. The joint is tapped, and the white cell count is 100,000/μL with more than 80 percent polymorphonuclear leukocytes. There are no crystals seen on the synovial fluid analysis. What is the likely cause of the knee pain and swelling?

(A) Gout

(B) Pseudogout

(C) Rheumatoid arthritis

(D) Septic arthritis

(E) Reiter's syndrome

The answer is Choice (D), septic arthritis. *Septic arthritis* involves a significantly elevated white blood cell count with a neutrophilic predominance in the joint. It can present clinically the same as gout and pseudogout; the key is in the synovial fluid analysis. A common cause of monoarticular joint sepsis is gonococcal infection, particularly in a younger adult. Other common causes of a septic joint are *Staphylococcus aureus* and *Streptococcus* species.

Because you see no crystals in the synovial fluid, this man has neither gout nor pseudogout. Rheumatoid arthritis can present with monoarticular arthritis, but it's rare, and you should see other features of this condition for Choice (C) to be right. The synovial fluid count would not show a left shift or bandemia in rheumatoid arthritis. The PANCE has questions that make you think, but the test-makers aren't interested in asking you something totally off the wall.

Reiter's syndrome, Choice (E), is a reactive arthritis and usually demonstrates the quatrad of arthritis, conjunctivitis, urethritis, and dermatitis. Lyme disease, which we cover in Chapter 19, can also present as an acute monarticular arthritis.

The polys: Affecting the proximal muscles

With rheumatologic conditions, test questions focus on discerning one condition from another. Two conditions that sound somewhat similar are polymyositis and polymyalgia rheumatica (PMR). Although both can affect the proximal muscles and have somewhat similar presentations, there are important differences between the two conditions.

Polymyositis

Polymyositis is muscle damage caused by an overexcited immune system. The muscle damage is significant enough that you can see elevated creatine phosphokinase (CPK) levels, usually in the thousands; this condition is called *rhabdomyolysis.* The main presenting symptom of polymyositis is weakness that gets worse throughout the day.

Patients with polymyositis or any form of muscle weakness can have difficulty using their muscles when switching body positions (for example, going from a lying to sitting position or from a sitting to standing position). At its extreme, patients with any form of proximal muscle weakness may demonstrate a positive *Gower's sign*, which means using the upper extremities to shift body positions. This is not specific to polymyositis — you see Gower's sign from other causes as well.

The treatment for polymositis is immunosuppressive therapy, including steroids or other immunosuppressive medications (which we discuss earlier in the section "Reading up on rheumatoid arthritis"). Exercise is crucial for maintaining strength and flexibility.

Polymyalgia rheumatica

Polymyalgia rheumatica (PMR) is an inflammatory condition that, like polymyositis, affects the proximal muscles. Unlike polymyositis, the presenting complaint with polymyalgia rheumatica is pain and difficulty with range of motion, particularly in the shoulder area. The patient may have type B constitutional symptoms as well, including fever, chills, weight loss, and drenching night sweats.

With polymyalgia rheumatica, the lab assessment can show an elevated sed rate and elevated white cell and platelet counts. Anemia due to inflammation can be present as well.

The treatment for polymyalgia rheumatica is steroids. Serial sed rates are followed to monitor response to therapy, and the steroid dose is tapered accordingly.

The sed rate is also important when you're comparing and contrasting polymyalgia rheumatica with fibromyalgia. Both can present similarly, with similar pain patterns, but polymyalgia rheumatica has an elevated sed rate, whereas fibromyalgia doesn't.

Which one of the following medical conditions is associated with polymyalgia rheumatica?

(A) Polymyositis

(B) Fibromyalgia

(C) Systemic lupus erythematosus

(D) Temporal arteritis

(E) Rheumatoid arthritis

The answer is Choice (D). Polymyalgia rheumatica and temporal arteritis are connected. *Temporal arteritis* is associated with a headache and tenderness on the temporal artery. There can also be ocular involvement, with eye pain and change in vision. The gold standard for the diagnosis of temporal arteritis is a temporal artery biopsy, although the biopsy is at risk of a sampling error and may not pick up the exact area of inflammation.

When the eye is affected, that's an emergency, and a sed rate is ordered. If the sed rate is high, the patient is started on steroids. Isn't this similar to the treatment of polymyalgia rheumatica?

Obsessing about Three Amigos: The Osteos

Co-author Rich is an osteopathic physician, and during his training, he dealt with the bones a lot. In this section, you read about three big bone disorders, namely osteoporosis, osteoarthritis, and osteomyelitis.

Winning over bone thinning: Osteoporosis

Osteoporosis, which is a loss of bone density, occurs most commonly in women after menopause. Risk factors for developing osteoporosis include age, hormonal status (post-menopause), lifestyle (exercise and muscle resistance training decrease osteoporosis risk), and alcohol and tobacco use (both increase risk).

The gold standard for the detection of osteoporosis is the DEXA (dual energy X-ray absorptiometry) scan. The DEXA scan is scored on the basis of a T-score, which compares a patient's bone density to the peak bone density of 30-year-old women (or men, if the patient is male).

Treatment for osteoporosis involves stopping smoking and drinking, increasing calcium and vitamin D intake, and increasing physical activity, especially muscle-strengthening exercises such as weight training. Prescription medications for treating osteoporosis include the bisphosphonates, such as alendronate (Fosamax) and ibandronate (Boniva).

For PANCE purposes, be aware of possible side effects of the bisphosphonates, including jaw necrosis and esophageal irritation. Avoid giving the patient bisphosphonates if advanced kidney disease (GFR < 30 mL/min) is present. In place of these medications, you may use calcitonin (Miacalcin) nasal spray.

Anti-estrogen therapy such as raloxifene (Evista) is also prescribed for osteoporosis. Common side effects are hot flashes, leg cramps, and (rarely) blood clots in the legs, lungs, or eyes. Other reactions can include leg swelling/pain, trouble breathing, chest pain, or vision changes.

Paining over osteoarthritis

Osteoarthritis (OA) is the most common cause of degenerative arthritis in the United States. It's characterized by "bone being on bone." Think of the joint cartilage as being the buffer or padding between two articular surfaces, like the meat in a sandwich. Lose the cartilage, and you develop a bad arthritis that can involve the back, hip, knees, and other weight-bearing joints. The more the person weighs, the worse osteoarthritis can get. Osteoarthritis can be debilitating and can affect quality of life.

Rheumatoid arthritis is an inflammatory arthritis; osteoarthritis is not. Remember that rheumatoid arthritis affects the MCP (metacarpophalangeal joints) and PIP (proximal interphalangeal joints) but spares the DIP (distal interphalangeal joints). Osteoarthritis affects the PIP and the DIP. Bony overgrowths that you see on the PIP are called *Heberden's nodes,* and those that you see on the DIP are called *Bouchard's nodes.* Know your nodes.

With osteoarthritis, radiologic studies show narrowing of the joint space and formation of osteophytes.

Treatment for osteoarthritis includes weight loss and pain relief. The first-line analgesics are acetaminophen (Tylenol) and nonsteroidals such as ibuprofen (Motrin). If this doesn't work, second-line therapy can involve the non-narcotic analgesic tramadol (Ultram). This med is an opioid but not a controlled substance. Glucosamine and chondroitin sulfate as well as methylsulfonylmethane (MSM) have been used in treating osteoarthritis.

Weight can worsen osteoarthritis, so exercise, weight loss, and physical therapy are important in regaining mobility and ambulation.

Bad to the bone: Opting out of osteomyelitis

During your hospital rotations, you may have seen someone with a history of diabetes who was admitted for evaluation of a worsening foot ulcer. The million-dollar question is always "Has the infection spread to the bone?" That is, is an *osteomyelitis* present? And if an osteomyelitis is present, is it occurring acutely, or has it being going on for a while (a chronic osteomyelitis)?

The diabetic foot ulcer is a common etiology of osteomyelitis. Vascular disease (reduced blood flow) and diabetes are typically associated with osteomyelitis. An osteomyelitis can also occur in the sacrum. What starts out as a soft tissue infection (sacral decubitus) can transform into an osteomyelitis. If you're asked about possible organisms on a diabetic foot ulcer, think about *Staphylococcus aureus* among Gram-positive organisms and *Pseudomonas aeruginosa* among Gram-negatives.

Common clinical presentations of osteomyelitis include fever, rigors, and erythema and tenderness around the area. If an open wound is present, it can be weeping. Use a cotton swab on examination to see whether the wound goes down to the bone. If possible, obtain a wound culture, but note that if it's not done the right way, you may just end up with normal skin flora and a subsequent false negative result.

You may see PANCE questions about imaging studies in the diagnosis of osteomyelitis. A radiograph is positive only if you have loss of bone that's greater than 50 percent. The radiograph may be revealing in the case of a chronic osteomyelitis (ongoing for more than 4 weeks); however, it's not likely to be revealing in an acute osteomyelitis.

The MRI is the test of choice for diagnosing an osteomyelitis. The MRI is better than a bone scan, which can pick up many bony abnormalities (including osteoarthritis) but may not be specific. However, if an MRI isn't possible, the bone scan is the next best test.

Treat osteomyelitis with intravenous antibiotics. They're often given for an average of 6 weeks, although the duration can change, based on the nature of the organism. Periodically check labs that test for inflammation, including the sed rate or C-reactive protein (CRP). In clinical practice, infectious-disease healthcare providers, who are often consulted initially for help in management, follow these patients.

With osteomyelitis, anything that can be done to improve vascular flow, especially to the lower extremities, is key, especially because antimicrobial therapy doesn't work as effectively if the blood flow to the area is compromised.

You're evaluating a 50-year-old man with a history of drug use who presents with fevers and rigors. Blood cultures are positive for *Staphylococcus aureus*. You obtain a transesophageal echocardiogram (TEE), and there's no evidence of valvular vegetation. In addition to starting antibiotics, which of the following would be your next step?

(A) Repeat blood cultures.

(B) Examine the body for possible injection sites.

(C) Examine the sacrum for a possible decubitus.

(D) Check a urine culture and sensitivity.

(E) Obtain an MRI of the spine.

The answer is Choice (E). *Staphylococcus aureus* is a bad bacterium. If someone is presenting with blood cultures positive for this organism, especially with a history of drug abuse, you need to think about two body areas that can be affected: the heart and the bones.

Staph aureus can cause valvular vegetations, and in someone with a history of intravenous drug abuse, it can cause right-sided endocarditis (vegetations on the tricuspid valve). *Staph aureus* can also cause an osteomyelitis. In this question, you're looking for a possible source. The TEE is negative, so you need to check out the spine, Choice (E).

Staph aureus is a true bacterium, so never treat it as a blood contaminant, Choice (A). This patient has no risk factors for a sacral decubitus, Choice (C) — he isn't nonambulatory or bed bound. Concerning Choice (D), patients who have indwelling Foley catheters are at higher risk for urinary colonization with *Staph.* They are not treated if they're asymptomatic. In this patient without urinary symptoms, you wouldn't need to check a urinalysis or culture.

We Got Your Back: Conditions of the Spine

Back pain is one of the most common, frequent, and ordinary reasons people visit healthcare providers. Even though co-author Rich is a kidney doctor, not a day that goes by that he doesn't hear someone say, "I threw my back out." Many cases of back pain are self-limiting; however, you'll likely see some special cases on the PANCE. In this section, we cover various causes of back pain.

Analyzing ankylosing spondylitis

Ankylosing spondylitis (AS), also called a *sacroiliitis,* is a rheumatologic condition that predominantly affects young men in their late teens to early 40s. It causes significant back pain and stiffness in the low back, particularly the iliosacral region.

Here are two key points to remember about ankylosing spondylitis:

- A radiograph of the lumbar spine can show a classic *bamboo spine*: The entire spine looks like a rigid stick of bamboo, pressing on nerves and causing increasing numbness in the lower part of the body. Over time, the spinal discs fuse, and the stiffness and pain get worse.

- Labwise, ankylosing spondylitis is associated with the antigen HLA-B27. Other medical conditions associated with the HLA-B27 antigen are inflammatory bowel disease (IBD), Reiter's syndrome (also known as reactive arthritis), and psoriatic arthritis.

The course of ankylosing spondylitis can be variable. In some people, it can remit spontaneously, and in others, it can worsen. At its worst extreme, it can cause fusion of the spine.

Because ankylosing spondylitis is a rheumatologic condition, it can affect more than the lower back. Other medical complications can include pulmonary fibrosis and uveitis. In uncommon cases, ankylosing spondylitis affects the aorta as aortitis.

Treatments for ankylosing spondylitis can include anti-inflammatories and immunosuppressive medications, if needed.

Dangerous curves: Seeing scoliosis

Scoliosis (from the Greek *skolios,* meaning "crooked") refers to a lateral curving of the spine. Most of the time, no one knows why someone gets scoliosis; hence, it's sometimes called *idiopathic scoliosis.* Both Rich and Barry remember being checked for scoliosis as little kids during their school physicals.

Scoliosis can be diagnosed at a very young age, before the child has symptoms of back pain. A doctor may suspect scoliosis if the shoulders aren't symmetrical. On exam, you ask the child to bend forward. The key is determining the degree of lateral curvature. If you suspect scoliosis on physical exam, you need a radiograph to further evaluate the scoliosis and determine the degree of lateral curvature.

Symptoms over time can include back pain and just plain fatigue. Treatment depends on the degree of the curvature, or *Cobb angle.* If the curve is mild (20 degrees or less), then the child can be followed with no acute intervention. If the curve is more than 20 degrees but less than 40 degrees, then the child needs to be evaluated for a back brace. If the curvature is greater than 40 degrees, surgical intervention is needed.

Don't be a slouch: Keeping up with kyphosis

Whereas scoliosis is a lateral curvature of the spine, *kyphosis* is a type of curving that can cause permanent slouching forward. You see it most often in older adults, due to acquired problems of the vertebrae and discs, including osteoarthritis of the back and osteoporosis. If osteoporosis is present, check for compression fractures. Also ask about any traumatic events in the past or any congenital problems.

You can identify kyphosis by physical examination (the person is usually hunched forward) and radiographic imaging. Recommendations include exercises to strengthen the musculature.

Severe curvature due to kyphosis can affect breathing. Pulmonary function tests (PFTs) can show a restrictive defect secondary to the kyphosis.

Helping herniated discs

A *herniated disc* (incorrectly called a "slipped disc") can be exceedingly painful — the condition has brought the best of men and women to their knees. *Disc herniation* occurs when the nucleus pulposus pushes through a weak area in the disc. It causes pain because of nerve compression.

The lumbar area is the most common area for a disc herniation to occur. The thoracic area isn't often affected. Herniated discs can also occur in the lower cervical area, but this isn't common.

The pain from a herniated disc can be extreme, and the person may experience numbness as well. Do a thorough neurological examination, especially if you have a high suspicion that a radiculopathy is present.

You may order imaging studies, including an MRI, especially if you find evidence of a neurologic disease. Treatment for a herniated disc is supportive and can include nonsteroidals, steroids, and physical therapy. Surgery may be indicated if conservative measures don't sufficiently improve symptoms.

Be aware of neurological emergencies involving the spine. One such emergency is *cauda equina syndrome* (CES), a significant compression of the nerves in the lumbosacral area of the spinal canal. If not acted on, it can lead to permanent loss of bowel and bladder function and lower extremity paralysis.

Causes of cauda equina syndrome are many and can include a herniated disc and spinal stenosis. Other causes are spinal trauma, epidural hematoma, infection, inflammation, and malignancy. Presenting symptoms can include back pain, paresthesias, and problems with the bowel and bladder. As symptoms get worse, the affected person may lose bowel and bladder tone (the sphincter can be affected) and experience a loss of reflexes. This is a surgical emergency and requires decompression of the affected area.

Sorting out spinal stenosis

Spinal stenosis is a common cause of back pain caused by a narrowing of the lumbar spine (*stenosis* means "narrow"). This condition involves both a narrowing of the spine as well as a narrowing of the *foramen,* which is where the nerves exit the spine. The most common cause is osteoarthritis that affects the spine. Prior spinal trauma and/or herniated discs also play a role in the development of spinal stenosis.

Spinal stenosis normally presents with low back pain that's worse with ambulation. As the condition worsens, the person may experience weakness associated with any type of weight-bearing. Other symptoms can include numbness and tingling.

Imaging studies include radiography and MRI. The MRI and/or CT scan is a more detailed test, but you can detect changes of osteoarthritis on a plain back radiograph.

A common PANCE question concerns evaluating whether pain in the low back and legs is due to vascular problems (for example, claudication symptoms) or whether it's a symptom of spinal stenosis. The key is that pain due to peripheral vascular disease stops when the affected person stops moving. However, pain associated with spinal stenosis continues as long as the person is bearing weight, whether standing or walking. The pain lessens when he or she sits down. This is one reason spinal stenosis is referred to as *pseudo-claudication.*

Treatment of spinal stenosis includes physical therapy, medications, and injections to help with pain. If these don't help, then the person may need surgery. You can refer the patient to an orthopedic physician at that point.

Pott's disease: Looking at TB of the spine

Tuberculosis (see Chapter 4) can affect organs in the body outside of the lung, including the spine. Tuberculosis as it affects the spine is called *Pott's disease,* named after the British surgeon Percivall Pott. It can affect the vertebrae as well as the intervertebral space. Presenting symptoms can include back pain, fever, weakness, and paresthesias. The treatment is medications used for the treatment of tuberculosis, as well as pain medication. Surgical intervention may also be needed.

Shouldering the Pain from Fractures

Pretty much everyone knows what it's like to hurt the shoulder or upper arm. Doing much of anything can be difficult, especially if the pain or injury affects the dominant arm. In this section, you read about different derangements of the shoulder and upper arm, namely fractures.

Getting clued in on collarbone fractures

Trauma is usually the only way that a clavicular fracture can occur. Either the person suffered a direct strike against the clavicle, or more commonly, the person fell on an outstretched arm or shoulder.

The affected person presents with pain and swelling, although sometimes you don't see much swelling. On examination, you can palpate the fractured area. Make sure you perform a thorough neurovascular examination as well. A radiograph is a good imaging study for identifying clavicular fractures.

Treatment of a fractured clavicle is generally conservative, consisting of the use of a sling and pain medication. Surgery may be required in a small percentage of cases — when you see multiple fractures on radiograph, when there's evidence of neurovascular compromise, or when the fracture isn't healing as it should, despite conservative treatment.

Securing the fractured scapula

A fracture of the scapula is uncommon. This fracture is usually associated with significant trauma to the thoracic area, such as from a high-impact motor vehicle accident.

On examination, as with any trauma, look for other associated injuries, including injuries to the arm, thoracic cage, and so forth. Closely associated injuries include pneumothorax, pulmonary contusion, and fracture of the clavicle.

Radiograph imaging can show a fractured scapula, although it's sometimes missed; a CT scan provides more detailed imaging. Understand that in many trauma situations, especially a motor vehicle accident, the person is first stabilized and then goes right down to the imaging center for a CT scan to look for traumatic injuries.

The treatment for a fractured scapula is usually conservative, involving a sling and pain medication. Physical therapy reduces the risk of a frozen shoulder.

Helping the fractured humerus

Fractures of the humerus, which are usually caused by trauma to the upper arm (usually related to falls), are most common in the elderly population. Underlying medical conditions that can affect bone health, including osteoporosis and renal osteodystrophy, place people more at risk for this fracture.

As with clavicle fractures, the most common cause of a fracture of the humerus is falling on an outstretched hand. Humerus fractures can also occur in the younger population, usually because of motor vehicle accidents. Sports injuries and auto accidents account for most humeral injuries in younger men.

A fracture can affect three areas of the humerus: the proximal humerus, the distal humerus, and the middle of the humerus (a mid-shaft fracture). On presentation, the person complains of pain in the affected area. He or she also usually has decreased range of motion. With a mid-shaft fracture, the person can complain of numbness of the dorsal aspect of the hand, which indicates damage to the radial nerve.

Most of the time, humerus fractures are treated conservatively without surgical intervention. Many times, the affected person is sent home with an arm sling or arm brace. If the radial nerve is significantly affected (a nerve palsy), then surgery may be indicated.

Forewarned, Forearmed: Advancing to the Elbow and Wrist

For the PANCE, you'd do well to remember the names and components of specific injuries and orthopedic conditions related to the elbow, forearm, and wrist. This is especially true of fractures.

Tennis, golfer's, and Little League elbow: Evaluating epicondylar injury

Epicondylar is a fancy way of saying, "let's look at the elbow for a second." The *epicondyles* are two bony areas found at the distal humerus; they are the medial epicondyle and the lateral epicondyle. Both can be inflamed, usually secondary to repetition or overuse. Here are some types of epicondylar injury:

✔ **Lateral epicondylitis (tennis elbow):** Lateral epicondylitis is an inflammation of the tendons at the lateral epicondyle. Specifically, it's an inflammation of the extensor carpi radialis brevis.

✔ **Medial epicondylitis (golfer's elbow):** Medial epicondylitis (ME) is an inflammation of the tendons that attach to the medial epicondyle. Golfer's elbow can also involve the ulnar nerve and lead to complaints of neuropathy affecting the middle and last two digits.

✔ **Medial epicondylar apophysitis (Little League elbow):** If children throw overhand, they can experience a valgus stress on the elbow joint. The repetitive motion can damage the structures of the elbow, resulting in an avulsion of the medial epicondylar apophysis (growth plate).

Presenting complaints for epicondylar injury can include pain over the affected area. Wrist extension can make the pain with lateral epicondylitis worse, and wrist flexion can make the pain with medial epicondylitis worse.

The treatments for both lateral and medial epicondylitis include stopping the underlying activity, a brief trial of nonsteroidals, alternating heat/ice treatments, and physical therapy. If someone fails to get better with conservative measures, surgery is an option, but it's rarely needed.

Elbowing nursemaids: A lift by the wrist

In children, a common elbow problem that you may be tested on is *nursemaid's elbow,* sometimes called *babysitter's elbow.* It occurs in the child, not the nursemaid. It can happen when someone grabs or pulls up the child by his or her wrist, causing slippage of the annular ligament.

On exam, the distal radius can be tender, and rotating the forearm can be difficult. The treatment is a closed reduction. In order to reduce the joint, the elbow has to be extended in combination with a pronated forearm.

Bettering bursitis

Recall that a *bursa* is a pocket filled with synovial fluid. Its job is to act as a kind of padding around the joints. In the elbow, the olecranon bursa can get inflamed, leading to *olecranon bursitis* (*student's elbow* or *baker's elbow*).

Normally, you shouldn't be able to feel a bursa. But when a bursa is inflamed, it's enlarged and erythematous. Most of the time, the treatment for bursitis is conservative, including anti-inflammatory medication and rest. The fluid doesn't need to be drained unless you suspect that an infection is present.

Noting numbing of the nerves of the forearm

Neuropathy is a problem that affects many people. The most common cause is diabetes — you may recall that diabetic neuropathy has a stocking-glove distribution. We cover many causes of peripheral neuropathy in Chapter 16, but for the purposes of this chapter, we focus on ulnar neuropathy and carpal tunnel syndrome.

Ulnar neuropathy

Recall that the *ulnar nerve,* which is the largest unprotected nerve in the human body, travels down the forearm to the medial aspect of the hand. The most common cause of ulnar neuropathy is nerve entrapment, such as from injury to the medial epicondyle. Other causes include connective tissue disease, diabetes, trauma, and tobacco use.

The most common presenting symptom of ulnar neuropathy is paresthesias involving the fourth and fifth digits. The person may also complain of elbow pain or a weak grip. Treatment can be nonsurgical or surgical. Indications for surgery include worsening weakness and muscle atrophy. Physical and occupational therapy, as well as conservative treatment, is recommended.

Carpal tunnel syndrome

Carpal tunnel syndrome (CTS) is an inflammation of the median nerve. Common presenting symptoms include paresthesias — weakness involving the thumb, first digit, and half of the second digit. Common causes of carpel tunnel syndrome include overuse and repetitive motion (such as typing at a keyboard incessantly, as Rich and Barry are doing), pregnancy, hypothyroidism, diabetes mellitis, sarcoidosis, and other connective tissue diseases.

Be aware of two physical exam signs concerning the diagnosis of carpal tunnel syndrome:

- ✔ **Phalen's sign:** Phalen's sign refers to holding the dorsal aspect of both hands together in flexion for 1 minute. If the person experiences pain or paresthesias with this maneuver, carpal tunnel syndrome may be present.

- ✔ **Tinel's sign:** Tinel's sign is tapping the wrist over the medial nerve, which you can do with a reflex hammer. Resulting pain and paresthesias suggest carpal tunnel syndrome.

The treatment of carpal tunnel syndrome can be conservative. It includes rest, anti-inflammatories, the use of wrist splints, and/or steroid injections. If these measures fail, consider surgery.

In any type of neuropathy, look for atrophy of the muscles innervated by that particular nerve. With regard to carpal tunnel syndrome, look for atrophy of the thenar eminence — that can be an indication for surgery.

Which of the following is associated with the development of carpal tunnel syndrome?

(A) Golfing

(B) Rheumatoid arthritis

(C) Hypertension

(D) Diabetes insipidus

(E) Hyperthyroidism

The answer is Choice (B), rheumatoid arthritis. Golfing, Choice (A), is associated with the development of medial epicondylitis. Hypertension, Choice (C), isn't associated with carpal tunnel syndrome. Diabetes mellitus and hypothyroidism are associated with the development of carpel tunnel syndrome, but diabetes insipidus and hyperthyroidism, Choices (D) and (E), are not.

Breaking a fall . . . and a wrist

Colles' fracture is a fracture of the distal radius, usually due to falling on an outstretched hand. Risk factors include underlying bone disease, including osteoporosis and renal osteo-dystrophy. (The kidney can be blamed for practically anything!)

Colles' fracture is diagnosed by a radiograph. The radius is shortened and angulated dorsally. The treatment depends on the degree of displacement. Options for mild displacement include casting and closed reduction. For more serious angulation and displacement, open reduction internal fixation (ORIF) may be necessary.

With a fracture of the distal radius, the ulna is usually involved.

Thumbing through Hand Injuries

In this section, we cover four conditions affecting the hand and wrist. They range from benign cysts to minor sprains to out-and-out fractures.

Going ganglionic: Ganglion cysts

A common soft tissue mass that you can see on the hands and wrists is a *ganglion cyst,* also known as a *bible cyst.* Like a lipoma, it's painless and moves about freely. This condition isn't malignant. Aspiration of the cyst fluid is a possible treatment. Note that these cysts tend to recur and that surgical intervention may be necessary.

De Quervain's tenosynovitis: Teasing tendons at the base of the thumb

Your arms contain many tendons, but you probably need to worry about only two, particularly if they get inflamed just before the PANCE. *De Quervain's tenosynovitis* is an inflammation of the two tendons around the bottom of the thumb. An initial irritation of the tendons then causes the synovium to become inflamed and edematous; hence, the term *tenosynovitis.*

Many of the causes mimic those of carpal tunnel syndrome and can include repetitive activity/overuse, pregnancy, and rheumatologic conditions like rheumatoid arthritis. Also, de Quervain's tenosynovitis is more common in older women.

Common presenting symptoms of de Quervain's tenosynovitis include pain over the thumb and wrist. The person may also experience swelling and restriction of movement.

Finkelstein's sign is linked to de Quervain's tenosynovitis. For this sign, the person essentially makes a fist, placing the thumb across the palmar aspect of the hand and then wrapping the fingers around the thumb. He or she then ulnarly deviates the fist downward, causing the wrist/thumb to be more in extension. If this maneuver causes pain around the thumb area, the person may have tenosynovitis.

The treatment for tenosynovitis can be conservative, including immobilization of the affected area and anti-inflammatories and pain medication. Steroid injections into the affected area have been used, with modest relief of the condition. Surgical intervention is warranted when conservative measures fail.

Thumbs up: Pointing out sprains and tears of the UCL

People can injure one of the ligaments of the thumb, namely the ulnar collateral ligament (UCL). A sprain of this ligament is called *skier's thumb*. (Such a sprain can also affect your ability to properly hitchhike.) What causes this sprain? Falling on an outstretched hand.

Usual presentation of skier's thumb includes pain and tenderness around the thumb's meta-carpophalangeal (MCP) joint. The patient can also have difficulty pinching things.

The treatment depends on whether you're dealing with a sprain or with a UCL tear. If a sprain is present, splinting and immobilization is recommended; if there's a tear, surgery may be needed.

Boxer's fracture: Giving metacarpels the old two-three

If you see a fist come flying at you, we recommend ducking — you'll be helping the person throwing the punch reduce his or her risk of fracturing a metacarpal. A *boxer's fracture* is a fracture of the second or third metacarpal, commonly seen among fighters and professional boxers. Besides having redness and swelling around the site of injury, the person may have trouble clenching and extending the affected digits.

A *bar room fracture* is a transverse fracture of the fourth or fifth metacarpal neck. That's what happens when an unskilled fighter throws a punch down at the honky-tonk.

Fractured metacarpals are diagnosed through a radiograph of the hand. The immediate treatment includes ice, rest, and the use of an ulnar gutter cast or support splint. Severe angulation generally requires surgery to put in a pin. The long-term treatment also involves directed hand strengthening exercises — and not hitting solid objects with the fists. Anger management may be needed.

Getting Hip to the Jive

Several hip-related conditions make regular appearances on the PANCE. In this section, you read about avascular necrosis, hip fractures, and the slipped capital epiphysis. In addition, we include a section on hip dislocation.

Asking about avascular necrosis (AVN)

When a person has a lack of blood supply to the head of the femur over a period of time, *avascular necrosis* (AVN) can result. Basically, *avascular* means "no blood." Something inhibits the blood supply to the head of the femur, which is bad because bones need blood. Ischemic changes lead to necrosis, and the necrosed head actually collapses.

The initial presentation of avascular necrosis is often groin pain, but you may also see pain in the knee, hip, or gluteal region. The pain is worse with walking or standing and is better with sitting. On exam, trying to elevate the leg while the affected person is lying down can cause a lot of pain.

One of the most recognized causes of avascular necrosis is long-term steroid use. Other medical conditions that have been linked to avascular necrosis include connective tissue disease, vasculitis, long-term ethanol use, and trauma.

Because avascular necrosis can affect both hips, both hips should be imaged, even if the pain affects only one side. Initial radiographs may be nondiagnostic, so the gold standard for diagnosing avascular necrosis is the MRI.

The treatment for avascular necrosis is comprehensive and usually involves the use of a cane or walker to reduce the degree of weight bearing. A range of surgical options is available, one being removal of the necrotic areas.

Which one of the following conditions is not associated with the development of avascular necrosis?

(A) Steroids

(B) Trauma

(C) Sickle-cell anemia

(D) Alcohol use

(E) Emphysema

The answer is Choice (E), emphysema. All the other choices — steroids, trauma, sickle-cell anemia, and alcohol use — are associated with the risk of avascular necrosis. You may be thinking to yourself, wouldn't someone with emphysema be on steroids? Although he or she can be, emphysema in and of itself hasn't been associated with the development of avascular necrosis. Don't read too much into the question.

Reviewing the slipped capital femoral epiphysis

In *slipped capital femoral epiphysis* (SCFE, or skiffy), the femoral head slips inferiorly through a weakened area in the *physis,* or growth plate. This condition primarily affects children and teenagers, more males than females. The clinical presentation can be similar to avascular necrosis: groin pain, knee pain, and/or hip pain. As with avascular necrosis, standing or walking can make the pain worse.

Determine the degree of slippage using radiography. You need radiographs of the pelvis and hips taken with an anterior-posterior view as well as a frog-lateral radiograph. Any displacement of 50 percent or greater is categorized as severe.

The treatment of SCFE is usually surgical, with physical therapy and not bearing weight on the affected leg and hip as long as necessary.

Determining the cause of the SCFE may require a medical workup. Consider an endocrine disorder, looking mainly at pituitary abnormalities and bone disorders such as osteomalacia. Bone disease secondary to kidney dysfunction is also in the differential diagnosis.

There's a small risk of SCFE developing into avascular necrosis (see the preceding section for details).

Helping hip fractures and dislocations

A hip fracture is something that healthcare professionals see in many elderly people admitted to the hospital after a fall. Elderly people may have bone-health problems such as osteoporosis, vitamin D deficiency, malignancy (usually metastatic to the bone), and/or renal osteodystrophy. Osteodystrophy increases the risk of a fracture.

If you examine someone who fell and fractured the neck of the femur, you see that the affected leg looks shorter than the opposite leg. The affected leg is also externally rotated. Order radiographs of the femur and pelvis to look for the severity and type of fracture.

Hip fracture is a generalized term, referring to fractures that can affect either the femur or trochanter. For test purposes, you need to know two types of hip fractures:

- ✔ **Femoral neck fractures:** These fractures are usually treated surgically. Because a femoral neck fracture can affect the blood supply to the head of the femur, the person has a risk of developing avascular necrosis. (See the earlier section "Asking about avascular necrosis [AVN].")

- ✔ **Intertrochanteric fractures:** These fractures, which occur between the greater and lesser trochanters, usually occur below the femoral neck. The majority of the time, they're treated surgically and have a good chance of healing well.

A hip fracture commonly involves the femoral neck, whereas a *dislocation* involves the head of the femur. With a dislocation, you see displacement of the femur's head from the acetabulum. The dislocation may be posterior (the most common type) or anterior. The most common cause of a hip dislocation is high-impact trauma, such as in a motor vehicle accident.

The hip is shortened in both a hip fracture and a dislocation. But unlike the femur neck fracture, where the leg is externally rotated, a dislocated hip is internally rotated. Imaging for a hip fracture includes radiographs of the hips and pelvis. If no fracture is present, then the hip simply needs to be reduced. This reduction often occurs in the emergency room, without surgery (a closed reduction). If the hip can't be reduced in the ER, then the patient may need to be taken to the OR for an open reduction.

Mending a Wounded Knee

Clinically, many health professionals see problems with knees in the older population. One of the most common causes is osteoarthritis. The more weight that a person is carrying, the more pain the person can feel and the more difficult walking can be.

Remember that many of the rheumatologic conditions, such as gout and rheumatoid arthritis, can affect the knee. We discuss those conditions earlier in "Reviewing the Rheumatologic Conditions." In this section, you read about some orthopedic conditions as they affect the knee.

Remember that high-yield PANCE questions often include identifying maneuvers that you can do on physical exam to delineate the type of injury. A good example maneuver is the McMurray test for a meniscal tear in the knee.

Observing Osgood-Schlatter syndrome

Osgood-Schlatter syndrome, which predominantly affects adolescent males, is an irritation of the patellar tendon at the tibial tubercle, or *tibial tuberosity.* Recall that the patella attaches the quadriceps to the tibial tubercle. Repeated stress causes small fractures along the patella tendon. In addition to chronic inflammation, this syndrome can cause changes in the tibial tubercle, including edema, pain, and increased bone growth.

Any type of strenuous activity can precipitate pain. The diagnosis of Osgood-Schlatter syndrome is made on physical examination. Radiograph findings can be variable.

The treatment is usually supportive, and it includes RICE (rest, ice, compression, and elevation). Stretching is key, especially for the quadriceps and hamstring muscles.

 On a test, you may be asked to differentiate Osgood-Schlatter syndrome from a closely related condition, *chondromalacia patella* (CMP). Although Osgood-Schlatter refers to pain at the tibial tubercle, chondromalacia is pain under the knee. It's actually irritation of the cartilage under the patella. The treatment again is conservative, including rest and temporarily refraining from strenuous physical activity.

Mulling over meniscal tears

The *menisci* are cartilaginous components that act to provide support for the knee during any type of valgus or varus stress. In the knee, you have both lateral and medial menisci. Tears to the medial menisci are more common.

You often hear about meniscal tears in the knees of professional athletes, especially basketball and football players. Think about the various medial and lateral stresses placed on the knee during a game, and you can easily see why these tears occur.

The affected person may say he or she feels pain on the affected side of the knee (that is, the lateral aspect of the knee if there's a lateral meniscus tear). As with most knee injuries, you see swelling and edema and pain on palpation. The patient also has trouble bearing weight on the affected side.

 For the PANCE, make the connection between meniscal tears and *McMurray's test.* In this maneuver, the knee is first flexed; with the opposite hand, a force is directed to stress the knee either medially or laterally. If you hear a clicking sound on the affected side when you begin to extend the leg, the test is positive. Pain can also be induced on the affected side.

The diagnosis of a meniscal tear is confirmed by an MRI. The treatment involves rest, refraining from strenuous physical activity, anti-inflammatory meds, and pain meds. Depending on the degree of meniscal tear, the patient may need arthroscopic surgery.

Considering cruciate tears

Ligaments in the knee include the anterior cruciate ligament (ACL) and posterior cruciate ligament (PCL). In addition, you have the medial collateral ligament and lateral collateral ligament.

ACL tears

Although you often hear about injuries related to an ACL tear in professional male athletes, ACL tears are actually more prevalent in women. The ACL tear is associated with a tear in the medial menisci, because both tears are caused by a twisting or sharp rotation of the knee. (See the preceding section for details on meniscal tears.)

As with meniscal tears, the person with an ACL tear reports having felt a pop before he or she went down. The pain can be excruciating, and bearing weight can be impossible.

 ACL tears can result in significant bleeding. You should be familiar with the *Lachman test* for diagnosing ACL tears. The leg is put in flexion at a 30 to 40 degree angle, with the leg externally rotated. You pull forward on the tibia, and if the ACL is intact, the ligament should hinder the forward movement of the tibia on the femur.

An MRI is needed to evaluate the ACL. The treatment can range from nonsurgical to surgical, depending on the person's age and the stability of the ligament. Conservative treatment consists of rest, temporarily refraining from strenuous physical activity, and taking anti-inflammatory meds and pain meds.

There's a triad of knee injuries that orthopedic providers don't like to see. Called everything from the "terrible triad" to the unhappy triad to "O'Donoghue's," this triad consists of an ACL tear, a medial meniscus tear, and injury (usually a significant tear) to the medial collateral ligament. In review studies done in the early 1990s, it was — fortunately — not found to be extremely common.

PCL tears

Tears to the posterior cruciate ligament (PCL) are a lot less common than tears to the ACL because the PCL is a heck of a lot stronger and can withstand a lot more punishment. Its main function is to keep the tibia and femur in line. Injuries to the PCL can occur when an anterior force is directed to a hyperextended knee or a posterior force is directed to a knee in the flexed position.

With mild injuries, range of motion is preserved, and there may not be a lot of swelling over the joint. The posterior drawer test can aid in the diagnosis of a PCL tear, and the diagnosis is confirmed by an MRI. Treatment includes intense physical therapy and rehabilitation.

Collateral ligament tears

Concerning the collateral ligaments, the medial collateral ligament (MCL) is the most commonly injured knee ligament. On physical examination, you test for possible injury to the MCL with a valgus stress test.

With an MCL tear, other ligaments, such as the ACL and the medial menisci, can be injured as well. Look for these other injuries, too.

Radiographs may be initially obtained to rule out a fracture of the nearby anatomy, especially the femur. The diagnosis is confirmed with an MRI. The treatment consists of rehabilitation for mild tears; note that if the ACL and/or medial menisci have been injured as well, then surgical intervention is needed.

Lateral collateral ligament tears are extremely uncommon. They're caused by an extreme varus stress on the knee. An MRI is the confirmatory test of choice. Mild tears are usually treated conservatively.

Which of the following is used to diagnose an anterior cruciate ligament (ACL) tear?

(A) Phalen's maneuver

(B) Lachman test

(C) McMurray's test

(D) Barlow's maneuver

(E) Ortolani's maneuver

The answer is Choice (B), the Lachman test. Note that an anterior drawer test that can also be used to assess for an ACL tear; however, this test isn't as sensitive or specific as the Lachman test. Phalen's maneuver is used in diagnosing carpal tunnel syndrome. McMurray's test is used in diagnosing meniscus tears. Choices (D) and (E) are used to test for congenital hip dislocations, not ACL tears.

Assessing Ankle Injuries

Injuries to the ankle are a common reason why people go to the emergency room. Many of these injuries are sports injuries or secondary to sports-related injuries. In this section, we look at typical problems that affect the ankle.

Studying the soft tissues of the ankle

The most common ankle injury is the ankle sprain. Sometimes you may see a diagnosis, especially in the ER, of an "ankle sprain and strain," but strains and sprains differ:

- ✔ **Strain:** In general, a *strain* is an injury to a muscle or tendon, usually caused by pulling or pushing or twisting the wrong way.

- ✔ **Sprain:** An ankle *sprain* refers to an injury that affects the ligaments. During an athletic competition or outdoor activity that involves running and jumping, the person lands on his or her ankle the wrong way, causing abnormal stretching and/or possibly a ligamentous tear, usually in the lateral ligaments. In the most common type of ankle injury, the ankle inverts — that is, the bottom of the foot turns inward, injuring the anterior talofibular ligament.

A radiograph is often ordered to evaluate an ankle injury for a possible fracture. However, the *Ottawa ankle rules,* which help clinicians determine whether a radiograph is needed, were designed to reduce unnecessary radiographs and to cut down on patient waiting time, especially in the ER. In short, you order a radiograph if the affected person

- ✔ Can't bear weight on the ankle immediately after the injury (or at the time of examination by a medical professional)

- ✔ Has bone tenderness in one of the following places:

    - Along the distal 6 cm of the posterior edge of the tibia or tip of the medial malleolus

    - Along the distal 6 cm of the posterior edge of the fibula or tip of the lateral malleolus

    - At the base of the fifth metatarsal

    - At the navicular bone

Just to make life even more difficult, there are three grades of ankle sprains — Grades 1, 2, and 3. The grading depends on the severity of the sprain (mild, moderate, or severe). Thus, Grade 1 is a mild sprain, and Grade 3 is a severe sprain. The more severe the sprain, the more rehabilitation the patient needs and the more time to recover. Most of the time, the treatment is temporarily not bearing weight on the ankle, applying intermittent ice and heat, and elevating the leg. An ankle splint and/or brace may be prescribed.

Testing Achilles

The Achilles tendon is vital because it connects the calf muscle to the heel. This tendon is important for walking, for activities like running and jumping, and for standing up on your tippy-toes. Achilles tendon injuries include strain and rupture. One of the most common patients to suffer with tendon injury is the *weekend warrior,* someone who's sedentary during the week and decides to go wild with athletics on the weekend. In addition to the lack of physical conditioning, failure to warm up, stretch properly, and wear proper footwear all play an important role in Achilles tendon injuries. The most common mechanisms of injury include sudden forced plantar flexion of the foot, unexpected dorsiflexion of the foot, and violent dorsiflexion of a plantar flexed foot.

Clinically, the most common presentation is the affected person's yelling "Ow!" and pointing to his or her calf area. The calf area right above the insertion site to the heel is tender. The MRI is the diagnostic test of choice. Treatment is conservative and consists of anti-inflammatories, pain medication, and rehabilitation. Surgery may be required for full-thickness tears.

The class of antibiotics called the fluoroquinolones has been reported to increase risk of tendon rupture. The Achilles tendon remains the most common site of quinolone-induced rupture.

Examining ankle fractures

Take an ankle and push, pull, rotate, invert, or evert it in any one significant direction, and you can fracture it. Most of the time, ankle fractures occur with ligamentous tears.

Presenting symptoms of an ankle fracture can include ecchymosis over the area of injury and an inability to bear weight. The ankle can be cold to palpation. The ankle can't be moved at all or can't be moved without significant pain (see the Ottawa ankle rules in the earlier section "Studying the soft tissues of the ankle").

Radiographs need to be done pronto. If the patient has a fracture, initial treatment can involve splinting and/or casting. The key is to avoid weight-bearing (by using crutches) and to keep the area as stable as possible. Some ankle fractures require immediate surgery.

Figuring Out the Foot

You should know about several medical conditions affecting the feet. Why? Because your feet are your friends — they get you where you need to go — and you should care about your friends. In addition, some of these conditions may pop up on the PANCE.

Studying the soft tissues of the foot

Sprains and strains of the foot are common, especially among athletes. For example, football players can sprain the first metatarsophalangeal (MTP) joint, a condition commonly known as "turf toe." Recall that the first MTP joint is the one most usually affected by gout.

You see chronic sprain and strains in the foot more often in the older population. Different grades of sprains affect the foot.

Ottawa rules for the foot state that a radiograph should be obtained in the following circumstances:

- ✔ The affected person feels pain in the middle of the foot and can't bear weight on the foot immediately after an injury (or at the time of examination by a medical professional).

- ✔ The affected person has tenderness either at the fifth metatarsal (the most lateral bone of the foot) or at the navicular bone (the most medial).

Stressing over stress fractures

Stress fractures are common causes of injury, especially for runners and people in sports like tennis and basketball. What do these sports have in common? A lot of running back and forth; sudden starts, stops, and pivots; and a lot of force and trauma to the foot and ankle with each step. Just having the foot strike the ground is a contributor. Playing on a hard surface doesn't help much, either.

Continued repetition and overuse, plus or minus bad footwear, contribute to the development of stress fractures. The most common location for stress fractures is the metatarsals, predominantly the second and third metatarsal. Other places can include the calcaneus and the navicular bones.

You need to order radiographs to evaluate the severity of a stress fracture in the foot. Depending on where the fracture is, the treatment can involve stabilization (immobilization) or surgery to reduce the fracture.

The bottom of the foot: Finessing fascia

A common medical problem affecting the bottom of the foot is *plantar fasciitis*. The affected person feels pain along the bottom of the foot, especially with the first few steps after long periods of rest, such as early in the morning. Common reasons for the inflammation include poor footwear (co-author Barry found out the hard way), flat feet, high arches, intense exercise (think of the marathoner), and obesity. Plantar fasciitis is more common in men than women. The patient usually has a point of maximal tenderness at the anteromedial region of the calcaneus.

The treatment for plantar fasciitis can involve losing weight, getting arch supports or better footwear, and taking anti-inflammatories and pain medication. Gentle massage to the area can help as well.

Practice Questions about Bones and Joints

These practice questions are similar to the ones you'll see on the PANCE about bones and joints.

1. Which of the following muscles is not part of the rotator cuff?

   (A) Supraspinatus

   (B) Infraspinatus

   (C) Subscapularis

   (D) Teres minor

   (E) Teres major

2. You're evaluating a 40-year-old woman who has a history of worsening morning stiffness and swelling of the fingers and hands. No facial rash is present. Which of the following labs is most specific for diagnosing this rheumatologic condition?

   (A) Erthryocyte sedimentation rate (ESR)

   (B) Rheumatoid factor

   (C) Anticitrullinate cyclic peptide

   (D) Antinuclear antibody (ANA)

   (E) Antiribonucleoprotein P (anti-RNP)

3. A radiograph showing chondrocalcinosis would be suggestive of which of the following conditions?

    (A) Gout

    (B) Pseudogout

    (C) Rheumatoid arthritis

    (D) Septic arthritis

    (E) Osteoarthritis

4. Which of the following medications is approved for the treatment of pain associated with fibromyalgia syndrome (FMS)?

    (A) Lyrica (Pregabalin)

    (B) Prednisone (Sterapred)

    (C) Carisoprodol (Soma)

    (D) Cyclobenzaprine (Flexeril)

    (E) Oxycodone (OxyContin)

5. Boxer's fracture is caused by an injury to which area of the hand or wrist?

    (A) First metacarpal

    (B) Scaphoid bone

    (C) Third metatarsal

    (D) Third metacarpal

    (E) Navicular bone

6. Which of the following is a potential side effect of colchicine?

    (A) Constipation

    (B) Edema

    (C) Leukopenia

    (D) Leukocytosis

    (E) Hyponatremia

Answers and Explanations

Use this answer key to score the practice questions about bones and joints from the preceding section. The answer explanations offer some insight into why the correct answer is better than the other choices.

1. **E.** The supraspinatus, infraspinatus, subscapularis, and teres minor are the four muscles of the rotator cuff. Whereas the teres minor externally rotates the humerus, the teres major, which is not part of the rotator cuff, internally rotates the humerus.

2. **C.** Anticitrullinate cyclic peptide (anti-CCP) antibodies are specific and sensitive to rheumatoid arthritis. The erthryocyte sedimentation rate (ESR) can be elevated in many conditions, including infection and inflammation. The rheumatoid factor is positive only 50 percent of the time in someone with rheumatoid arthritis. The antinuclear antibody (ANA) test can be positive in many autoimmune conditions, including systemic lupus erythematosus (SLE). Anti-RNP (antiribonucleoprotein) is specific for mixed connective tissue disease. The clinical presentation marks this condition as rheumatoid arthritis.

3. **B.** Pseudogout is characterized by a "chalk line" on a radiograph. Osteoarthritis causes more joint destruction, and the classic radiograph appearance for rheumatoid arthritis is joint space narrowing and erosive arthritis.

4. **A.** The FDA approved lyrica (Pregabalin) for the treatment of pain in fibromyalgia syndrome (FMS). The other listed meds aren't indicated in the treatment for fibromyalgia.

5. **D.** Injury to the third metacarpel is the classic finding in a boxer's fracture.

6. **C.** Colchicine can cause myopathy, diarrhea, and leukopenia. Its dose needs to be adjusted in the setting of kidney disease. It doesn't cause leukocytosis, which is one of the side effects of steroids like prednisone, nor does it cause hyponatremia, constipation, or edema.

Part III
Reviewing Surgical Topics and Other Organ Systems

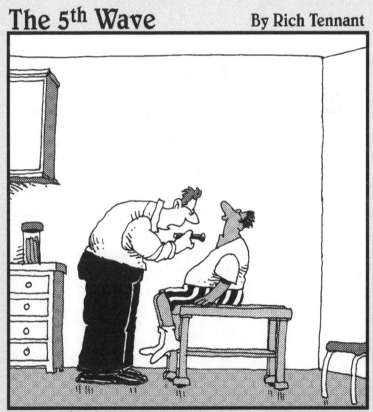

The 5th Wave   By Rich Tennant

"I see what's blocking your airway. Apparently, someone said something at some point that just stuck in your craw."

In this part . . .

*P*art III has four high-yield chapters about topics that you can't avoid on the test. It begins with Chapter 7 (surgical) and goes on to detailed discussions of eye, ear, nose, and throat conditions (Chapter 8), reproductive medicine (Chapter 9), and the genitourinary system (Chapter 10).

Chapter 7

Checking Out Common Surgical Topics

· ·

In This Chapter

▶ Reviewing surgical signs and symptoms

▶ Evaluating the patient pre-op and post-op

▶ Getting on with the gallbladder

▶ Investigating common intestinal surgeries

· ·

*W*hen you're preparing for recertification by taking the PANRE, you have the opportunity to select an exam that's focused on surgery. Sixty percent of the test is still general in nature, but the other 40 percent focuses on surgery. As for the PANCE, many of the topics concerning the gastrointestinal system appear on both the medicine and surgical portions of the examination, because you see significant overlap with certain conditions.

To do well on the PANCE or PANRE, you need a good sense of broad-based surgical concepts, not encyclopedic knowledge about a specific topic. One vital area is the surgical signs and symptoms that you'd focus on when performing a history and physical (H&P). You need to know the essentials of a thorough pre-operative assessment (including pre-operative risk) and how to care for the post-operative patient.

In this chapter, you read about the fundamental aspects of general surgery, including fluid management. Given the breadth that surgery encompasses, we review further surgical evaluation and management in the anatomic chapters. For example, you find info about the gastrointestinal tract in Chapter 5 and orthopedics in Chapter 6.

Reviewing Surgical Signs and Symptoms

Doing a thorough history and physical (H&P) is important. Any medical professional should be able to pick up more than 90 percent of the information needed to diagnose the underlying medical condition from the H&P. The key is asking the patient the right historical questions and paying close attention to detail on the physical examination.

For testing-taking purposes, understand the clinical scenario presented and pay attention to the clues in the questions. In clinical practice, pay attention to the H&P. Sometimes the symptoms presented and your physical examination can point you in a totally different direction than you first thought.

Asking the right questions about symptoms

Whether you work in the surgical arena or have been through a surgical rotation, you know the importance of asking the right questions. A common reason for a surgical consultation, especially in the emergency room, is to evaluate abdominal pain. The basic question is whether the person needs to go to the operating room (OR) immediately or should simply be kept under close observation.

When you're asking questions about the etiology of pain, remembering the alphabet can help you, especially the letters O, P, Q, R, S, and T:

- ✔ **O — onset:** Did the pain begin suddenly or gradually?

- ✔ **P — provocation or palliation:** For example, can the person pinpoint what may have caused the pain in the first place? In the case of a hernia, was the person lifting something heavy and/or employing improper lifting techniques? Does anything make the pain better (lessen it) or worse (increase it)? With some forms of abdominal pain, especially a duodenal ulcer, the affected person may say that eating makes the pain better.

- ✔ **Q — quality:** Is the pain cramping (as with gastroenteritis), sharp (diverticulitis, peritonitis, or perforation), crushing (myocardial infarction), or ripping (aortic dissection)? Is the pain dull, or does it burn (dysuria and urgency secondary to a urinary tract infection)?

- ✔ **R — region or radiation:** Where is the pain located? Does the pain stay in one spot, or does it travel somewhere else? Pancreatitis, for example, often radiates to the back. Symptoms of _cholecystitis_ (inflammation of the gallbladder) can include radiation to the right shoulder.

- ✔ **S — severity, usually on a scale of 1 to 10:** If someone is bent over double in pain, some badness is going on. A pain scale allows the affected person to give an assessment of his or her own pain. Remember that _pain_ is subjective; _tenderness_ is a finding obtained on physical examination.

- ✔ **T — time:** When did the pain begin? Is the pain constant or intermittent? What was the person doing when the pain began?

Focusing on the patient's medical history

Past medical problems that you're presented with in a clinical scenario are important. Knowing whether hypertension, diabetes, or coronary artery disease is present provides insight into pre-operative risk as well as into the etiology of the person's pain. For example, if someone has a history of coronary artery disease, carotid disease, or peripheral vascular disease and is presenting with intermittent abdominal pain after a meal, you may think about mesenteric angina or mesenteric ischemia. If the person has a history of multiple surgeries, especially abdominal surgeries, and is presenting with nausea/vomiting, you may suspect that adhesions (scarring) from prior bowel surgeries may be causing a bowel obstruction. And if the person fell or was involved in a motor vehicle accident and is complaining of pain pointing to the left side of the abdomen, you may be dealing with a splenic injury.

Knowing the patient's medication regimen is crucial. Before surgery, you need to know if a person is on a blood thinner, such as aspirin, clopidogrel (Plavix), or warfarin (Coumadin). With warfarin, for example, you may need to reverse the prothrombin time/INR with fresh frozen plasma (FFP) prior to taking the patient to the OR. If the person has a metal valve replacement, you need to know how soon you can restart anticoagulation after surgery. Pay attention to all medications a person is taking, both prescription and nonprescription.

Social and family history is important as well. A person who smokes may have diminished lung function or peripheral circulation present. If a person drinks and has drunk alcohol recently, that can interfere with anesthesia. If cirrhosis is present, you may see a clotting problem. You need to know if a patient has a family history of a bleeding diathesis or a clotting problem.

Performing the physical exam

Test-makers can and will transform many physical exam signs into great test questions, especially in the field of general surgery. Many test questions about a physical examination give you a sense of the person's hemodynamic stability. For example, are his or her vital signs okay? If the person has abdominal pain, has a barely palpable blood pressure, and is tachycardic, then the person is in shock and likely needs to go to the OR emergently. If the vitals are stable and if you see no red flags on physical examination, then maybe the patient simply requires close observation.

What are some of the red flags on examination? The biggest is one that says a surgical emergency may be present — that is, an acute abdominal emergency. This means evidence of peritonitis or perforation. If on examination you see evidence of rebound tenderness, then that's a surgical emergency, too. It suggests that a perforation may be spilling intestinal contents into the peritoneal space, causing *peritonitis.* A laundry list of conditions can cause an abdominal perforation, including intestinal malignancy, inflammatory bowel disease (IBD), acute appendicitis, and peptic ulcer disease (PUD), to name a few (we cover abdominal conditions in detail in Chapter 5).

In the emergency room, you're evaluating a 74-year-old woman who presented with abdominal pain. She states it began abruptly and radiates to her back. On physical examination, she is moaning and in pain. Blood pressure in the right arm is 160/90 mmHg, whereas blood pressure in the left arm is 82/60 mmHg. You notice decreased pulses in the lower extremities. Which one of the following is your next immediate step in management?

(A) Admit to the ICU for observation.

(B) Obtain a stat CT scan of the thorax and abdomen with IV contrast.

(C) Call a general surgeon for consultation.

(D) Perform an ultrasound of the left upper extremity.

(E) Perform an ECG stat.

The correct answer is Choice (B). This patient most likely has an aortic dissection, so she needs a CT scan of the abdomen and pelvis with intravenous contrast to determine whether an aortic dissection is present. The question contains important clues — sudden onset of pain with radiation to the back, differential blood pressure measurements in the upper extremities, and decreased pulses in the lower extremities. None of the other answers make sense.

Evaluating the Pre-Op Patient

Suppose the surgical team has assessed the patient, and you decide that the patient needs to go to the operating room. This may be an emergent situation or an elective surgery, such as an elective laparoscopic cholecystectomy. Well, in addition to the H&P you've already done, you need to order some baseline labs and also assess how risky it is to take this patient to the OR. In other words, will the patient likely survive the surgery?

Looking at the labs

If the patient was initially seen in the emergency room, he or she may have already drawn most of the labs you need. The PANCE/PANRE may ask you which additional labs you need to confirm or deny a particular diagnosis. For example, if someone has abdominal pain radiating to the back, you may need to order an amylase and/or lipase in order to confirm that pancreatitis is present. You get the idea.

Here are some labs you may encounter on the test:

- **Complete blood count (CBC):** The CBC is a common lab test — don't leave home without it. An elevated white blood cell count can indicate either a stress response or an infection. If you see a left shift or bandemia, then an infection is likely present. Significantly elevated hemoglobin/hematocrit levels may mean significant volume depletion, especially in the setting of an individual who has recurrent nausea/vomiting and poor oral intake. Anemia can point you in the direction of a chronic bleeding problem from the GI tract or a developing hematoma somewhere (if a trauma or fall occurred). Remember that the platelet count can be high in infections, inflammation, and iron deficiency, all of which can happen in a surgical patient (or someone with a GI bleed).

- **Chemistry panel:** A chemistry panel is extremely useful. If the person has been experiencing N/V/D (nausea/vomiting/diarrhea), then knowing the serum sodium and potassium is important; the potassium may be low. If the person has a history of diabetes, you need to know the blood glucose level as well as the kidney function. Make sure you know the kidney function of anyone who's going to undergo some type of imaging study that uses intravenous dye.

- **Levels:** If the person is on a medication that requires some type of therapeutic monitoring, such as warfarin (Coumadin), theophylline (Theo-Dur), lithium (Eskalith), and/or digoxin (Lanoxin), then levels may need to be drawn. Volume depletion and kidney disease can really affect lithium and digoxin levels. Any type of bowel process has the potential to dramatically affect the INR. If the person has an active GI bleed, the blood urea nitrogen (BUN) level can be really elevated as compared to the creatinine level. It's generally recommended you obtain baseline coagulation studies (PT/INR and PTT) prior to any surgery.

- **Liver function tests (LFTs):** Whether you obtain liver function tests (LFTs) should depend on the history as well as the clinical presentation. If someone presents with right upper-quadrant (RUQ) pain, then obtaining LFTs is essential. If the person has icterus on examination, obtaining LFTs is important. If the surgery isn't related to the abdomen and the person has no history of liver disease or any significant past medical history, LFTs aren't likely needed.

Which of the following can elevate the blood urea nitrogen (BUN) levels?

(A) Saline administration

(B) Bleeding due to diverticulosis

(C) Malnutrition

(D) Penicillin

(E) Bleeding due to a duodenal ulcer

The correct answer is Choice (E), bleeding due to a duodenal ulcer. Saline administration would lower the BUN levels, because volume depletion can be a cause of an elevated BUN. A lower GI bleed would not cause an elevation in the BUN, so Choice (B) is wrong. An upper GI bleed, especially a slow upper GI bleed, would. Malnutrition, Choice (C), would cause someone to have a low BUN level due to the low protein stores in the body. Tetracycline, not penicillin, increases BUN levels, so Choice (D) is incorrect.

Assessing the perioperative risk

Be able to stratify your surgical patient's risk of morbidity and mortality. The H&P is vital in identifying risk factors. Significant risk factors include coronary artery disease, diabetes, kidney disease, and active/ongoing cardiac issues. These include a recent myocardial infarction or history of congestive heart failure or valvular problems (examples being significant aortic stenosis or mitral regurgitation).

If a person has significant cardiac risk, the patient may need further testing and clearance from the cardiologist before being allowed to proceed with surgery. We discuss cardiovascular conditions in Chapter 3.

Of course, the type of surgery is also important in determining the surgical risk. For example, the guidelines from the American College of Cardiology (ACC) stratify risk based on cardiac versus noncardiac surgery. Another important criterion often cited is the Goldman criteria for surgery, which evaluate cardiac risk in patients for noncardiac surgery.

Caring for the Post-Op Patient

When the patient gets out of the OR, your first consideration is ensuring that the patient is hemodynamically stable. Pay attention to the vital signs. If the blood pressure is low, then he or she needs volume resuscitation to ensure adequate tissue perfusion. Pressors may or may not be needed. Sometimes you need to monitor the patient closely, and a central venous pressure (CVP) monitor or a Swan-Ganz catheter may be necessary.

Over the next several days, the goal is to get the patient eating, sitting up, and walking as soon as possible (as long as it's safe to do so). Complications can occur post-operatively. In particular, maintaining adequate deep venous thrombosis (DVT) prophylaxis is important for as long as the patient isn't walking around.

In this section, we cover post-operative fever, DVT risk, and the basics of fluids and nutrition management.

Monitoring for fever

A high-yield surgical topic on the PANCE/PANRE is the etiology of fever in the patient post surgery. Not all fever is related to infection. Common causes of fever in the post-surgical patient can include atelectasis as well as DVT, which we cover in the next section — yet another reason DVT prophylaxis is so important! Using the incentive spirometer frequently after surgery prevents atelectasis.

The timing of the fever is important in determining the etiology:

- **1 to 2 days after surgery:** Atelectasis is a very common cause of fever the first day or two after surgery.

- **3 days after surgery:** If the fever persists after 3 days, then examine the surgical sites for any wounds that may be infected. Does the person have a decubitus ulcer (pressure ulcer or bedsore)? Look at the sacral area to make sure a sacral decubitus isn't present. Also look at the urinary tract as a possible source of the fever, and make sure you're not dealing with a DVT. If you have a high clinical suspicion of a DVT, you may need to order a Doppler ultrasound of the lower extremities.

✔ **More than 3 days after surgery:** If the fever persists for more than 3 days, then you need to dig even deeper. Look at the medications the person is on. Do you see a rash or peripheral eosinophilia? Sometimes these can be signs that the fever is due to a medication. If nothing turns up there, again look at the surgical site. You may need to order imaging studies such as a CT scan, or the patient may need to go back to the OR.

Remember the five *w*'s of the causes of the post-operative fever: wind (think of the air in the lungs or atelectasis), water (urinary tract infection), wound (surgical infection), walking (or lack thereof — the DVT), and wonder drugs (drug or medication fever).

Reducing the clot risk

Most surgical patients are going to be flat on their backs for at least 24 hours after surgery, depending on the procedure. It may take several days before they're sitting in a chair, let alone walking around. You need to make sure your patient doesn't get blood clots. Be aggressive in reducing the risk of a deep venous thrombosis (DVT) in your patient.

Different surgeries have different types of DVT risk. Orthopedic procedures such as hip or knee surgery have a very high risk. The risk also increases with

✔ The person's age (the older the person, the higher the risk)

✔ The seriousness of the surgery

✔ History of a clotting disorder

✔ History of cancer

For more information about DVT prophylaxis, see Chapter 6.

In general, for any hospital patient, unfractionated heparin 5,000 units is usually administered subcutaneously every 8 hours as a standard of care to prevent a DVT from forming. Other medications for DVT prophylaxis include enoxaparin (Lovenox) and fondaparinux (Arixtra). Remember that enoxaparin needs to be dose-adjusted in kidney disease, and if the kidney disease is severe, fondaparinux can't be used.

Understanding fluids and nutrition

Knowing the principles of managing fluids and nutrition is important not only for test-taking purposes but also for taking care of patients. We begin with a brief review of fluid management for the post-op patient.

If the blood pressure is low, then 0.9 percent saline (also known as *isotonic* or *normal* saline) is usually the first fluid you administer to the patient. It fills the vascular space and can help restore blood pressure but doesn't provide any free water content.

If after a few days of normal saline you obtain blood work and notice a rising sodium level, switch the saline to a more hypotonic fluid to give more free water, especially if the patient is still NPO (nothing by mouth) or has a nasogastric tube and is being suctioned. If the patient can't drink water, you need to provide it intravenously. Examples of more hypotonic solutions include 0.45 percent saline and D5W. Think of the 0.45 percent saline as a hybrid bag, providing half sodium and half free water. D5W is a very dilute solution providing only free water (with 5 percent dextrose as well). Think of it as the equivalent of water you'd drink from the tap.

Surgeons love using *lactated Ringer's solution,* or LR. It's a very comprehensive IV fluid, containing potassium, calcium, and lactate. It's also a little more dilute than normal saline but more concentrated than 0.45 percent saline. However, if the patient has kidney problems or a high potassium level to begin with, you may not want to use this fluid.

Nutrition is especially important in the post-operative period. Many patients don't eat well prior to coming to the hospital, especially if they have abdominal complaints. If the patient is unable to take nutrition PO, then your options are to either administer tube feedings or to provide intravenous nutrition (TPN/total parenteral nutrition). Here are two key points about providing nutrition:

- Remember the law of the gut: If you have it, use it.

- Patients after surgery are catabolic and have greater caloric needs and protein requirements. When you prescribe TPN, make sure you're meeting that person's caloric needs and providing the optimal number of calories from protein, calories, and lipids. Without nutrition, the patient won't be able to heal properly.

You are on the surgical service and are evaluating a 55-year-old man in the ICU admitted with acute upper gastrointestinal bleeding. On admission, his vitals are the following: blood pressure 82/40 mmHg, heart rate 120 bpm. The monitor shows sinus tachycardia. You're waiting for blood to be brought up from the blood bank. Given the above vital signs, which of the following would you do next?

(A) Administer a beta blocker for the tachycardia.

(B) Give a fluid bolus with normal saline.

(C) Administer D5W to provide for free water needs.

(D) Give 0.45 percent saline at 70 mL/hr with no bolus.

(E) Give intravenous dextran.

The correct answer is Choice (B). This patient is in hypovolemic shock. You need to give isotonic (normal) saline to fill the vascular space. You wouldn't give a beta blocker because the tachycardia is compensatory for the acute blood loss. If the patient were hypernatremic, then you'd administer D5W, but it has no role in volume repletion. Intravenous dextran isn't used much, if at all; if anything, it can increase bleeding risk. The 0.45 percent saline, although it provides some volume, isn't aggressive enough for volume resuscitation for a patient in hypovolemic shock.

Getting on with the Gallbladder

Gallbladder surgery is one of the most common types of surgery medical professionals are exposed to during their training. In this section, you review common indications for surgery: gallbladder inflammation and gallstones.

Hot and bothered: Gallbladder inflammation

Anyone who has experienced gallbladder pain knows it can be debilitating. We commiserate! Presenting symptoms can include abdominal pain with eating. Recall that the risk factors for gallbladder inflammation are the five *f*'s: female, fat, fertile, fair, and forty. Classic gallbladder pain often radiates to the right upper quadrant (RUQ), although midepigastric pain can be present. Pain can also radiate to the right shoulder.

On physical examination, in addition to midepigastric tenderness, you may find tenderness to palpation in the right upper quadrant. Specifically, a positive Murphy's sign indicates that cholecystitis may be present.

Various laboratory and imaging studies can be helpful in diagnosing cholecystitis. On a CBC, a leukocytosis may be present, with or without an accompanying left shift. You may also see elevation in the hepatic function tests, particularly the alkaline phosphatase and bilirubin levels. Amylase can be elevated but is relatively nonspecific.

Ultrasonography is the imaging study of choice for further evaluating right upper-quadrant pain. Common findings can include gallbladder dilatation, thickening of the gallbladder wall, gallbladder sludge, and/or pericholecystic fluid. A CT scan with contrast may be ordered, but it's less sensitive to issues concerning the right upper quadrant.

You can order a hepatobiliary iminodiacetic acid (HIDA) scan to see how well the gallbladder is functioning. Just as an echocardiogram can show the ejection fraction of the heart, the HIDA scan can show the ejection fraction of the gallbladder. If other imaging studies of the gallbladder are normal and you want to find out how well the gallbladder is working, this scan is the one to order.

When the patient is admitted to the hospital, he or she is initially made NPO, with intravenous fluids and antibiotics being administered.

Surgeons previously used an open surgical approach to treat the inflamed gallbladder, but because of laparoscopic techniques, the number of post-operative days patients spend in the hospital has decreased.

Stoned: Gallbladder stones

Gallstones are a common cause of cholecystitis, but they can also cause nonspecific pain, such as biliary colic. Gallstones actually come in two types:

- ✔ **Cholesterol stones:** Cholesterol stones are the most common kind. They contain a lot of cholesterol and a little bit of calcium.
- ✔ **Pigment stones:** You can find pigment stones in states of chronic hemolysis, including sickle-cell disease.

Gallstones can be present and completely asymptomatic, in which case the treatment is watching and reducing risk factors that contribute to their formation. The treatment includes diet modification, specifically avoiding fatty foods, and minimizing the use of medications that increase the risk of gallstones, including hormonal therapy that's estrogen-based. One medication that's been used to try to reduce the risk of gallstones is ursodeoxycholic acid (ursodiol).

A life-threatening complication of gallstones is gallstone pancreatitis, the management of which we talk about in Chapter 5.

Investigating Common Intestinal Surgeries

Every medical professional should know about some common abdominal surgeries. In this section, you review evaluating and managing appendicitis, diverticulitis, hernias, volvulus, and spleen problems. In Chapter 5, we cover hemorrhoids, which can be a pain in the you-know-what.

Apprehending the inflamed appendix

For test-taking purposes, you need to know a lot about evaluating and managing acute appendicitis. Acute appendicitis is a common cause of emergent surgery, especially in the younger population. It typically causes pain in the right lower quadrant (RLQ). Inflammation of this organ, either via obstruction from lymph glands or fecalomas (fecaliths) can be life-threatening if not recognized. Perforation and/or abscess formation are serious complications of acute appendicitis.

For testing-taking purposes, you should recognize the typical clinical presentation: pain that begins in the mid-abdomen and migrates into the right lower quadrant. Fever, nausea, vomiting, and anorexia are usually also present.

On physical examination, the affected person can be toxic-looking and febrile. Pertinent physical examination findings include tenderness along *McBurney's point*. This point is on the right side of the abdomen, one-third the distance from the anterior superior iliac spine (ASIS) to the umbilical area.

Other common clinical signs of acute appendicitis include the following:

- ✓ **Rovsing's sign:** Rovsing's sign occurs when left lower-quadrant (LLQ) palpation causes right lower-quadrant tenderness.

- ✓ **Psoas sign:** Psoas sign relates how flexion or extension of the hip causes right lower-quadrant pain. Appendicitis can, in certain people, cause an inflammation of the psoas muscle. If the affected person is supine, flexion of the right hip causes rip-roaring right lower-quadrant pain. If the person is lying on his or her left side (in left lateral recumbent position), then extension of the right hip can elicit pain.

- ✓ **Obturator sign:** In obturator sign, rotating the hip internally and externally elicits pain.

- ✓ **Blumberg's sign:** In Blumberg's sign, slow compression and rapid release over a specific site of the abdomen elicits pain. It's a sign of peritonitis.

Dieulafoy's triad deals with an acute appendicitis and consists of abdominal tenderness, skin hypersensitivity, and contraction of the muscle at Mcburney's point. We cover Dieulafoy's triad in Chapter 22.

Abnormal lab findings for a person with acute appendicitis can include a leukocytosis on a CBC, and you may see abnormal electrolytes, depending on how significant the nausea, vomiting, and anorexia are. Imaging studies can include an ultrasound or CT scan of the abdomen. However, the key to recognizing acute appendicitis is in the history and the findings on physical examination.

An inflamed appendix is often approached surgically, using laparoscopic technique. Preoperatively, intravenous fluids and antibiotics can be started.

Dealing with diverticulitis

Many people, especially older adults, have *diverticulosis,* an outpouching in the wall of the large intestine. If Rich had a nickel for the number of times he's seen diverticulosis on a CT scan of the abdomen ordered for a completely different reason, he'd have a lot of nickels. *Diverticulitis,* or inflammation of this outpouching, is a common cause of left lower-quadrant (LLQ) pain.

A significant risk factor for the development of diverticulitis is the American diet, which is deficient in fiber and high in processed and refined foods. The most common clinical presentation is intense left lower-quadrant pain associated with fever. Constipation and/or diarrhea may be present. On physical examination, you find left lower-quadrant tenderness, and peritoneal signs may be present.

A CT scan with oral contrast is often done to evaluate for possible abscess or fistula.

Because of the increased risk of perforation, a colonoscopy should never be performed during an acute attack of diverticulitis.

The affected person is admitted to the hospital, made NPO, and given intravenous hydration, antibiotics, and pain medication. After the first attack, a change in diet is recommended, including an increase in fiber content.

On a test, you may be asked for antibiotic choices concerning the treatment of diverticulitis. A combined approach is metronidazole (Flagyl) and a fluoroquinolone, such as ciprofloxacin (Cipro).

One episode of diverticulitis is not enough to warrant surgical intervention unless an abscess or fistula is present. The expression "the third time's the charm" rings especially true for diverticulitis: If someone has a third attack, he or she may require colonic surgery.

Intestinal twists: Straightening out volvulus

Volvulus is the intestine's version of Twister: The intestine literally twists on itself. The most common area for volvulus to occur is the sigmoid colon, although it can occur in other areas as well, including the cecum.

Depending on where the volvulus is, the typical presentation is sudden onset of abdominal pain. Physical examination reveals decreased or absent bowel sounds, focal tenderness, and even peritoneal signs. A volvulus needs be recognized and treated immediately; an intestine that remains twisted is at risk for decreasing its own blood supply, which can lead to a necrotic, gangrenous bowel — not a good thing.

Radiographic signs are important in identifying a volvulus. On a plain radiograph, you can see distended sections of large bowel, especially if a sigmoid volvulus is present.

In most cases, decompressive surgery/therapy is needed. A rectal tube may be used to decompress the affected area of intestine.

Helping people with hernias

Hernias are a common surgical problem. If the abdominal wall is weak enough, sometimes a tear or open area becomes large enough for some part of the intestine to slide into places it doesn't belong. Surgical intervention is needed to treat any hernia.

One of the most common types of hernia is the inguinal hernia. Such hernias can be either indirect or direct:

- **Indirect:** An indirect hernia, which is the more common type, refers to a failure of the inguinal ring to close during development. This hernia occurs when the intestine and/or other abdominal contents travel through the deep inguinal ring into the inguinal canal.

- **Direct:** With the direct hernia, the intestine travels through a weakened area in the inguinal triangle. Direct hernias don't commonly go into the scrotal area.

If you can remember going to the doctor and being instructed to "turn your head and cough" (and Barry remembers this from his Boy Scout camp physical every summer), the doctor was checking whether a hernia was present.

Femoral hernias, which are more common in women, can cause a bulging in the mid-thigh area as the intestine pushes its way through an opening in the femoral canal. On physical examination, the inguinal ligament is medial to the femoral hernia protrusion.

On examination, check whether the hernia is reducible. If the intestinal contents are not able to go into their original position, this is a surgical emergency. The intestine is at risk of strangulation and ischemia.

Removing the spleen

The spleen is an integral part of the lymph system, and of course maintaining a healthy immune system is important. When the spleen is no longer working, you're at risk for infection with encapsulated organisms (see Chapter 18 for details).

Why remove this organ? The most common reason is trauma — the spleen is often injured in motor vehicle accidents. Splenic trauma is a surgical emergency. Other causes include various hematologic malignancies, such as lymphoma, polycythemia vera and other myeloproliferative states, hereditary spherocytosis, and other spherocytosis.

Common labs that are monitored pre- and post-surgery are the blood counts as well as the coagulopathy profile. Imaging procedures can include obtaining a CT scan, especially in the case of trauma.

Practice Questions on Surgical Topics

These practice questions are similar to the PANCE/PANRE surgical questions.

1. You're preparing a patient to go into surgery for emergent cholecystectomy. The patient presented with a fever of 38.9°C (102°F) and acute right upper-quadrant pain. Ultrasound demonstrates ductal dilatation, thickening of the gallbladder wall, and pericholecystic fluid. The patient is made NPO and started on intravenous fluids. Which antibiotic would be appropriate to administer?

   (A) Vancomycin (Vancocin)

   (B) Gentamicin (Garamycin)

   (C) Metronidazole (Flagyl)

   (D) Ampicillin-sulbactam (Unasyn)

   (E) Azithromycin (Zithromax)

2. Which one of the following statements concerning deep venous thrombosis prophylaxis is true?

   (A) Intravenous heparin administered every 8 hours is acceptable for deep venous thrombosis prophylaxis.

   (B) Hip surgery for repair of a fracture would be considered a moderate risk for the development of deep venous thrombosis.

   (C) The dose of fondaparinux (Arixtra) must be reduced if kidney disease is present.

   (D) A full-strength aspirin can be used solely for deep venous thrombosis prophylaxis.

   (E) The efficacy of fondaparinux (Arixtra) can be followed by measuring partial thromboplastin time (PTT) levels.

3. You're evaluating a 65-year-old woman who presents with fever and acute lower left-quadrant pain. She states that it began last night and won't let up. She says that it began in the back and radiates to the lower left-quadrant area. She denies nausea, vomiting, or diarrhea. She has no history of diverticulosis. Her temperature is 38.9°C (102°F). There is lower left-quadrant tenderness and left costovertebral tenderness. She admits to dysuria and urinary frequency. The urinalysis is pending. What is the most likely diagnosis?

    (A) Diverticulitis

    (B) Volvulus

    (C) Ovarian torsion

    (D) Pyelonephritis

    (E) Ulcerative proctitis

4. Which medical condition is associated with Grey-Turner's sign?

    (A) Acute appendicitis

    (B) Ulcerative colitis

    (C) Emphysematous pyelonephritis

    (D) Hemorrhagic pancreatitis

    (E) Acute cholecystitis

5. An older gentleman with a history of alcoholism and chronic pancreatitis presents with pain radiating to the back. He states the pain is much worse than before. He has a mild fever. His white blood cell count is normal, but you note that his hemoglobin level is 8.5 mg/dL. You look at the lab values in his medical record and note that it was 10.5 on a prior hospitalization. Lab values, including liver function tests, amylase, and lipase, are normal. What is your next step?

    (A) Send the gentleman home because the lipase is normal.

    (B) Obtain a CT scan with intravenous contrast if able.

    (C) Obtain an outpatient gastrointestinal consultation.

    (D) Obtain an abdominal ultrasound.

    (E) Repeat the labs because there may be a mistake.

6. Which of the following conditions causes left lower-quadrant pain?

    (A) Acute appendicitis

    (B) Meckel's diverticulum

    (C) Volvulus

    (D) Diverticulitis

    (E) Regional enteritis

Answers and Explanations

Use this answer key to score the practice surgical questions from the preceding section. The answer explanations provide insight into why the correct answer is better than the other choices.

1. **D.** Ampicillin-sulbactam (Unasyn) is a good choice for intra-abdominal surgeries because it has good Gram-positive, Gram-negative, and anaerobic coverage. The flora of the biliary tract are predominantly Gram-negative and anaerobic. Vancomycin (Vancocin) covers Gram-positive organisms, and gentamicin (Garamycin) is predominantly Gram-negative. Metronidazole (Flagyl) is anaerobic in its coverage. Azithromycin (Zithromax) is not indicated to treat biliary infections. It's used in treating community-acquired pneumonia (CAP).

2. **C.** Fondaparinux (Arixtra) is administered in a standard dose of 2.5 mg per day. The dose needs to be adjusted for kidney disease, usually requiring a decrease in dosing. A heparin infusion, Choice (A), is usually given for the treatment of a documented pulmonary embolism or deep venous thrombosis. It wouldn't be used for DVT prophylaxis; subcutaneous dosing of 5,000 units every 8 hours is the recommended regimen for DVT prophylaxis. Hip surgery, Choice (B), or any orthopedic surgery below the waist is considered to be high-risk, not moderate-risk, for deep venous thrombosis. Note that full-strength aspirin, Choice (D), can't be used for DVT prophylaxis; it's prescribed for the prevention and treatment of coronary artery disease (CAD). Concerning Choice (E), factor Xa levels, not a partial thromboplastin time (PTT), are measured in patients taking fondaparinux (Atrixa). This lab value is measured in anyone receiving intravenous heparin.

3. **D.** Part of being on a surgical rotation is the evaluation and identification of abdominal pain. The pattern of the pain is important here. Pyelonephritis, Choice (D), usually presents with back pain. The patient may have had a kidney stone that passed, but she has positive costovertebral tenderness on examination and urinary symptoms, too. And in the question, you're told that she has no history of diverticulosis. In the end, this isn't a surgical case at all, but her presentation may look surgical, and you should know the differential.

4. **D.** *Grey-Turner's sign,* which is ecchymoses and bruising located in the flank areas, is a sign of hemorrhagic pancreatitis. Cholecystitis, Choice (E), is associated with Murphy's sign. Appendicitis, Choice (A), is associated with Rovsing's sign, psoas sign, obturator sign, and Blumberg's sign.

5. **B.** Even if you weren't sure of the answer, this question includes enough red flags to signal you to order the CT scan: the patient's report that the pain has worsened and the decrease in hemoglobin. The reasons to obtain a CT scan in this case are several: The gentleman may have hemorrhagic pancreatitis, he may have some abdominal trauma (he may be too drunk to remember), or he may have a pseudocyst.

   You may be asking yourself, "Isn't his lipase level normal?" In chronic pancreatitis, the lipase levels may not rise like they do in acute pancreatitis. An ultrasound isn't likely to show you much. This gentleman needs a CT scan.

6. **D.** Diverticulitis commonly presents as left-sided abdominal pain. All the other choices — acute appendicitis, Meckel's diverticulum, volvulus, and regional enteritis — present as right-sided pain. Meckel's diverticulum is a cause of right lower-quadrant pain in a young child.

Chapter 8

Exploring Problems of the Eyes, Ears, Nose, and Throat

. . . .

In This Chapter

▶ Picking on nose conditions

▶ Being down in the mouth (and throat)

▶ Considering ear conditions

▶ Watching for eye problems

. . . .

This chapter is all about getting in your face — the eyes, ears, nose, and throat. Unfortunately, many, many medical conditions can affect the face. From sinusitis to orbital cellulitis, there's a plethora of disorders, and any one of them can surface on the PANCE/PANRE. We begin this chapter with a prominent topic, the nose.

Knowing Facts about the Nose

Your nose isn't on your face just to hold piercings and keep your eyes apart. This protuberance is a vital component of the respiratory mechanism, and it houses cells that are part of the olfactory system. A variety of conditions can affect the nose. In this section, you read about sinus problems, nasal polyps, allergic rhinitis, bleeding disorders, and foreign bodies.

Airing your grievances: Sinus problems

The sinuses are spaces in the head, and they're filled with air. *Sinusitis* is an inflammation of the sinuses. It's a common reason people go to see the primary care provider. The pain of a sinus headache can be debilitating.

Be aware of the anatomy. Each person has four major sinus cavities in the osteomeatal complex: frontal, maxillary, ethmoid, and sphenoid. The osteomeatal complex (OMC) is the area where all the sinuses except the sphenoidal sinus drain. (The sphenoidal sinus drains into the sphenoethmoidal recess.) Note that the osteomeatal complex is important for ventilation as well.

Just like bronchitis, sinusitis comes in acute and chronic forms:

✔ **Acute sinusitis:** Although acute sinusitis can be either bacterial or viral, many cases are viral in nature. If the PANCE asks about common bacterial causes of acute sinusitis, think of the big three, which are also causes of otitis media (an inflammation of the middle part of the ear — see the later section "Ear inflammation: Observing otitis of all types"). Those bacterial creatures are *Haemophilus influenzae*, *Moraxella catarrhalis*, and *Streptococcus pneumoniae*.

Some of the most common presentations of acute sinusitis involve the maxillary sinus. This condition can present with acute tooth pain. Common clinical presentations of acute sinusitis can also include facial pain, fever, sinus congestion, Eustachian tube dysfunction, and/or a leaky nose.

✓ **Chronic sinusitis:** Sinusitis is chronic if the symptoms have persisted for more than 12 weeks. In the common clinical scenario, the person still has sinus congestion, facial pain, and rhinorrhea (runny nose) despite rounds of antibiotics. He or she isn't getting better. This is where you start looking for anatomic problems. Obtaining a CT scan isn't unreasonable, because you want to look at the osteomeatal complex. The use of multiple antibiotics may change the flora in the sinuses and increase the risk of fungal overgrowth, although this idea is somewhat debatable.

If symptoms persist, you may need to consult an ear, nose, and throat (ENT) specialist for further investigation. Causes of chronic sinusitis can include nasal polyps, anatomic issues (a deviated nasal septum), a blocked osteomeatal complex, allergy, and trauma to the nasal area. Sometimes sinus surgery may be recommended.

One consequence of recurrent sinus infections or chronic sinusitis is dysfunction of the Eustachian tube. When this happens, a patient may have decreased hearing as well as pressure in the ears. Everyone knows the feeling of opening his or her mouth wide, hoping the ears will pop, in the setting of a cold, sinus infection, upper respiratory infection, or change in altitude.

Acute and chronic sinusitis may be accompanied by a thick nasal discharge, which is usually green in color and may contain pus (indicating a purulent infection) or blood.

What is *snot?* Don't laugh! Someone's going to ask this question in clinical practice. Snot is another term for *nasal mucus.* When foreign particles (dust, sand, pollen, smoke, fungi, and germs) are trapped in the nose hairs, they're surrounded by mucus. Note to PAs working in pediatrics: You can tell your young patients that boogers are dried mucus and bad foreign stuff. When a person gets a cold, more mucus forms and the nose gets stuffed up.

Sometimes on the PANCE, questions about treating a medical condition differ from what you may have seen on your clinical rotations. This can be true for sinusitis. The first-line treatment recommended for an acute bacterial sinusitis is amoxicillin (Amoxil). This is fine for a test question, but clinically, you may see a lot of resistance to this antibiotic. Other reasonable first-line treatments include the addition of clavulanic acid to the amoxicillin (Augmentin) or the use of a macrolide antibiotic like azithromycin (Zithromax). If you're asked on the test for a second-line treatment for otitis media, sinusitis, or acute bacterial pharyngitis, think erythromycin (Robimycin). And we think it's pretty likely that you'll see this type of question in one form or another.

Nosing around nasal polyps: Mucosa gone wild

In someone who has recurrent sinusitis or chronic sinusitis, you need to make sure that the person doesn't have nasal polyps. *Nasal polyps* are actually just the nasal mucosa gone wild, forming polyps. In addition to sinus symptoms and recurrent sinus infections, other symptoms can include headaches and a loss of smell.

For test purposes, when you think about nasal polyps, also think about *Samter's triad* — a combination of nasal polyps, asthma, and aspirin sensitivity. In this case, the patient, usually a young adult, presents with sinus-type symptoms that don't go away. Asthma symptoms aren't far behind. You need to have a high clinical suspicion, but if you have an asthmatic patient and look up the schnoz with a schnozoscope and see polyps, you need only add aspirin sensitivity to have the triad.

Be aware of other conditions that can increase the risk of nasal polyp formation. One big example is cystic fibrosis, which you read about in Chapter 4.

Although the treatment of nasal polyps can include steroids, it usually involves consulting an ENT about surgical removal.

Assessing allergic rhinitis

Allergies can be a real pain. Sneezing, watering eyes, and rhinorrhea, especially during certain seasons of the year, affect some people big time. Usually, there's a trigger. An allergen such as ragweed, pollen, mold, or dust may bring on these symptoms. Sometimes people complain of *anosmia.* (They don't smell bad; they smell *badly.*)

In addition to trying to identify the potential allergen based on history, you can order allergy tests. Testing can include allergy skin testing or blood tests called RAST (immunoassay) testing. You may order an immunoglobulin E (IgE) level to assess the "allergy level" of the body.

The first-line treatment for allergic rhinitis is an intranasal steroid to relieve inflammation and swelling. An example of this is fluticasone propionate (Flonase). Antihistamines, such as loratadine (Claritin) and cetirizine (Zyrtec), can also be used. ***Caution:*** Many older antihistamines can be sedating.

Be aware that allergic rhinitis sometimes presents as a persistent cough. Other differential diagnoses for a persistent cough can include cough-variant asthma and gastroesophageal reflux disease (GERD). You can see how many of these symptoms can overlap.

You're evaluating a 45-year-old man who presents with recurrent sneezing, watery eyes, and nasal congestion. He says he has these symptoms every spring. You initially put him on a nasal steroid, which has helped his symptoms somewhat, but they persist. Which one of the following would you add next to help alleviate his symptoms?

(A) Oseltamivir (Tamiflu)

(B) Loratadine (Claritin)

(C) Amoxicillin/clavulanic acid (Augmentin)

(D) Famciclovir (Famvir)

(E) Prednisone (Sterapred)

The correct answer is Choice (B), loratadine. The second-line treatment for allergic rhinitis after the use of an inhaled steroid is an antihistamine. Choice (A), oseltamivir, is used to treat influenza A and B. Choice (C), amoxicillin, is a first-line treatment for otitis media and bacterial sinusitis. Choice (D), famciclovir, is an oral medication used to treat herpes simplex. Choice (E), prednisone, wouldn't be used in combination with a nasal steroid, although sometimes steroids have been given for cases of refractory chronic sinusitis to help alleviate the pain, swelling, and inflammation. Prednisone can also be given for an acute case of bronchitis.

Stopping nosebleeds: Epistaxis

During your clinical rotations, you've likely come across someone with *epistaxis* — the person's nose won't stop bleeding. Here are several points about epistaxis you should be aware of:

✔ Know your anatomy. People can have anterior nosebleeds or posterior nosebleeds. About 90 percent of nosebleeds happen at Kiesselbach's plexus (Little's area), a venous plexus that's affected during an anterior nosebleed. For a posterior nosebleed, the acute symptoms can involve swallowing and spitting up blood.

✔ Epistaxis has multiple causes. A major cause is uncontrolled high blood pressure. Other causes include nose picking, intranasal steroids, and/or chronic oxygen use. The latter two can dry out the nasal mucosa big time. Other causes include getting hit in the beak (trauma) or inhaling a nasal irritant (such as street drugs).

✔ For an anterior nosebleed, the initial treatment is to gently squeeze the anterior aspect of the nose to see whether the blood will clot. Make sure you instruct the affected person to lean his or her head forward to avoid obstructing the airway.

If the person has an underlying coagulopathy (such as liver disease), is on warfarin (Coumadin), or is on an antiplatelet agent such as clopidogrel (Plavix), pinching the nostrils together may not stop the nosebleed. You may need to stop the blood-thinning agent or correct the coagulopathy (in the case of warfarin).

✔ Subsequent treatment for an anterior nosebleed is nasal packing. You may need to call an ENT, who may use a topical cauterizing agent like silver nitrate.

Removing stuff stuck up the nose

Don't shove things up your nose! There! Your mother told you, and now a board-certified doctor is telling you.

Little kids like to shove things like toys up their noses. Some adults do, too, but it's not as common, unless you're dealing with someone who has psychiatric issues or is developmentally delayed. Boys tend to put things up their noses more commonly than girls, and the right nostril is often the nasal orifice of choice. The foreign object usually settles out into one of the nasal turbinates, usually the middle one.

The issue with a foreign body in the nose comes from possible complications, including infection or perforation. The sinuses, ears, and/or ophthalmic areas can become infected. Physical damage can occur, depending on the nature of the foreign body.

Symptoms can include pain, unilateral drainage, headache, loss of smell, and/or fevers. A radiograph or CT scan can sometimes help in localizing and identifying the foreign body. However, nothing beats direct visualization. Removing a foreign body should be done by an experienced professional, usually an ENT.

Looking at the Mouth and Throat

In this section, you get to read about the exciting world of the pharynx, the larynx, and other aspects of the mouth. Fasten your seatbelts, because our brief, fast ride down the Grand Canal is about to get wild!

Soothing the sore throat

Acute pharyngitis (called "strep throat" by the common folk) can be painful. It can also be a source of test questions, which can also be painful. Acute pharyngitis, like sinusitis, can be bacterial or viral. It affects kids a lot.

A common cause of acute bacterial pharyngitis is Group A beta-hemolytic strep (GABHS), which can be diagnosed by a rapid strep test (RST) in the office. Clinical signs and symptoms can include difficult and painful swallowing, anterior cervical adenopathy, and fevers. The patient may have other associated upper respiratory infection symptoms. On physical examination, you can see an exudative pharyngitis with increased pharyngeal injection. The initial treatment for an acute bacterial *(Strep)* pharyngitis is penicillin, usually amoxicillin (Amoxil). For someone who is penicillin-sensitive, the next treatment of choice is erythromycin.

Recall the complications of a strep pharyngitis infection, including the risk of rheumatic fever and post-streptococcal glomerulonephritis. With each diagnosis that you read about, see whether you can make connections with other disease processes to help you on the test.

A very common cause of viral pharyngitis is mononucleosis via the Epstein-Barr virus. (You read about Epstein-Barr virus in Chapter 19.) Splenomegaly can be present with Epstein-Barr virus, and the affected kid (it's usually a young person) can't play contact sports for several weeks until the splenomegaly resolves. Other viral causes of pharyngitis include adenovirus, influenza, and the rhinovirus (the cause of the common cold).

On a PANCE question, the difference between bacterial and viral causes of pharyngitis may depend on the type of cervical adenopathy. Anterior cervical adenopathy is more associated with a bacterial form of pharyngitis (GABHS), whereas posterior cervical adenopathy is more associated with a viral infection.

Connecting oral ulcers to other conditions

Oral aphthous ulcers (canker sores) can be very painful. A test question may ask you about conditions that can predispose someone to oral aphthous ulcer formation. A big one is systemic lupus erythematosis (SLE). In fact, oral ulcers are one of the diagnostic criteria for SLE.

You can see mouth ulcers with Crohn's disease as well as with herpes (cold sores or fever blisters). Women are affected more than men.

The treatment is supportive, and it can include topical steroids and pain medication, such as oral lidocaine. Evaluating for the underlying cause is also important.

Feeling around for inflamed glands

For the PANCE, you should have some familiarity with the salivary glands. If you remember your anatomy, you'll recall that you have major and minor salivary glands. For the purposes of the test, focus on the two major salivary glands: the parotid gland and the submandibular gland.

Parotitis: The parotid gland

Parotitis is a condition in which the parotid gland is inflamed. One of the most common viral causes, which you read about in Chapter 19, is mumps. A bacterial infection can cause parotitis as well. For test-taking purposes, one of the most common causes of bacterial parotitis is *Staphylococcus aureus*.

The clinical presentation of parotitis is asymmetric swelling of one cheek, especially with a mumps parotitis. The affected area can be erythematous. The person may experience a dry mouth and have pain over the affected area, especially when trying to open the mouth. Food may taste bad as well.

Which of the following is a cause of parotitis?

(A) Measles

(B) Fifth disease

(C) Hypercalcemia

(D) Sjögren's syndrome

(E) Sickle cell anemia

The correct answer is Choice (D). Parotitis is a complication of *Sjögren's syndrome,* an auto-immune disease characterized by dry eyes and dry mouth. Concerning Choice (A), mumps, not measles, is a cause of parotitis; measles are associated with Koplik spots. Fifth disease is an example of a viral exanthema in children (remember the "slapped-cheek" appearance). Hypercalcemia (Choice [C]), especially caused by hyperparathyroidism, is a cause of kidney stones. Sickle cell anemia, Choice (E), is a cause of gallstones, usually pigment stones secondary to a hemolytic anemia.

Sialadenitis: The salivary gland

Sialadenitis is a fancy term just meaning an inflamed salivary gland. This term encompasses parotitis as well as inflammation of the submandibular gland. Here are three key points about sialadenitis:

- ✔ The treatment of a bacterial infection includes an antibiotic, usually a penicillin derivative.

- ✔ Just as the kidney can have kidney stones, so, too, can the salivary glands (well, not kidney stones but something similar). The parotid and submandibular glands can both get salivary duct stones. The treatment is pain relief and adequate hydration.

- ✔ The ingestion of foods to increase saliva production is encouraged. Go suck on a lemon!

A complication of an infected gland can be an abscess. Often, imaging needs to be done — a CT scan is usually first-line.

Managing Malignancies of the Head and Neck

Malignancies of the head and neck include cancer that can affect the mouth, nasal cavity, throat, larynx, sinuses, and salivary glands. Cancers that affect the head and neck often begin in these areas and can spread via the lymphatic system to other areas.

Other than occuring in the same general place, oral and throat cancers have three things in common:

- ✔ Risk factors include smoking cigarettes and chewing tobacco.

- ✔ The most common histologic cell type is squamous cell cancer.

- ✔ Treatment is a multifaceted approach, including surgery, chemotherapy, and/or radiation, depending on the extent of metastasis.

Open wide for a look at oral cancer

As the name implies, *oral cancer* refers to malignancies that affect the mouth, including the lips, palate, and tongue.

✔ Symptoms can include dysphagia and/or odynophagia.

✔ A hard "lump" or oral ulceration can be an initial sign of a malignancy.

Oral leukoplakia are white patches found in the mouth. Risk factors for the development of leukoplakia are the same as for head and neck cancer: tobacco use. Leukoplakia should be biopsied, as they can develop into a malignancy.

✔ The diagnosis is confirmed by tissue biopsy findings.

Talking about throat cancer

Throat malignancies primarily involve the pharynx and the larynx. Here are some key points to be familiar with:

✔ Initial symptoms can include hoarseness, if the larynx is affected.

✔ Presenting symptoms can consist of neck pain, dysphagia, a palpable neck mass, weight loss, and other type B constitutional symptoms, including fever, chills, and night sweats.

✔ Other symptoms can be present, depending on other areas that may be affected. For example, ear pain (otalgia) can be a symptom of a malignancy of the head and neck.

✔ Human papillomavirus (HPV) is a risk factor for many cancers of the pharynx and of the oral cavity as well.

Examining the Ear

A lot of medical conditions can affect the ear. From infection to inflammation, from vertigo to tinnitus and hearing loss, you get an earful in this section.

Ear inflammation: Observing otitis of all types

Otitis (inflammation of the ear) comes in two kinds: otitis externa and otitis media. Although the two conditions share the word *otitis,* they're quite different.

Otitis externa (external otitis)

Otitis externa (also called *external otitis*), as the name suggests, affects the outer ear. You see it in two common scenarios. The first is *swimmer's ear,* which you see in someone who does a lot of swimming. Kids are infected more than adults. The other clinical scenario is in someone who's relatively immunocompromised, such as a person with uncontrolled diabetes.

Otitis externa is very painful. The outer ear is red and inflamed and looks nasty. You may see skin irritation that mimics dermatitis on the ear.

The most common bacterial organism causing otitis externa is *Pseudomonas aeruginosa,* especially in someone with uncontrolled diabetes. Note that *Staphylococcus aureus* is also a common cause of otitis externa. Fungal organisms can also be responsible.

If you see a test question concerning either otitis externa or osteomyelitis (see Chapter 6) in someone with diabetes, *Pseudomonas* is going to be a high-yield answer.

Treatment for otitis externa is antibiotics to relieve the infection and steroids to relieve the inflammation. These are topical solutions.

Otitis media

Otitis media is an inflammation of the middle part of the ear, usually seen in children, although it can also occur in adults. Otitis media has both acute and chronic forms.

This condition is caused by a bacterial infection, the three most common being *Streptococcus pneumoniae, Moraxella catarrhalis,* and *Haemophilus influenzae.* Concerning clinical presentation, the person feels significant pain in the ear, especially if you gently pull on the tragus of the ear. Fever can be present, and the child usually looks toxic. The child may be in tears because the ear pain is so bad.

On physical examination, you often notice a lack of the "cone of light" reflex when you look at the tympanic membrane with an otoscope. If you were to do air insufflation of the tympanic membrane in someone with otitis media, that would elicit some pain as well. A lot of pressure is behind the eardrum, which can be painful. In addition, the tympanic membrane can be angry and erythematous.

The treatment of otitis media is antibiotics; the first choice is usually amoxicillin (Amoxil).

Repeated ear infections may mean that myringotomy tubes are needed. These tubes should help over the long haul. Complications of otitis media, if untreated, include mastoiditis, abscess, or meningitis. Over time, repeated infections can affect a kid's hearing.

The chronic form of otitis media actually involves a rupture of the tympanic membrane. This is a result of an infection that has persisted for several weeks.

Another complication of chronic otitis media is a *cholesteatoma,* a cyst-like structure filled with squamous epithelium that can destroy surrounding structures. It can occur in the middle ear or in the mastoid bone. Common initial symptoms can include pain, ear drainage, and hearing loss. On otoscopic examination, you can see a lot of scar material that doesn't get better with antibiotics. The best imaging study is a CT scan of the head to look further at the bone. The treatment is primarily to remove the cholesteatoma surgically.

Bracing for vertigo

If you've ever had vertigo, you know how debilitating the sensation of the room spinning can be. Vertigo can occur by itself, or it can accompany other symptoms, such as decreased hearing or even tinnitus. You should be aware of several causes of vertigo for the test.

Benign positional vertigo

Benign paroxysmal positional vertigo (BPPV) is the most common form of positional vertigo and is probably the most common disorder involving vertigo. It's an affliction of the inner ear. In the most common clinical scenario, when the patient changes the position of the head, he or she feels that the room is spinning. The person may experience significant nausea as well. The diagnosis is confirmed by the Dix-Hallpike test. Treatment involves a maneuver such as the Epley maneuver to help retrain the inner ear.

Experts attribute benign paroxysmal positional vertigo to the buildup of calcium within the posterior semicircular canals of the inner ear. The utricular sac — the balancing equipment of the inner ear — actually contains crystals. The role of the semicircular canals is the detection of rapid changes in head movement, and with the buildup of calcium crystals, things in the inner ear get a little messed up, causing the sensation of being on a merry-go-round.

Note that the terms "dizzy" or "lightheaded" are nonspecific. You often need to tease out whether the person's symptoms are from vertigo or from orthostatic hypotension. With *orthostatic hypotension,* the dizziness or lightheadedness occurs when the person is switching positions (for example, going from lying down to either a sitting or a standing position).

Ménière's disease

Ménière's disease usually affects one ear and can cause dizziness, vertigo, tinnitus, or decreased hearing in the affected ear. It's caused by an increased amount of fluid in the inner ear. The build-up of this extra fluid in the inner ear is referred to as *endolymphatic duct obstruction.*

There's no gold standard for diagnosing of Ménière's disease — the diagnosis is made by ruling out other potential causes of vertigo. Unfortunately, there's no cure. Treatment is supportive. Low-sodium diets (to discourage the buildup of fluid) are advocated. Meclizine (Antivert) is recommended to help with the vertigo. Perhaps 20 to 30 percent of patients go on to develop bilateral disease.

Schwannomas

Schwannomas (or *acoustic neuromas*) are rare, slow-growing brain tumors that can affect cranial nerve VIII. Symptoms can include hearing loss and balance problems. You also see vertigo and tinnitus with these tumors. They're diagnosed with brain imaging, usually a CT scan or MRI of the brain with intravenous contrast. Options for treatment are often surgical, but radiation can be used as well.

Labrynthitis

Labrynthitis can cause vertigo. A classic presentation is a person who had a cold or sore throat a week or so ago that has resolved but who several days later presents with significant vertigo. These symptoms can sometimes persist for months. The gold standard treatment is vestibular rehabilitation therapy (VRT), usually in an outpatient unit.

Does tinnitus ring a bell?

With *tinnitus,* people often report hearing a ringing sound or a buzzing in their ears. Tinnitus is a symptom, not a disease. Many conditions can cause tinnitus. It can be associated with other symptoms, including decreased hearing and vertigo.

The most common type of tinnitus is subjective, in which the person doesn't have any objective hearing problems but complains of a buzzing noise. The treatment for tinnitus depends on its cause. For some causes (consider the mechanic who's been around loud noises all his life), the use of a low masking sound may help. We counted 29 suggested treatments!

Minding the mastoids

Mastoiditis is an inflammation of the mastoid bone. It's usually the result of an untreated middle ear infection or bad middle ear infections that persist despite treatment. Symptoms can include fever and pain in the mastoid area. You may see swelling and redness. In the setting of an acute otitis media, there may be purulent ear drainage (yuck).

The treatment involves antibiotics as well as consideration of surgery (typically a mastoidectomy) if the person remains symptomatic despite aggressive antibiotic treatment. Imaging studies of the head, including an MRI, are often done.

Evaluating ear trauma

Some things can cause trauma to your wonderful ears. Just as kids sometimes shove things up their noses, kids also shove foreign objects in their ears. In addition, barotrauma, which is due to changes in air pressure, can affect the ears.

A foreign body in the ear is a pretty common condition. Toys and other things may be shoved in the ear, or insects can fly into it. In his running days in high school, Rich hated it when insects would fly in his mouth or his ear.

Symptoms depend on the object as well as on how deep it is in the ear canal and how long it's been there. The deeper it is, the higher the risk of perforating the tympanic membrane.

If the person tries to take the object out (usually without knowing what he or she is doing), that can cause further irritation. If the tympanic membrane isn't perforated, a medical professional looks in the ear and tries to remove the object. The doc or PA may even try irrigation. Sometimes the person has to see an ENT for the removal. Barry knows one story where a smart doc used a magnet to coax a ball bearing out of a child's ear.

If the person has a bug in his or her ear, the insect needs to be dead before removal. The person shouldn't try to smash his or her ear with the hand in the hope of killing the bug. All he or she will get is a concussion. Instead, a good dose of mineral oil in the ear should be used to kill the bug.

Barotrauma is injury of the ear due to sudden changes in pressure (think SCUBA divers). The changes in pressure can be enough to cause damage to the ear — typically decompression sickness (also known as *the bends*). The most common area to be affected by changes in pressure is the middle ear. Symptoms can include hearing and balance problems. The best treatment is prevention, and a SCUBA diver should be familiar with how to equalize pressure during ascents

Waxing eloquent

The body makes many odd substances, and *cerumen* — ear wax — leads the list. Excessive cerumen may impede the passage of sound in the ear canal, causing conductive hearing loss. An article in the *Journal of the American Academy of Audiology* says cerumen is the cause of 60 to 80 percent of hearing aid faults.

Treatment of excessive ear wax is with carbamide peroxide (Debrox), and the patient can use the ear drops at home. If that doesn't work, a medical professional tries syringing and *should* (but sometimes doesn't) inspect the ear canal afterward. The gold-standard treatment is an ear pick or curette *used by a medical professional,* which guarantees physical removal of the wax.

Homing in on hearing loss

Different medical conditions can contribute to hearing loss. The two kinds of hearing loss are conduction hearing loss and sensorineural hearing loss. *Conduction hearing loss* most commonly refers to problems with sound being transmitted from the outer ear to the middle ear. Causes include ear wax buildup, a foreign body in the ear, or a narrowing of the ear canal.

Sensorineural hearing loss occurs farther in. The problem is with the hair cells in the organ of Corti and/or with the nerves in the inner ear. Cranial nerve XIII can be affected, and sometimes the brain function is affected, too. Medications that cause ototoxicity can cause sensorineural deafness. Other causes include schwannomas and Ménière's disease.

Eye, Eye, Captain: Looking at Eye Conditions

Although the eyes don't take up much physical space, they're prone to countless conditions. You need to be aware of how the internal and external structures of the eye function and what can interfere with the function. Diseases such as diabetes can affect the eyes, and the eyes can also be early indicators of health problems such as multiple sclerosis. The old saying is "The eyes are the window to the soul," but you could also say that the eyes are the windows to your health.

Clearing up lens conditions

The lens of the eye can be affected by several conditions, including cataracts, corneal trauma, and foreign bodies. In this section, you read about these common conditions, which you've likely seen in your clinical rotations and/or clinical practice. The latter two conditions you likely saw during your time in the ER.

Cataracts — partly cloudy

Cataracts, or cloudy areas, are a very common condition that affects the lens. Over time, the affected person loses the ability to see. Many systemic conditions can cause cataracts, common ones being hyperparathyroidism and diabetes. Steroids can cause them as well. Astronauts who have left Earth orbit have a high incidence of cataracts, possibly due to cosmic rays. One big cause is just getting older. The treatment is usually surgical, often using a laser.

Scratching the surface on cornea trauma

The cornea is the outermost part of the eye, and it's susceptible to trauma. By *trauma,* we refer to anything that scratches the eye. Signs can include increased lacrimation, a sensation of fullness in the eye, eye itching, and pain.

A regular ophthalmoscope may miss a small corneal abrasion. You need a slit lamp and fluorescein dye to get a really detailed look at the eye. The treatment of a corneal abrasion is usually conservative, although sometimes topical antibiotics may be prescribed.

A *corneal ulcer* is a bacterial infection of the cornea. There are a variety of causes, including *Staph*, *Strep*, and *Pseudomonas*. The diagnosis is confirmed with fluorescein angiography. The treatment is topical antibiotics and/or antifungals. One viral infection that you can't forget is herpetic keratitis. Herpes simplex keratitis commonly presents with a dendritic ulcer.

Eyeing foreign bodies

When Rich was little, there was a child's oath: "Cross my heart, hope to die, stick a needle in my eye." We're not sure why anyone would want to stick a needle in his or her eye, except to show sincerity.

The eye can be subject to trauma from objects flying into it. For many activities — carpentry, machining, welding, or target shooting, for example — wearing eye protection is vital. The treatment for eye trauma depends on how much of the eye is affected. Foreign objects can cause significant injury. The ophthalmologist needs to see the person pronto to do a slit-lamp examination to determine the extent of the damage. This is a full examination to make sure that the person has no bleeding in the eye or problems with the pupil.

Covering external eye structures

In this section, you read about issues affecting the conjunctiva, common medical conditions affecting the eyelid and tear ducts, and problems of the orbit, including infection and orbital trauma. You can see a lot of orbital trauma (in an ER or trauma rotation) as a result of motor vehicle accidents.

Conjunctivitis

Conjunctiva are thin membranes that blanket and protect the surfaces of both eyes. *Conjunctivitis* (pinkeye) is an irritation/infection of the conjunctiva. The most common cause of conjunctivitis is a virus, such as adenovirus. Bacterial conjunctivitis is caused by *Streptococcus pneumoniae, Moraxella catarrhalis,* or *Haemophilus influenzae.* Other causes of conjunctival irritation are allergic and fungal. Common presenting symptoms include redness, eye tearing, and pain. There's also an eye discharge.

Watch out! Viral or bacterial conjunctivitis is contagious! You treat bacterial conjunctivitis with topical antibiotics if it doesn't resolve on its own in about 3 days.

Pinkeye isn't the only thing that can happen to the conjunctiva. *Pterygium* ("surfer's eye") refers to a benign growth on the conjunctiva. The etiology isn't known, but it may be a reaction to the weather, including excessive sun or wind exposure. The symptoms are like those of other eye conditions, namely tearing, redness, and itching. The treatment is usually conservative. However, if the growth begins to cover a significant amount of the eye, then surgical intervention is warranted.

Bumps around the eyelid

Two eye conditions that have to do with sebaceous glands are often thought of as similar, but they have significant differences. One is the chalazion; the other is the stye.

The *chalazion* is a cyst-like structure that forms because of a blockage of the *meibomian gland,* a special type of sebaceous gland in the eye. Rich has had a couple of these, and although they're painless, they're a pain in the butt. He constantly felt like he had something in his eye. He teared a lot, and because the chalazion is in the eyelid itself, even looking at it was difficult. The affected eye is often tender and swollen and very, very photosensitive.

Chalazions often resolve on their own, especially if they're small. Interventions can include the use of warm compresses to soften the area and promote drainage. If they continue to enlarge or fail to settle within a few months, then smaller lesions may be injected with a corticosteroid, or larger ones may be surgically removed using local anesthesia.

A *stye* (a hordeolum) derives from an infected sebaceous gland. It differs from a chalazion, which comes from a *blocked* sebaceous gland. If untreated, a stye can develop into a chalazion. Rather than being in the eyelid itself, styes are on the lid margin. The treatment is topical warm compresses and topical antibiotics when needed.

Inflammation of the tear duct and eyelid

Dacryoadenitis refers to an inflamed tear duct that may become blocked. The most common cause is infection, either viral or bacterial. A common bacterial cause is *Staphylococcus aureus*. The upper eyelid is swollen and erythematous, and it can be painful. The treatment often is supportive and involves antibiotics in the case of a bacterial infection.

Blepharitis is inflammation of the eyelids. The lids can be red and swollen, and the skin can be crusty and/or flaky. One of the most common causes is a bacterial infection secondary to your old friend *Staph aureus*. The treatment is warm compresses and antibiotics.

Orbiting the eye

When you read about the orbit, we aren't talking about orbiting the Earth. Rather, we're talking about the *orbit* around the eyeball — the eye socket and related structures.

The *blowout fracture* is a fracture of the orbit, usually as a result of a traumatic event, such as a car accident or a blunt trauma. Basically, the supporting structures of the bone are fractured. The dreaded complication of an orbital fracture is paralysis of the extraocular muscles. A CT scan gives you a more detailed look at the orbit. Any paralysis of the extraocular muscles is an indication for surgery because there's likely nerve entrapment. Other significant symptoms include double vision and eye swelling.

Orbital cellulitis is an infection, usually bacterial, of the tissues orbiting the eye, which can include the lid and cheek. The person may also have very significant eye swelling and loss of vision in the affected eye as well as significant pain. The treatment is intravenous antibiotics, although sometimes surgical intervention is necessary.

In clinical practice and on the PANCE, you must differentiate between *orbital* cellulitis and *periorbital* cellulitis. Periorbital cellulitis is an infection in front of the orbital septum, whereas orbital cellulitis occurs behind the orbital septum. In addition, the person with periorbital cellulitis doesn't present with vision loss or pain. The eye isn't bulging, either. You may see erythema and swelling around the eye, however.

Focusing on the retina

The retina is a multi-layered structure in the eye, with cones, rods, and blood vessels. A lot of things can affect the retina, including diseases, occlusions, and aging.

Diseases of the retina

Retinopathy is a general term that refers to some form of noninflammatory damage to the retina of the eye. Two of the biggest diseases that can cause retinopathy are hypertension and diabetes mellitus, although there are many others. *Cytomegalovirus retinitis* is an inflammation of the retina.

The retina is visible through an ophthalmoscope (fundoscope). In someone with a history of diabetes or hypertension, on clinical exam you should take a stab (ouch!) at looking into his or her eyes to check the retina and the blood vessels. With diabetic retinopathy, you see hemorrhages as well as "cotton-wool" exudates. As for hypertensive retinopathy, there are four stages:

✔ **Stage I:** Narrowing of the arterioles, often named "silver wiring"

✔ **Stage II:** More arteriovenous narrowing

✔ **Stage III:** Hemorrhages; on an eye exam, you can see cotton-wool exudates

✔ **Stage IV:** Papilledema

The stages of hypertensive retinopathy don't always progress from I through IV. For example, someone who's admitted to the hospital with a new onset hypertensive emergency (see Chapter 3) may exhibit papilledema (Stage IV) without having the other stages.

In advanced retinopathy, blood vessels become fragile and can rupture. The treatment of choice is usually laser photocoagulation surgery.

Retinal detachment

The retina is a multi-layered structure. The retina can detach from its support network. Symptoms can include having a loss of central vision or seeing floaters (little specs of debris within the eye's vitreous humor, which is normally transparent). Note that although floaters may be indicative of retinal detachment, often they're not. The degree of vision loss and other symptoms depends on how much of the retina is detached.

Risk factors for retinal detachment include being nearsighted, a history of eye trauma, or cataract surgery. Inflammation of the uvea (uveitis) and conditions such as diabetic retinopathy can predispose someone to retinal detachment. Retinal detachment needs to be treated urgently.

Retinal vascular occlusions

The first of the retinal vascular occlusions is occlusion of the retinal artery, which causes vision loss. If the central retinal artery becomes acutely blocked, the person experiences a painless, total loss of vision in the affected eye. If a branch retinal artery is blocked, the person experiences only a partial loss of vision in that eye. The eye exam will include a pupillary defect and, on fundoscopic exam, a pale fundus with a "cherry red spot" near the fovea.

Be aware of risk factors for this occlusion. Emboli from either a clogged carotid artery or a clot in the left atrium from atrial fibrillation are leading causes. Giant cell arteritis (also known as *temporal arteritis*) is another huge risk factor.

The key in treatment is looking for the underlying cause. Often an ophthamologist is consulted, but there's no magic bullet to make retinal vascular occlusions better. Sometimes the vision loss is permanent. Panretinal photocoagulation (PRP) with an argon laser may be effective.

Not only can the retinal arteries become occluded, but so can the retinal veins. Hypertension and diabetes are risk factors. The presentation can be similar to a retinal artery occlusion: a loss of vision. The occlusion may be in a central or branch retinal vein. Here are the key points:

- ✔ Experts think that atherosclerosis and a low blood flow state contribute to the formation of a small clot within the vein, more so than this being an embolic phenomenon.

- ✔ When the retinal vein is blocked, the macula swells, leading to an increase in ocular pressure. A form of acute glaucoma can result due to the buildup of intraocular pressure. After all, the vein is the sole source of drainage for the retina.

- ✔ Part of the workup for a central venous occlusion is looking for a hypercoagulable state, given the thrombus formation. The treatment is similar to treatment of arterial occlusion: laser photocoagulation.

Macular degeneration

Age-related macular degeneration (AMD) is the leading cause of adult blindness in industrialized countries. The main clinical symptom is loss of central vision with sparing of peripheral vision. When the *macula* (the central portion of the retina) degenerates, the main portion of the retina is essentially knocked out, so the person has no more central vision.

Macular degeneration may be dry or wet (exudative). The wet version is a more severe form, although it accounts for only 10 to 15 percent of cases. Both forms can lead to detachment of the retina if left untreated.

Researchers think that the pathogenesis of macular degeneration is related to significant deposition of cholesterol deposits, called *drusen.* You can see these yellow flecks on a fundoscopic (ophtalmoscopic) examination.

The main treatment for the wet type of macular degeneration is injections of angiogenesis inhibitors, such as bevacizumab (Avastin) and aflibercept. Effective specific therapies are intravitreous injection of a VEGF inhibitor, possibly thermal laser photocoagulation (in selected patients), and photodynamic therapy. For the dry form, the use of antioxidants and certain minerals, including a combination of zinc, vitamin C, vitamin B$_6$, and/or beta carotene, can be beneficial. Laser coagulation may also help improve the condition and prevent further loss of vision in someone with dry macular degeneration.

Looking deep into the eyes

Some eye conditions can become medical emergencies if not treated. In this section, you read about papilledema, glaucoma, and hyphema, as well as optic neuritis.

Papilledema: Under intracranial pressure

Papilledema is swelling of the optic disc due to increased intracranial pressure. Rich has seen this condition in people who present to the hospital with hypertensive emergencies.

The diagnosis is made with an ophthalmoscope. Papilledema has many causes, including a brain malignancy (primary or metastasis, usually with elevated intracranial pressure and midline shifting when severe), bleeding in the brain, benign intracranial hypertension, and malignant hypertension. On ophthalmic examination, the optic disc looks blurred because you're no longer able to see the margins.

The treatment is to lower the intracranial pressure in the brain. For a hypertensive emergency, this means a gradual lowering of the blood pressure. For a brain tumor, it may mean high-dose steroids, mannitol, and/or neurosurgery.

Glaucoma: Lowering the intraocular pressure

Glaucoma is defined as damage to the optic nerve secondary to a very elevated intraocular pressure. If left untreated, this condition can result in permanent blindness. Be aware of two big types of glaucoma:

- ✔ **Open-angle glaucoma:** This type, which is the most common, is often hereditary and painless. The affected person can describe a gradual loss of vision. On examination, the ophthalmologist often sees damage to the optic nerve.

- ✔ **Angle-closure glaucoma:** Angle-closure glaucoma, which is a medical emergency, is characterized by the triad of a fixed and dilated pupil, severe eye pain, and loss of vision. The intraocular pressure is very high. This form of glaucoma is treated surgically.

A variety of eye drops are used to treat glaucoma by lowering the intraocular pressure. Although marijuana (cannabis) may lower intraocular pressure, this effect lasts for only a few hours and isn't as effective as other medications.

Hyphemas — my eye bleeds for you

A *hyphema* is blood in the anterior chamber of the eye. The most common cause is trauma. Another significant risk factor is any type of coagulopathy. This condition usually affects one eye, not both. Clinical symptoms can include eye pain and photosensitivity.

Many hyphemas resolve on their own, but the medical professional often recommends avoiding strenuous physical activity, avoiding further trauma, and avoiding rubbing or touching the eyes. Correcting any coagulopathies is a good idea, too.

Being aware of optic neuritis

Optic neuritis is the inflammation of the optic nerve, and it causes acute vision loss and pain in the eye. It can be the initial symptom of multiple sclerosis. On examination, you see an abnormality in the optic nerve. The immediate treatment (because of the acute inflammation) is either intravenous hydrocortisone or the more commonly used methylprednisolone sodium succinate (Solu-Medrol). The key is looking for the underlying cause, because this condition can be associated with many other autoimmune and rheumatologic disorders.

Tracking eye movements and muscle conditions

Various conditions affect the ability of the eye to move as it should. In this section, you read about conditions such as strabismus and nystagmus.

Pointing the eye in the right direction

Strabismus is a disorder of the muscles of the eyes, preventing both eyes from focusing on the same object at the same time. The extraocular muscles don't work in synchrony, so each eye essentially does its own thing. Here are two types of strabismus, based on the direction of deviation:

- ✔ **Esotropia:** Esotropia (deviation of the eye toward the nose) is a form of strabismus in which the person is cross-eyed.

- ✔ **Exotropia:** Exotropia is the opposite of esotropia. The eyes deviate outward, so the person is walleyed.

If strabismus is left untreated, the muscles of the weaker eye can become even weaker, leading to *strabismic amblyopia* ("lazy eye"). Amblyopia leads to vision loss in the affected eye because the two eyes aren't working in synchrony. The child with amblyopia needs a full ophthalmic examination and full medical evaluation.

Studies show that approximately 3 percent of children suffer from amblyopia, and it needs to be detected by age 4. Although a vision screen for young children can be difficult, the Blackbird Vision Screening system is very effective, mainly because it's a fun test and kids like to take it.

Strabismus has many causes, from cranial nerve lesions to medical conditions such as hyperthyroidism and myasthenia gravis. Treatment of strabismus involves treating the underlying cause. Sometimes interventions are done to strengthen the weaker eye. With amblyopia, this typically involves putting an eye patch over the stronger eye to force the muscles of the weaker eye to work harder, making them stronger.

Flipping out over eyelids

Ectropion refers to an eyelid that's turned outwards. You can see it in certain genetic disorders because it's a weakness in collagen framework. You can also see it with Bell's palsy. With ectropion, the affected person can have really dry eyes that can be painful and irritated.

Conjunctival irritation is common, and treatment is directed at giving artificial tears to those with keratoconjunctivitis sicca (dry eyes) as well as surgery if necessary.

Entropion is an eyelid that's turned inward. When this happens, the eyelashes turn in as well and can rub against the eye. As with an ectropion, the eye can become infected and irritated over time. Treatment again involves the use of artificial tears to help keep the eye lubricated as much as possible. If the eyelashes are rubbing against the eye, surgery is usually indicated.

Knowing nystagmus

Nystagmus is involuntary eye movement. It may be physiologic (normal) or pathological (bad), with variations within each type. The key is the way the eyes normally move. The eyes can move horizontally (side to side), they can move vertically (up and down), and just to keep things interesting, they can also rotate (parents hate this eye movement). Pathological nystagmus involves three basic characteristics of abnormal eye movement: too slow, too fast, and too jerky.

Causes of nystagmus include congenital disorders, acquired or central nervous system disorders, toxicity, pharmaceutical drugs, and alcohol. Actually, we counted 53 possible causes of nystagmus.

Although nystagmus was previously considered untreatable, several drugs have been identified for treatment in recent years. Think of memantine (typically for treating Alzheimer's), levetiracetam (an anticonvulsant), amifampridine (for rare muscle diseases), dalfampridine (for multiple sclerosis), and acetazolamide (for epileptic seizures).

Practice Questions on the Eyes, Ears, Nose, and Throat

These practice questions are similar to the PANCE questions you may see about eye, ear, nose, and throat conditions.

1. You're evaluating a 34-year-old woman who presents with dizziness, vertigo, and tinnitus in the right ear. She is also complaining of drainage in the right ear. She denies any prior cold, upper respiratory infection, or focal weakness. Which one of the following is her likely diagnosis?

   (A) Salicylate toxicity

   (B) Labrynthitis

   (C) Benign paroxysmal positional vertigo

   (D) Ménière's disease

   (E) Acute sinusitis

2. Which of the following medications is ototoxic?

   (A) Gentamicin

   (B) Doxycycline (Vibramycin)

   (C) Cefazolin (Ancef)

   (D) Metronidazole (Flagyl)

   (E) Clarithromycin (Biaxin)

3. You're evaluating a 67-year-old man who was involved in a motor vehicle accident. On physical examination, you notice a significant restriction of right eye movement. Which of the following would you order next?

   (A) Radiograph of the orbit

   (B) CT scan of the orbit

   (C) MRI of the head without gadolinium

   (D) Skull radiograph

   (E) PET scan

4. Which of the following muscles is innervated by cranial nerve IV?

   (A) Superior oblique

   (B) Lateral rectus

   (C) Eyelid

   (D) Forehead

   (E) Trapezius

5. Which one of the following conditions is a complication of acute otitis media?

   (A) Sinusitis

   (B) Pharyrngitis

   (C) Meningitis

   (D) Peritonsillar abscess

   (E) Dacryoadenitis

6. Which one of the following would be a cause of sensorineural hearing loss?

   (A) Cerumen impaction

   (B) Flying in a plane at high altitude

   (C) Otitis externa

   (D) Ménière's disease

   (E) Otitis media

Answers and Explanations

Use this answer key to score the practice questions from the preceding section. The answer explanations give you some insight into why the correct answer is better than the other choices.

1. **D.** This woman has multiple symptoms affecting one ear, and they point to Ménière's disease as the likely diagnosis. Choice (B), labrynthitis, is usually due to a prior upper respiratory infection. Choice (C), benign paroxysmal positional vertigo, would present with vertigo-like symptoms but not the accompanying symptoms. Choice (E), acute sinusitis, would present with sinus congestion, fever, Eustachian tube dysfunction, rhinorrhea, and so forth.

2. **A.** Gentamicin is an aminoglycoside antibiotic. The two main classes of medications that are ototoxic are loop diuretics and aminoglycoside antibiotics, which are both nephrotoxic and ototoxic.

3. **B.** This man who suffered a motor vehicle accident has a blowout fracture. If the extraocular muscles are restricted, which is a possible effect, then you should order a CT scan of the orbit. None of the other choices apply in this situation.

4. **A.** Expect to see some questions about the cranial nerves on the PANCE. The superior oblique muscle, Choice (A), is an extraocular muscle innervated by cranial nerve IV. The lateral rectus, Choice (B), is innervated by cranial nerve VI. The eyelid, Choice (C), is innervated by cranial nerve VII to close the eyelid. The forehead, Choice (D), is innervated by cranial nerve VII, too. The trapezius, Choice (E), is innervated by the cranial nerve XI.

5. **C.** Meningitis is a complication of acute otitis media. Peritonsillar abscess, Choice (D), can be a complication of pharyngitis. Dacryoadenitis, Choice (E), is blockage of a lacrimal duct because of a bacterial infection.

6. **D.** On a test, be able to differentiate between conductive hearing loss and sensorineural hearing loss. Cerumen impaction, flying in a plane at high altitude, otitis externa, and otitis media — all the choices except Choice (D) — are causes of conductive hearing loss. Think of conductive hearing loss as beginning in the outer part of the ear up to the middle part of the ear. Sensorineural hearing loss concerns problems that affect the inner ear, such as Ménière's disease, Choice (D).

Chapter 9

Reviewing Reproductive Medicine

. . . .

In This Chapter

▶ Understanding menstrual disorders

▶ Looking at problems of the breast

▶ Observing the uterus, ovaries, and cervix

▶ Looking at problems of the vulva and vagina

▶ Going over pregnancy, contraception, and abortions

. . . .

*R*eproductive medicine is a broad topic that covers many obstetric and gynecologic issues. Read this chapter to understand common issues in reproductive medicine, including pregnancy and its complications, birth control, basic gynecologic issues, sexually transmitted diseases (STDs), and breast health.

Managing Menstrual Disorders

Menstruation, or shedding of the endometrium, is part of a 28-day cycle, and it's a normal physiologic process. *Menarche* is the name for the first menstrual period, and it usually takes place between the ages of 10 and 16, with the median age being 12 or 13 years. The PANCE/PANRE may ask about the range of starting ages as well as about abnormalities in a woman's menstrual cycle. In this section, you read about amenorrhea, dysmenorrhea, and premenstrual syndrome.

Missing periods: Considering primary and secondary causes of amenorrhea

Amenorrhea is the absence of menstrual periods in a woman of reproductive age. Amenorrhea can have primary and secondary causes. *Primary amenorrhea* is the failure of menses to start by the age of 16 years in the presence of normal growth and secondary sexual characteristics. If by age 13 menses has not started and the onset of puberty is absent, a workup for primary amenorrhea should start. Primary amenorrhea can be due to problems with the organs themselves — problems with the uterus (congenital absence of one) or the ovaries. Alternatively, it can be due to a problem with the hypothalamus-pituitary axis.

Secondary amenorrhea is defined as the early cessation of menses. In this case, the body or a particular organ isn't making the necessary hormones for a woman to have menstrual cycles. Some experts diagnose secondary amenorrhea only after a woman hasn't had a menstrual cycle for 6 months or more; others believe that 90 days marks the minimum time requirement.

Common causes of amenorrhea include hypothyroidism, prolactinoma, and polycystic ovarian syndrome (PCOS). Dramatic changes in weight, either significant gain or loss, can also be causes of amenorrhea. Some marathon runners are so calorically deprived that they develop a secondary amenorrhea. Eating disorders, such as anorexia or bulimia, can also be causes.

On clinical presentation, you want to look for physical changes. Does she have more facial hair than before? Hirsutism may be a sign of polycystic ovarian syndrome or Cushing's. Does she have any nipple discharge? You see discharge with pituitary tumors. If her weight has changed, does she have an underlying eating disorder, has she had recent surgery, or is a malabsorption syndrome causing changes in weight?

The workup for amenorrhea includes the measurement of various hormone levels, including TSH, FSH, LH, and prolactin. Don't forget the good old β-hCG, because you don't want to miss a pregnancy, which is the most common cause of secondary amenorrhea. The treatment depends on investigation of the underlying problem.

Painful periods: Diagnosing dysmenorrhea by process of elimination

Dysmenorrhea is defined as a painful menstruation. Most commonly, this occurs when women first start menstruating and again in women in their late 30s and early 40s. When a woman has dysmenorrhea, think of two basic processes: endometriosis and chronic pelvic pain, which you usually see in someone with a history of pelvic inflammatory disease (PID), although this condition can have other etiologies.

The workup for dysmenorrhea involves exclusion of other disorders, such as an STD or cervicitis. Women sometimes need pelvic ultrasounds and surgical interventions for you to exclude other causes. The treatment includes evaluating the underlying cause as well as symptomatic pain relief, which means the use of nonsteroidals and analgesics as needed.

Premenstrual syndrome

Premenstrual syndrome (PMS) is a constellation of various symptoms, both physical and psychological, that are connected with the menstrual cycle. These symptoms, which can be debilitating, occur before or during menses.

Symptoms of PMS include labile moods, irritability, gastrointestinal upset, insomnia, anorexia or a ravenous appetite, and myalgias. The woman may have dysmenorrhea as well.

The cause of PMS isn't known. Nutrient deficiencies, in addition to hormonal alterations during the menstrual cycle, may play a role. The treatment includes lifestyle changes, such as beginning an exercise regimen (to increase endorphins), as well adopting more of an anti-inflammatory diet in case the condition is triggered by a specific food group. Avoiding caffeine, correcting nutrient deficiencies, and getting an adequate ingestion of vitamins and minerals may help. As always, anti-inflammatories and analgesics can be important for symptomatic management.

You're evaluating a 25-year-old woman who states that she has regular menstrual periods. However, they're associated with heavy flow and usually last about 6 to 8 days without significant pain. Which one of the following defines this young woman's medical condition?

(A) Amenorrhea

(B) Dysmenorrhea

(C) Menorrhagia

(D) Oligomenorrhea

(E) Endometrial cancer

The correct answer is Choice (C). *Menorrhagia* is defined as periods that occur regularly and are on schedule but have heavy flows and last a little longer than a normal menses. *Amenorrhea* means the absence of a menses. *Dysmenorrhea* refers to painful menses. *Oligomenorrhea* is menses in a cycle that's greater than 30 days. When you're evaluating a question concerning vaginal bleeding, you should assess cancer risk. You see endometrial cancer, Choice (E), in an older woman, usually postmenopausal, who presents with vaginal bleeding. The woman in this example question has no known risk factors for endometrial cancer.

Homing in on Problems of the Breast

From infection to malignancy, many medical problems can affect the breast. In this section, you read about some breast-related medical conditions and their evaluation and management.

Blocked milk ducts: Managing mastitis

Mastitis is a bacterial infection in the milk ducts. The most common cause is *Staphylococcus aureus*. Other bacteria, including *Streptococcus,* can also cause mastitis. The most significant risk factor for developing mastitis is breastfeeding. Women who are immunocompromised, including those with HIV, are also at significant risk of developing mastitis.

You obtain the culture via a sample of breast milk. For a simple infection, the treatment is a first-generation cephalosporin. Other medication classes can include penicillin or macrolide antibiotics. The treatment of a breast abscess includes incision and drainage (I&D) of the abscess plus the use of antibiotics.

If the infection is left untreated, a possible complication is abscess formation. Determining whether you're dealing with a simple infection or with an abscess can be difficult. In that case, you may need an ultrasound to make the diagnosis.

Leaking milk: Controlling prolactin to treat galactorrhea

Galactorrhea is the leaking of breast milk in someone who isn't postpartum. The most common cause of galactorrhea is increased secretion of prolactin. If you see a PANCE question concerning the cause of galactorrhea, the answer is a pituitary tumor or prolactinoma until proven otherwise. Profound hypothyroidism can also cause this condition, but that's not as common as an elevated prolactin level. Therefore, the prolactin level is the first test you order for anyone with galactorrhea.

Any medication that acts as a dopamine antagonist also increases the risk of galactorrhea. Why? Because dopamine can inhibit the production of prolactin. Giving a medication that blocks the action of dopamine can cause more prolactin to be secreted.

The treatment of galactorrhea is treating the prolactinoma. Depending on the size of the prolactinoma, treatment options include just careful monitoring of symptoms; the use of dopamine agonists, including bromocriptine (Parlodel), which inhibits the production of prolactin; and/or surgical and radiation treatments.

Man boobs: When hormone imbalance leads to gynecomastia

Gynecomastia is the one breast-related condition that affects men rather than women. To use the vernacular, it means the development of "man boobs." Medically, it refers to the enlargement of the breast due to a glandular hyperplasia of the breast cells.

In addition to testosterone, all men have estrogen in their bodies. These hormones normally exist in a homeostatic balance, so men typically don't develop the man boob. But the body can actually convert testosterone into estradiol, and whenever the body makes less testosterone with more estradiol, you have the perfect setup for gynecomastia.

What conditions can cause gynecomastia? Liver failure and alcohol abuse are two biggies. Any conditions that can affect testosterone production and cause hypogonadism can increase the risk for gynecomastia. Mumps, which you read about in the infectious diseases chapter (Chapter 19), can cause orchitis; in turn, the orchitis can increase the risk of developing hypogonadism, which also increases the risk of developing gynecomastia.

Gynecomastia increases the risk of breast cancer in men. Men with gynecomastia may need to have mammograms done.

Distinguishing the fibros

Fibroadenoma and fibrocystic breast disease are two separate conditions, but they overlap in one respect: They're benign conditions.

Fibroadenoma

Fibroadenomas are benign breast lumps that occur in young women, usually in their early 20s. The lumps are painless and freely movable. The first step in diagnosis is to do a breast examination. Then you order imaging studies to look at the breast. Options include a mammogram and ultrasound. In a younger woman, the ultrasound may be recommended first because the mammogram is unreliable because her breasts have more fatty tissue. The gold standard for confirmation that the mass isn't breast cancer is a core biopsy, not a fine needle aspiration.

Because fibroadenomas are benign, surgery usually isn't required. They're often related to a woman's menstrual cycle and may come and go in a pattern.

Fibrocystic breast disease

Fibrocystic breast disease usually occurs in women in their late 30s and 40s. With fibrocystic breast disease, the main complaint is that one or both breasts hurt. Usually both breasts are affected.

The diagnosis is first suggested by a breast examination, palpating breast lumps. That can be painful. An imaging study such as a mammogram may be ordered, but the gold standard of diagnosis is the breast biopsy.

Fibrocystic breast disease is a benign condition, but it does increase the risk of developing breast cancer down the line. With fibrocystic breast disease, you use biopsies to look for the presence of atypical cells, which occur less than 5 percent of the time.

Which one of the following would be recommended for treating fibrocystic breast disease?

(A) Morphine

(B) Not wearing a bra for a short period of time

(C) Caffeine products

(D) Yearly ultrasounds

(E) Ibuprofen

The correct answer is Choice (E). Fibrocystic breast disease can be painful, and ibuprofen has a role in helping with the pain. Morphine, Choice (A), is kind of strong for this condition. If anything, the woman with fibrocystic breast disease wants the support of a good bra, making Choice (B) wrong. She should refrain from caffeine because it can worsen the condition, so Choice (C) is wrong. Choice (D), ultrasound, isn't recommended, although routine clinical breast exams and patient self-examinations are.

Beating breast cancer

The top two causes of death for women are heart disease (see Chapter 3) and breast cancer. The PANCE will likely include several questions about breast cancer.

Risk factors for breast cancer include a family history of breast cancer, usually in a first-degree relative (that is, one's mom or sibling). Others factors are older age, nulliparity (not having given birth to viable offspring), early menarche, and late menopause. Obesity is also a risk factor for the development of breast cancer, as is bottle-feeding (as opposed to breast-feeding). Other risk factors include a sedentary lifestyle and excessive alcohol intake.

Another big risk factor is testing positive for the breast cancer genes, breast cancer type 1 susceptibility protein (BRCA1) or BRCA2. Women who test positive for this genetic mutation have an increased risk for both breast and ovarian cancer.

Here are the screening guidelines for breast cancer:

✔ Women between the ages of 50 to 74 should have a mammogram at least every 2 years.

✔ Having a screening before the age of 50 is a decision between a patient and her medical professional. They assess the woman's risk factors and family history. That being said, the American Cancer Society does endorse mammogram screening beginning at age 40.

Finding a breast lump on clinical breast exam or seeing a lump on a mammogram often first suggests the diagnosis. On the breast examination, you're looking for changes in size and shape (asymmetry in one breast compared to another). Dimpling, peau d'orange, and nipple retraction are also signs of a possible malignancy. The breast should be separated into quadrants, and each quadrant should be palpated carefully. Examining the axillary area for the presence of lymphadenopathy is mandatory.

If the mammogram confirms a mass, sometimes an ultrasound can confirm whether the mass is cystic or solid. The standard of care is a breast biopsy to determine the type of abnormality you're dealing with.

Here's a brief review of types of breast cancer (yup, there are several):

✔ **Infiltrating ductal carcinoma:** Infiltrating ductal carcinoma is the most common type of invasive breast cancer, accounting for more than 70 percent of all breast malignancies. It usually doesn't have a great prognosis.

✔ **Lobular carcinoma:** This form usually occurs in the upper outer quadrant of the breast. Lobular carcinoma often responds to hormonal treatment.

✔ **Ductal carcinoma in situ (DCIS):** This is the most common cause of noninvasive breast cancer.

The treatment of breast cancer is multifactorial. For ductal carcinoma in situ, the treatment is usually lumpectomy plus radiation. For the other two, it's often mastectomy with concomitant chemotherapy and radiation.

Tamoxifen (Nolvadex) is commonly used for treating breast cancers that are estrogen and progesterone positive. Note that this drug increases the risk of developing endometrial carcinoma.

Understanding the Uterus

Without the uterus, reproduction couldn't occur. Several medical problems can affect the uterus. The organ may move out of place, bleed, or contain abnormal tissue growth.

Uterine prolapse: Slipping into the vagina

The uterus and other pelvic structures are supported by pelvic muscles and ligaments. As these muscles weaken from prior pregnancies, obesity, pelvic surgeries, or menopause, the uterus may slip into the vagina. Be aware that uterine prolapse occurs in stages.

Common presenting symptoms of uterine prolapse can include dyspareunia (painful sexual intercourse), pelvic pain, and abdominal pain. The patient may also have significant urinary symptoms, including urgency, frequency, and burning, and the risk for urinary tract infections increases. A vaginal discharge may be present.

On physical examination, you need to do a pelvic examination so you can see the degree of uterine prolapse into the vagina. Treatment can include placing a pessary to help support the uterus. Kegel exercises, which strengthen the pelvic floor musculature, may also be prescribed. In certain cases, the woman may need surgery.

With weakening of the pelvic floor musculature and ligaments, a uterine prolapse may not be all that you see on pelvic examination. In addition, you may see bladder prolapse into the vagina (cystocele) and/or rectal prolapse into the vagina (rectocele). We address both of these conditions later in "Recognizing protrusions: Things ending in -cele."

Ruling out causes for dysfunctional uterine bleeding

Bleeding from the uterus has many causes. *Dysfunctional uterine bleeding* (DUB) is bleeding from the uterus without an identifiable anatomic cause. That is, no tumor or other source of bleeding is present. The most common reason for dysfunctional uterine bleeding is a change in the hormonal milieu. Basically, estrogen sticks around too long, which causes changes in the uterine lining that promote bleeding.

Note that dysfunctional uterine bleeding is diagnosed after other causes are excluded. A full clinical workup is indicated — look for bleeding disorders and chemistries and check a β-hCG level to rule out pregnancy. You also need to check thyroid levels and hormonal levels. Be sure the woman doesn't have polycystic ovary syndrome (see the later section "Looking at ovarian cysts and PCOS"). From an anatomic standpoint, make sure the woman doesn't have a leiomyoma (fibroid) or endometrial cancer before saying that she has dysfunctional uterine bleeding. This testing can involve a pelvic ultrasound and a dilation and curettage (D&C) to make sure she doesn't have an abnormality of the uterine lining.

The treatment of dysfunctional uterine bleeding consists of oral contraceptives to try to bring the body's hormones back into balance.

Leiomyomas: Bleeding from uterine fibroids

A *fibroid* is a benign neoplasm of the uterus. It's actually an overgrowth of the uterus's smooth muscle. Fibroids (leiomyomas) are a common cause of bleeding in women. They can grow in many places in the uterus; the two most common places are in the submucosa and within the muscular layer of the uterus. Risk factors include being African-American, being obese, and having had early menarche.

You can find fibroids on physical examination. The initial presentation can also be irregular bleeding. Other symptoms include abdominal pain and increased pelvic and abdominal pressure. You can confirm the diagnosis by a pelvic ultrasound. The treatment is usually surgical, including a myomectomy or a hysterectomy, depending on the number and extent of the fibroids. Newer, less invasive techniques include uterine artery embolization.

A not-so-silver lining: Evaluating endometriosis

Endometriosis is the abnormal spread or growth of endometrial tissue into other areas of the body, especially the pelvic area. The tissue can go anywhere and stick itself where it shouldn't, including the ovaries, the Fallopian tubes, and even the intestine.

Symptoms of endometriosis can include significant pelvic pain, pain during intercourse, and dysmenorrhea. If that constellation of signs and symptoms is present, the diagnosis is often confirmed through a diagnostic laparoscopy. The treatment is usually pain relief, with the use of nonsteroidals and/or analgesics. In addition, medications to change the hormonal milieu of the body are often prescribed. These meds include oral contraceptives, androgens, and gonadotropin-releasing hormone-like medications. The goal is to decrease the size of the ectopic endometrial tissue. Surgery is sometimes indicated in addition to or instead of medical therapy.

Treating endometrial cancer

Endometrial cancer is a cancer of the uterine lining that you see most often in postmenopausal women. The most common initial symptom is vaginal bleeding. Other symptoms can include a vaginal discharge and dyspareunia, but unexplained vaginal bleeding is the predominant symptom.

Risk factors for endometrial cancer include being nulliparous, having had early menarche, and having late menopause. Other factors include older age and using tamoxifen (Nolvadex).

To diagnose endometrial cancer, you need tissue. The first step is an endometrial biopsy. Sometimes you may need a D&C to further confirm the diagnosis. Other modalities, including transvaginal ultrasound, have also been used. The treatment of choice is often surgical, including a total abdominal hysterectomy and bilateral salpingo-oophorectomy (TAH-BSO). The affected woman may also need chemotherapy and/or radiation, depending on the degree of metastases.

Examining the Ovaries

The two big medical conditions that can affect the ovaries are ovarian cysts and ovarian cancer. Ovarian cysts can cause abdominal and pelvic discomfort in women, and ovarian cancer is a cause of increased morbidity and mortality in older women. You don't want to miss these conditions.

Looking at ovarian cysts and PCOS

Ovarian cysts can be painless and asymptomatic. On the other hand, they can cause abdominal pain and bloating. Most of the time, the ovarian cyst goes away spontaneously without any surgical intervention. A simple ovarian cyst, if it's painful, can usually be treated with oral contraceptives. Larger cysts, on the order of 10 cm, may need surgical removal.

One major cause of cysts on the ovaries is *polycystic ovarian syndrome* (PCOS), also called *Stein-Leventhal syndrome*. PCOS is a disorder of anovulation, and you usually see it in women in their late 20s and early 30s. This condition is characterized by amenorrhea, hypertension, impaired fasting glucose (or full-blown diabetes mellitus), obesity, and hyperlipidemia. Often, the components of metabolic syndrome are present. Hirsutism and other features that may resemble Cushing's syndrome, including the presence of abdominal striae, can also be present. A pelvic ultrasound can confirm the presence of ovarian cysts.

The treatment of PCOS includes weight loss. The diabetes medication metformin (Glucophage) may help with weight loss by decreasing insulin resistance and help alleviate some of the PCOS symptoms. You can also use hormonal therapy.

Reviewing ovarian cancer

Ovarian cancer is a leading cause of morbidity and mortality in older women. Risk factors for ovarian cancer include being of an older age (you usually see this cancer in postmenopausal women), using tobacco, being obese, being nulliparous, and undergoing hormonal therapy.

Note two other risk factors for ovarian cancer: If someone has a BRCA genetic mutation, she has an increased risk not only for breast cancer but also for ovarian cancer. Another risk factor for ovarian cancer is tamoxifen, which is used to treat estrogen- and progesterone-receptor positive breast cancer.

Signs and symptoms of ovarian cancer can include abdominal and pelvic pain and/or abdominal distention. Until proven otherwise, the presence of abdominal ascites in an older woman in the absence of liver disease/cirrhosis is ovarian cancer. Unfortunately, ovarian cancer is often silent until it's well advanced.

Most of the time, you initially see the ovarian cancer on a pelvic ultrasound. Other radiologic studies, including a CT scan of the abdomen and pelvis, are used to stage the cancer after diagnosis. Laparoscopic surgery is often needed to confirm the diagnosis and obtain a tissue biopsy. At the time of diagnosis, there is often evidence of metastatic spread.

The treatment is often multifactorial and can include surgery (debulking surgery to remove as much tumor as possible) in combination with chemotherapy and radiation. The chemotherapy can be administered intravenously or intra-peritoneally.

The tumor marker CA-125 (MUC16) is used as a surveillance marker to detect reoccurrence of ovarian cancer. It's not used to diagnose ovarian cancer.

Surveying the Cervix

Problems with the cervix often occur in younger women. Examples include cervical incompetence during pregnancy, cervicitis, cervical dysplasia, and cervical cancer. For cervical incompetence, prompt diagnosis and management is important. For the latter conditions, especially cervical cancer, routine screening is vital to detect the problem early. Convincing a younger person of the importance of screening is sometimes hard.

Dealing with an incompetent cervix

Cervical incompetence refers to the cervix's dilating and effacing prematurely before a pregnant woman's expected due date. Risk factors for cervical incompetence include a history of prior cervical surgeries or a history of miscarriages.

If the condition isn't corrected, the baby can be born much sooner than he or she is supposed to be. The treatment is a surgical intervention known as a *cerclage.* It's usually performed around the 13-week mark of pregnancy. With a cerclage, the cervix is sewn shut to prevent premature birth.

Treating an inflamed cervix

Cervicitis refers to an inflamed cervix, usually caused by the same organisms that cause a sexually transmitted infection (STI). Other causes include instruments used for birth control and foreign objects that may be placed in the vagina, such as tampons.

Initial symptoms can be nonspecific and include dysuria, dyspareunia, pelvic irritation, and pruritus in the affected area. Left untreated, cervicitis can lead to *pelvic inflammatory disease* (PID).

You diagnose cervicitis by doing a pelvic examination. You're assessing for cervical motion tenderness (the "chandelier sign"). You also do a Pap smear to assess for cervical cancer, and test for *Chlamydia/Gonococcus* and other causes of STIs. As always, you need to assess for high-risk behaviors and keep HIV in the back of your mind.

Sorting out sexually transmitted infections

Vaginitis, urethritis, and cervicitis can all be symptoms of a sexually transmitted infection (STI). Additionally, each STI has symptoms that are unique to the specific condition. Realize that STIs can be a cause of pelvic inflammatory disease (PID) if left untreated. This can manifest in several forms, including *salpingitis* (inflammation of the Fallopian tubes) and tuboovarian abscess. Pelvic inflammatory disease increases the risk of infertility big time. Here are some STIs to know for the test. We discuss a few others, such as syphilis and HIV, in Chapter 19.

Trichomoniasis

Trichomoniasis is caused by the single-celled protozoa *Trichomonas vaginalis*, a bacterium that can also cause cervicitis, vaginitis, and urethritis. The classic description of trichomoniasis is the presence of a frothy, yellowish-green vaginal discharge. Punctate hemorrhages may be visible on the vagina and cervix ("strawberry cervix"). The treatment is metronidazole (Flagyl). Both the affected woman and her partner should be treated, even if the partner isn't exhibiting any symptoms.

Gonorrhea and chlamydia

Gonorrhea is a common STI that can produce symptoms in both men and women. Common symptoms include burning, a vaginal discharge (urethral discharge in men), and cervicitis or an inflamed penile area. There also can be the urinary symptoms of dysuria, urgency, and frequency.

The key to diagnosis is to obtain a urethral swab in men or a cervical culture in women. A Gram stain is often done, although you can also do specialized DNA testing to test for *Neisseria gonorrhea.* The high-yield test-taking phrase is "Gram-negative intracellular diplococci." The treatment for gonorrhea is usually 1 g of ceftriaxone (Rocephin), which can be given intramuscularly.

Many people who have gonococcus also have concomitant infection with *Chlamydia trachomatis*. In addition to ceftriaxone, there two treatment regimens that are used for *Chlamydia:* a single 1 g dose of azithromycin (Zithromax) or a 7-day course of doxycycline (Vibramycin), taken twice a day.

Gonococcus can affect other areas of the body as well, especially if left untreated. These conditions can include gonococcal pharyngitis and arthritis. A person may also have a disseminated gonococcal infection, which in rare cases can be a cause of meningitis.

Human papillomavirus

Human papillomavirus (HPV) is associated with unprotected sexual relations. Complications of cervical dysplasia occur in young women, and rectal cancer may occur in both men and women. The virus is a cause of genital warts.

You need to be aware of certain serotypes because some types of HPV put the affected woman at increased risk of developing cervical cancer. Here are the serotypes commonly asked about on tests:

- HPV serotypes 6 and 11 increase the formation of condyloma acuminata, or genital warts.
- HPV serotypes 16, 18, and 31 increase the risk of developing cervical cancer.

Gardasil is a vaccination that women and men can get in their early teen years to mid-20s to help prevent acquiring certain cancer-causing HPV serotypes. The diagnosis of human papillomavirus can be confirmed by Pap smear.

Understanding cervical dysplasia and carcinoma

You need to be aware of cervical cancer screening as well as the cancer's evaluation and management. *Cervical dysplasia* refers to premalignant changes that require very close follow-up. Cervical dysplasia and cervical cancer are caused by the human papillomavirus (HPV).

Cervical cancer usually occurs in younger women. Risk factors for the development of cervical cancer include multiple sexual partners, sex at a younger age, and HIV.

Diethylstilbestrol (DES) is a synthetic estrogen used years ago to prevent miscarriage. Women who were exposed to DES in-utero have a dramatically increased risk of developing cervical or vaginal cancer. The histology is clear cell adenocarcinoma. Given the number of women in the 1950s–1970s who were given this medication, you'll likely see a test question on this aspect.

Many times, the woman has no symptoms to signal that cervical cancer may be present. Some symptoms are nonspecific and can include vaginal discharge and vaginal bleeding.

Here are the screening recommendations for cervical cancer:

✔ All women should get a Pap smear every 3 years, starting at age 21.

✔ Women over the age of 65 don't need to be tested anymore if their three most recent Pap smear results were normal.

Order a colposcopy if the Pap smear gives you concern for dysplasia or atypical cells. After the colposcopy, depending on the results of the biopsy findings, additional procedures may be necessary. One option includes the loop electrosurgical excision procedure (LEEP).

Reviewing Vulvas and Vaginas

In this section, you read about infections, tissues that enter the vaginal canal when they shouldn't, and cancer that affects the vulva.

Treating vaginal infections

Bacterial vaginosis (BV) is caused by bacterial overgrowth, most commonly *Gardnerella vaginalis.* The main tipoff for bacterial vaginosis is the presence of a thin, grayish white discharge that smells "fishy" with the addition of KOH (potassium hydroxide). Other high-yield test-taking tips include a vaginal pH that's greater than 4.5. "Clue cells" are present on the wet mount as well. The treatment is with metronidazole (Flagyl).

Candidal vulvovaginitis is a common form of vaginitis in women. Risk factors include diabetes and multiple rounds of antibiotics. On pelvic examination, you can see what looks like a "cottage-cheese" or "yogurt-like" discharge. The woman usually complains of severe itching. The treatment is one dose of fluconazole (Diflucan) 150 mg or topical antifungals like Monistat.

Recognizing protrusions: Things ending in -cele

Besides uterine prolapse, which we discuss earlier in the chapter, two medical conditions that can affect the vagina are the rectocele and the cystocele. The *rectocele* is rectal tissue that protrudes into the vaginal wall. A *cystocele* is a weakness in the pelvic structures that causes the bladder to protrude into the vaginal wall.

Risk factors for these conditions include multiple pregnancies as well as prior pelvic surgeries. Each of these, over time, can cause a weakening of the pelvic floor musculature. Treatment includes the use of a pessary and Kegel exercises. Surgery is indicated in severe cases.

Visiting cancer of the vulva

The most common presenting symptom of cancer of the vulva is a lump or sore on the vulva that causes pruritus or is painful. Another presenting symptom can be acyclic vaginal bleeding. Risk factors include age as well as having a history of multiple sex partners or prior HPV infection. Tobacco use is a risk factor, as it is for nearly every type of cancer.

The workup includes a pelvic examination. If you suspect a lesion of being cancerous, you further examine the lesion with a colposcopy. The treatment is mainly surgical, although chemotherapy and radiation may be done as well.

Managing the Normal Pregnancy

Pregnancy is an important topic for PANCE questions. In this section, you read about the standard of care for pregnant women as well as about normal labor and delivery. Later in the chapter, we address some of the complications that can occur during pregnancy.

Understanding prenatal screening

You can find many guidelines for prenatal screening. For the PANCE, think of the screening recommendations in terms of each trimester of the pregnancy. The focus is on the big-ticket items, such as screening for Down syndrome. If the pregnancy is high-risk (because of advanced age, significant family history, and so on), a closer follow-up with an OB/GYN is needed, but here's a general rundown of prenatal screenings by gestation week:

✔ **Initial visit:** The initial visit to the obstetrician is a complex one, which includes a thorough history and physical. Start the woman on folic acid/prenatal vitamins if she's not taking them already, because they reduce the fetus's risk of neural tube defects like spina bifida.

  After the initial visit, assuming that she has an uncomplicated pregnancy, you usually schedule follow-up visits at 4-week intervals until 28 weeks, at 2- to 3-week intervals between 28 and 36 weeks, and weekly thereafter.

✔ **At 10 to 12 weeks gestation:** If the parents have a family history of certain genetic disorders, you may do a chorionic villus sampling (CVS) to look for chromosomal or genetic disorders in the fetus. The chorionic villus sampling doesn't look for neural tube defects, which is done with an amniocentesis.

✔ **At 14 to 18 weeks gestation:** Order a genetic screen, often referred to as a *triple screen*. It includes testing for alpha-fetoprotein (AFP), β-hCG, and estradiol (E2):

  • **AFP:** Low levels of AFP may mean that the fetus is at risk of developing Down syndrome. AFP levels may be elevated for a number of reasons; elevated levels are associated with spina bifida.

  • **β-hCG:** Low hCG levels indicate a risk that the fetus may develop Trisomy 18 (T18).

  • **Estradiol:** Low levels of estradiol increase the risk of developing Down syndrome and/or Trisomy 18.

  Perform an amniocentesis between 15 to 18 weeks if you find an abnormality on the triple screen, such as high levels of AFP in the maternal serum. An amniocentesis allows you to further evaluate the fetal amniotic fluid. An older maternal age is another indication to have an amniocentesis performed.

✔ **At 20 weeks gestation:** You'll usually have ordered a fetal ultrasound to look at Junior and to make sure all the parts are intact and that they're developing okay.

✔ **At 24 to 28 weeks gestation:** Rh testing is done. If the mom is Rh negative and hasn't been previously sensitized, then give her Rh immune globulin (RhoGAM). The oral glucose tolerance test is given during this time to screen for gestational diabetes (see the later section "Watching gestational diabetes").

✔ **At 35 to 37 weeks gestation:** Testing for Group B *Strep* via vaginal culture occurs late in the third trimester, between 35 and 37 weeks of gestation — just prior to expected delivery.

Moving through the stages of labor and delivery

Labor and delivery (L&D) is the process by which the baby (along with the placenta) comes out of the mom. Labor and delivery involves four stages, which you see in Table 9-1.

Table 9-1	Stages of Labor and Delivery	
Stage	**Beginning**	**End**
1	The stork arrives (okay, actually the first stage begins when the cervix begins to dilate)	Full cervical dilation
2	Full dilation of the cervix	Delivery of the baby
3	After delivery of the baby	Delivery of the placenta
4	After delivery of the placenta	Immediate postpartum period

Dealing with Pregnancy Complications

All is well when the pregnancy proceeds normally without any complications. Unfortunately, complications can and do happen in pregnancy. In this section, you read about some of these conditions, from uncontrolled hypertension to emergent bleeding disorders.

Gestational bleeding problems

Three bleeding-related complications that can occur include placenta previa, abruptio placentae, and post-partum hemorrhage.

Placenta previa

Placenta previa is an uncommon cause of bleeding that's potentially life-threatening to both mom and baby. In this condition, the placenta is located at the lowest part of the uterus and covers much of the cervix. The initial presentation is painless bleeding that occurs late in the second trimester. This condition is diagnosed by a pelvic ultrasound.

Sometimes placenta previa can simply be watched to see whether the affected placenta migrates up the uterine wall. Cesarean section is the preferred method of delivering the infant before the onset of labor in cases of placenta previa. In emergent cases where you see evidence of fetal distress, a C-section is done.

This condition increases the risk of sepsis and bleeding post-partum.

Abruptio placentae

Abruptio placentae is a life-threatening medical condition for both mother and fetus. Here, the placenta detaches from the uterus before delivery. This condition presents with acute abdominal and back pain, as well as vaginal bleeding. There are different grades of abruptio placentae, but its most severe form involves significant hemorrhage. Other symptoms include significant uterine contractions, which can harm the fetus.

Aggressive volume resuscitation and transfusion of blood and/or blood products (to correct any underlying coagulopathy) is vital. If the fetus is still viable, a C-section may be done.

Postpartum hemorrhage

Postpartum hemorrhage, which occurs after delivery, is defined as more than 0.5 L of blood loss following a spontaneous vaginal delivery. If the mother had a C-section, then double that amount, 1.0 L, is considered to be significant blood loss. Postpartum bleeding has many causes, but the most common one is *uterine atony:* The uterus fails to fully contract after delivery of the baby.

If the uterus isn't contracting, you first massage the uterus to enable it to contract. Treatment then includes volume and blood resuscitation, as well as correcting any underlying coagulopathy. If this doesn't help, then emergent surgical intervention, including hysterectomy, is warranted.

Ectopic pregnancy: Attaching in the wrong place

Sometimes when a sperm sweeps an egg off its feet and the two make a home together, they set up house in the wrong neighborhood.

Ectopic pregnancy is a pregnancy outside of the uterus. The most common place for an ectopic pregnancy to occur in the ampullary portion of the Fallopian tube, and the next most common place is in the abdominal area. Ectopic pregnancy is a potentially life-threatening situation for the mother if it's not treated emergently. The embryo will not survive. Risk factors include tobacco use, advancing maternal age, and a history of pelvic inflammatory disease.

Common presenting symptoms include acute onset lower-quadrant abdominal pain with elevated β-hCG. Other signs can include bleeding, especially vaginal bleeding. The diagnosis is confirmed by an ultrasound.

Treatment of an ectopic pregnancy can be either medical or surgical. Methotrexate (Rheumatrex) has been used in the treatment of an ectopic pregnancy, because it can end the pregnancy. If medical treatment isn't warranted, then she needs emergent surgical intervention.

Sharing spaces with tumors: Gestational trophoblastic disease

Sometimes the fetus winds up sharing the uterus with unexpected tumors. *Gestational trophoblastic disease* (GTD) refers to abnormal cells growing in the uterus that form a mass. They form grapelike clusters and can form a *hydatidiform mole,* which is not malignant. The usual presentation is vaginal bleeding late in the second trimester.

On examination, the fundal height of the uterus is a lot higher than you'd expect for gestational age. In addition, the β-hCG level is super high. The mother can also present with symptoms reminiscent of hyperthyroidism. You can see "grape-like clusters" on the ultrasound; however, tissue is required to make a diagnosis.

Treatment, which is always necessary, is evacuation of the pregnancy. Suction curettage is the preferred method.

A *choriocarcinoma* is a form of GTD that is a rapid-growing, intrauterine malignancy. Presenting symptoms can include uterine swelling, vaginal bleeding, and abdominal pain. Physical examination can reveal uneven swelling of the uterus. Like a hydatidiform mole, the serum β-hCG is super high. The mainstay of treatment is usually chemotherapy.

Treating blood pressure problems in pregnancy

Hypertension frequently occurs during pregnancy. You need to be able to diagnose and tell the difference between pre-eclampsia and gestational hypertension:

✔ **Pre-eclampsia:** In pre-eclampsia, hypertension arises and you see significant proteinuria on or after the 20th week of gestation. The blood pressure is usually greater than 140/90 mmHg and as high as 160/110 mmHg. The proteinuria needs to be in excess of 300 mg/dL in a 24-hour period for pre-eclampsia to be diagnosed. There can also be increased serum uric acid and lactate dehydrogenase (LDH) levels.

✔ **Gestational hypertension:** Gestational hypertension, or pregnancy-induced hypertension, is high blood pressure that occurs after the 20th week of pregnancy without proteinuria being present.

The gold standard of treatment for pre-eclampsia is delivery of the fetus via C-section. If this can't be done, the patient needs to be closely monitored, sometimes in the hospital. Medications that can help control blood pressure during pregnancy for both pre-eclampsia and gestational hypertension — that is, meds that aren't toxic to the fetus — include methyldopa (Aldomet), labetalol (Normodyne), hydralazine (Apresoline), and amlodipine (Norvasc).

Potential complications of pre-eclampsia include the following:

✔ **Eclampsia:** Eclampsia is a bad, bad complication characterized by seizures. Patients with pre-eclampsia are given magnesium sulfate for eclampsia prophylaxis. The treatment of choice is delivery of the baby via an emergent C-section.

✔ **HELLP syndrome:** HELLP syndrome is characterized by hemolysis, elevated liver enzymes, and low platelets. It can also be associated with disseminated intravascular coagulation (DIC) and acute kidney injury (AKI). The treatment is delivery of the baby.

Watching gestational diabetes

Gestational diabetes is elevated blood glucose levels that occur during pregnancy, usually diagnosed by a positive oral glucose tolerance test. This screening occurs between the 24th and 28th weeks of pregnancy. In addition to the results of the oral glucose tolerance test, pay attention to the blood glucose levels before and after meals. If they're elevated, the mother may need insulin therapy in addition to monitoring the diet closely.

If gestational diabetes is left untreated, a potential complication is *fetal macrosomia*. This means that the baby is large and is at risk for complications such as *shoulder dystocia*. In this situation, the baby's head is deliverable but the shoulder is unable to move below the mother's pubic bone. Shoulder dystocia can be fatal because the umbilical cord can get squeezed in the process. A variety of maneuvers are done to try to squeeze the baby through, but often a C-section is necessary.

Touching on other complications

When a baby has Rh-positive blood and the pregnant mom has Rh-negative blood, the mother's body can make antibodies to the Rh-positive blood, leading to *Rh incompatiblity*. This is not good. A hemolytic anemia can develop. At its worst, Rh incompatibility can result in fetal death due to the buildup of bilirubin. An *Rh immune globulin* shot is given to Mom at the 24- to 28-week mark to prevent Rh incompatibility.

In the movies, you've seen where the mother's water breaks and she's rushed to the hospital. *Premature rupture of membranes* occurs before 37 weeks gestation. The treatment is the use of antibiotics to avoid infection. Infection can be a trigger for delivery, and the goal of antibiotic treatment is to avoid infection and forestall delivery. Depending on the estimated gestational age (EGA), the fetus may not be viable for extrauterine life, with the lungs being the last to mature.

Avoiding Unwanted Pregnancy

In your career, you'll be called upon to advise women about the "best" choice of contraceptive. This isn't an easy task, because there are at least 31 contraceptive variants. Here are some you should know:

- ✔ **Abstinence:** The most effective way to prevent unwanted pregnancy is abstinence, because even the best contraception isn't 100 percent effective. Of course, abstinence is honored more in the breach than the observance.

- ✔ **Condoms:** A condom with spermicide decreases the risk of pregnancy or STI compared to a condom alone. We're talking about a latex condom, not sheepskin.

- ✔ **Oral contraceptives (the pill):** The pill is a very common method of contraception. Oral contraceptives may be combination estrogen-progesterone formulations or progestin-only formulations, which contain synthetic progestins. A variety of formulations are available, and you need to discuss them with your patients on a case-by-case basis.

  Oral contraceptives work several ways to prevent pregnancy. In addition to preventing ovulation, they increase the thickness of the cervical mucus (blocking the uterine entry of sperm) and decrease the thickness of the uterine lining (decreasing the chances of fertilization).

  Be aware of the side effects of the oral contraceptives, specifically the ones that contain estrogen. They can cause hypertension as well as cholestatic-liver disease. In conjunction with the pill, smoking can dramatically increase the risk of developing a deep venous thrombosis (DVT) or a pulmonary embolism (PE).

- ✔ **Intrauterine device (IUD):** An IUD is an object placed in the uterus to immobilize sperm on the way to the Fallopian tubes and/or to prevent implantation. The IUD may be a metal (usually copper) type or a hormonal type. The metal type increases the risk of menstrual bleeding, but the big advantage with this type of contraception is that once it's in, it's in. Some IUDs can stay in for an average of 5 to 10 years. Who should not get an IUD? A woman in a committed, monogamous relationship who, already having children, doesn't want any more children anytime soon or who is not ready for permanent sterilization. Note that an IUD does not protect against STIs.

✔ **Diaphragm:** A diaphragm is a way to prevent fertilization. It may offer some protection against STDs; however, additional protection is recommended. The woman has to know how to put the device in its proper position with each and every episode of intercourse, and the diaphragm should remain in place for at least 6 hours after the last episode of intercourse. Using a diaphragm increases the risk of a bacterial infection.

Understanding Spontaneous and Elective Abortions

Abortion can be a very difficult topic to deal with and talk about. *Abortion,* which is the termination of a pregnancy, may be spontaneous or elective. On the PANCE, spontaneous abortion questions appear more often than elective abortion questions.

Spontaneous abortions occur primarily in the first or second trimester. The most common cause of a spontaneous abortion is genetic or chromosomal abnormalities; these typically occur in the first trimester. Other causes of spontaneous abortions include the presence of other medical conditions such as diabetes mellitus and rheumatologic disease. You may recall that the anti-phospholipid antibody syndrome is a cause of second-trimester miscarriages.

An elective abortion may be medically necessary, such as when the health of the mother would be at significant risk if she were to deliver the baby. In your clinical life, you'll need to discuss options openly and honestly with someone dealing with an unwanted pregnancy. Helping her understand all her options, including adoption, is important.

Practice Reproductive Medicine Questions

These practice questions are similar to the reproductive medicine questions you may encounter on the PANCE.

1. Which one of the following is true concerning the evaluation of ovarian cysts?

    (A) They are seen in polycystic kidney disease.

    (B) They are always painful.

    (C) They are a precursor to ovarian carcinoma.

    (D) They almost always need to be removed surgically.

    (E) They can be part of a syndrome that includes hypertension and diabetes.

2. Which one of the following conditions can present with fever, tachycardia, heat intolerance, and hyperdefecation?

    (A) Hypothyroidism

    (B) Hydatidiform mole

    (C) Placenta previa

    (D) Endometriosis

    (E) Vaginitis

3. You're evaluating a 65-year-old woman who presents with abdominal distention and bloating. An abdominal ultrasound confirms the presence of ascites. Which one of the following is she most likely to have?

    (A) Adrenal cancer

    (B) Renal cell carcinoma

    (C) Ovarian carcinoma

    (D) Cervical cancer

    (E) Liver cancer

4. The use of tamoxifen increases the risk of which type of cancer?

    (A) Breast

    (B) Ovarian

    (C) Cervical

    (D) Endometrial

    (E) Liver

5. Untreated hyperglycemia during pregnancy increases the risk of which one of the following?

    (A) Macrosomia

    (B) Spina bifida

    (C) Renal agenesis

    (D) Low birth-weight babies

    (E) Down syndrome

6. Which of the following is a risk factor for vulvar cancer?

    (A) Anorexia

    (B) Vitamin B$_{12}$ deficiency

    (C) Human papillomavirus

    (D) Epstein-Barr virus

    (E) Adenovirus

Answers and Explanations

Use this answer key to score the practice reproductive medicine questions from the preceding section. The answer explanations offer insight into why the correct answer is better than the other choices.

1. **E.** You see ovarian cysts with polycystic ovarian syndrome (PCOS), which is characterized by hypertension and diabetes as well as amenorrhea, obesity, and hyperlipidemia. You don't see them with polycystic kidney disease, Choice (A). Ovarian cysts can be painful but are usually painless, making Choice (B) incorrect. They aren't a precursor to ovarian carcinoma, Choice (C). They can be watched unless they cause significant pain, in which case they need to be surgically removed, so Choice (D) is wrong.

2. **B.** A hydatidiform mole is an example of gestational trophoblastic disease (GTD). It can present with symptoms that mimic hyperthyroidism. Choice (A), hypothyroidism, would present with the opposite symptoms, including cold intolerance and constipation. Choice (C), placenta previa, presents with painless bleeding. Choice (D), endometriosis, can present with abdominal and pelvic pain, especially around the menses. Choice (E), vaginitis, presents with a vaginal discharge. Depending on the type of vaginitis, a fever and pelvic pain may also be present.

3. **C.** With the presence of ascites in an older woman, think about ovarian cancer. Adrenal cancer, Choice (A), is very rare. The adrenal glands are common sites of lung metastasis. Renal cell carcinoma, Choice (B), can present with hematuria, and usually a renal mass is found incidentally. It commonly spreads to the lung and the bones, and it isn't known to cause ascites. You most often see cervical cancer, Choice (D), in younger females in their 40s. Liver cancer, Choice (E), can cause ascites, but the question says "most likely." In a 65-year-old woman with ascites, ovarian cancer is the first thing you'd think of and try to rule out.

4. **D.** The use of tamoxifen (Valodex) can increase the risk of endometrial cancer. It does not increase the risk of breast, ovarian, cervical, or liver cancer.

5. **A.** Gestational diabetes is associated with the development of a big baby (fetal macrosomia), not a low birth-weight baby, Choice (D). One significant risk as a result of macrosomia is shoulder dystocia. Spina bifida, Choice (B), is related to folic acid deficiency, which is why women of childbearing age need to take prenatal vitamins even before becoming pregnant. ACE inhibitors should never be taken during pregnancy because they can cause babies to be born with the congenital absence of kidneys, Choice (C). Down syndrome, Choice (E), is associated with advanced maternal age.

6. **C.** HPV isn't just associated with cervical cancer; it's also a risk factor for the development of vulvar cancer. Anorexia, Choice (A), is associated with electrolyte abnormalities and amenorrhea, not with vulvar cancer; obesity, on the other hand, is a risk factor for just about every cancer you read about in this chapter. Vitamin B$_{12}$ deficiency, Choice (B), is not a risk factor for the development of vulvar cancer; a deficiency of this important vitamin can have many effects, including neuropathy, diarrhea, and dementia. Choice (D), Epstein-Barr virus, is associated with mononucleosis, hepatitis, and an increased risk of lymphomas in the organ-transplant patient. Choice (E), adenovirus, is a viral cause of pharyngitis and conjunctivitis.

Chapter 10

Understanding the Genitourinary System

· ·

In This Chapter

▶ Understanding urinalysis and urinary abnormalities

▶ Considering kidney conditions

▶ Exploring the electrolytes and acid-base

▶ Touching base on prostate and testicle problems

▶ Looking at bladder and kidney cancer

· ·

The genitourinary (GU) system is composed of the kidneys, ureter, and bladder. Because the kidneys are one (really, two) of the workhorses of the body, we spend a lot of time on them in this chapter. The primary functions of these complex organs include filtering and eliminating toxins, maintaining blood hemoglobin and electrolyte levels, and regulating both fluid and acid-base balance.

In this chapter, you review high-yield points for GU system topics, including urinary abnormalities, acute renal failure, and electrolyte and acid-base balance. In addition, you review the myriad medical conditions that can affect all parts of the GU system, including the male sex organs (for information on conditions that affect female sex organs, see Chapter 9, which covers reproductive medicine). The GU system accounts for 6 percent of PANCE questions, and you might as well answer those questions correctly.

Although the GU system can be complex, it's actually pretty easy to get a handle on. Instead of trying to memorize thousands of facts, aim to understand basic principles and recognize key words or phrases in the test questions.

Analyzing Urinary Abnormalities

In many questions about kidney disease, the *urinalysis* (UA) can guide you toward the right answer. Abnormalities of the urine, especially hematuria and proteinuria, are typical question fodder on the PANCE/PANRE. Understanding such urinary abnormalities is vital in differentiating among causes of nephritis as well as in analyzing causes of kidney disease.

Using urinalysis

In evaluating any kidney problem — whether it's acute kidney failure, chronic kidney disease, hematuria, or proteinuria — understanding how to interpret a urinalysis is vital.

The urinalysis has two basic components: the dipstick and the examination of urine sediment under the microscope:

✔ **Dipstick test:** A dipstick is a urine test strip. It contains chemicals that react with a urine sample. When you look for abnormalities on the dip, you look for chemicals that react with the strip testing positive.

✔ **Urine sediment examination:** Abnormalities in the sediment include the presence of red cells, white cells, and/or different types of urinary casts. *Urinary casts* are a combination of a certain type of cell and Tamm-Horsfall protein, a protein made in the kidney tubules. For example, a red cell plus Tamm-Horsfall protein is a red cell cast, and a white cell plus Tamm-Horsfall protein is a white cell cast. You get the idea.

Here's how to interpret the results of the urinalysis:

✔ **The urine dips positive for blood:** Hematuria is present (see the later section "Handling hematuria: Blood in the urine"). Now consider whether red cells are present on the urinalysis microscopic:

• If red cells are present on the urinalysis microscopic, the differential diagnosis is huge and includes malignancy (bladder or kidney cancer), a kidney stone, kidney infarction, infection, and glomerulonephritis (GN).

• If the urine dips positive for blood but red cells are not present on the urinalysis microscopic, then consider the diseases associated with myoglobinuria.

✔ **The urine dips positive for protein:** Proteinuria is present (see the section "Watching for proteinuria"). The urine dip can be 1+ to 4+ for protein. Depending on the degree of proteinuria, this result can be a sign of diabetic nephropathy (if a person has diabetes), nephrotic syndrome, or glomerulonephritis.

If urinalysis is positive for both blood and red cells in addition to protein, then glomerulonephritis is in the differential diagnosis.

✔ **The urine dips positive for glucose and for protein:** This is an early clue that the person has diabetic-related renal disease or diabetic nephropathy. The next step is testing for *microalbuminuria,* in which the kidney leaks small amounts of albumin into the urine.

✔ **The urine dips positive for nitrites and leukocyte esterase:** You're dealing with a urinary tract infection (UTI). The urine sediment should also show *pyuria,* a predominance of white cells. A urine culture of > 10^5 is diagnostic of a urinary tract infection. Note that unless the patient is pregnant, asymptomatic bacteriuria is never treated.

✔ **The urine dips positive for leukocyte esterase and nitrites as well as a count greater than 50 WBC/HPF (white blood cell count in high power field magnification):** You're likely dealing with a classic presentation of a *pyelonephritis.* This patient will present with fever and flank pain.

Here are some other notes on urinary abnormalities:

✔ Hyaline casts can be a sign of dehydration. Another potential clue to dehydration is an elevated specific gravity. A reading of > 1.020 is a sign of dehydration, whereas 1.010 is close to normal.

✔ Squamous epithelial cells are not a sign of kidney disease; they represent a contaminated urinary specimen. The best way to avoid getting these cells in the urine is to obtain a midstream urinary collection.

✔ On a test, anytime you see muddy brown granular casts, think acute tubular necrosis (ATN).

✔ If the urinalysis is positive for red cells, dysmorphic red cells, and/or red cell casts, think vasculitis and/or glomerulonephritis (GN).

Pyuria means having white cells in the urine. However, the WBC can mean different things, depending on the clinical scenario:

✔ Think urinary tract infection (UTI) if the person has pyuria, the dip is positive for nitrites and leukocyte esterase, and the person has symptoms of dysuria and urinary frequency. Often, for a urinary tract infection to be present, more than 10,000 colonies of a causative organism need to be in the urine culture.

✔ Think acute interstitial nephritis (AIN) if the person has pyuria but the urinalysis dips negative for nitrites and leukocyte esterase and if the urine is positive for eosinophils.

You are evaluating a 25-year-old woman who is admitted to the hospital with a fever of 38.3°C (101°F), tachycardia, and left-sided flank pain of 24 hours duration. Urinalysis is positive for 1+ blood and 2+ protein, and it's positive for nitrites and leukocyte esterase as well. Microscopic evaluation reveals > 50 WBC/HPF. Which of the following is the most likely diagnosis?

(A) Acute glomerulonephritis

(B) Acute interstitial nephritis

(C) Pyelonephritis

(D) Renal infarction

(E) Diabetic nephropathy

The answer is Choice (C), pyelonephritis. The key to answering this question correctly is not only in the clinical presentation but also in the urinalysis. A finding of nitrites and leukocyte esterase on the urine dip as well as significant pyuria with a WBC > 50 in combination with the unilateral flank pain and fever is a classic presentation for pyelonephritis.

Acute glomerulonephritis, Choice (A), isn't the right answer because it almost never presents with unilateral flank pain. Also, with acute glomerulonephritis, the predominant finding on urinalysis is hematuria, which can include red cells, red cell casts, and/or dysmorphic erythrocytes.

Acute interstitial nephritis (AIN), Choice (B), can present with a fever, but it usually doesn't present with unilateral flank pain.

The classic presentation of an acute renal infarction, Choice (D), is an abrupt onset of unilateral flank pain. However, red cells are usually predominant in the urinalysis on microscopic examination. Other causes of unilateral flank pain (not included in the possible answers) include an acute hydronephrosis or a kidney stone. With a kidney stone, you'd expect to see primarily red blood cells on examination of the urinary sediment. (For details on kidney stones, see the later section "Eliminating Kidney Stones: Pass/Fail.") Diabetic nephropathy, Choice (E), can have proteinuria, but pyuria isn't a standard finding in diabetic nephropathy.

Handling hematuria: Blood in the urine

Hematuria, which means blood in the urine, is a very common clinical problem. Being able to evaluate this condition is important because the causes are many and they affect people of any age or gender. Not fully evaluating the cause of hematuria can have dire consequences for the patient — for example, you may miss a potential cancer or nephritis.

Hematuria can be gross (macroscopic) or invisible to the naked eye (microscopic). Microscopic hematuria is diagnosed by urinalysis, with blood dipping positive.

The key to answering test questions about hematuria is figuring out where the hematuria originates. The clinical presentation and urinalysis are vital in determining this. Ask yourself the following questions:

✔ **Is the hematuria coming from the glomerulus itself?** When the source of the hematuria is the glomerulus, the urinalysis dips positive for blood and, in most cases, protein. The microscopic examination can show red cells, dysmorphic red cells, and/or red cell casts.

✔ **Is the hematuria coming from somewhere along the GU tract (for example, the bladder, ureters, or somewhere in the kidney, as you might see in a renal cell carcinoma)?** Causes of bleeding where the urinalysis is positive for blood and the microscopic evaluation shows red blood cells include cystitis, kidney or bladder cancer, infection, or a kidney stone.

✔ **Is the hematuria due to another process?** *Rhabdomyolysis* is caused by any process that damages muscle enzymes, causing excess release of creatine phosphokinase (CPK) from the damaged muscle. Common causes include trauma or crush injuries as well as the side effects of medications, including statins used in the treatment for cholesterol. These muscle enzymes overwhelm the kidney and can cause acute renal failure, usually secondary to acute tubular necrosis (ATN). Treatment includes aggressive hydration, usually with intravenous saline.

Hematuria can occur by a mechanism where the urinalysis dips positive for blood but the urine sediment doesn't show any red blood cells. The urinalysis-dip false positive is due to the presence of the myoglobin. Rhabdomyolysis and intravascular hemolysis are two important causes of such hematuria.

Watching for proteinuria

Proteinuria, or protein in the urine, is the single most significant prognostic factor in determining the risk of future kidney disease. The cause of the proteinuria is important, as is the quantity of protein that the kidney excretes.

When evaluating a question concerning proteinuria, keep these points in mind:

✔ In a test question, tipoffs that proteinuria may be present include the appearance of frothy or bubbly urine and/or presence of edema seen on the patient's exam.

✔ Proteinuria is present if a urinalysis dips positive for protein. If hematuria is also present, think about glomerulonephritis or vasculitis.

✔ If a person has diabetes, screen for microalbuminuria by ordering an albumin/creatinine ratio. A normal level is 30 or less.

✔ Along with the amount of protein, the age of the person and the kidney function (indicated by creatinine level) are clues to help you figure out what may be causing the proteinuria.

✔ The first-line treatment for proteinuria of any cause is to use an angiotensin-converting enzyme inhibitor (ACE inhibitor) or angiotensin receptor blocker (ARB).

A test question about proteinuria typically concerns either what may be causing the proteinuria or what the first-line treatment should be.

Delineating proteinuria by degrees

If proteinuria is present on urinalysis, the next step is quantifying the amount of protein in the urine through a 24-hour protein collection or random/spot urine to obtain a protein/creatinine ratio. Here's how to classify the type of proteinuria:

- ✔ A normal protein/creatinine ratio is 0.2 or less, corresponding to 200 mg or less of total protein in the urine.

- ✔ More than 200 mg of total protein but less than 3,500 mg is considered *tubular-range proteinuria.*

  A cause of tubular-range proteinuria in teenagers and young adults is *benign orthostatic proteinuria.* This is tubular-range proteinuria in the range of 1 to 2 grams. It's purely positional: The protein is elevated when the person is sitting or standing but goes away when the patient is lying down. There's no definitive treatment for it — the proteinuria will go away as the person gets older.

- ✔ More than 3.5 grams (3,500 mg) of protein in a 24-hour urinary collection is *nephrotic-range proteinuria.* See the next section for details on nephrotic syndrome.

Tests may also tell you what the serum albumin is. A normal amount of albumin excreted in the urine in 24 hours is 150 mg or less. A normal albumin/creatinine level is 30 mg or less.

Identifying nephrotic syndrome (NS)

Nephrotic syndrome is an important clinical condition that you need to be familiar with. Among other abnormalities, a significant amount of protein is being excreted. Here are the four components of nephrotic syndrome; they all need to be present for the diagnosis:

- ✔ Greater than 3.5 grams of protein in a 24-hour urine collection (nephrotic-range proteinuria)

- ✔ Hyperlipidemia

- ✔ Edema

- ✔ Low serum albumin (hypoalbuminemia)

In nephrotic syndrome, the urinalysis shows only proteinuria, not hematuria (blood in the urine). This point is important because for the most part, the various causes of nephrotic syndrome differ from the causes of glomerulonephritis, which you review in the later section "Getting it about glomerulonephritis (GN)."

For PANCE purposes, here are the four causes of nephrotic syndrome you need to know:

- ✔ **Minimal change disease (MCD):** Minimal change disease is the most common cause of nephrotic syndrome in young children. Minimal change disease is also associated with certain cancers, particularly non-Hodgkin lymphoma, and with certain drugs like NSAIDs and lithium. The first-line treatment for minimal change disease is ACE inhibitors/ARBs and prednisone.

- ✔ **Focal segmental glomerulosclerosis (FSGS):** You can divide this condition into primary and secondary causes. HIV and obstructive sleep apnea (OSA) are common secondary causes. Again, the first-line treatment is ACE inhibitors/ARBs and prednisone.

- ✔ **Membranous nephropathy:** Membranous nephropathy is the most common cause of nephrotic syndrome in older adults. Membranous nephropathy can be divided into primary and secondary causes. Common secondary causes include lupus, hepatitis B, and solid organ cancers. On a test, a common complication of membranous nephropathy is renal vein thrombosis.

✔ **Diabetic nephropathy (DN):** Diabetic nephropathy is the most common cause of proteinuria and chronic kidney disease (CKD) in the United States. Here are some points concerning diabetic nephropathy:

- You screen for albumin in the urine by ordering an albumin/creatinine ratio. A normal level is 30 mg or less. *Microalbuminuria* is defined as an albumin level of 30 to 300 mg. A level greater than 300 mg is termed *macroalbuminuria.* You screen for microalbuminuria annually in anyone who has diabetes.

- The first line of treatment for diabetic nephropathy is using an ACE inhibitor or ARB.

- The goal blood pressure is < 125/75 mmHg for someone with more than 1 g total protein in the urine.

You are seeing a 5-year-old child in the office who presents with significant edema. The urinalysis shows 3+ protein but no blood. The serum albumin is 2.3 mg/dL. You order a 24-hour urine collection, and it shows 5 grams of protein. What is the most likely cause of proteinuria in this young child?

(A) Membranous nephropathy

(B) Focal segmental glomerulosclerosis (FSGS)

(C) Minimal change disease (MCD)

(D) Benign orthostatic proteinuria

(E) Transient proteinuria

The answer is Choice (C). Minimal change disease is the most common cause of nephrotic-range proteinuria in young children. Membranous nephropathy, Choice (A), and focal segmental glomerulosclerosis, Choice (B), represent common causes of idiopathic nephrotic-range proteinuria in older adults. Benign orthostatic proteinuria, Choice (D), is a distinct condition. It usually occurs in teenagers, and the range of proteinuria is usually in tubular range, on the order of 1 to 2 g. The child in question has nephrotic-range proteinuria, not tubular-range proteinuria. Transient proteinuria, Choice (E), is a temporary type of proteinuria that can present during illness, stress, or exercise. It resolves when the aforementioned problems resolve and requires no treatment.

Exploring Acute Kidney Failure: It Isn't Cute

Acute renal failure (ARF) (or *acute kidney injury* — AKI) is defined as an abrupt rise in the creatinine (Cr) level or an abrupt decrease in the glomerular filtration rate (GFR) from baseline. Common causes of acute renal failure that you'll be tested on include prerenal azotemia, acute tubular necrosis (ATN), acute interstitial nephritis (AIN), obstruction, glomerulonephritis (GN), and vasculitis. We discuss all these causes in this section.

Starting out simply: Prerenal azotemia

The easiest kidney-failure-related condition to diagnose is prerenal azotemia. With *prerenal azotemia,* the blood urea nitrogen (BUN) can be elevated (BUN/Cr ratio > 1), and the urinalysis is negative for blood or protein. You may see hyaline casts on the urinary sediment. Clinically, acute renal failure from prerenal azotemia improves with volume repletion.

In evaluating causes of acute renal failure, an important diagnostic tool (in addition to the urinalysis) is the *fractional excretion of sodium* (FENa). The kidney can detect subtle changes in perfusion, for example, secondary to volume loss (such as profound diarrhea) or gastrointestinal bleeding. In those situations, the job of the kidney is to hold on to all the sodium it can in order to maintain kidney perfusion. That's why in prerenal azotemia or volume depletion, you see a low FENa. Other states where you can see a low FENa include glomerulonephritis and certain forms of acute tubular necrosis (see the next section).

Analyzing acute tubular necrosis (ATN)

Acute tubular necrosis (ATN) is the most common condition of acute of acute kidney failure in the hospital setting. This type of acute renal failure is often diagnosed by looking at the clinical setting. You should recognize both the causes of acute tubular necrosis and what you can do to prevent the acute renal failure in the first place.

Common causes of acute tubular necrosis are shock, low blood pressure, dye nephropathy related to contrast studies, and medications, including chemotherapy agents like cisplatin (Platinol), the antifungal agent amphotericin B, and aminoglycoside antibiotics. Medications like these cause a *nephrotoxic* acute tubular necrosis. Acute tubular necrosis related to low blood pressure or low perfusion states is called *ischemic* acute tubular necrosis.

Important lab findings that can help in diagnosing acute tubular necrosis are the urinalysis and the fractional excretion of sodium (FENa). On urinalysis, the most common reported finding is muddy brown granular casts. In many cases, the urinalysis is completely normal. Most causes of acute tubular necrosis cause an FENa of > 3. The exceptions are contrast nephropathy and rhabdomyolysis, where it's < 1.

Contrast-induced nephropathy (CIN) is defined as a rise in the serum creatinine by 25 percent, or 0.5 mg/dL, which usually occurs 24 to 48 hours after an interventional study such as a cardiac catheterization or an angiogram. This is a common etiology of acute tubular necrosis in the hospital setting. Risk factors for contrast nephropathy include diabetes, volume depletion, underlying kidney disease, and multiple myeloma. The only proven therapy for the prevention of contrast-induced nephropathy is administering isotonic saline at least 12 hours prior to the intended procedure. N-acetylcysteine (Mucomyst) is an antioxidant that's also used in preventing contrast-induced nephropathy.

An important clinical distinction is the difference between atheroembolic renal disease (AERD) and contrast nephropathy. Although both can occur after an interventional study, there are subtle differences:

- ✔ Atheroembolic renal disease usually occurs several weeks after an interventional study, whereas contrast-induced neuropathy occurs 24 to 48 hours after an interventional study.

- ✔ With atheroembolic renal disease, you see digital infarcts (blue toes) and livedo reticularis on physical exam.

In a common test question scenario, a patient had an interventional study and now presents with acute renal failure. The time course is the clincher: If the acute renal failure occurred 24 to 48 hours after the study, the answer is contrast-induced neuropathy. If the kidney function worsened 2 to 3 weeks after the study, the answer is atheroembolic renal disease.

Assessing acute interstitial nephritis (AIN)

Many commonly prescribed medications can cause a type of inflammatory response in the kidney, leading to *acute interstitial nephritis* (AIN).

Recognize clues and buzzwords in a PANCE question that make you think of acute interstitial nephritis. For example, think about acute interstitial nephritis if you see antibiotics and acute renal failure together in the same question.

With acute interstitial nephritis, someone generally develops acute renal failure a few days after being placed on an offending medication — common causes are antibiotics, including penicillins and cephalosporins. Other medications that can cause acute interstitial nephritis are trimethoprim/sulfamethoxazole (Bactrim), fluoroquinolones (Cipro), proton-pump inhibitors (PPIs), and NSAIDs.

Pertinent physical exam findings for acute interstitial nephritis can include a fever, and sometimes a skin rash is present. Important labs are an abnormal urinalysis, including pyuria and urine eosinophils. Tubular-range proteinuria may be present. The key to treatment is to withdraw the offending medication. Sometimes prednisone may be used.

The triad of fever, skin rash, and eosinophiluria occurs only about 10 percent of the time in people who have acute interstitial nephritis. If the urinalysis is negative for any white blood cells or eosinophils, then even if the person has taken an antibiotic, acute interstitial nephritis is not your answer. Remember, pay attention to the urinalysis.

Getting it about glomerulonephritis (GN)

Glomerulonephritis (GN) is an inflammation of the *glomerulus,* which in essence is a network of capillaries responsible for kidney filtration. When they get inflamed, bad things can happen. Although glomerulonerphritis isn't very common clinically — it causes only about 3 to 5 percent of kidney disease in the United States — the condition is distinct enough to be terrific fodder for test questions. In addition, some types of glomerulonephritis can worsen kidney function quickly if not properly diagnosed.

Glomerulonephritis has myriad causes. The clinical presentations of glomerulonephritis can vary greatly, depending on the individual. There can be either macroscopic or microscopic hematuria. Proteinuria is almost always present, and the creatinine can be normal or abnormal.

When dealing with questions concerning glomerulonephritis, pay attention to two main points in the question:

- **What's the age of the patient?** There are distinct causes of glomerulonephritis, depending on the age of the person in the question. For example, *post-streptococcal glomerulonephritis* (PSGN) is seen in young children.

- **Are the complements normal or low?** *Complements* are pro-inflammatory proteins of the immune system that can be produced or consumed, depending on the medical condition.

To remember glomerulonephritis with normal complements, say "HI" to Henoch-Schoenlein purpura (HSP) and IgA nephropathy:

- **Henoch-Schoenlein purpura:** Henoch-Schoenlein purpura is cause of glomerulonephritis in a young person, who can present with arthritis, abdominal pain, acute renal failure, and purpura, usually on the lower extremities. The treatment is observation, although prednisone can be used as well.

✔ **IgA nephropathy:** IgA nephropathy is often preceded by a prior pharyngitis and can present with gross hematuria. The time course of the pharyngitis to the development of the hematuria is often a few hours to a few days.

If the complements levels in the blood are low (meaning they're being consumed), then think about one potential group of conditions that can cause glomerulonephritis. Causes of glomerulonephritis with low complements include the following (***Tip:*** Think S&M: two *S*'s and two *M*'s — strep, systemic, membranoproliferative, and mixed):

✔ **Post-streptococcal glomerulonephritis (PSGN):** This type of glomerulonephritis is seen in young children a few weeks after a strep throat or skin infection (for example, impetigo). The child has a low C3 level that will normalize after 6 weeks. Antibody tests used in the diagnosis of post-strep glomerulonephritis include antistreptolysin (ASO) titer and anti-DNase B titer.

Being able to differentiate between IgA nephropathy (IgAN) and post-streptococcal glomerulonephritis (PSGN) is high-yield on any test. With IgA nephropathy, the complements are normal, whereas they're low in post-streptococcal glomerulonephritis. Also, the time period between sore throat and glomerulonephritis is shorter in IgA nephropathy than it is in post-streptococcal glomerulonephritis.

✔ **Systemic lupus erythematosus (SLE) causing glomerulonephritis:** There are actually six different classes of lupus nephritis. They have low complements, and you can use anti-dsDNA antibody to help diagnose and gauge how active it is.

✔ **Membranoproliferative glomerulonephritis (MPGN):** You may see a scenario on the test where a young person has a low C3 that doesn't normalize after 6 weeks but rather stays persistently low. If so, think membranoproliferative glomerulonephritis. The answer isn't post-streptococcal because in that case, you'd expect the low C3 to normalize. Membranoproliferative glomerulonephritis is common in young people. In older adults, the most common cause is hepatitis C.

✔ **Mixed cryoglobulinemia:** A *cryoglobulin* is a protein that precipitates at cold temperatures and dissolves when the temperature warms up. There are three types of cryoglobulins: I, II, and III. For the purpose of glomerulonephritis, we're talking about Type II. Hepatitis C is a big cause of mixed cryoglubulinemia.

You are seeing a 16-year-old boy for hematuria. He had a sore throat 1 week ago, and now he has developed gross hematuria. Urinalysis is positive for 3+ blood and 2+ protein. His creatinine is 1.6 mg/dL. You order complement levels and note that both C3 and C4 are within normal limits. What is the likely diagnosis?

(A) Post-streptococcal glomerulonephritis

(B) IgA nephropathy

(C) Henoch-Schönlein purpura (HSP)

(D) Minimal change disease (MCD)

(E) Membranous nephropathy

The answer is Choice (B). IgA nephropathy is often preceded by a prior pharyngitis and can present with gross hematuria. The time course of the pharyngitis to the development of the hematuria is often a few hours to a few days.

In contrast, with post-streptococcal glomerulonephritis, Choice (A), the pharyngitis can precede the development of the glomerulonephritis by a few weeks. Another key point in this question is that the complements are normal. They're normal in IgA nephropathy but low in post-streptococcal glomerulonephritis.

Henoch-Schönlein purpura, Choice (C), is a cause of glomerulonephritis in a young person that can present with arthritis, abdominal pain, acute renal failure, and purpura, usually on the lower extremities. Like IgA, Henoch-Schönlein purpura also has normal complements.

Minimal change disease, Choice (D), is a cause of nephrotic syndrome in kids and does *not* present with hematuria. It presents only with proteinuria and/or the nephritic syndrome. Membranous nephropathy, Choice (E), is a cause of nephritic syndrome in older adults. Hematuria is not present in this condition.

Blood vessels of the kidney: Getting inflamed over vasculitis

Vasculitis is the inflammation of the small blood vessels of the kidney. The three causes of vasculitis that you'll see in some fashion on the PANCE are Wegener's granulomatosis, Goodpasture's disease, and Churg-Strauss syndrome. Recognize that because these conditions inflame blood vessels in addition to the kidney, they can affect other body systems as well.

- **Wegener's granulomatosis:** Wegener's granulomatosis is associated with the triad of sinusitis, hemoptysis (lung involvement), and kidney involvement (with hematuria, proteinuria, and kidney failure). It has a positive anti-neutrophilic cytoplasmic antibody (c-ANCA) more than 80 percent of the time. On kidney biopsy, it shows a "pauci-immune necrotizing vasculitis." Note that this is a key phrase you may see on the test to help clue you in to the diagnosis.

- **Goodpasture's disease:** Goodpasture's disease presents with both hemoptysis and acute kidney failure. It's associated with a positive antiglomerular basement membrane (anti-GBM) antibody. On kidney biopsy, Goodpasture's shows "linear deposition of IgG along the kidney basement membrane" — this is a key phrase you may see on the test. The treatment can involve steroids and cyclophosphamide (Cytoxan); in addition, plasmapheresis is used.

  Although either Wegener's granulomatosis or Goodpasture's syndrome can cause both hemoptysis and renal failure (the pulmonary-renal syndromes), a key difference is in the antibody tests.

- **Churg-Strauss syndrome:** The typical presentation for Churg-Strauss syndrome is an asthma that keeps relapsing after the patient has finished a course of treatment with steroids. Also, expect a very high serum eosinophil count. In addition to the kidneys and lungs, Churg-Strauss can affect the heart.

Obstructive uropathies: Obsessing about urinary blockages

Obstructive uropathies are very common causes of acute kidney disease, especially in the older male population. Understanding the basic approach to evaluating and treating an obstructive process is important. Here are a few general points concerning the causes and evaluation of an obstructive process:

- The most common cause of obstruction in men is benign prostate hyperplasia (BPH). We discuss this condition later in "Shrinking benign prostatic hyperplasia (BPH)."

✔ The most common cause of obstruction in a young woman is cervical cancer. In an older woman, think about ovarian cancer as the cause. We cover cervical and ovarian cancer in Chapter 9.

✔ You can diagnose an obstruction by kidney ultrasound (the most common approach), CT scan, or MRI.

If a test question gives you a scenario concerning acute renal failure in a patient whom you think has an obstruction, don't choose a CT scan with contrast.

✔ If you see a bilateral hydronephrosis on ultrasound, your next step is to have a Foley catheter placed.

As an imaging modality, the kidney ultrasound is important in a number of ways other than determining whether an obstruction is present. Consider the following points:

✔ If both kidneys are small, are echogenic, or show cortical thinning, think of chronic kidney disease.

✔ If one kidney is small compared to the other, the difference can be congenital (the person was born with a small kidney), unilateral renal artery stenosis, or unilateral reflux nephropathy (usually in a young woman with a history of recurrent urinary tract infections).

✔ If both kidneys are large by ultrasound criteria, think about HIV, diabetes, polycystic kidney disease, multiple myeloma, and/or amyloidosis.

Persisting about polycystic kidney disease (PKD)

Polycystic kidney disease (PKD) is the most common hereditary cause of kidney disease in the United States. It's characterized by cysts that can grow so large they can overwhelm the kidney and other organs, including the liver and pancreas. Here are some key points about this condition:

✔ Polycystic kidney disease is inherited in an autosomal dominant fashion. This means that if one parent has the condition, a son or daughter has a 50 percent chance of inheriting the condition. There's also an autosomal recessive form that affects very young children and can affect the liver big time.

✔ The diagnosis of polycystic kidney disease is confirmed by kidney ultrasound.

✔ If the blood pressure is elevated, the treatment is to use an ACE inhibitor or ARB.

✔ Polycystic kidney disease can affect the brain. Screening for berry aneurysms is important, especially if the patient has a family history of these aneurysms. Magnetic resonance angiography (MRA) with contrast is the diagnostic procedure of choice to diagnose the aneurysms.

Confronting Chronic Kidney Disease (CKD)

Chronic kidney disease (CKD) is a significant health problem in the United States. More than 31 million people have been diagnosed with chronic kidney disease, and the problem is getting worse. For both the PANCE and in practice, you need to be aware of the stages of chronic kidney disease, issues with anemia and bone health, and indications for dialysis.

Seeing the stages of chronic kidney disease

Chronic kidney disease has six stages, each more advanced than the previous one:

✔ Stage I means that the glomerular filtration rate (GFR) is okay but proteinuria is present. Even if the kidney function is normal, someone can have early stage kidney disease just by having proteinuria.

✔ Stage II means mild kidney disease with a GFR of 60–89 mL/min.

✔ Stage III refers to moderate kidney disease. The GFR is 30–59 mL/min. At this stage, you usually begin to see abnormalities in blood and bone metabolism.

✔ Stage IV is advanced kidney disease with a GFR of 15–29 mL/min.

✔ Stage V is advanced kidney disease with a GFR of 15 mL/min or less.

✔ At Stage VI, someone is on or needs to start dialysis.

Test questions often ask absolute indications for dialysis, which include the following:

✔ Fluid overload refractory to diuretic therapy

✔ A positive pericardial friction rub, which is suggestive of uremic pericarditis

✔ Very high potassium with ECG changes

✔ A toxic ingestion of a substance removed by dialysis; examples include lithium and the toxic alcohols (ethylene glycol, methanol, and rubbing alcohol) — see Chapter 14 for information on toxic ingestions

At which stage of chronic kidney disease (CKD) should a patient be seen for transplant evaluation and discussion regarding placement of permanent access for dialysis?

(A) Stage I

(B) Stage II

(C) Stage III

(D) Stage IV

(E) Stage V

The answer is Choice (D), Stage IV. Obtaining a transplant evaluation and obtaining a permanent access for dialysis (a fistula) are things that should be done at this stage of kidney disease. The first three stages are too early, and the last one is too late.

Understanding how kidney disease affects the blood and the bones

Kidney disease, unfortunately, doesn't exist in a vacuum; it affects the bones and the blood, too. A major cause of anemia in kidney disease is due to the kidney's decreased production of erythropoietin. You begin to see reductions in blood hemoglobin levels as early as Stage III chronic kidney disease (see the preceding section for details on staging).

Here are some test-taking points concerning anemia in chronic kidney disease:

✔ Other causes of anemia other than the decreased production of erythropoietin in chronic kidney disease include the three *i*'s: iron deficiency, inflammation (which can have a direct suppressive effect on the bone marrow), and infection.

✔ If the hemoglobin level is < 10 mg/dL, erythropoietin stimulating agents (ESA) are prescribed.

✔ Recognize that iron levels need to be adequate for ESAs to work. Iron deficiency is the most common cause of ESA resistance. The iron can be given intravenously or orally.

Concerning bone changes, you can begin to see changes consistent with *secondary hyper-parathyroidism* as early as Stage III. Bone disease in chronic kidney disease is important not just from a bone perspective — elevated parathyroid hormone (PTH) levels can have adverse effects on other organs, including the heart. In addition to an elevated PTH level, other changes include an elevated phosphorous level (the kidneys can begin having trouble getting rid of the extra phosphorous). In advanced stages of kidney disease, you may expect to see low calcium levels.

Here are some test-taking points concerning bone disease in chronic kidney disease:

✔ The pattern of secondary hyperparathyroidism in chronic kidney disease is high phosphorous, low calcium, and elevated intact PTH.

✔ For Stage III chronic kidney disease and higher, many patients are prescribed a low-phosphate diet and phosphate binders to bind dietary phosphorous in the intestine.

Eliminating Kidney Stones: Pass/Fail

Kidney stones (renal calculi) cause pain and hematuria. They commonly occur in young and middle-aged men. Here are several big payoff areas dealing with renal calculi.

Searching for signs and symptoms of kidney stones

Many kidney stones pass through the GU tract on their own. For a stone to wreak havoc, it usually has to be bigger than 5 mm. Here are two key points concerning the presentation of an *acute kidney stone flare,* also known as *renal colic*:

✔ The pain is rapid onset and is usually a unilateral, sharp, stabbing flank pain with radiation to the inguinal region (groin area) on the same side. The pain can be so debilitating that it makes a grown man cry.

✔ Hematuria, either macroscopic or microscopic, can be present. The urinalysis dips positive for blood and shows many RBC/HPF (red blood cells per high power field) in the microscopic sediment. The presence of gravelly or sandy urine is indicative of small crystals.

Diagnosing kidney stones with imaging studies

When evaluating someone with acute flank pain, you'll likely need to choose a radiologic modality to further evaluate the cause of the pain. You have these choices:

- ✔ **Radiograph:** A KUB (kidneys, ureter, bladder) radiograph can detect the presence of many types of stones, except uric acid stones. The radiograph cannot evaluate for a hydronephrosis or a pyonephrosis — you need a more definitive study for that. A radiograph is often used to follow the size of a stone chronically but has limited use acutely.

- ✔ **Renal ultrasound:** A renal ultrasound can detect stones higher up in the GU tract (that is, in the kidneys and proximal ureters) but can't fully evaluate the lower GU tract.

- ✔ **Spiral CT scan without contrast:** A spiral CT scan of the abdomen and pelvis *without* contrast is the gold standard not only for evaluating for kidney stones but for evaluating the whole GU tract.

An intravenous pyelogram (IVP) is currently much less popular for evaluating kidney stones because it requires the administration of contrast dye. Other techniques, such as ultrasonography, frequently provide similar or more detailed information. An MRI is not indicated.

Categorizing kidney stones by type

You should know about four types of kidney stones: calcium oxalate, calcium phosphate, uric acid, and magnesium ammonium phosphate (struvite). We take a closer look at each one in this section and include some specific treatment info. We cover general treatment in the next section.

Calcium oxalate

Calcium oxalate stones are the most common type of kidney stone. Patients with calcium oxalate stones often have elevated urinary levels of calcium and oxalate and lower levels of urinary citrate. Medical conditions that can be associated with these types of stones include the following:

- ✔ **Primary hyperparathyroidism:** Recall the triad of hyperparathyroidism: elevated serum calcium, elevated PTH, and increased 24-hour urine calcium.

- ✔ **Absorptive (idiopathic) hypercalcinuria:** The cause of absorptive hypercalcinuria is unknown, but experts think that the affected person has increased intestinal absorption of calcium.

Calcium phosphate

Calcium phosphate stones are the second most common type of kidney stone. You can see this type of kidney stone in combination with calcium oxalate or on its own. Here's the most common clinical presentation:

- ✔ It's common in young women.

- ✔ A nongapped metabolic acidosis is present.

- ✔ Hypokalemia is predominant.

The treatment is administration of potassium citrate.

Uric acid

Uric acid stones usually occur in acidic urine, with a pH of 6.0 or lower. Here are two big points about uric acid stones:

- ✔ Uric acid stones can be associated with other medical conditions, including gout, diabetes, obesity, and malabsorptive states such as chronic diarrhea and Crohn's disease.

- ✔ A uric acid stone is *radiolucent,* meaning it can't be seen via radiograph. Even Superman with his X-ray vision would likely miss a uric acid stone.

The treatment is hydration (as is true for all stones), alkalinization of the urine (to a pH of 6.5 or greater), and allopurinol (but only if a 24-hour urine demonstrates an overproduction of uric acid).

Struvite

The struvite kidney stone consists of magnesium ammonium phosphate. The usual presentation is a young woman with a history of recurrent urinary tract infections, usually with a urease-positive organism (urease produces an alkaline urine pH). You can also see this type of stone in anyone with altered GU anatomy or who has either a chronic Foley catheter or requires frequent catheterizations.

Treating kidney stones

Here's the basic treatment for chronic kidney stones of all types:

- ✔ Increase fluid intake to ≥ 2 liters (about 8 cups) a day.

- ✔ Where urine citrate concentration is low, increase it with potassium citrate.

- ✔ For calcium-based stones — all the main types except uric acid stones — prescribe a low-sodium, low-oxalate diet and add the diuretic hydrochlorothiazide (HCTZ) to lower calcium excretion.

If a patient has an acute stone attack, you're likely to be evaluating him or her in the emergency room. IV fluids and analgesics for pain are first-line. The results of a CT scan concerning the size of the stone indicate what to do next:

- ✔ If the stone is ≤ 5 mm, it should pass on its own.

- ✔ If the stone is > 5 mm, surgical intervention may be needed. The stone can be extracted via a procedure called a *ureteroscopy.* Extracorporeal shock wave lithotripsy (ESWL) can be used as well to break up the stones so they can pass.

Getting Excited about Electrolytes

The kidneys, of course, regulate electrolyte concentrations. If you work in a hospital setting, no matter what your specialty, you're interacting with patients who have electrolyte abnormalities, including abnormalities of sodium balance (hyponatremia and hypernatremia) and potassium balance (hypokalemia and hyperkalemia). In fact, these four electrolyte abnormalities are the most common ones seen in a hospital setting, especially among older people. This section covers high-yield points about abnormalities of sodium and potassium.

Hyponatremia: Not enough sodium

Hyponatremia is defined as a serum sodium of < 135 mEq/L and a serum osmolality of < 280 mOsm/kg.

Pseudohyponatremia means that the serum sodium level is < 135 mEq/L but the serum osmolality is 280–300 mOsm/kg; true hyponatremia involves a low serum osmality as well. Examples of pseudohyponatremia include multiple myeloma and very, very high triglyceride levels of > 1,000 mg/dL.

High blood glucose levels, as in diabetic ketoacidosis (DKA) or in a hyperosmolar state hyperglycemic hyperosmolar nonketotic coma (HHNKC), can cause a low serum sodium level with an elevated serum osmality that's > 300.

On a test question concerning hyponatremia, look at the serum osmolality and blood glucose first. If the serum osmolality is normal, think pseudohyponatremia. If the glucose level is high and the serum osmolality is high, the patient doesn't have true hyponatremia. Don't let the serum osmality trip you up on the test.

To further evaluate hyponatremia, the next two steps after obtaining the serum osmolality are to obtain the urine osmolality and to evaluate the person's volume status. In addition to findings on physical examination, the urine sodium level is important. After you've established that the patient has true hyponatremia, you assess the patient's volume status so you can identify and treat the hyponatremia:

- ✔ **Hypovolemic hyponatremia:** Think diuretics like hydrochlorothiazide, furosemide (Lasix), and decreased oral intake. The treatment is salt repletion, usually with intravenous normal saline. Diuretics often cause hyponatremia and hypokalemia together. The urine sodium in a hypovolemic hyponatremia is < 25 with a fractional excretion of sodium (FENa) that's < 1.

  If the urine sodium is obtained while the person is on a diuretic, it may be falsely high. For test-taking purposes, however, assume that in a scenario where someone has hyponatremia after taking a diuretic, the urine sodium level in the test reflects a volume-depleted state.

- ✔ **Euvolemic hyponatremia:** Think hypothyroidism, adrenal insufficiency, and the syndrome of inappropriate antidiuretic hormone hypersecretion (SIADH). The urine sodium is > 25, and the FENa is > 3. For SIADH, the first line of treatment is water restriction.

- ✔ **Hypervolemic hyponatremia:** Think congestive heart failure, kidney disease, and cirrhosis. The urine sodium is < 25, or the FENa is < 1. Although there's excess volume on board, the kidney isn't being perfused adequately, leading to low urine sodium levels. For congestive heart failure, the treatment is fluid restriction and diuretics. The same is true for cirrhosis and kidney disease.

On the test, you choose to give *hypertonic saline* (3 percent saline) to someone with hyponatremia only if the sodium dropped quickly or the person is confused.

Hypernatremia: Too much sodium

Hypernatremia is defined as a serum sodium > 145 mEq/L. It commonly refers to losses of water in excess of sodium. Here are two commonly encountered scenarios:

✔ A patient has increased free water losses and isn't getting enough free water replacement. Examples include a patient who has had a cerebrovascular accident (CVA) and isn't able to ask for water when thirsty or a person with increased insensible losses (from fever or diaphoresis) who isn't meeting his free water requirements.

✔ A person has ongoing urinary losses, perhaps from pure water loss (that is, diabetes insipidus), an osmotic diuresis (the effect of high glucose causing urinary losses of free water), or judicious use of diuretics like furosemide (Lasix).

In problems concerning hypernatremia, you often need to calculate a *free water deficit* and decide on the best type of fluid replacement. Here's the equation for calculating the free water deficit:

$$\text{Free Water Deficit} = \text{Total Body Water} \times \left(\frac{\text{Current Sodium}}{\text{Desired Sodium}} - 1 \right)$$

First calculate the *total body water* (TBW), which is the patient's weight in kilograms multiplied by the percentage of the body that is water. Depending on age and gender, it can vary from 50 to 60 percent. Suppose you're dealing with an elderly woman who weighs 72 kilograms with 50 percent total body water content. Here's her total body water:

$$\text{Total Body Water} = 72 \text{ kg} \times 0.5 = 36 \text{ kg}$$

To calculate her free water deficit (in liters), plug the total body water, current sodium, and desired sodium into the formula. The woman's current sodium is 154, and the desired level is 140:

$$\text{Free Water Deficit} = \text{Total Body Water} \times \left(\frac{\text{Current Sodium}}{\text{Desired Sodium}} - 1 \right)$$
$$= 36 \times \left(\frac{154}{140} - 1 \right)$$
$$= 3.6$$

The free water deficit is 3.6 L.

The type of fluid to give depends on the clues in the question. If the person has visible signs of volume depletion, including tachycardia and hypotension in addition to hypernatremia, he or she may require 0.45% saline. If the vital signs are stable, then you can replace free water only, using a fluid such as D5W. For the elderly woman we describe in this section, if her vital signs are stable, the logical choice is D5W.

Hypokalemia: Not enough K

Hypokalemia (a low potassium level) is a common electrolyte abnormality that can derive from a variety of causes, such as diuretics and diarrhea.

A great acronym for remembering the causes of hypokalemia is RIG:

✔ **R = renal losses:** This includes diuretic use, osmotic diuresis (from high blood glucose levels), and forms of renal tubular acidosis.

✔ **I = intracellular shift:** This means things that will push potassium into the cells. Note that the causes of hypokalemia in this category — intravenous insulin, albuterol nebulizers, bicarbonate, and so on — are also treatments for acute *hyper*kalemia, which we discuss next. Other causes of hypokalemia include B_{12} supplementation and filgrastim

(Neupogen). Filgrastim is granulocyte-colony stimulating factor (G-CSF) used to build up the white blood cell counts after chemotherapy in neutropenic patients.

✔ **G = gastrointestinal losses:** This includes vomiting, diarrhea, and malabsorption.

A low potassium level can have a detrimental effect on the heart. It can make the heart irritable and can predispose someone to cardiac arrythmias. On an ECG, significantly low potassium levels (less than 3 mg/dL) can cause widening of the QT interval. When the levels of potassium are very low, you can also see a U wave on an ECG.

If you're dealing with a potassium level that doesn't normalize despite potassium replacement, check the magnesium level. It's likely to be low, and replacing that will help normalize the potassium level. When replacing the potassium, you usually don't want to replace more than 10 mEq/hour

Hyperkalemia: Too much K

Hyperkalemia, defined as a potassium level > 5.0 mg/dL, can be very dangerous. High levels of potassium can cause significant heart problems. PANCE questions concerning hyperkalemia usually expect you to recognize the causes, clinical signs and symptoms (including ECG changes), and treatment of hyperkalemia.

Looking at causes and symptoms of hyperkalemia

Common causes of high potassium are advanced kidney disease, cell turnover states (hemolysis and rhabdomyolysis), adrenal insufficiency, and renal tubular acidosis (Type 4). Hyperkalemia may be caused by certain classes of meds, such as ACE inhibitors, potassium-sparing diuretics, heparin, and NSAIDs.

The symptoms of hyperkalemia can be nonspecific, depending on the potassium level. For levels ≤ 6.0 mEq, there may not be any symptoms. Higher than this, and the person can experience weakness, dizziness, bradycardia, and even syncope if he or she is having an arrhythmia. High potassium levels increase the risk of sudden death.

Here are ECG changes that can occur at higher-than-normal potassium levels:

✔ At 5.5–6.0 mEq/L, you may begin to see peaked T waves.

✔ As you approach 7.0 mEq/L, you may see widening of the QRS and widening of the PR intervals as well.

✔ As the potassium gets higher, you see further widening of all complexes until all form is lost. In some patients, the complexes widen so much you lose all sense of the complex and get the dreaded sine wave, which doesn't support a good prognosis.

Treating hyperkalemia

If the potassium is > 5.5 mg/dL or if peaked T waves are present on the ECG, then sodium polystyrene sulfonate (Kayexalate) can be given for hyperkalemia. This med is an osmotic diarrheal agent used to rid the body of excess potassium via the GI tract (and the patient has to deal with the taste). Sodium polystyrene sulfonate can take 3 to 4 hours to work, so it doesn't act quickly enough to lower the potassium if the patient has significant ECG changes.

If the patient has ECG changes, including QRS widening and PR interval widening, take the following steps:

1. **Give calcium gluconate intravenously first to stabilize the heart.**

2. **Give 10 units regular insulin and 1 ampule of D50 glucose intravenously to shift the potassium into the cell.**

An albuterol nebulizer also works to force potassium into the cell (via beta-2 receptor activation). However, it isn't as effective as insulin and glucose. Sodium bicarbonate is given intravenously as well, particularly if a metabolic acidosis is present.

Touching Base with Acid-Base

An important function of the kidneys is maintaining acid-base balance. Acid-base isn't as daunting as it may first seem. You just have to get back to the basics. Questions about acid-base are actually pretty easy when you know a few important principles.

Reviewing some base-ics

If you understand the three eternal truths of acid-base, the rest is a piece of cake. To make a determination, start with an arterial blood gas (ABG) and a blood chemistry (a basic metabolic panel, often referred to as the CHEM-7). Then look at the three maxims:

✔ A normal pH means the patient has either of the following:

- A normal blood gas

- Two completely separate acid-base disorders

✔ You can never compensate to a normal pH; it's impossible to do physiologically.

✔ The kidney compensates for the lung, and the lung normally compensates for the kidney.

Interpreting the arterial blood gas results

You can evaluate the ABG using the following three steps:

1. **Look at the pH.**

   A pH > 7.4 is a sign of an alkalosis. When you see this pH, you can already eliminate respiratory and metabolic acidosis from your choices.

2. **Calculate the anion gap.**

   The *anion gap* represents the difference between the unmeasured anions and unmeasured cations. You calculate it by taking the sodium minus the sum of the chloride and bicarbonate:

   $$\text{Anion gap} = Na^+ - (Cl^- + HCO_3^-)$$

   A normal anion gap is usually ≥ 12. An elevated anion gap clues you in that a metabolic acidosis is present.

3. **Identify the primary disorder.**

   Say the patient in question has an alkalosis. Now you need to figure out whether the alkalosis is respiratory or metabolic. Look at the bicarbonate level. If it's elevated (for example, 35 mEq/L), the combination of an elevated bicarbonate level plus a pH > 7.4 points to a metabolic alkalosis.

Table 10-1 gives you the rundown on four acid-base disorders.

Table 10-1		Classifying Acid-Base Disorders	
Condition	*pH*	*ABG and Ions*	*Causes*
Respiratory alkalosis	pH > 7.4	Low pCO_2 level	Hypoxemia (pneumonia, pulmonary embolism, or congestive heart failure), pain, anxiety, liver disease, early Gram-negative sepsis, and pregnancy (physiologic)
Respiratory acidosis	pH < 7.4	Elevated pCO_2 level	Pain medications (opiates/narcotics), alveolar hypoventilation (the blue bloater), and neuromuscular disorders
Metabolic alkalosis	pH > 7.4	Elevated bicarbonate level	Vomiting, nasogastric (NG) suctioning, and diuretic use
Metabolic acidosis	pH < 7.4	Low bicarbonate level	For a metabolic acidosis without an anion gap, think **CRUD:** C = carbonic anhydrase inhibitor (Diamox), R = renal tubular acidosis, U = ureteral diversion, and D = diarrhea; for a gapped metabolic acidosis, think **MUDPILES:** M = methanol, U = uremia, D = DKA (diabetic ketoacidosis), P = paraldehyde, I = INH (isoniazid) or idiopathic, L = lactic acidosis, E = ethanol or ethylene glycol, S = salicylate

You are in the ICU and are asked to interpret the following arterial blood gas (ABG) findings:

pH	7.28
pCO_2	68
pO_2	65
HCO_3	28 (assuming a normal level of 24–26)

What is the acid-base disorder?

(A) Respiratory acidosis

(B) Respiratory alkalosis

(C) Metabolic acidosis

(D) Metabolic acidosis

(E) Normal acid-base status

The answer is Choice (A), respiratory acidosis. The pH is less than 7.4, which means you're dealing with an acidosis. The next step is to figure out whether you're dealing with a metabolic acidosis or a respiratory acidosis. The pCO_2 level here is elevated, which indicates the condition is respiratory. An elevated pCO_2 level and a pH less than 7.4 point to a respiratory acidosis. This is not a normal-acid base status.

Putting Up with the Problematic Prostate

The three basic prostate problems you should be familiar are benign prostatic hyperplasia (BPH), prostatitis, and prostate cancer.

Shrinking benign prostatic hyperplasia (BPH)

Benign prostate hyperplasia (BPH) occurs because the prostate gets so big it can block urinary flow by squashing the urethra. You see this condition in older men. Signs and symptoms include the following:

- Difficulty initiating urinary flow
- *Nocturia* (getting up several times a night to use the facilities)
- Straining to go and leakage after voiding (the dreaded dribble)
- Complete bladder retention if the blockage is severe enough

The treatment of benign prostatic hyperplasia varies, depending on symptom severity:

- Medical treatment can include alpha blockers like terazosin (Hytrin), tamsulosin (Flomax), and finasteride (Proscar), which inhibit the enzyme 5-alpha reductase.
- If the symptoms are severe, then urological intervention is needed, including a transurethral resection of the prostate (TURP).

Kidney obstruction secondary to benign prostatic hyperplasia is the most common cause of kidney failure in older men.

Not passing on prostatitis

Prostatitis, or inflammation of the prostate gland, can present with a wide range of symptoms. Know whether you're dealing with acute or chronic prostatitis:

- **Acute prostatitis:** Acute prostatitis is usually caused by a bacterial process, most notably Gram-negative rods. A man with acute prostatitis presents with shaking chills, high fevers, back pain/perineal pain, and dysuria/urinary urgency. Laboratory abnormalities include significant pyuria. You would *not* perform a prostatic massage. Give antibiotics quickly after obtaining a urine culture.
- **Chronic prostatitis:** Chronic prostatitis can be bacterial or nonbacterial. The nonbacterial form is thought to be a more inflammatory type of condition. This chronic form can also present with urinary urgency and/or dysuria, but it's less likely to have the toxic presentation of the acute condition. Chronic recurrent prostatitis that does not get better may require surgical intervention.

Prostate cancer

Prostate cancer is a common form of cancer among older men, and you usually see it in men older than 40. The most common presentation consists of difficulty voiding. Suspect the condition if you see an elevated prostate-specific antigen (PSA) blood test. On digital rectal examination (DRE), the prostate may be big or asymmetric. The medical practitioner may or may not feel a nodule.

The gold standard of treatment for prostate cancer is *prostatic biopsy,* which can produce important histologic information, including the Gleason score. The Gleason score, which gives you a sense of the severity of the prostate cancer, is somewhat subjective. The pathologist evaluates the biopsied tissue and assigns a primary grade for the most affected tissue area and then gives a secondary grade for the next most affected area. The grades go from

Gleason Pattern 1 to Gleason Pattern 5. The first pattern means that the cancerous tissue is pretty normal, and Pattern 5 means that the prostate glandular tissue itself is difficult to identify. This is not good.

The primary and secondary grades are added up to give a Gleason score, which can range from 2 to 10. Generally, the higher the Gleason score, the more aggressive the cancer is. Higher grades require consideration of more invasive treatment than do the lower grades.

In addition to getting the Gleason score, staging prostate cancer is important. Staging can include CT scans of the chest, abdomen, and pelvis as well as a bone scan. Prostate cancer commonly metastasizes to bone; on lab work, one big tip-off to this is an elevated alkaline phosphatase.

The treatments for prostate cancer can vary. They can include external beam radiation treatments or brachytherapy seed implants. Hormonal therapy can also be done generally in widely metastatic disease. Surgical options include removal of both testes and prostatectomy.

Investigating Urinary Incontinence

Urinary incontinence, a person's inability to hold his or her urine, can be awful to live with. Depending on the type and severity of the incontinence, it can affect the person's quality of life. You need to be aware of four basic types of urinary incontinence:

- **Functional incontinence:** This means that the person has some type of ambulatory dysfunction and can't get to the facilities fast enough.

- **Stress incontinence:** This refers to a loss of urine experienced during coughing or sneezing, Valsalva maneuver (bearing down), or any physical activity. It's very common in women. The treatment involves performing exercises that strengthen the pelvis floor (Kegel exercises).

- **Urge incontinence:** In this case, the loss of urine is involuntary and is not brought on by physical exercise. In men, benign prostate hyperplasia can cause urge incontinence — see the earlier section "Shrinking benign prostatic hyperplasia (BPH)." Other causes include any spinal injury or neurological disease. The treatment involves using anticholinergic medication that can help relax the bladder, such as tolterodine (Detrol) and oxybutynin (Ditropan).

- **Overflow incontinence:** With overflow incontinence, people complain of dribbling or leaking all the time. The affected person has a problem with the bladder detrusor muscle, and the bladder is always filled to capacity. Neurologic diseases or anything that can block the urethra can worsen the symptoms.

Don't give someone with overflow incontinence anticholinergic meds; you'll only make the problem worse. The patient may require chronic or intermittent Foley catheterization.

Testing the Testes and Surrounding Anatomy

A lot of health conditions can affect the testes. Not only are the conditions important clinically, but they're also high-yield for tests. From torsion to cancer to infection, be aware of these conditions. You don't want to feel like you've been kicked in the you-know-whats when you encounter testicle questions on the PANCE.

Tales of the twisted testicle: Torsion

Testicular torsion is a condition you wouldn't wish on your worst enemy. Here, the testis is literally twisted around the spermatic cord, cutting off the blood supply. Testicular torsion usually occurs in young males. Risk factors include *cryptorchidism* (an undescended testicle), which is also a risk factor for testicular cancer.

A typical presentation involves sudden onset acute unilateral testicular pain and scrotal swelling. You can use a Doppler ultrasound to evaluate for torsion. Testicular torsion is a surgical emergency because the blood supply is compromised.

Seeking testicular conditions ending in -cele

You should be aware of three terms ending in *cele* that affect the testes: hydrocele, varicocele, and spermatocele. *Cele* comes from the Greek word meaning "tumor."

- ✔ **Varicocele:** A varicocele is simply a varicosity within the spermatic vein. The most common presentation is a left-sided nontender mass. A classic description is that of a "bag of worms." It increases in size with positive intra-abdominal pressure and reduces in size with lying down or scrotal elevation. Ultrasound is the diagnostic test of choice, and surgical intervention can be curative if the patient feels pain or is infertile.

   The sudden appearance of a left-sided varicocele in an older gentleman should prompt you to evaluate for possible renal cancer causing occlusion of the spermatic vein. A right-sided varicocele warrants consideration of possible vena cava obstruction.

- ✔ **Spermatocele:** A spermatocele is just that: a mass that contains sperm. Spermatoceles are small and can be diagnosed by ultrasound. The usual treatment is just observation.

- ✔ **Hydrocele:** A hydrocele is a soft fluid-filled mass that contains the remnants of the tunica vaginalis. A hernia may also be present. The treatment can be observation or surgical intervention.

Hydroceles and spermatoceles transilluminate, whereas varicoceles do not. You may see this point in a test question as a clinical clue to diagnosing these conditions.

Priapism: Erections that won't go away

Priapism is basically an erection that's maintained for several hours, usually greater than 4 hours. This is a medical emergency, and it's not associated with sexual stimulation.

In any African-American patient presenting with priapism, do a hemoglobin electrophoresis to evaluate for sickle-cell disease, which can be a cause. Hematologic malignancies like leukemia and clotting disorders (thrombophilic states) can cause priapism as well. Medications associated with priapism include antihypertensives, antipsychotics, antidepressants, PDE5 inhibitors, and anticoagulants.

You direct treatment at the underlying cause. In many cases, this requires an emergency urologic referral, because priapism is a urologic emergency for decompression of the corpus cavernosa. In cases of sickle-cell disease, the patient needs IV hydration, oxygen, administration of a beta-2 agonist to the affected area, and exchange transfusions.

Evaluating erectile dysfunction (ED)

In *erectile dysfunction* (ED), the affected person is unable to maintain a sufficient erection in the face of sexual stimulation. This failure to perform can be psychological in origin, although a medical evaluation should be done, especially in a middle-aged or older man.

Common medical conditions can predispose someone to erectile dysfunction, including hypertension (because the side effect profile of many classes of antihypertensive medications includes erectile dysfunction), diabetes, hypothyroidism, low testosterone levels, high cholesterol, peripheral vascular disease, and tobacco and/or excessive alcohol use. Other causes include prior trauma, either to the affected area or any type of spinal injury or surgery that could have affected nerve supply to the area.

Sildenafil (Viagra) is a vasodilator used in the management of erectile dysfunction. The medication increases blood supply to the area. It can lower blood pressure, especially if it's given with nitroglycerin. In addition to sildenafil, other treatments for erectile dysfunction include treating the underlying medical condition. Counseling is recommended, especially for men in whom the cause may be less physiological and more psychological.

Inspecting for infection: The -itises

Common infections that affect the testicle and surrounding anatomy include *orchitis, epididymitis*, and *urethritis*:

- ✔ **Orchitis:** Orchitis refers to an infection of the testicular area, and the cause is commonly bacterial. The affected person presents with fever, pain, and swelling. An ultrasound can be diagnostic, and the urinalysis can show signs of an infection. The empiric antibiotic therapy for orchitis is similar to that of epididymitis (see the next bullet). Scrotal elevation is also recommended.

  Testicular torsion and orchitis can have similar presentations, so make sure you rule out testicular torsion. You can evaluate for torsion with an ultrasound.

- ✔ **Epididymitis:** Epididymitis is an infection of the epididymis. Infection spreads via the vas deferens. The onset is sudden, and the epididymis is swollen and tender to touch. The urinalysis can show positive pyuria.

  The treatment is specific, depending on the age of the person. If he's younger than 35, he gets ceftriaxone (Rocephin) and doxycycline for 10 days, because the etiology is epidemiologically more likely to be an STI, either gonorrhea or chlamydia. If he's older than 35, he receives ciprofloxacin (Cipro) for 10 days.

- ✔ **Urethritis:** Urethritis is the inflammation of the urethra. Pain with urination and urethral discharge are common presenting signs and symptoms. Urethritis is primarily associated with STIs in a male who is sexually active. The diagnosis of urethritis is made by obtaining a urethral culture (the dreaded swab). A urinalysis with culture and wet prep can also be obtained.

  The treatment of urethritis is primarily antibiotic treatment. This includes ceftriaxone (Rocephin) and doxycycline (Doryx). Remember the importance of treating the partner as well, if possible.

  The triad of Reiter's syndrome (reactive arthritis) includes arthritis, conjunctivitis, and urethritis. Balanitis (infection of the glans penis) may be present as well.

  If you see a multiple-choice question and both gonorrhea and chlamydia are choices, they'll often cancel each other out because both are the commonest causes of STI (after HPV), including urethritis. *Chlamydia trachomatis* is the most common cause of bacterial STI, followed by *Neisseria gonorrhea*.

Testicular tumors

Cyclist Lance Armstrong suffered from and conquered testicular cancer. Tumors of the testicle commonly occur in the younger age group. The majority of testicular tumors are germ cell tumors, the most common being a seminoma. They don't secrete anything, meaning you don't use the tumor markers β-hCG and alpha-fetoprotein to diagnose them. A significant risk factor for the development of a seminoma is cryptorchidism (an undescended testicle). Although patients with seminonas present with testicular enlargement, some present with no symptoms. Physical examination can determine the presence of a testicular mass.

If you suspect a testicular mass, look for signs of potential metastatic spread, including back pain and the presence of lymph nodes and unilateral lower extremity edema (lymphatic obstruction of venous drainage).

After diagnosing testicular cancer, staging is done, including a CT scan of the abdomen/pelvis with contrast. Treatment depends on the type of cancer. Seminomas are very responsive to radiation. Surgical intervention depends on the extent of tumor spread.

Considering Kidney and Bladder Cancer

Two conditions you don't want to miss are kidney cancer and bladder cancer. You need to be aggressive in your investigation of possible malignancy because, many times, it presents rather insidiously. Here we review the key points you need to be aware of concerning renal cell carcinoma and bladder cancer. Hematuria, which we discuss earlier in "Handling hematuria: Blood in the urine," is present in both conditions.

Reeling in renal cell carcinoma (RCC)

When you think about kidney cancer, the most common histological cell type you see is *renal cell carcinoma* (RCC). Although experts can't name a definitive cause, renal cell carcinoma is linked to specific risk factors, including the following:

- ✔ Cigarette smoking
- ✔ Von Hippel-Lindau (VHL) disease
- ✔ Acquired cystic kidney disease (This condition occurs over time. The cysts that form have a tendency to become malignant.)

Most of the time, the initial presentation of renal cell carcinoma is painless hematuria, either macroscopic or microscopic. Renal cell carcinoma is called the *internist's tumor* because internists often found the carcinoma when it presented the class triad of unilateral flank pain, hematuria, and palpable mass. The triad occurs in people with renal cell carcinoma less than 10 percent of the time, however.

The best diagnostic test for renal cell carcinoma is a CT scan with intravenous contrast. To trace a local tumor to the surrounding vessels, undertake a study to look at the blood vessels, such as a CT angiogram dedicated to the area or an angiogram of the renal vessels. The initial line of treatment is surgical (that is, nephrectomy). Depending on the area and degree of spread, sometimes a partial nephrectomy can be performed instead of a total nephrectomy.

Paraneoplastic phenomena associated with renal cell carcinoma include high calcium levels, polycythemia, and hypertension.

Beating bladder cancer

The two most common cell types of bladder cancer are *squamous cell carcinoma* (SCC) and *transitional cell carcinoma* (TCC), with transitional cell carcinoma being the more common.

Common presentation of bladder cancer includes hematuria, either gross or microscopic. Risk factors include smoking and certain jobs related to dye-making, rubber, or chemicals. The diagnosis is made by cystoscopy.

A history of recurrent urinary tract infections and catheterization points toward squamous cell carcinoma. The treatment is based on the degree of tumor invasion. Options for the treatment of bladder cancer include *intravesical* therapy (put into the bladder itself) such as bacillus Calmette-Guérin (BCG) instillation, surgery (cystectomy), and/or chemotherapy.

Practice Genitourinary System Questions

The practice questions here give you a sense of what to expect of PANCE genitourinary questions.

1. You're evaluating a 32-year-old man who was found on the ground after a drug overdose. It's not known how long he was there, but from the history, you suspect it may have been several hours. On admission, his creatinine level is 4.5 mg/dL. Urinalysis is strongly positive for blood, but the microscopic evaluation reveals only 0–2 RBC/HPF. Which of the following is the likely cause of hematuria and acute renal failure in this patient?

   (A) Wegener's granulomatosis

   (B) Acute glomerulonephritis

   (C) Rhabdomyolysis

   (D) Acute interstitial nephritis

   (E) Minimal change disease

2. You're seeing a 65-year-old man in the primary care office who presents with worsening lower extremity edema. He has a history of Type 2 diabetes. On physical exam, he has a blood pressure of 150/86 mm Hg. His albumin/creatinine ratio is 160. His creatinine is 1.2 mg/dL. Which of the following medications would you prescribe for treating this patient?

   (A) Lisinopril (Zestril)

   (B) Diltiazem (Cardizem)

   (C) Amlodipine (Norvasc)

   (D) Hydrochlorothiazide (Microzide)

   (E) Terazosin (Hytrin)

3. You're seeing a patient who will be undergoing a cardiac catheterization in the next 24 hours. He has Stage III chronic kidney disease (CKD) with a creatinine level of 1.5 mg/dL. Which of the following interventions should be instituted at this time?

   (A) Encourage the patient to drink plenty of fluids the night before the procedure.

   (B) Administer a dose of furosemide prior to the procedure.

   (C) Order intravenous normal saline and oral N-acetylcysteine (Mucomyst).

   (D) Rehydrate with an oral bicarbonate-based solution.

   (E) Administer a dose of hydrochlorothiazide before the procedure.

4. Which one of the following statements concerning post-streptococcal glomerulonephritis is true?

   (A) The mainstay of treatment requires the use of steroids like prednisone.

   (B) It is characterized by normal complement levels.

   (C) The glomerulonephritis occurs two to four days after the development of pharyngitis.

   (D) It is characterized by low complement levels that persist for months after diagnosis.

   (E) It is a self-limiting condition.

5. You're treating a 62-year-old man for benign prostatic hyperplasia (BPH). He has an American Urological Association (AUA) symptom score of 7, denoting mild BPH symptoms. He also has hypertension, so you elect to start terazosin (Hytrin). What would you advise this patient concerning potential side effects of this medication?

   (A) There are no side effects he needs to be aware of.

   (B) He should get up slowly and notify you if he has lightheadedness or dizziness.

   (C) He should call you if his blood pressure increases.

   (D) He needs blood work to monitor potassium levels.

   (E) He needs to watch for edema and constipation.

6. You are in the ICU and are asked to interpret the following arterial blood gas (ABG) findings:

pH	7.52
pCO_2	48
pO_2	65
HCO_3	33 (assuming a normal level of 24–26)

   What is the acid-base disorder demonstrated in this patient?

   (A) Respiratory acidosis

   (B) Respiratory alkalosis

   (C) Metabolic acidosis

   (D) Metabolic alkalosis

   (E) Normal acid-base equation

Answers and Explanations

Use this answer key to score the practice genitourinary system questions from the preceding section. The answer explanations offer insight into why the correct answer is better than the other choices.

1. **C.** The history fits the clinical picture of rhabomyolysis and muscle damage causing the acute kidney failure. Wegener's granulomatosis, Choice (A), is an example of a vasculitis that affects the sinuses, lungs, and kidneys. You'd expect to see red blood cells in the urinary sediment. With acute glomerulonephritis, Choice (B), you'd expect to see red blood cells and/or red blood cell casts in the urine. Acute interstitial nephritis, Choice (D), usually causes white blood cells, urine eosinophils, and/or white cell casts in the urine. Minimal changes disease, Choice (E), is a cause of nephrotic syndrome in adults and wouldn't cause hematuria.

2. **A.** Lisinopril is an example of an ACE inhibitor, which is the first line of treatment for proteinuria. The man in this question has diabetic retinopathy and neuropathy. He also has an elevated blood pressure and microalbuminuria, on the basis of his albumin/creatinine ratio. Concerning Choice (E), terazosin (Hytrin) would be a good choice if benign prostatic hyperplasia were present; however it's not the best choice for diabetic nephropathy.

3. **C.** The only proven therapy for the prevention of contrast-induced nephropathy is the administration of isotonic saline at least 12 hours prior to the intended procedure. N-acetylcysteine (Mucomyst) is an antioxidant that's also used to prevent contrast-induced nephropathy. Choice (A) is wrong because drinking plenty of fluids isn't as effective as intravenous hydration in preventing contrast-induced nephropathy. Giving a diuretic like furosemide (Lasix), Choice (B), would be counterproductive and could actually worsen kidney function. Oral-based solutions, whether they contain bicarbonate or not, haven't been proven to be of any benefit, so Choice (D) is wrong. You wouldn't want to give hydrochlorothiazide (HCTZ), Choice (E), prior to a contrast dye procedure. It would worsen kidney function.

4. **E.** Post-streptococcal glomerulonephritis occurs in young children, usually a few weeks after a pharyngitis. It's characterized by a low complement level C3 that usually stays low for 6 weeks and then normalizes. This condition is self-limiting and doesn't require steroid or other immunosuppressive treatment. Antistreptolysin titers (ASO) are elevated early in the condition, and anti-DNase B titers rise later on.

5. **B.** The patient is on terazosin (Hytrin), which is an alpha blocker. A main side effect of alpha blockers is postural hypotension, so the patient needs to get up slowly and notify you if he experiences any lightheadedness or dizziness. You may need to adjust the dose or discontinue the medication if the symptoms are severe.

   Alpha blockers serve double duty: They're used to treat both benign prostatic hyperplasia and hypertension. This medication won't increase blood pressure, Choice (C), nor is this medication a diuretic or ACE inhibitor, which can affect potassium levels, Choice (D). Edema and constipation, Choice (E), are common side effects of calcium channel blockers, not alpha blockers.

6. **D.** This patient has metabolic alkalosis. To understand this question, you need to understand the patterns of acid-base disorders. First, the pH is > 7.4, so you're dealing with an alkalosis. The next step is to figure out whether you're dealing with a metabolic alkalosis or a respiratory alkalosis. The bicarbonate level here is elevated, and an elevated bicarbonate level plus and elevated pH points to a metabolic alkalosis. So what about the elevated pCO_2? This is the respiratory compensation for the metabolic alkalosis. Remember, the pH tells you the primary process that's going on.

Part IV
Pursuing Primary Care, Pharmacology, and Behavioral Health

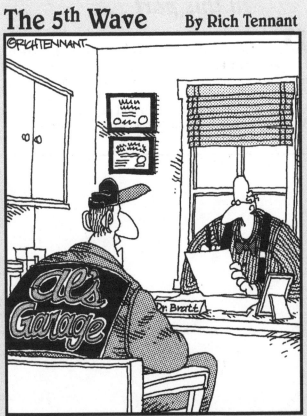

The 5th Wave   By Rich Tennant

"There's a 'thbump, thbump' when I walk upstairs, and then I hear a low 'ka-chink, ka-chink' going around corners, and I'm having trouble getting my horn to work."

In this part . . .

Part IV deals with special medical topics that are high-value for the PANCE — you can be sure that they'll be on the test. In four chapters, we cover pediatrics (Chapter 11), health maintenance and medical ethics (Chapter 12), behavioral health and psychiatry (Chapter 13), and pharmacology and toxicology (Chapter 14).

Chapter 11

Prepping for Pediatrics

· ·

In This Chapter

▶ Examining a newborn after delivery

▶ Knowing childhood milestones

▶ Looking at vaccinations for infants

▶ Knowing some pediatric medical conditions

▶ Understanding causes of child mortality

· ·

We sprinkle a lot of words about pediatric conditions throughout this book, especially in the cardiology chapter (congenital heart disease; see Chapter 3), the infectious diseases chapter (viral exanthems; see Chapter 19), and the pulmonary chapter (bronchiolitis; see Chapter 4). Here, we give you brief snapshots of pediatric topics not covered in other chapters. These topics should be high-value for the PANCE and PANRE.

Performing a Newborn Examination

After the third stage of labor, which is *delivery,* the baby needs to be examined. The first part of the general examination is getting a good look at the newborn. By *look,* we don't mean seeing how cute the baby is. We mean looking at the newborn with a medical eye. For example, does the baby have a good pinkish skin color? Is the baby premature or small in stature, or is he or she a good size? Does the baby have a good cry?

Pay attention to posture — not your own but the newborn's. The baby should have more of a flexed posture. Then check the newborn's body and reflexes, as we explain next. We also cover the APGAR score, which gives you a pretty good indicator of how the newborn is doing.

Examining the baby's body

After the general examination, start at the baby's noggin and work your way down:

1. **Check the newborn's head.**

   On the head, the child may have mild scalp bruising or mild scalp edema. This is normal and is often a result of the childbirth process. Also pay attention to the fontanelles.

   A bulging fontanelle can be a sign of a central nervous system infection (meningitis), increased intracranial pressure (hydrocephalus), or even a subdural hematoma. Note that crying can also cause the fontanelle to bulge. In that case, the bulging should go away when the baby stops crying.

2. **From the head, work your way down, focusing on the eyes, ears, mouth, and tongue. Then look at the neck, shoulders, and clavicles.**

   Here you're looking for symmetry. Any asymmetry can be a sign of a congenital problem.

3. **Do a good heart and lung examination.**

   Be aware that the "normal" for newborns and infants is different from what it is for adults. For a newborn, the normal respiratory rate is 40 to 60 breaths per minute, and the normal pulse is 120 to 160 beats per minute.

4. **Examine the abdomen.**

   On abdominal examination in a newborn, you should be able to palpate a liver edge (this isn't pathologic, as it is in adults). The spleen tip shouldn't be palpable. Concerning the umbilical cord, the normal anatomy is one vein and two arteries. The skin should be inspected for any lesions.

5. **Work your way down from the abdomen to the hips.**

   Concerning the hips, you want to be sure that the newborn doesn't have a congenital hip click. Hip maneuvers are likely topics of a test question.

   You can use Barlow's maneuver and the Ortolani test to detect a congenital hip dislocation. Usually, Barlow's maneuver is done first. It tests for hips that are original in position but may be dislocated out of position. If a hip click is present, then do Ortolani's maneuver as a confirmatory test. Ortolani tests are for already dislocated hips that may be put back in place.

Checking reflexes

The reflexes present in a newborn are pretty good to know for the PANCE. If these reflexes are absent, some badness going on, and you need to investigate more.

The sucking reflex is present at birth for obvious reasons. The grasping reflex is present as well. Put something in the hands of a newborn, and the baby will put his or her fingers around it and not let go. This reflex can last for several months after birth.

The *Moro reflex,* or startle reflex, is present in the newborn but goes away after a few months. Say the newborn is surprised or startled for some reason. The head goes back and the legs extend forward. The hands go up straight, almost like the baby is being arrested. You may see flexion of the thumb and digits, which then can become clenched fists. (Parents should be thankful that this reflex goes away after a couple of months. Could you picture a 16-year-old flailing like this?) If the Moro reflex is completely absent, it suggests possible damage to the brain or central nervous system.

Assigning a score: APGAR, Not AEIOU

An APGAR score is given to a child immediately after birth. The number indicates how well the newborn is doing at 1 minute and then at 5 minutes after the birth. You look at five factors:

- Skin color (should be pinkish)
- Pulse (should be 140 to 160 beats per minute)
- Reflexes

✔ Muscle tone

✔ Respiration (whether the neonate is having any breathing difficulties)

Although the score is named after Dr. Virginia Apgar, APGAR makes a great acronym: appearance, pulse, grimace, activity, respiration.

For each factor, the infant is assigned a score of 0 to 2. For example, if the infant's heart rate is less than 100 beats per minute, he or she gets a score of 1 for the pulse category. If it's greater than 100 beats per minute, the newborn gets a score of 2 for that category. No pulse at all merits a 0.

A total score of 7 or greater means that the infant is in good shape, and a score of less than 7 means that the infant is in trouble.

Reviewing Childhood Milestones

We remember our firsts — the first date, the first car, the first serious love interest, the first marriage, the first divorce. In the world of pediatrics, there are many firsts, and pediatricians call them *milestones*. Milestones are things that kids and infants should be doing at certain ages to show that they're developing well.

Any childhood development chart shows pediatric milestones at regular, defined intervals. Over the first year, milestones occur every 3 months. Here are very common developmental milestones from birth to 1 year of age:

✔ **At birth:** Newborns should cry and cry and cry some more. The bonding process with the mother begins at this time. Concerning body parts, newborns are unable to raise their heads by themselves.

✔ **At 3 months:** The kids become kleptos, grasping and holding onto anything put in their little hands. These babies cry in different inflections to indicate different needs.

✔ **At 6 months:** By the half-year mark, babies begin to make syllables. Now they can raise their heads and like to put toys in their mouths.

✔ **At 9 months:** Babies can sit by themselves. They can pick up objects using their fingers.

✔ **At 1 year:** They can stand with assistance. They can say two or three words at a time.

Other milestones occur at 15 and 18 months, and then there are annual milestones up to the age of 6. For details, we encourage you to look for a pediatric milestone chart in one of your textbooks.

Vaccinating the Infant

An infant needs a lot of vaccinations, many of which we cover in the pulmonary and infectious disease chapters (Chapters 4 and 19, respectively). In this section, we briefly review some of the vaccinations likely to be in PANCE questions.

✔ The MMR is the vaccination to prevent measles, mumps, and rubella. You can read about these viral exanthems in Chapter 19. A child receives this vaccination between 12 and 15 months of age and a repeat booster between the ages of 4 and 6 years.

✔ The *Haemophilus influenzae* type B vaccination, given between the ages of 2 and 6 months, prevents epiglottitis.

✔ The hepatitis B vaccine is initially given to newborns, with a follow-up vaccination between the ages of 1 and 2 months. A third vaccination is given at around 6 months of age.

✔ The varicella vaccine (against chickenpox) is given at 1 year, with a follow-up recommended before the age of 4 years. (*Note:* The varicella vaccine can also be given as a single dose for anyone over the age of 60.)

Reviewing Some Pediatric Medical Conditions

In this section, we review jaundice, rotavirus, Reye's syndrome, and other medical conditions specific to pediatric care that we don't cover in other chapters. They may appear on the PANCE.

Jaundice: Heeding the warning of yellow skin

You may see a question or two on the test concerning neonatal jaundice. The cause of icterus and jaundice in the neonate is the buildup of bilirubin in the body. This happens in most newborns and is referred to as *physiologic jaundice.* Very high levels of bilirubin can cause *kernicterus,* a type of toxic neurologic encephalopathy. The most common type of therapy for physiologic jaundice is the use of phototherapy (light therapy), which helps the bilirubin break down into metabolites that are easier for the body, especially the kidneys, to eliminate.

Reducing the runs: Rotavirus and diarrhea

The *rotavirus* is the commonest cause of infectious diarrhea in the pediatric population. People transmit it by touching stool and then not washing their hands. Then they contaminate everything they touch. Think about children in daycare. If you're a healthcare professional dealing with diapers and you don't wash your hands, you can become a mode of transmission.

The clinical presentation of rotavirus can mimic that of other infectious diarrheas. It includes nausea, vomiting, and (of course) diarrhea. The treatment is supportive, including aggressive intake of fluids to prevent dehydration. We cover other causes of infectious diarrhea in Chapter 19.

Infants can get a vaccine (RotaTeq or Rotarix) to prevent rotavirus. This vaccination is administered to babies beginning at 2 months of age.

Keeping up with Kawasaki's disease

Kawasaki's disease (also called *mucocutaneous lymph node syndrome*) is a rheumatologic disorder that can affect the heart. It's such a profound clinical syndrome that we include it in this chapter. You see Kawasaki's in a higher percentage of children of Asian descent. The initial presentation can include a very high fever for several days. In addition, the child may have a characteristic "strawberry tongue" and a skin rash. The rash typically begins as perineal erythema and desquamation, followed by macular, morbilliform, or targetoid skin lesions of the trunk and extremities. There's significant adenopathy. If Kawasaki's is left untreated, a possible side effect is vasculitis or aneurysm, especially of the coronary arteries. The treatment is prednisone.

Assessing childhood avascular necrosis

Legg-Calvé-Perthes syndrome (Perthes disease) is a form of avascular necrosis in children. No one's certain why it occurs, but there's a problem with the blood flow to the head of the femur. The clinical presentation for a child is similar to an adult's, where you see pain in the hip, the inguinal area, or even the knee. The child may present with a limp. You can make the diagnosis by radiograph, but if it's questionable, the MRI is a much better study. The treatment is to maintain strength and mobility in the joint. Extensive physical therapy is mandatory. Orthopedic surgery is done only when medical therapy doesn't work.

Preventing Reye's syndrome

One pediatric medical emergency that you can count on seeing on the test is *Reye's syndrome.* This clinical syndrome can cause liver failure and brain injury. It can occur when a child takes aspirin or other salicylate derivatives in the setting of a viral illness. Diagnosing Reye's early is important. In the worst-case scenario, Reye's can result in encephalopathy, coma, and even death. The key is prevention.

Keeping an Infant or Child Safe

Infants' and children's lives aren't cut short by heart attacks, diabetes, chronic obstructive pulmonary disorder (COPD) exacerbations, or strokes. Kids tend to die from congenital stuff, accidents, and trauma. Here's a brief overview of causes of infant and child mortality:

✓ **Newborns and infants (12 months of age or less):** The leading causes of mortality are congenital (hence the need for a really good newborn examination) and sudden infant death syndrome (SIDS).

Sudden infant death syndrome (SIDS) is alarming because no one knows what really causes it. Sleeping on the abdomen and exposure to secondhand smoke seem to be risk factors. The kicker is that there's no forewarning — people think the baby is just sleeping. Babies should always be put to bed on their backs or sides.

✓ **Ages 1 to 4:** The leading cause of death is accidents. Congenital problems run a close second.

✓ **Age 5 to the early teen years:** The leading cause of death is accidents. Homicide is also an important cause of death in this age group.

✓ **Teenage years to young adulthood:** Suicide is a big cause of death in addition to accidents.

Be aware of signs of child abuse and/or child neglect. Signs can include unexplained bruising or bite marks. In addition, the child may have problems in the classroom as well as a fear of others, especially adults. Don't forget to look for signs of depression and abnormal behaviors, including changes in eating habits and an unkempt appearance.

Practice Questions for Pediatrics

These practice questions are similar to the ones you may see on the PANCE about pediatric development and conditions.

1. Which one of the following is a risk factor for sudden infant death syndrome (SIDS)?

   (A) Advanced maternal age

   (B) Newborn lying on his or her side

   (C) Exposure to cigarette smoke

   (D) Newborn lying on his or her back

   (E) Macrosomia

2. Which one of the following is a risk factor for developing testicular cancer?

   (A) Cryptorchidism

   (B) Varicocele

   (C) Hydrocele

   (D) Paraphimosis

   (E) Hypospadias

3. Which one of the following is true concerning the characteristics of childhood autism?

   (A) Kids with autism do well with changing routines.

   (B) Childhood autism is usually diagnosed before the age of 3 years.

   (C) Females are more affected than males.

   (D) Environmental factors likely do not play a role in this condition.

   (E) Benzodiazepines are a mainstay of treatment.

4. You're evaluating a 4-month-old infant who presents with a fever of 39.4°C (103°F) and tonic-clonic seizure. There's no prior history of seizures or epilepsy. A lumbar puncture is unrevealing. Which one of the following is the likely cause of this infant's seizures?

   (A) Meningitis

   (B) Encephalitis

   (C) Malignancy

   (D) Fever

   (E) Epilepsy

5. Which of the following is a risk factor for the development of Down syndrome?

   (A) Gestational diabetes

   (B) Maternal alcohol use

   (C) Advanced maternal age

   (D) Folate deficiency during pregnancy

   (E) Lead poisoning

6. In addition to physical examination, which one of the following is most useful in diagnosing congenital hip dysplasia in the newborn?

   (A) Radiograph

   (B) Ultrasound

   (C) CT scan

   (D) MRI

   (E) Bone scan

Answers and Explanations

Use this answer key to score the practice pediatrics questions from the preceding section. The answer explanations give you insight into why the correct answer is better than the other choices.

1. **C.** Exposure to cigarette smoke is considered to be a risk factor for the development of SIDS. Lying on the stomach is the risk factor, but lying on the side or the back, Choices (B) and (D), is not. Choices (A) and (E), advanced maternal age and macrosomia, are wrong as well; the risk if SIDS increases with a younger mother or a low birth weight.

2. **A.** *Cryptorchidism* is an undescended testicle, and it increases the risk of testicular cancer. The other choices — varicocele, hydrocele, paraphimosis, and hypospadias — are not known risk factors. Choice (E), *hypospadias,* is a genetic condition where the urethral opening is in the wrong place on the penis.

3. **B.** Childhood autism is diagnosed before the age of 3 years. Autistic kids are usually better with a fixed routine, making Choice (A) incorrect. Males are way more affected with autism than females, so Choice (C) is incorrect. Environmental factors, Choice (D), likely play a huge role in this condition. Benzodiazepines, Choice (E), are used as adjunctive therapy for panic disorder and generalized anxiety disorder in adults.

4. **D.** This infant is having febrile seizure (a fever fit). A normal lumbar puncture rules out meningitis and encephalitis, Choices (A) and (B). It would be very highly unlikely for a malignancy, Choice (C), to be a cause of a fever and seizure in an infant this age. The question says that the child has no history of epilepsy, making Choice (E) incorrect.

5. **C.** Advanced maternal age is a risk factor for the development of Down syndrome in the child. Choice (A), gestational diabetes, increases the risk of macrosomia, and Choice (B), alcohol use, increases the risk of a low birth-weight baby and the development of fetal alcohol syndrome. Choice (D), folate deficiency, increases the risk of spina bifida in the newborn. Choice (E), lead poisoning, can cause basophilic stippling and a microcytic anemia. It can also cause peripheral neuropathy in addition to other symptoms.

6. **B.** Many PANCE questions concerning congenital hip dysplasia in the newborn focus on the Barlow and Ortolani maneuvers. The best imaging study for the newborn is the ultrasound. In the first few months of life, much of the joint may not be well visualized on standard radiologic imaging.

Chapter 12

Managing Health Maintenance and Medical Ethics

*T*he PANCE includes key concepts concerning basic health maintenance and issues in medical ethics. Having an understanding of preventive medicine, medical screening, and important topics in medical ethics is vital not only for answering test questions correctly but also for your career as a healthcare professional.

In this chapter, you get an overview of basic concepts in epidemiology with a review of terms you see in medical literature. Concerning medical ethics, understanding when and how to treat as well as when and how to stop treatment are difficult issues that everyone involved in patient care struggles with. Healthcare is filled with moral dilemmas and ethical questions. Again, expect to see a couple of questions about this topic on the exam.

Recalling Preventive Medicine Guidelines

What is *health,* anyway? In 1946, the World Health Organization (WHO) defined health as "a state of complete physical, mental, and social well-being and not merely the absence of disease or infirmity."

That's a tough order to fill. As a healthcare professional, you may be evaluated on how well you adhere to preventive medicine guidelines. In this section, you read about types of prevention and review some preventive medicine guidelines. You may have seen some of these guidelines already. In Chapter 4, for example, you read about obtaining annual flu shots.

Categorizing prevention types

Benjamin Franklin said it best when he said, "An ounce of prevention is worth a pound of cure." Health maintenance involves different types of prevention, namely primary, secondary, and tertiary prevention.

✔ **Primary prevention:** The goal of primary prevention is to use measures that prevent disease or illness from occurring in the first place.

- ✔ **Secondary prevention:** Secondary prevention means a medical condition may be present, but screening catches the condition early, before the person develops symptoms.

- ✔ **Tertiary prevention:** Tertiary prevention focuses on limiting further progression of a disease process or on rehabilitation to help improve a significantly disabling condition (in other words, restoring a person's functioning).

As an example in primary prevention, suppose a person does *not* have a diagnosis of coronary artery disease (CAD) but takes steps to reduce risk factors for developing CAD. These steps can include exercising; adhering to an eating plan low in saturated fat and high in fruits, vegetables, and whole grains; keeping cholesterol levels and blood pressure low; and never starting smoking. Secondary prevention includes lowering the cholesterol to goal and adhering to strict blood pressure guidelines. Aspirin therapy is also indicated, as the person has documented CAD. Tertiary prevention is treating someone who has CAD as diagnosed by a cardiac catheterization. Steps to reduce further progression could include the use of beta blockers, ACE inhibitors, statin therapy, and exercise therapy. Note the overlap between secondary and tertiary prevention as it relates to CAD; the difference is that with secondary prevention, you're trying to intervene before the person develops the symptoms of CAD. With tertiary prevention, the person has established CAD (with a catheter and multiple stents placed), and you're trying to prevent the condition from getting any worse.

Broadly, primary prevention can include the following:

- ✔ **Lifestyle choices:** Physical exercise reduces the risk for many conditions and is good for total body health. Stopping smoking, limiting alcohol use, and following a healthy diet are all examples of primary prevention.

- ✔ **Vaccines:** A vaccine prevents a disease from occurring in the first place. Examples include vaccines intended to prevent measles, mumps, smallpox, and influenza.

- ✔ **Condoms and safe sexual practices:** The goal is to prevent the spread of sexually transmitted disease (STI), especially HIV/AIDS. Some practices can prevent pregnancy as well.

- ✔ **Safety gear:** Other examples of primary prevention include using a helmet when riding a bike and wearing a seatbelt.

Examples of secondary prevention can include cancer screening and prophylaxis of deep venous thrombosis (DVT) in a hospital setting. Some medical conditions are prevalent in the population, and screening for them reduces the risk of acquiring them. Also, if a cancer is caught early, you've reduced the risk of potential complications. The same goes for DVT prophylaxis. Someone who's bedridden and not moving is at high risk for developing of a deep venous thrombosis. The goal is to minimize the risk with prophylaxis, such as anticoagulation therapy.

Examples of tertiary prevention include aggressive rehabilitation to restore functionality in a person who has suffered a stroke. In someone diagnosed with diabetes, tertiary prevention includes screening for eye and renal problems.

You're evaluating a 55-year-old male with a history of asthma, which has been well controlled on his current asthma regimen. He notes that recently at work he's been having "asthma flares." Your goal is to identify potential allergens at his workplace that are worsening his asthma. Which of the following would this be an example of?

(A) Primary prevention

(B) Secondary prevention

(C) Tertiary prevention

(D) Occupational health prevention

(E) Global Initiative for Chronic Obstructive Lung Disease (GOLD) criteria

The correct answer is Choice (C). This man's asthma was stable before an exposure at work that has caused an exacerbation. Looking for potential allergens to prevent worsening of his condition is an example of tertiary prevention. An example of secondary prevention, Choice (B), is the use of a steroid inhaler in someone who's been having asthma exacerbations and for whom an as-needed albuterol inhaler isn't enough. Primary prevention, Choice (A), would be eliminating risk factors that could foster the development of asthma and/or lung disease, including not smoking in the house and reducing exposure to second-hand smoke and other lung irritants. Given that this issue is taking place at work, occupational health may be called in, but there is no such concept as occupational health prevention, Choice (D). The GOLD criteria, Choice (E), refers to the Global Initiative for Chronic Obstructive Lung Disease and is a way of staging and raising awareness about COPD, not asthma.

Screenings: Following preventive medicine guidelines

For test-taking purposes, you should be familiar with routine health prevention screening measures. Several of them are here, and we cover some screens in the chapters about various organ systems. For example, we give details about colon cancer screening in Chapter 5, which covers the digestive system. You also read about pediatric vaccinations in Chapter 11.

Many of the cancer screening recommendations, especially for breast and prostate cancer, have been debated. Here, we present the current general preventive medicine guidelines for cancer and other conditions:

- **Breast cancer screening:** Women under 40 should have a breast examination performed every 3 years by a licensed medical professional and annually after they turn 40. Between ages 40 and 49, based on a consultation with a medical professional who knows their health history, mammograms should be obtained every 1 to 2 years. For women aged 50 to 74, a mammogram should be done every 2 years.

- **Prostate cancer screening:** African-American men aged 40 to 45 should be screened for prostate cancer with a digital rectal examination (DRE) and a prostate-specific antigen (PSA) test. If a man has a family history of prostate cancer, especially in a family member younger than 65, he should also discuss screening between the ages of 40 and 45 with his healthcare provider. If any man is known or likely to have the BRCA1 or BRCA2 mutations, he should discuss prostate cancer screening at ages 40 to 45.

  All men over 50 should speak with their healthcare provider concerning their risk of acquiring prostate cancer and whether they should be tested. It's debatable whether men over the age of 74 should be tested for prostate cancer on an annual basis.

- **Cervical cancer screening:** Women should start getting cervical cancer screenings at the age of 21 or 3 years after the onset of sexual activity, whichever is earlier. The woman should have a Pap smear done annually until the age of 30. If the woman has had normal Pap tests 3 years in a row, this examination can be done every 3 years. The general recommendation is that screening can stop after the age of 70, although some recommend that it stop after the age of 65.

- **Aneurysm screening:** A man who has a history of smoking should have an abdominal ultrasound done once between the ages of 65 and 75. It's not recommended that women be screened for any type of abdominal aneurysm.

- **Osteoporosis screening:** Screening for osteoporosis should begin for women over age 65 with no risk factors via a DEXA scan (which you read about in Chapter 6). If a woman has other risk factors (such as prior steroid use), then the screening should begin by age 60.

You're evaluating a 38-year-old female who has a family history of cancer. She asks you about testing for breast cancer because her friend was just diagnosed. Her breast self-examinations have been normal. Which of the following would you recommend?

(A) Mammogram

(B) Breast ultrasound

(C) Breast examination by a medical professional

(D) PET scan

(E) CA 27.29 level

The correct answer is Choice (C). The current recommendations state that unless there's a significant family history of breast cancer, mammography should begin after the age of 40. The recommendation of a breast examination by a medical professional every 3 years still stands in this case. Choice (B), breast ultrasound, would be used as an adjunctive test to evaluate an abnormal finding as seen on a mammogram or in a young patient with concerning findings. Choice (D), PET scan, is used for evaluating the activity of malignancies after they've been diagnosed. Choice (E) is a tumor marker for breast cancer. A tumor marker is almost never used as part of screening; it's used only to measure disease activity after diagnosis.

Population Patterns: Reviewing Epidemiology

Epidemiology is the branch of medicine that helps people figure out patterns concerning disease and other health-related conditions as they affect the population at large. For example, epidemiologists work to find the cause or source of epidemics of infectious disease. They seek to discover health-determinant patterns in a society.

In the Bad Old Days, tracing the origin and dissemination of a disease like bubonic plague was relatively easy. Travel routes were limited to sailing ships and poor roads. In the modern world, people travel a lot and move fast. The important work of the epidemiologist has therefore become more difficult.

When you take the PANCE, your task is to recognize common terms used in epidemiology and to interpret some simple population-based data. You won't see many questions in this subject area, but the more you know, the better you'll do. This section briefly looks at some fundamentals the test may ask you about.

Identifying conditions with lab tests: Being positive and negative, sensitive yet specific

Specificity and *sensitivity* are words you see in the epidemiologic world big time. They both relate to the reliability of a laboratory test for a given medical condition.

Before we review specificity and sensitivity, we need to explain two other concepts: positivity and negativity. A *positive test* reveals the presence of the condition or disease for which the test is being done. Say you're dealing with someone who comes to your office presenting with a fever and productive cough. You order a chest radiograph, which shows a lobar infiltrate in the right lower lobe. His imaging study shows that pneumonia is present. This is a true positive test because not only does he have symptoms of pneumonia, but his chest radiograph shows that as well.

As you would expect, a *negative test* result doesn't show the specific condition or disease for which the test is being done. Test results may be false. For example, you're evaluating a person with diabetes who says she feels "funny" and is sweating and tachycardic. You suspect hypoglycemia, but the person's glucometer reports a normal blood glucose reading. You send a blood sample to the lab, and it shows a blood glucose level of 30. The glucometer reported that the blood glucose level was normal when in fact it was low. If the glucometer reading and the lab results were similar, this would be a true negative. However, because the glucometer differed from the blood test, the glucometer gave a false negative result. The person needs a new glucometer.

Concerning false positive testing, say you're called about a lab value for a potassium level that is 8.0 mEq/L. If the potassium level were really this high, you'd expect to see changes in the vital signs, including bradycardia and an abnormal heart rhythm. You would also expect to see ECG changes. You rush to see the patient, and the vital signs are normal, as is the ECG. You call the lab and find out this was a hemolyzed specimen. This is a false positive result.

In the medical profession, no diagnostic test is 100 percent foolproof. The ideal test would be both specific and sensitive.

- ✔ *Specificity* deals with how reliable the test is in detecting a certain medical condition while minimizing the likelihood of false positive results.

- ✔ *Sensitivity* deals with the probability that a test says a person has a certain medical condition.

You want a test to accurately pick up those who have a certain medical condition (having a good sensitivity) and minimize the number of people who falsely test negative for a certain condition (having a good specificity).

What's our vector, Victor?

You must watch *Airplane* at least once in your life. You get lines like "We have clearance, Clarence" and "What's our vector, Victor?" This sidebar is about disease vectors.

In epidemiology, a *vector* is any person, animal, or microorganism that carries and transmits an infectious agent — and there are plenty of vectors. Different vectors contribute to human disease, animal disease, and plant disease. Here are some animal stars of the vector world:

- ✔ The *Anopheles* mosquito is responsible for transmitting human malaria. It's the king of vectors. However, a new vaccine looks promising — we should see it in 2015.

- ✔ The *Aedes* mosquito can spread dengue fever and yellow fever.

- ✔ Fleas can spread many diseases, of which bubonic plague is the most famous. Some estimates say that the plague has killed more than 200 million people.

- ✔ In the United States, ticks of the genus *Ixodes* get special attention because they pass on the bacterium for Lyme disease.

- ✔ In Africa, the tsetse fly is a scourge. It's the vector of human African trypanosomiasis (sleeping sickness).

- ✔ Here, kitty, kitty! House cats are the vector for *Toxoplasma gondii,* which causes toxoplasmosis, and for *Bartonella henselae,* which causes cat scratch fever.

The concept of vectors extends reasonably to two other areas: people and water.

- ✔ Remember Mary Mallon, also known as Typhoid Mary? She was the first person in the United States identified as an asymptomatic carrier of the typhoid fever pathogen (*Salmonella enterica,* serovar Typhi). Her score: 53 people infected and 3 people dead.

- ✔ If you lived near Broad Street in Soho, London, in 1854, dying of typhoid fever was easy. Contaminated water was the delivery vehicle. The physician who figured this out noted occurrences of the disease on a map that showed water wells. The doctor was John Snow, considered to be one of the fathers of epidemiology.

For an example, consider the Lyme test. The confirmatory test to truly diagnose Lyme disease is a Western blot. If a Western blot demonstrates that Lyme is present, then Lyme disease is highly likely to be present. This is a highly specific test. The number of people testing falsely positive for Lyme disease with the Western blot is low.

Consider another example. The RPR, or rapid plasma reagin, is a screening test for syphilis. However, other medical conditions, especially vasculitis and other rheumatologic conditions, can cause an RPR to be positive. This test has a high sensitivity — it would detect almost all patients with syphilis — but it also has a lot of false positives. Thus, it has a high sensitivity but low specificity for syphilis.

Looking at the numbers: Incidence and prevalence of a condition

A common test question involves understanding the difference between incidence and prevalence:

- **Incidence:** For any health-related condition or illness, *incidence* refers to the number of people who've newly acquired this condition.

- **Prevalence:** Prevalence concerns the number of people who have this condition over a defined time interval.

Remember, because these are *epidemiologic* terms, they're dealing with the population at large.

For example, say you wanted to investigate the number of cases of tuberculosis (and who wouldn't want to do that?) in all people over the age of 65. Incidence is the number of new cases diagnosed in the past year, and prevalence is the number of people diagnosed who were over the age of 65.

Studies and trials: Evaluating epidemiological studies

You should be aware of the differences among the types of epidemiologic studies. The first step is to recognize whether the study is a retrospective study or a prospective study:

- **Retrospective:** A retrospective study means that you're looking into the past to figure out what happened. For example, a retrospective study may involve looking at patient charts. Or it may involve searching medical databases and registries, such as the Cochrane Library, for specific conditions.

- **Prospective:** A prospective study means that you're looking to the future to see whether a specific outcome will happen. A classic example of a prospective study is the large clinical trials to evaluate a medication and its effects on treating a medical condition.

In this section, we cover several types of retrospective and prospective studies.

Randomized controlled trials

Clinical drug trials are often randomized controlled studies, the best kind of clinical research trials. The *randomized controlled study* includes two groups of people: one control and one intervention, or variable (the group being tested). The distribution of participants between the control group and intervention group is random and avoids allocation bias.

This type of study is the best because it's usually double-blinded — in plain English, this means that both the investigator and those being tested walk around wearing big goggles. Seriously, *double-blinded* means the study is designed so neither the investigator nor the participant knows upfront which treatment is being given to which person. This blinding prevents bias. Bias, of course, is a bad thing in the research community.

Case-control studies

A *case-control study* is a type of retrospective analysis where you're comparing a control group (those who are healthy) with another group that has a certain medical condition. This study is purely an observational analysis and depends on looking up patient data. As a researcher, you'd look at some factor or characteristic in both groups to see whether there's any link between the specified characteristic and the disease.

For example, in a case-control study, you may compare people who've had myocardial infarctions (MI) with those who haven't, comparing the prevalence of diabetes in each group. You'd find that diabetes is more prevalent in the MI group. Of course, we now know that diabetes increases the risk of an MI.

Cohort studies

A *cohort study* follows a group of people (a cohort) over a period of time, sometimes years. Here, you first identify persons who've been exposed to Factor X. You follow these people over a defined time interval and see whether they develop either certain symptoms or the actual condition you're studying.

For example, perhaps you're watching a select population who may have been exposed to a pesticide during childhood. They may have had different levels of exposure, but you watch them for the development of any symptoms.

Cross-sectional studies

If a cohort study is following people over time, a *cross-sectional study* is just the opposite: It's looking at a medical condition and the population at the same time. In other words, a cross-sectional study tries to tell you the incidence or prevalence of a certain medical condition, depending on what you're looking for.

Say you wanted to know the incidence of people with three eyeballs within a population. If you were to find out that many of the children who developed three eyeballs had been exposed to a certain pesticide, then you'd need to study this population specifically. Maybe someday you'll do this study. We'll keep an eye out for you.

You want to study the potential link between exposure to a pesticide and the development of three eyeballs. You have identified a group of people who have been exposed to a certain pesticide. You decide that you want to watch them over a period of five years to see whether they develop a third eyeball. Which type of study would you be conducting?

(A) Randomized controlled study

(B) Case-control study

(C) Cohort study

(D) Retrospective study

(E) Cross-sectional study

The correct answer is Choice (C). This is an example of a cohort study. You're going to follow this same group of people over time to see whether they develop that third eyeball. For a randomized controlled study, Choice (A), you'd need to have two groups of people:

one group who had been exposed to a certain measure of the pesticide and one group who hadn't. Neither the investigator nor the participants would know whether a particular participant had been exposed to the pesticide or to a harmless substance. (*Note:* If you think this randomized controlled study of a pesticide seems like a good idea, we'd like you to read the later section "Meeting Up with Medical Ethics" very carefully.) A case-control study, Choice (B), would involve looking at people who developed three eyeballs and people who hadn't and comparing the exposure to pesticides in each group. The cross-sectional study, Choice (E), would be looking the exposure of a pesticide and the development of three eyeballs that had already occurred over a given period of time. You aren't following people over time with this type of study.

Seeking statistical significance

We invite you to say the above phrase very quickly three times. You can't, can you? Luckily, on a test, all that you're likely to be asked is whether something is statistically significant. *Statistically significant* means that the research often has significant clinical relevance and the ability to change how medical professionals take care of patients. As you read medical literature that reports different kinds of research being done, look for statistical significance.

You need to be aware of the *p-value* in the study. *P* stands for *probability:* the lower the *p*-value, the more significant the value is.

When statisticians do their calculations, if the *p*-value is less than 0.05, then the study is felt to be statistically significant, and everyone is happy. For testing purposes, be aware of this numerical value.

A high *positive predictive value* (PPV) means that a positive test accurately reflects the underlying condition being tested. A high *negative predictive value* (NPV) means that a negative result is also accurate, indicating that a condition isn't present.

Dealing with Domestic Violence

In your professional career, you'll likely see patients who've suffered domestic violence. This is such a hot topic that you need to recognize it and be able to deal with it appropriately. Be aware that domestic violence concerns not only spousal abuse but also child abuse.

On physical examination, look for evidence of physical abuse, including bite marks and bruises. This requires doing a full physical examination, including looking closely at the extremities and hidden areas, especially if you're considering that sexual abuse may have occurred.

The clinician first needs to ask whether domestic violence is occurring. Too often, this question isn't asked. The patient needs to know that she (it's almost always a woman) can talk to you about anything. Provide the patient with information about where she can go to report and escape the abuse. These places can include a local shelter and the police department.

For child abuse, federal law requires a practitioner to report any known or suspected abuse to Child Protective Services.

For both PANCE and clinical purposes, be aware that domestic violence doesn't deal with just physical abuse. It takes many forms, including physical aggression (hitting, kicking, biting, shoving, restraining, slapping, throwing objects) or threats thereof, sexual abuse, emotional abuse, verbal abuse, controlling/domineering behavior, intimidation, stalking, passive/covert abuse, neglect, and economic deprivation. With economic deprivation, one partner doesn't allow the other to be in control of the other partner's finances and/or refuses to provide monetary support when needed.

In the many forms of abuse, the central issue is one of control. If one partner has the power to strip away the other's self-esteem, he or she then has the element of control. Both physical and verbal abuse may be employed to maintain that control.

Which of the following statements is true concerning domestic violence?

(A) Episodes of violence rarely occur more than once.

(B) Domestic violence is present only if you see signs of physical abuse.

(C) Withholding finances is considered a form of abuse.

(D) Only young women between the ages of 18 and 35 should be screened for domestic violence.

(E) Healthcare professionals don't need to be educated in how to deal with domestic violence issues.

The answer is Choice (C). Because domestic violence is so important, medical professionals need to be educated and trained in dealing with these situations. Domestic violence happens repeatedly, and there are many forms of violence outside of physical abuse. In addition, you may not see obvious signs of physical abuse on examination (remember, you need to do a head-to-toe examination). Concerning Choice (D), you need to have a high index of suspicion for all people when it comes to domestic violence.

Meeting Up with Medical Ethics

Medical ethics is a hot-button issue in medicine. Many books have been written about the subject, including *Medical Ethics For Dummies,* by Jane Runzheimer, MD, and Linda Johnson Larsen (Wiley). As a healthcare professional, you deal with ethical issues every day. This section describes some basic principles of medical ethics that you should be aware of and may see on the PANCE.

Practicing ethical principles

Medical ethics come into play with every patient you see. Most of the time, what constitutes ethical behavior is pretty straightforward; occasionally, situations get messy, but these principles can help you do the right thing:

- ✔ **Doing no harm (nonmaleficence):** The basic principle that all health professionals abide by is the principle of not doing harm to the patient. This is the principle of *nonmaleficence* (in Latin, *Primum non nocere* — "First, do no harm"), and it's part of the Hippocratic Oath that all physicians take.

- ✔ **Benefiting the patient (beneficence):** Although not performing certain actions or participating in certain activities that could harm the patient is important, you also want to do your best to benefit the patient. This is the principle of *beneficence* (in Latin, that's *Salus aegroti suprema lex*).

✓ **Determination by the patient, not for the patient (autonomy):** Medicine has changed in a lot of ways. A key change is patient autonomy. *Autonomy* is the ability to decide and think for oneself. In the case of medicine, the patient has the right to refuse treatment or choose his or her treatment *(Voluntas aegroti suprema lex)*. The relationship between patient and medical professional should be one that promotes autonomy, not paternalism. In *paternalism,* one person tells someone else what to do or makes decisions for him or her.

Promoting patient autonomy (or self-determination) means that as a medical professional, you need to explain options to a patient. The patient needs to be properly informed to make the best decisions possible about his or her care. With this knowledge, the patient can provide *informed consent,* which is vital for good patient care. For any procedure or proposed medical treatment, you tell the patient the benefits (the "why" of doing the procedure) in addition to the risks. For example, a cardiac catheterization is very beneficial in helping identify and treat symptomatic blockages of the coronary arteries. One potential risk is that the dye used may affect the kidneys, especially if risk factors such as diabetes and kidney disease are present.

The patient must also be aware of other treatment options that may exist. He or she has the right to refuse any procedure or proposed medical treatment as well. The patient needs to know the consequences of not having a procedure done. As you can see, in addition to knowing your medical stuff, you need to be a good communicator.

Abiding by patients' rights

The patient is a partner in medical care and has rights that you must respect and abide by. These take the form of a "bill of rights" that healthcare professionals know and follow. A bill of rights includes many of the principles you read about in the preceding section, including promoting patients' autonomy.

Where can you find a patient's bill of rights? Walk into any hospital or healthcare center, and you can (and should) see a patient's bill of rights, usually at the entrance. It's also provided to each patient when he or she is admitted. The bill of rights should also be given to any patient who is establishing a new relationship with a doctor.

A patient's bill of rights typically includes the following principles:

✓ The patient should be fully informed about any procedure and/or proposed medical treatment as well as about his or her condition.

✓ The patient should know that his or her medical information is confidential, a concept known as *patient-provider privilege*. Health professional–patient confidentiality is vital to good patient care.

✓ The patient has the right to be treated by the provider he or she chooses. This includes consultations with medical specialists.

✓ The patient has the right to refuse a medical treatment even if it's highly recommended.

✓ The patient has the right to be treated by the same provider and/or to change providers if he or she isn't satisfied with the treatment.

For the PANCE, you should be familiar with the terms presented here. In many cases, you'll be given different scenarios and asked to either identify the principle being described or pick the best answer for that situation.

Practice Health Maintenance and Medical Ethics Questions

These practice questions are similar to the PANCE questions you may see about preventive medicine, epidemiology, domestic violence, and ethics.

1. You're seeing a 19-year-old woman who has been sexually active for the past two years. You spend much of the office visit convincing her to practice safe sex. What kind of prevention is this an example of?

   (A) Primary prevention

   (B) Secondary prevention

   (C) Tertiary prevention

2. Your patient is a 19-year-old woman who has been sexually active for the past two years. At what age would you recommend that she receive a Pap smear?

   (A) 19

   (B) 20

   (C) 21

   (D) 22

   (E) 23

3. Which of the following has the lowest evidence of study bias?

   (A) Retrospective study

   (B) Case-control study

   (C) Cross-sectional study

   (D) Randomized controlled study

   (E) Cohort study

4. Which condition does the *Haemophilus influenzae* B vaccine prevent?

   (A) Croup

   (B) Legionella pneumonia

   (C) Epiglottitis

   (D) Influenza

   (E) Rhinovirus

5. You have been studying Condition X for five years. You have identified a number of people who have Condition X. You have also identified a blood test that can identify that Condition X is present when the blood test is positive. What term describes the ability of the blood test to detect those in the population who indeed have Condition X?

   (A) Sensitivity

   (B) Specificity

   (C) Incidence

   (D) Prevalence

   (E) Statistical significance

6. A 25-year-old woman presents wearing sunglasses. She's sporting a huge black eye. When you question her, she states that she "ran into a door." You suspect spousal abuse. What do you do next?

   (A) Call the police.

   (B) Call Child Protective Services.

   (C) Keep quiet and just treat that shiner.

   (D) Lecture her and tell her to move out.

   (E) Assure her of confidentiality and remind her about counseling services and shelters.

Answers and Explanations

Use this answer key to score the practice questions from the preceding section. The answer explanations give you insight into why the correct answer is better than the other choices.

1. **A.** The use of safe sexual practices to prevent the spread of disease is an example of primary prevention. Remember that with primary prevention, the goal is to use measures that prevent disease or illness from occurring in the first place.

2. **B.** A young woman should obtain a Pap smear either at age 21 or 3 years after the onset of sexual intercourse, whichever is earlier. With this patient, sexual relations began at the age of 17, so she is due at the age of 20 to get a Pap smear.

3. **D.** The randomized controlled study has the lowest incidence of study bias because both the subject and the experimenter are double-blinded. The experimenter doesn't know who has been assigned a certain medication or test, and the subject doesn't know which treatment has been rendered.

4. **C.** *Haemophilus influenzae* B vaccine is used to prevent (or reduce the risk of) getting epiglottitis. It's usually recommended to give this vaccine to children starting at 2 months of age.

5. **A.** The *sensitivity* of a test is its ability to correctly identify those who have Condition X through a positive test. *Specificity* focuses more on whether the blood test is negative in people who don't have Condition X. *Incidence* refers to the number of new people in whom Condition X was detected in a certain time period, such as the past month. *Prevalence* is the number of people diagnosed with Condition X in a population, such as the elderly.

6. **E.** It's important to build trust with the person, or she may not share future incidents. At the same time, she should be aware of counseling services (often anonymous hotlines) and the availability of shelters. Otherwise, your intervention is limited.

Chapter 13

Tending to Behavioral Health

*B*ehavioral health is an important component of overall health, so you'll see some questions on the PANCE/PANRE concerning behavioral disorders. Abnormal behaviors can be difficult to assess and to treat. Nevertheless, you need to know some essential symptoms and likely treatments.

In studying the field of psychiatry, you should be familiar with the bible of behavioral health, the *Diagnostic and Statistical Manual of Mental Disorders (DSM)*. The current version of the *DSM* is the *DSM-IV-TR,* a text revision of the 4th edition. It contains 943 sizzling pages of behavioral and psychiatric disorders. The book provides a well-ordered approach to diagnostic criteria, describing a minimum of 297 disorders. A new edition, the *DSM-5,* is planned for May 2013. It proposes to add, modify, and reorganize some diagnoses.

In this chapter, we give you a broad picture of behavioral health and provide some sample questions that mirror what may appear on the test.

Getting Specific about Anxiety Disorders

Anxiety is a very broad term. Generally, it concerns how people react to stress. Everyone has anxiety from time to time in response to a particular stressor. Examples include anxiety brought on by the loss of a job, financial worries, or an upcoming certification exam. Another significant cause of anxiety is fear. However, with anxiety disorders, the emotional reaction to a perceived fear seems rational only to the person who is having that reaction. You may see both physical and emotional symptoms of anxiety. In this section, we introduce you to generalized anxiety disorder, panic disorder, phobias, and related conditions.

Watching for panic attacks: A perceived reason to panic

A *panic disorder* involves an anxiety-evoked response to a perceived fear. People with a panic disorder experience many of the following symptoms in the form of *panic attacks:* nausea, stomachache, palpitations, tension, hypertension, fatigue, weak muscles, headache, chest pain, and/or shortness of breath. Profound diaphoresis and tachycardia often accompany a panic attack, and many times, the person experiencing a panic attack thinks that he or she is having a heart attack because of the overlapping symptoms. A full medical evaluation is necessary to exclude other "organic" causes of the symptoms, such as acute coronary syndrome (ACS; see Chapter 4) and hyperthyroidism.

Panic attacks can occur spontaneously. Often, a noticeable change in behavior accompanies the recurrent attacks.

Panic disorder may occur with *agoraphobia,* which literally means "fear of the market" or "public place fear." The person worries about future panic attacks and therefore avoids places or events where escape would be embarrassing or impossible. That leads to a fear of going outside — the person is literally afraid of leaving home. Agoraphobia is a big topic, and you can expect to see a question or two about it on the PANCE.

When you're evaluating someone with a panic disorder, you need to investigate for a possible medical etiology. Perform a thorough past medical history, including documenting prescription meds — think dimethylxanthine derivatives like theophylline (Theo-Dur) and over-the-counter meds. Don't ignore street drugs, such as cocaine and methamphetamine, or herbs, such as ephedra (ma huang). All these substances can mimic or be a possible contributory factor to a person's anxious symptoms. Medical problems such as hyperthyroidism, catecholamine excess states (think pheochromocytoma), or excess serotonergic states (think carcinoid) can contribute to anxiety. A plain old heart attack can also be an anxiety-provoking event.

If the PANCE asks about the "best treatment" for panic and many of the anxiety disorders, the main answer isn't anti-anxiety medications like benzodiazepines. Although they may be effective, the main source of treatment (in addition to a full medical evaluation) is cognitive or behavioral therapy to try to figure out what's causing the panic attacks in the first place.

You're evaluating a 45-year-old woman for a possible panic disorder. Which of the following medical conditions can be associated with panic disorder?

(A) Hypothyroidism

(B) Hypercalcemia

(C) Mitral valve prolapse (MVP)

(D) Hyperglycemia

(E) Hypokalemia

The answer is Choice (C) — mitral valve prolapse can be associated with panic disorder. Hyperthyroidism, not hypothyroidism, is associated with symptoms resembling a panic attack. Hypercalcemia causes lethargy, not anxiety. Although the symptoms of hypoglycemia trigger anxiety-type symptoms, hyperglycemia doesn't; hyperglycemia can cause lethargy and confusion, especially if the levels are high enough (think diabetic ketoacidosis). Hypokalemia isn't associated with panic symptoms, although it can cause or trigger arrhythmias, which can then cause panic!

Generalized anxiety disorder: Experiencing general, ongoing worry

Generalized anxiety disorder (GAD) is literally being anxious about everything for a long time. The symptoms can overlap many of the symptoms of a panic disorder (see the preceding section). Tension, fatigue, nausea, trouble sleeping, feeling "pain all over" — all of these can be related to anxiety. Usually, for a diagnosis of generalized anxiety disorder, the symptoms have to have been occurring for about 6 months or more.

As with panic disorder, the treatment for generalized anxiety disorder is mainly behavior-based therapy, although medications such as the "benzos" (benzodiazepines) often need to be used in conjunction. Realize that the causes or triggers of generalized anxiety disorder are often difficult to pinpoint.

For the PANCE, you need to know about the side effects of medications commonly prescribed for generalized anxiety disorder, including the benzodiazepines. Examples include clonazepam (Klonopin) and lorazepam (Ativan). Here are a few key points about benzodiazepines in general:

✔ They can cause sedation and lethargy as side effects. You need to be careful of the dosing in someone who has liver disease or cirrhosis, because these conditions increase the half-life of many benzodiazepines.

✔ Stopping benzodiazepines abruptly can cause a withdrawal reaction. Withdrawal reactions cause the opposite symptoms of what the medication is supposed to do. For the benzos, this can mean agitation and excitability. Physical manifestations can include tachycardia and even hypertension.

✔ A person can become so sedated on a benzo that it can cause respiratory depression. The antidote for a benzodiazepine overdose is flumazenil (Romazicon).

Naming other anxiety disorders

The following brief descriptions get you into the world of anxiety disorders. It's by no means complete, because a person can develop a fear of practically anything at any time, and medical science may then discover and report it. Here are a few anxiety disorders you're likely to see on the test:

✔ **Post-traumatic stress disorder (PTSD):** Anyone can develop PTSD after a traumatic experience. You see the condition more than ever in soldiers returning home after serving in one of America's two recent wars. The stressor that causes PTSD is significant. Examples of traumatic events include war, rape, domestic violence, a devastating illness, a major accident, natural disasters, the sudden death of someone close, or seeing someone else severely hurt or killed. The symptoms can occur as early as a few months after the traumatic event, although this can vary from person to person.

The person with PTSD keeps reliving parts of the traumatic event over and over. Experiencing momentary flashbacks is not uncommon. The affected person often has trouble sleeping due to the recurrent nightmares. In addition, he or she seeks to avoid potential triggers for those bad memories. The person becomes angry and anxious and can exhibit physical signs of extreme anxiety, including sweating, palpitations, and tachycardia. The person may have a history of substance and/or alcohol abuse as a way to try to cope with the memories.

✔ **Obsessive-compulsive disorder (OCD):** Here, the affected person develops *obsessions* (repetitive thoughts that won't go away) and *compulsions* (repetitive behaviors, such as excessive hand-washing, always starting a walk on the same foot, or using only one "special" drinking glass) to deal with anxiety.

Serotonin selective reuptake inhibitors (SSRIs) are used in treating OCD. You may also see the medication clomipramine (Anafranil), which is a tricyclic antidepressant, used in the treatment of OCD.

✔ **Separation anxiety disorder (SAD):** Separation anxiety disorder is the name for recurring distress when a person fears separation from parents, children, a significant other, or home. Note that this SAD isn't the same as another SAD — seasonal affective disorder.

Figuring out phobias

Phobia is the Greek word for "fear." If you want to split hairs, fear isn't exactly anxiety. *Fear* is a healthy emotional response to a perceived danger. Fearing a charging lion is quite rational. By contrast, look at the phobias. A fear of bananas isn't rational and surely isn't healthy.

A *phobia* is a fear of something that isn't thought to be a danger. Phobias can be significant enough to interfere with a person's social functioning, and they often don't go away without therapy. Phobias are classified as anxiety disorders.

An irrational fear of anything is possible. Here are some common ones you should know:

- ✔ *Agoraphobia* literally means "public place fear." It's a fear of places or events where escape would be embarrassing or impossible.
- ✔ *Acrophobia* is an irrational fear of heights.
- ✔ *Arachnophobia* is an irrational fear of spiders and other arachnids, such as scorpions.
- ✔ *Nyctophobia,* fear of the dark, is a common fear. It's right up there with fear of monsters under the bed and fear of monsters in the closet. Fear of the dark is common among children and can be seen in adults to varying degrees.
- ✔ *Pedophobia* is an irrational fear of infants or children.

In various lists, we've counted 179 phobias, including *dentophobia* (the fear of dentists and dental procedures), *ephebiphobia* (the fear of young people), and *turophobia* (the fear of cheese).

The diagnostic criteria for phobias are outlined in the *DSM-IV-TR* in sections on social and specific phobias. In general for the diagnosis, look for a "marked and persistent fear that is excessive or unreasonable." Treatments are highly varied.

Scrutinizing Schizophrenia

Schizophrenia is a psychosis in which the person has significant problems with thinking. The symptoms become so bad they can overtake a person's life, and the person experiences a detachment from reality. In addition to confused thinking, the affected person often experiences delusions and/or hallucinations. The most common hallucinations are auditory. Even though the Greek word *schizophrenia* means "split mind," schizophrenia isn't the same as dissociative identity disorder (multiple personalities), which we cover later in this chapter.

Paranoia may be present. Broadly, *paranoia* is an irrational belief in a threat or conspiracy directed against the person, the idea that "they're out to get me."

What causes schizophrenia? Welcome to the wonderful medical term *multi-factorial* — a combination of DNA, environmental exposures, and/or social stressors seem to contribute. In addition, the variety of symptoms that can be present have produced a debate about whether a diagnosis of schizophrenia represents a single disorder or a number of different syndromes.

Distinguishing between delusions and hallucinations

You need to know the difference between a delusion and a hallucination. A *delusion* is a false belief that the patient is absolutely convinced is true. For example, a person believing he or she can fly has a delusion. Delusions are associated with many mental illnesses, including schizophrenia and even Alzheimer's disease.

Here are a few examples of delusions:

- ✔ **Persecutory:** Persecutory delusions are common in schizophrenia. The person may think that harm is happening right now or that it's going to come soon from a persecutor. Wearing an aluminum foil hat to fend off the mind-controlling rays of space aliens likely falls into this category.

- ✔ **Grandiose:** Grandiose delusions (delusions of grandeur) are delusions in which the sufferer believes he or she has special powers or talents. This is the arena where thinking you're Napoleon resides. It's a grandiose delusion unless, of course, you *are* Napoleon.

- ✔ **Delusions of love:** In this delusion, the affected person thinks that someone or some people are in love with him or her. The affected person believes that he or she is the special recipient of messages, signs from the lover that only the affected person can see. The person with delusions of love may give gifts or send messages of love to that unsuspecting person. This delusion can be seen with schizophrenia as well as with manic-depressive disorder.

A *hallucination,* by contrast, is a sensory perception in which the person sees or hears things that aren't there. That is, there's no external basis for the perception. Actually, any sense can be the vehicle for hallucination — sight, hearing, touch, smell, or taste. The hallucinations in schizophrenia are mostly auditory. For example, a person may claim that "the television is sending me messages."

Diagnosing schizophrenia

There are different types of schizophrenia, and the diagnosis is in the clinical presentation. The affected person needs to have at a minimum two symptoms present for at least 6 months. Symptoms can include the following:

- ✔ **Delusions alone:** Delusions may be enough for you to make a judgment, especially if the delusions strike you as really strange. Remember, evaluating diseased minds is often a highly subjective process.

- ✔ **Hallucinations alone:** Hallucinations may be enough to help you render a judgment, especially if the person describes the voice (or voices) as not his or her own and if the voice speaks from outside of his or her head.

- ✔ **Disorganization of speech or behavior:** Disorganized speech patterns such as incoherence, flight of ideas, word salad, and frequent derailment may be clinical signs that illustrate the thinking and cognitive problems present in schizophrenia. Basically, what comes out of the person's mouth doesn't make sense. Disorganized behavior, such as dressing in a bizarre manner, can also be a symptom.

- ✔ **Problems with activities of daily living (ADL):** Schizophrenia can affect the ability of the affected person to do routine everyday tasks, to hold down a job, to engage socially with peers and colleagues, and to be in a relationship. As the condition continues, it negatively impacts the patient and leads to a downward social drift.

- ✔ **Negative symptoms:** Negative symptoms can include lack of motivation, social withdrawal, and diminished affective responsiveness, speech, and movement. People with catatonic schizophrenia, for examples, can exist in an almost permanent stupor.

Treating schizophrenia

In addition to behavioral or cognitive therapy, the use of antipsychotic medications is inherent in the treatment of schizophrenia. In general, antipsychotics may be typical or atypical. The typical meds are used sparingly in deference to the newer atypical antipsychotics. Here are the main side effects you should know:

- **Typical antipsychotics:** Typical antipsychotics, such as haloperidol (Haldol) and thioridazine (Mellaril), are called *typical* because of the extrapyramidal side effects associated with them. These side effects occur when you block the dopamine receptors in the brain. A common example of an extrapyramidal side effect is tardive dyskinesia, or lip-smacking. For test-taking purposes, you should be familiar with the side effects of these commonly prescribed medications.

- **Atypical antipsychotics:** Here are some of the atypical antipsychotics the PANCE may ask you about:

  - Clozapine (Clozaril) is a very effective medication for treating psychoses. You'll likely be asked about clozapine's bone marrow effects, particularly agranulocytosis.

  - Olanzapine (Zyprexa) has the common side effect of weight gain. It can also cause hyperglycemia and can affect cholesterol and triglyceride levels.

You're evaluating a 30-year-old man with a history of delusions, hallucinations, and "weird thinking patterns" that have been occurring over the past 3 months, according to the patient's wife. What psychiatric condition does this person likely have?

(A) Schizophrenia

(B) Schizoaffective disorder

(C) Schizophreniform disorder

(D) Bipolar disorder

(E) Generalized anxiety disorder

The answer is Choice (C), schizophreniform disorder. The key to this question is being aware of time. *Schizophreniform disorder* has the same features as schizophrenia but requires only 3 months of symptoms for a diagnosis to be made, whereas schizophrenia, Choice (A), requires 6 months for a diagnosis. As for the other choices, *schizoaffective disorder,* Choice (B), has the features of schizophrenia combined with the features of a mood disorder (see the later section "Meeting the Mood Disorders" for info on mood disorders). Choice (D), bipolar disorder, is a mood disorder, not a psychotic disorder. Generalized anxiety disorder, Choice (E), is an anxiety disorder, and hallucinations and delusions aren't features of generalized anxiety disorder.

Probing Personality Disorders

Everyone has a personality (except maybe some of Barry's previous co-workers). However, not everyone is afflicted with a personality disorder. One of the marks of a personality disorder is behaviors or thought processes that are very different from societal norms. The person isn't making it in life. In addition, the person doesn't see the behaviors as inappropriate.

Diagnosing and treating personality disorders

When evaluating someone for a personality disorder, you're looking for patterns of behavior. In many cases, the affected person has demonstrated a certain pattern of behavior over a long period of time, but it may have gone unrecognized. If someone has a personality disorder in childhood, the odds are pretty good that it will continue into his or her adult life.

Diagnosis of a personality disorder is subjective, and it consists of observing and discovering "patterns of disorder." A personality disorder can be thought of as a type of psychosis, as the person can deviate from societal norm. Here are some areas to pay attention to in your evaluation:

✔ An inability to fully function in society

✔ Rigid and dysfunctional patterns of feeling and thinking

✔ Rigid and inflexible patterns of behavior

✔ Lack of emotional response or abnormal emotional response

The gold standard of treatment for personality disorders is behavioral and/or cognitive therapy. Counseling is vital. This can manifest as individualized counseling sessions or even group sessions involving a family member or significant other. Medications are utilized only when needed; the mainstay of treatment is intense counseling or psychotherapy.

Reviewing common personality disorders

Personality disorders come in several forms. The *DSM* lists 10 disorders in three groups in Axis II, and the list tends to evolve over time. Personality disorders are behaviors that differ prominently from social expectations. Mildness or severity is subjective, depending on the degree of impairment. In this section, you read about a few of the more common ones that you may be asked about on the PANCE.

Defining borderline personality disorder

Borderline personality disorder is a common example of a personality disorder. The person may have significant issues with low self-esteem and can experience the extremes of moods. He or she can either really like or really hate someone. The affected person can also have a tendency toward self-mutilation — for example, the affected person may make cuts in his or her arms with a razor blade. The patient has a tendency to exhibit impulsive, high-risk activities such as alcohol/drug abuse, unsafe sex practices, gambling, or other reckless behaviors.

Borderline personality disorder is commonly diagnosed in young people, females more often than males. Identification of this condition and intense psychotherapy are so important in the treatment of this personality disorder.

Being antisocial

Antisocial personality disorder refers to a pattern of behavior in which the affected person doesn't care about others or about laws and/or societal norms. This person tends to engage in criminal acts, for example, and not feel remorse for his or her actions. This type of behavior usually occurs for years.

Many people with antisocial personality disorder have a history of conduct disorder that began when they were children or in their teenage years. *Conduct disorder* can include behaviors such as bullying, picking fights, and showing cruelty to animals. Again, the issue is recognizing a pattern of behavior.

Feeling divided over split personality

Dissociative identity disorder (DID) is a condition in which the person displays multiple distinct identities, or personalities. The condition isn't prevalent in the general population but may be more prevalent in people diagnosed with another mental illness.

Dissociative identity disorder is not schizophrenia. Although a person with schizophrenia experiences confused thinking, delusions, and/or hallucinations, he or she has only one identity. What complicates things is that dissociative identity disorder is often comorbid with other disorders.

Causes of dissociative identity disorder include a history of abuse, particularly both severe sexual and physical abuse in childhood. The affected person tries to disconnect from his or her environment by forming other personalities. The goal of therapy is to try to merge the various personalities into a singular identity. This can be difficult and requires intense psychotherapy.

Which of the following statements is true concerning personality disorders?

(A) The behaviors associated with personality disorders often occur acutely over a period of weeks to months.

(B) Symptoms of personality disorders include delusions and hallucinations.

(C) Self-harm is a component of borderline personality disorder

(D) Giving someone a wedgie could be a sign of a social phobia.

(E) The treatment of personality disorders involves the use of multiple medications.

The correct answer is Choice (C). Self-harm is one important criterion used in the diagnosis of borderline personality disorder. Regarding Choice (A), personality disorders involve patterns of behavior that have likely been occurring over a period of years, not acutely over weeks to months. Delusions and hallucinations, Choice (B), are seen more often with psychotic disorders, such as schizophrenia, than with personality disorders.

Concerning Choice (D), don't confuse social phobia with antisocial personality disorder. *Social phobia* is a fear of social events and social situations. An example of a social phobia is a fear of speaking in public. Although the person with social phobia may exhibit *avoidance behavior* (avoiding high-profile public events), he or she doesn't engage in criminal or abusive behavior, which is the hallmark of antisocial personality disorder.

As for Choice (E), the main treatment of personality disorders is psychotherapy. Medications can be adjunctive, but they're not the primary means of therapy.

Meeting the Mood Disorders

In addition to personality disorders and psychoses (see the preceding sections), you should be familiar with the evaluation and treatment of some major mood disorders for the PANCE. Mood disorders involve major changes in a person's emotions. You're not simply dealing with a "moody individual." In this section, you deal with the extremes of emotional states.

Overcoming major depression and dysthymia

Depression is a very common mood disorder, and it's one of the main complaints elicited during outpatient visits to one's primary care provider. Major depressive disorder (MDD) has 14 entries in the *DSM-IV-TR*.

With *major depressive disorder,* someone experiences depressed mood and/or *anhedonia,* the inability to feel any joy in anything. The person can be barely interested in life itself or the activities of daily living. He or she often doesn't feel good about himself or herself, either. Here are some points concerning depression:

✔ The symptoms can vary from sleeping all the time to having trouble sleeping.

✔ Sufferers often hate themselves and have very low self-esteem.

✔ Sufferers can have weight gain or weight loss.

✔ The affected person, especially one with a full-blown depression, is often disheveled and odoriferous. The person is so depressed he or she doesn't care about himself or herself at all, which can result in poor hygiene and an unkempt appearance.

✔ The periods of depression often last a long time. By diagnostic criteria, they need to last for at least 14 days.

If a healthcare provider feels that someone may be depressed, the provider often uses a formalized questionnaire, such as the Beck Depression Inventory (BDI), to get a sense of the patient's psyche.

When you're doing an evaluation for depression, consider (and rule out) other medical conditions that can mimic depression. Common examples include hypothyroidism, adrenal insufficiency, anemia, advanced kidney disease, and electrolyte abnormalities, including hyponatremia, hypernatremia, and hypercalcemia.

When you're seeing elderly patients, don't mistake depression for dementia. The conditions can and often do present the same way. In fact, the conditions present so similarly that depression can be called *pseudo-dementia* in the elderly.

The treatment for depression includes not only psychotherapy and a full medical evaluation but also medications, namely serotonin selective reuptake inhibitors (SSRIs) and tricyclic antidepressants. Common side effects of the SSRIs can include weight gain and insomnia or hypersomnia. What a mix! Some of the SSRIs can cause hyponatremia. Tricyclic antidepressants can cause anticholinergic side effects as well as increase the risk of cardiac arrhythmias by prolonging the QT interval.

Before treating anyone with depression, make sure he or she doesn't have bipolar disorder (we cover bipolar disorder in the next section). Starting a bipolar person on depression meds or increasing the antidepressant dose can trigger a manic event. As you may surmise, the treatment for depression differs from the treatment for bipolar disorder.

Dysthymia is a milder form of depression. People who are affected have many of the same symptoms of depression, including changes in eating habits, changes in sleep patterns, feelings of low self-worth, and/or feeling fatigued; however, these symptoms are milder. Before you can make a diagnosis of dysthmia, the person has to have had many of these depressive symptoms for at least 24 months. The treatments for dysthymia and depression are similar.

You're evaluating a 30-year-old woman who states that she has difficulty wanting to "get out of bed in the morning." She says she just wants to be alone in the dark, away from everyone. You question her a little further and discover that 2 months ago, she gave birth to a son. What psychiatric condition are you most likely dealing with?

(A) Hypothyroidism

(B) Dysthymia

(C) Cyclothymia

(D) Panic disorder

(E) Post-partum depression

The correct answer is Choice (E), post-partum depression. The key to answering this question is paying attention to the time period. The symptoms of post-partum depression can begin 30 days after giving birth. Some experts feel they can last several months.

As for the other choices, there's no evidence of hypothyroidism on physical examination. Concerning dysthymia, the woman's symptoms are pretty severe; by contrast, with dysthymia, the person is able to function nearly fully in society. As for cyclothymia, the question mentions no cycling of symptoms between hypomania and dysthymia; this person is really depressed. Finally, this person is having the symptoms opposite those of panic disorder.

Understanding bipolar disorder and cyclothymia

Bipolar disorder used to be called manic-depressive disorder. The dictionary definition of *bipolar* is "having or relating to two poles or extremities" (think of the two poles of a magnet). The patient with bipolar disorder goes through tremendous mood swings, from a manic phase to a depressive phase, usually with a little bit of "normal" mood in between:

- **Manic phase:** Clinically, elevated moods are called *mania,* which comes from the Greek word for madness. During a manic phase, you can expect to see symptoms such as decreased need for sleep, aggression, quick decision-making, and/or an unlimited supply of energy. In addition, the affected person can be delusional. For example, the person may think he or she can buy everything and therefore go on lavish shopping sprees, nearly emptying the bank account in the process.

- **Depression phase:** The body is geared toward balance, so after the manic high, the affected person can come crashing down into a deep depression. The symptoms can be exhaustive and can include hopelessness, anorexia, social isolation, and sadness. A major depressive episode can last from 2 weeks to over 6 months.

As you may expect, bipolar disorder interferes with functioning. Unfortunately for the clinician, symptoms can vary quite a bit — and you can't order a lab test for bipolar disorder. Some people demonstrate features of both mania and depression at the same time. And some people have *rapid cycling,* with no normal mood between manic and depressive episodes. As with many conditions, the exact causes of bipolar disorder aren't clear. Bipolar patients are at risk of suicide in both the manic and depressed phases.

So how do you treat or at least manage bipolar disorder? The first-line approach is medication. The most common medication is lithium carbonate (Eskalith). It's approved by the FDA for treating depression, but it isn't without side effects, which can include thyroid abnormalities, leukocytosis, and a benign tremor. The big-time side effect of lithium carbonate is kidney disease. Many people who've used this med for years have stabilization of their bipolar disorder, but their kidney function is affected. However, lithium is still one of the best medications out there for this condition.

Other medications used commonly clinically include lamotrigine (Lamictal) and divalproex sodium (Depakote). Lamotrigine can be associated with a skin rash that goes away with discontinuation of therapy. It's very good for mood stabilization, preventing depressive episodes. Divalproex sodium can cause an increase in the liver function tests.

You can order psychotherapy after the person is initially stabilized with medication. Of course, it's essential that he or she be receptive to treatment. Behavioral-based therapy can help identify potential triggers of manic and/or depressive behavior. In cases where a person poses a danger to himself or others, consider an involuntary commitment to the hospital.

Cyclothymia is a milder form of bipolar disorder in which the affected person alternates between periods of dysthymia and hypomania. Think of *dysthymia* as a milder form of depression and *hypomania* as a milder form of manic disorder. The key here is recognizing that many people with cyclothymia are functional, unlike those with bipolar disorder, who often aren't able to fully function in society.

Understanding Substance Abuse

You're sure to see substance abuse questions on the PANCE. Substance abuse is a form of substance-related disorder (which is a little like saying the same thing twice). Many substances — from opiates to chocolate milkshakes — have legitimate and beneficial uses. However, an excessive or off-purpose use of a substance can be classified as abuse. In many cases, the result is dependence or addiction. In some cases, the result is degeneration of the abuser, leading to illness and death.

Drug abuse is an important topic because of its frequent occurrence and negative impacts. It's not just an individual clinical problem but a societal issue as well. The popular drugs to abuse are opioids (opium, morphine, and heroin), methamphetamine, amphetamines, barbiturates, cocaine, marijuana, and hash. Both street drugs and prescription drugs can be abused. Tobacco and alcohol tend to fall into their own categories.

In this section, we cover the difference between dependence and addiction and then discuss the abuse of specific substances in more detail. For information on overdoses, see Chapter 14.

Distinguishing between dependence and addiction

Make sure you understand the difference between dependence and addiction. *Physical dependence* refers to how a person's body gets used to or handles a particular drug. For any medication you prescribe, whether it's pain medication or diabetes medication, the person's body needs to be able to adapt to it. For example, a person on insulin depends on that medication to keep his or her blood sugar low.

The hot topic for drug dependence is pain medication, more so than street drugs. People on pain meds (after a motor vehicle accident, for example) come to physically depend on them to help relieve their pain. They may even develop a tolerance to the meds and require a higher dose. The resolution involves talking with their healthcare providers and agreeing on a plan to meet an intended goal: to reduce and eliminate use of the meds.

Addiction is more of a psychological issue. The addicted person may take the pain medication even when it's not scheduled. He or she may sneak extra doses and begin to crave the medication. His or her whole life starts to revolve around the medication. The addiction can take over the person's life.

To eliminate abuse, the substance abuser first has to acknowledge that a problem exists. After that, he or she often needs to be treated and monitored closely at a dedicated treatment center because drug withdrawal can occur. The *withdrawal reaction* often involves precisely the opposite of what the drug usually does. For example, withdrawal may cause tremors, anxiety, perceptual disturbances, dysphoria, psychosis, and seizures.

Realize that there are other types of addiction besides drug addiction. Examples can include gambling, food, sex, texting, and using the Internet. The comparison is not inappropriate, because these behaviors can take on an importance that, like drugs, degrades the sufferer's lifestyle. And like heroin, these habits can be hard to kick.

Looking at common forms of substance abuse

Recognizing signs of substance abuse is important. The person who "uses" may often miss work, miss family obligations, and neglect others in the family. He or she may have a police record for recurrent substance use. In addition, drug abusers may "abuse themselves" (use the drug) before or during work. An example is the forklift driver who has three beers each morning before work or has a brewski or pops a narcotic pill or two during his or her break.

Alcohol, tobacco, and other drugs are common substances that are abused by many people. In this section, you read more about these disorders and how to best manage and treat them.

Alcohol abuse

Alcohol — that is, the relatively nonpoisonous ethanol — is America's favorite legal addictive drug.

You can use questionnaires to gauge someone's use of alcohol. A popular one you should know about is the CAGE questionnaire. Ask your patients four questions to screen for alcohol abuse:

- ✔ **C — cut down:** Has the affected person — or anyone else — ever felt the need to reduce the amount that person drinks?

- ✔ **A — angry or annoyed:** Does the person become angry or annoyed when asked about his or her drinking habits?

- ✔ **G — guilt:** Does he or she feel guilty about excessive drinking?

- ✔ **E — eye-opener:** Does the person need an *eye-opener,* the famous first drink in the morning to help with a hangover?

If a person answers two or more of these questions in the positive, he or she may have a problem with alcohol.

For anyone with a substance abuse problem, the key is to recognize that there *is* a problem. That's often the hardest step. The long-term key is to abstain. Note that someone who abuses alcohol often abuses other substances as well, including tobacco and other drugs.

You need to be aware of several points concerning alcohol use, especially overuse. As a clinician, you often first meet the person who is abusing alcohol in the emergency room. We include information on "dealing with the drunk" here. Here are some high-yield facts:

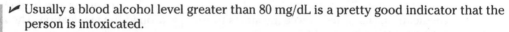

- ✔ Usually a blood alcohol level greater than 80 mg/dL is a pretty good indicator that the person is intoxicated.

- ✔ If a patient presents with the odor of alcohol, you need to be guarded in your diagnosis and treatment plan. The history of the presenting illness may not be reliable. Further, don't be too swift to blame findings on the alcohol. Your findings may actually be related to another condition.

- ✔ Patients who abuse alcohol may present to the hospital with a change in mental status. Besides inebriation, other differential diagnoses include hypoglycemia and electrolyte abnormalities, alcoholic hepatitis, hepatic encephalopathy, Wernicke's encephalopathy, infection/sepsis, and/or a subdural hematoma. If a person with suspected alcohol abuse is found down and is unresponsive, the person may have hit his or her head and could have a subdural hematoma.

- ✔ The initial treatment for alcohol intoxication includes the *banana bag,* an IV solution that includes magnesium, thiamine, folic acid, and a multivitamin. Many people suffering from alcohol abuse have multiple nutritional deficiencies.

- ✔ Do not give glucose without first giving thiamine. You could precipitate Wernicke's encephalopathy.

Recognize the signs of alcohol withdrawal. The symptoms of *delirium tremens* (the legendary DTs) usually occur about 48 to 72 hours after drinking stops. This is acute withdrawal, and symptoms can include very high blood pressure, tachycardia, and even a fever. The treatment is benzodiazepines. When someone comes into the hospital with a history of alcohol abuse, benzodiazepines such as oxazepam (Serax) need to be started around the clock to prevent abrupt alcohol withdrawal.

Other meds can be used to treat alcoholism, although they're rarely used anymore. One example is disulfiram (Antabuse). Anyone taking it experiences violent nausea and vomiting after drinking alcohol. You should be aware that other medications can cause a disulfiram-like reaction; these include oral sulfonylureas used to treat diabetes and the antibiotic metronidazole (Flagyl).

Nicotine abuse, primarily smoking

You can get a sense of how much someone smokes — and that person's subsequent risk of smoking-related conditions — by estimating *pack years*. For example, if someone has been smoking 1 pack a day for 30 years, he or she has 30 pack years. That's a lot of cigarettes. There are 20 cigarettes in most packs of cigarettes. If you talk with someone who smokes a pipe, ask whether the pipe is filtered or unfiltered. In addition, ask whether the person smoked cigarettes before starting on the pipe.

Stopping smoking can be very hard, and the treatment is often multidimensional. For the purposes of the PANCE, be aware of the five *a*'s of quitting smoking:

✔ **Ask:** Talk to your patient about his or her smoking with every interaction.

✔ **Advise:** Encourage your patient to quit smoking.

✔ **Assess:** Does your patient really want to quit?

✔ **Assist:** For example, help the patient pick a "quit day."

✔ **Arrange:** For example, help the patient pick a smoking cessation class.

In conjunction with other measures, such as cessation classes, the prescription medication bupropion (Zyban) has been used to help people quit smoking. One main side effect of bupropion is that it can lower the seizure threshold.

Some sort of nicotine replacement is often required to prevent withdrawal. Note that the person isn't supposed to smoke while using the nicotine patch or the gum. Nicotine is a vasoconstrictor, and the combination can cause chest pain and/or hypertension.

Drug abuse

You should be able to recognize some of the main side effects and potential risks of many drugs that are commonly abused, especially the stimulants. Here we're talking about both prescribed medications and illegal substances. Realize that drug abuse is a widespread problem, especially among younger generations and teenagers.

In Chapter 14, you can read about the many of the physiologic side effects of drug use, especially stimulant use. We cover overdoses of cocaine, meth, and other substances. Also see Chapter 3 for ways these drugs can affect heart health and cause hypertensive emergencies.

In many cases, the person who abuses drugs needs some form of inpatient treatment for substance use, especially given all the medical comorbidities with the condition.

Evaluating Eating Disorders

Eating disorders are very prevalent in society. You don't want to miss them or some of the clinical signs that can go along with them. This knowledge is valuable both for your clinical practice and for the PANCE. Here we focus on the eating disorders that you'll likely be asked about on the test. Please note that although these disorders are predominant in women, men can also be affected.

Recognizing anorexia

Anorexia nervosa (AN) often occurs in younger women. The affected person often has a distorted image of self; she feels that she's "too fat" when she's actually below a healthy weight range for her age and height. Here are the key points for recognizing and treating anorexia:

✔ People with anorexia often severely restrict the amount of food they eat and are severely malnourished. This is the type of anorexia nervosa most people are familiar with.

Although purging behaviors are often associated with bulimia (see the next section), they can occur with anorexia as well. Behavior may include excessive exercise and the use of laxatives as part of the purging.

✔ The affected person may be adrenally insufficient as well as amenorrheic. She often needs intensive treatment, usually in a hospital, to attend to her medical needs. Consultation with a nutritionist/dietitian is vital.

✔ The treatment for anorexia involves intense psychotherapy to change the patient's self-image, particularly (mis)perceptions about her body.

Beating bulimia

Like anorexia, *bulimia nervosa* (BN) often occurs in younger women. Again, the affected person has a distorted sense of self and an abnormal self-image. Here are a few key points about bulimia:

✔ Most commonly, the affected person engages in binging and purging behavior. The key to PANCE questions concerning bulimia is to pay attention to physical exam clues in the questions. The fingers go into the mouth to induce vomiting, so look at the knuckles and fingers for scratches, calluses, and/or discoloration. In addition, you may see *parotid gland hypertrophy* (an enlargement of the salivary glands) and loss of enamel in the teeth because of recurrent gastric exposure due to vomiting. The person may also have many dental problems, including cavities.

✔ Pay attention to blood work. Because of the excessive vomiting, a metabolic alkalosis may be present. Often, the affected person is profoundly hypokalemic (vomiting blows out your potassium) and has low to undetectable magnesium levels. See Chapter 10 for info on electrolytes and acid-base disorders.

✔ In addition to a nutrition consultation, the affected person needs intense psychotherapy.

Practice Behavioral Health Questions

These practice questions are similar to the PANCE behavioral health questions.

1. You're examining a 35-year-old man who is exhibiting acute psychotic behavior. He also has delusions and hallucinations. He has a history of a hypertrophic cardiomyopathy as well. Which of the following medications would you be very hesitant to give this man?

   (A) Haloperidol (Haldol)

   (B) Olanzapine (Zyprexa)

   (C) Lithium carbonate (Lithobid)

   (D) Oxazepam (Serax)

   (E) Diazepam (Valium)

2. You're seeing a 35-year-old woman for evaluation of major depressive disorder. You want to begin treatment with an antidepressant. Which of the following conditions do you need to exclude before you treat her?

   (A) Panic disorder

   (B) Seasonal affective disorder

   (C) Borderline personality disorder

   (D) Bipolar disorder

   (E) Dementia

3. You're seeing a 25-year-old man in the ER who was recently started on metoclopramide (Reglan). He presents with a very high fever and a change in mental status. On physical examination, his muscles are rigid. His body temperature is 40.0°C (104°F). You obtain a stat CPK level, and it is 50,000. This man is in severe trouble. What is the most likely diagnosis?

   (A) Serotonin syndrome

   (B) Tyramine reaction

   (C) Neuroleptic malignant syndrome (NMS)

   (D) Drug overdose

   (E) Bacterial infection

4. You're going to school with a colleague who swears that he has every medical condition you are studying. In school, you're currently studying the GI system. He's having some diarrhea and fears he may have colon cancer. He beseeches the physicians to allow him to have a colonoscopy. This behavior could be an example of what psychiatric condition?

   (A) Malingering

   (B) Factitious disorder

   (C) Somatoform disorder

   (D) Hypochondriasis

   (E) Social phobia

5. You are evaluating a 55-year-old man who comes to the clinic complaining of a fever. You take his temperature, and it is 39.4°C (103°F). You find out that this person may have somehow heated the thermometer with a lighter to induce a false reading. This behavior could be an example of what psychiatric condition?

   (A) Malingering

   (B) Factitious disorder

   (C) Somatoform disorder

   (D) Hypochondriasis

   (E) Social phobia

6. What's the most immediate treatment needed in a patient suffering from neuroleptic malignant syndrome?

   (A) Intravenous diuretics

   (B) Intravenous haloperidol (Haldol)

   (C) Intravenous metoclopramide (Reglan)

   (D) Warming blanket

   (E) Dantrolene sodium

Answers and Explanations

Use this answer key to score the practice behavioral health questions from the preceding section. The answer explanations give you insight into why the correct answer is better than the other choices.

1. **A.** Haloperidol (Haldol) is a typical antipsychotic that can cause cardiac arrhythmias, specifically by prolonging the QT interval. You wouldn't give it to someone with a hypertrophic cardiomyopathy. A good choice to use for this patient would be olanzapine (Zyprexa), Choice (B). Choice (C), lithium carbonate, is used for bipolar disorder. Choices (D) and (E), oxazepam and diazepam, are used for anxiety and panic disorders. These other meds may be used adjunctively (although the person still needs to be given a medication to control his or her psychotic behavior).

2. **D.** In anyone you think has major depressive disorder, make sure you consider that the person may have bipolar disorder. By giving a bipolar person an antidepressant, you can unmask a manic episode. Choice (A), panic disorder, wouldn't be a concern here, and Choice (B), seasonal affective disorder, makes no sense. Nothing in the question suggests that her depression is related to seasons of the year (for example, better in June than in January). Note that Choice (C), borderline personality disorder, can be associated with depression. The woman in the question is typically too young to have dementia, Choice (E), and nothing in the question makes you think that she does.

3. **C.** This man has neuroleptic malignant syndrome (NMS), which you usually see after someone takes a neuroleptic or antipsychotic. This person took metoclopramide (Reglan). He presents with fever and a change in mental status. His muscles are rigid because of the medication. A person with neuroleptic malignant syndrome has an elevated CPK level.

   Choice (A) is wrong because serotonin syndrome (SS) occurs with medications that can cause excessive serotinergic activity. Examples of such medications include SSRIs, tricyclics, certain over-the-counter medications, and anti-Parkinson's medications. Symptoms can include confusion, fever, and tachycardia. You usually see Parkinson's and hyperactive reflexes with SS, as compared to the muscle rigidity you seen in neuroleptic malignant syndrome.

   A tyramine reaction, Choice (B), concerns the interaction of a MAO inhibitor with anything that contains tyramine, such as wine and cheese. Choice (D), a drug overdose, is nonspecific, and the question gives no evidence of a bacterial infection, Choice (E).

4. **D.** This colleague has a textbook case of hypochondriasis.

5. **B.** This person is actively trying to mess with the equipment to cause the healthcare provider to think a disease or medical condition is present when it really isn't. Therefore, he has factitious disorder, Choice (B). This condition differs from Choice (A), malingering, in which the person is making up symptoms or acting sick. With malingering, the person isn't trying to sabotage medical equipment or do something illegal. Concerning Choice (C), a somatoform disorder is a mental disorder causing physical symptoms; a somatoform disorder is not a syndrome that's purposely made up. With Choice (D), hypochondriasis, the affected person thinks that he or she has every medical condition. With Choice (E), the person is afraid of a particular aspect of society, such as when someone is afraid to go on stage or be seen in public places.

6. **E.** The immediate choice for the treatment of neuroleptic malignant syndrome (NMS) is Choice (E) — you need to do something to stop the muscle rigidity, so you give dantrolene sodium. Bromocriptine can also be given. Concerning Choice (A), the treatment of choice is intravenous fluids, not diuretics. You don't want to dehydrate this person. Choices (B) and (C) would be contraindicated: You would not give a neuroleptic to someone with neuroleptic malignant syndrome. Concerning Choice (D), you'd use a cooling blanket, not a warming blanket, because the person would be hyperthermic.

Chapter 14

Focusing on Pharmacology and Toxicology

*A*s a student, you probably spent some time in the emergency room (ER) — maybe during a scheduled ER rotation or a medicine or critical care service — and you needed to admit someone to the hospital. You've likely seen and evaluated patients with toxic ingestions, fatal or near-fatal drug overdoses, or drug-drug interactions that adversely affected their health.

You see questions about these topics on the PANCE/PANRE, so this chapter reviews some principles of pharmacology, as well as common toxic ingestions and medication interactions. Of course, we also include the basics of identifying and treating conditions you see in "real life" as well as "test life."

Reviewing Basic Pharmacological Principles

Before we get into the nitty-gritty of nasty medication side effects, drug-drug interactions, and toxic ingestions, you need to review some basic pharmacological principles. The body processes a medication in four basic ways: absorption, distribution, metabolism, and elimination. If any of these processes is altered in some way, then bad things can happen.

Absorbing the medication

For a medication to work in the body, it has to be absorbed. Medications given orally (the most frequently used route of administration) require an intact gastrointestinal (GI) tract for proper absorption. In Chapter 5, we discuss conditions related to low nutrient levels in certain malabsorption syndromes (for example, inflammatory bowel disease). Such conditions can cause malabsorption of oral medications, too.

Other factors can impact a medication's absorption as well, one being its *bioavailability* (how much medication is absorbed in the GI tract). Different medications are made differently and absorbed differently by the intestine; for example, you sometimes see significant differences in bioavailability when comparing a brand name medicine to its generic counterpart.

Certain medications can also affect the absorption of others. For example, many oral iron preparations must be taken separately from other medications because iron can decrease their absorption. Usually, the medication levothyroxine (Synthroid) is taken separately from other meds because the interaction can affect its absorption. Less of it is absorbed when it's not taken on an empty stomach apart from other medications.

Distributing the medication

After a medication is absorbed, it has to go somewhere. Different medications have different volumes of distribution. For example, medications that are *lipophilic* (fat-loving) are found in higher concentrations in adipose tissue than those that are *hydrophilic* (water-loving). Some medications can achieve a therapeutic blood concentration, and others build up in the body tissues. For example, fluoroquinolones are used in treating many genitourinary (GU) infections because they have good tissue penetration into that area. They're used for treating lung infections such as bronchitis and pneumonia for the same reason. Although the aminoglycoside antibiotics likewise have good GU penetration, they wouldn't be good choices for treating a lung infection because they don't penetrate the lung tissue very well.

If you understand how the body handles a medication or class of medications, you can better understand how to treat a toxic ingestion or a significant drug interaction. Some medications, like digoxin (Lanoxin), bind to plasma proteins such as albumin. These medications can stick to these proteins like glue, which becomes problematic if they reach a toxic level. For drugs such as this, you need to know how much of a medication is protein-bound and how much is the unbound (active) portion. If a medication is highly protein bound, it cannot be removed by dialysis.

Metabolizing the medication

How the body metabolizes a medication is a biggie in terms of drug-drug interactions. The majority of medications are metabolized in the liver (meaning they're *hepatically metabolized*), usually via various cytochrome pathways. For example, cytochrome P450 (CYP) is a common metabolic pathway for many medications, including antiseizure meds. As the liver's metabolic machinery processes the medications, they can act as either enzyme inhibitors or enzyme activators:

- **Enzyme inhibitors:** Inhibit the metabolism of other medications
- **Enzyme activators:** Increase the metabolism of other medications, thus lowering drug levels

A common example of an enzyme inhibitor is cimetidine (Tagamet). This H2 blocker can inhibit the metabolism of many medications processed by the same metabolic pathway so they have a longer half-life in the body.

Increasing or decreasing the half-life of some medications can have dramatic results. One of the most dramatic examples of this is warfarin (Coumadin), which you read about later in this chapter. Any medication that's an enzymatic inhibitor can increase the half-life of warfarin. This can thin the blood and increase the risk of bleeding. Too low of a warfarin level can increase the risk of clots. Being on warfarin means following the blood levels and the prothrombin time (PT/INR) closely.

On the PANCE, you should be familiar with the mechanism of action of commonly prescribed medications. Following is an example question on mechanism.

Which of the following medications works by increasing the pancreatic secretion of insulin?

(A) Metformin (Glucophage)

(B) Acarbose (Precose)

(C) Glucagon (GlucaGen)

(D) Glimepiride (Amaryl)

(E) Cosyntropin (ACTH)

The answer is Choice (D). Glimepiride (Amaryl) belongs to the class of medications called sulfonylureas, which increase pancreatic secretion of insulin. Metformin (Glucophage) decreases liver production of glucose and increases peripheral utilization of glucose. Acarbose (Precose) inhibits carbohydrate absorption. Glucagon isn't even applicable here; it's used to treat life-threatening hypoglycemia. Cosyntropin (ACTH) is used to evaluate for adrenal insufficiency.

Eliminating the medication

After the body processes the medication, the med needs to leave the body somehow. The main medication or its metabolites are eliminated either by the GI tract or more commonly via the kidney. Kidney disease can extend the half-life of many medications, such as insulin.

Examining Common Medication Side Effects

The average person over age 60 takes about nine prescription medications and sees a minimum of four different healthcare providers. The potential for someone to experience the side effects of these medications is huge, as is the potential for significant drug-drug interactions.

On the test, you have to recall the side effects of commonly prescribed medications. This section reminds you of those side effects as well as how to manage toxic levels of a prescribed medication. Many of these medications are cardiac-related, which is no surprise because chest pain and congestive heart failure are the most common reasons people are admitted to the hospital.

Coughing up the ACE (inhibitor)

Angiotensin converting enzyme (ACE) inhibitors such as lisinopril (Zestril) and ramipril (Altace) are commonly prescribed not only for treating hypertension but also for diabetic nephropathy.

Say you encounter a test question about a newly prescribed medication and the person is experiencing a nonproductive cough. Among the answer choices, look for an ACE inhibitor. In addition to a cough, a common laboratory finding in someone taking an ACE inhibitor is hyperkalemia (see more about evaluating and managing hyperkalemia in Chapter 10).

In addition to a cough and hyperkalemia, a major and potentially life-threatening side effect of ACE inhibitors is *angioedema,* an anaphylactic reaction that occurs after taking an ACE inhibitor. The initial management includes remembering the ABCs: securing the *airway* (the tongue can swell big time and obstruct the airway), checking for *breathing,* and supporting the *circulation* if needed (for example, administering intravenous fluids and pressors). It's also important to treat the underlying anaphylaxis, using epinephrine, histamine blockers, and intravenous steroids.

Unusual side effects of hyperkalemia-causing meds

Two other medications besides ACE inhibitors that can cause hyperkalemia have unique effects. Potassium-sparing diuretics like spironolactone (Aldactone) can do more than cause hyperkalemia; they can also cause breast tenderness (actually, nipple tenderness) in some people, especially in higher doses. Rich has had to decrease the dose or even stop the medication in certain instances. Trimethoprim/sulfamethoxazole (Bactrim) is a commonly prescribed antibiotic. Not only can it raise potassium levels, but it can also cause pseudo–renal failure by erroneously raising creatinine levels.

Dealing with digoxin

Physician assistants usually prescribe digoxin (Lanoxin) to help patients who have systolic heart failure. Because it works on the atrioventricular (AV) node, it's also given to help with rate control in treating atrial fibrillation.

Digoxin depends on the kidney for excretion, and you can monitor the medication by checking the digoxin level in the blood. Be aware of medications that can raise digoxin levels. Calcium channel blockers, macrolide antibiotics, and other antiarrythmic agents can increase the blood levels of digoxin and increase the risk of digoxin toxicity. Furthermore, hypokalemia and hypercalcemia can make digoxin toxicity worse.

Be aware of signs of digoxin toxicity, especially in the older population. Signs include nausea, vomiting, blurry vision, or seeing a halo. The person may also experience confusion, hallucinations, and lethargy. In addition, you can see many types of cardiac arrythmias, including atrial and ventricular arrythmias (for example, junctional rhythm).

The treatment for digoxin toxicity is to administer digoxin antibodies (Fab fragments). Because digoxin is heavily bound to plasma proteins, you can't remove it through dialysis.

Sorting out the statin side effects

The statins are one of the most commonly prescribed medications to treat hyperlipidemia. Examples include atorvastatin (Lipitor) and simvastatin (Zocor). These medications aren't without their side effects, including elevated liver enzymes (LFTs) and myalgias.

The LFTs should be measured before prescribing a statin, at least once a month for the first 3 months, with any elevation, and periodically thereafter.

The myalgias are less common, but you may see them with higher doses of statins. The patient may have muscle pain, usually in the proximal muscle areas, with or without elevated CPK levels. Treatment can include decreasing the dose of the medication, stopping the medication, or changing to another statin. Some data suggest that supplementing with ubiquinol (coenzyme Q_{10}) may help decrease some of the myalgia symptoms.

A significant consequence of statin-induced muscle damage is rhabdomyolysis, whose evaluation and management we discuss in Chapter 10.

Bashing the blockers' side effects

A slowing of the heart rate is a side effect of both beta blockers, such as propranolol (Inderal), and calcium channel blockers (CCBs), including diltiazem (Cardizem). Beta blockers work on the sinoatrial (SA) node and AV node. Certain calcium channel blockers, like diltiazem, can affect AV nodal conduction. The dosage of these medications is usually slowly titrated, with both the blood pressure and heart rate being watched carefully. If the heart rate gets too low or if the blood pressure drops (symptomatic bradycardia), then urgent treatment is needed. Here are some key points on monitoring and treatment:

- ✔ Before talking about specific antidotes for beta blockers and calcium channel blockers, don't forget your ABCs. Having good IV access and starting IV fluids is crucial, especially if hypotension is present. Cardiac monitoring is a must, and you may need to place a transcutaneous pacer on the patient.

- ✔ Symptomatic bradycardia is first treated with atropine, no matter the cause. Atropine won't be effective if a third-degree heart block is the cause of the bradycardia.

- ✔ Symptomatic bradycardia due to beta-blocker toxicity is usually treated initially with high-dose glucagon.

- ✔ Symptomatic bradycardia due to calcium channel blockers is initially treated with intravenous calcium and epinephrine.

   Insulin and glucose aren't just for treating diabetes or hyperkalemia; you can also use them in managing a calcium channel blocker overdose that remains refractory to calcium and epinephrine therapy. Insulin and glucose infusions are given along with potassium to manage the toxicity. The many uses of insulin are just amazing!

Which one of the following is true concerning calcium channel blockers?

(A) Diltiazem (Cardizem) is commonly used for the treatment of systolic heart failure.

(B) Diltiazem (Cardizem) has a negative ionotropic effect.

(C) Amlodipine (Norvasc) can be used for the treatment of atrial fibrillation.

(D) Common side effects can include diarrhea and polyuria.

(E) Amlodipine (Norvasc) cannot be used in the treatment of congestive heart failure.

The answer is Choice (B). The calcium channel blockers, especially the nondihydropyridines such as diltiazem (Cardizem) and verapamil (Calan), have a negative ionotropic effect (they can decrease the contraction of the left ventricle, which is why they're used in the treatment of hypertrophic cardiomyopathy). This is why diltiazem and varepamil can't be used in treating systolic heart failure. The other answers in the question are incorrect. Amlodipine (Norvasc) is fourth-line in the treatment of heart failure (used cautiously), but it's not used to treat atrial fibrillation because it has little or no effect on the AV node. The side effects of calcium channel blockers include constipation and edema. Diuretics can cause polyuria.

Treating toxic theophylline

Theophylline (Aerolate JR) is an older medication used in treating asthma and chronic obstructive pulmonary disease (COPD). Watching the side effects of this medication is important.

As with digoxin, you can measure theophylline by measuring a blood level. A normal level is 10 to 20 mcg/mL; however, even at physiologic doses, you can see side effects. Theophylline is a dimethylxanthine, so it has a diuretic effect and can cause electrolyte abnormalities, including hypokalemia. It can also cause hypercalcemia and hypomagnesemia (see Chapter 10 for details on electrolyte imbalances).

Symptoms of acute toxicity include nausea, vomiting, tachycardia, cardiac arrythmias, and seizures at high doses. Treatment includes activated charcoal, supportive measures, and dialysis if the levels are super high.

Although theophylline can elicit any kind of cardiac arrhythmia, one of the most common (and one you're likely to see on the test) is multifocal atrial tachycardia (MAT).

Eliminating excess lithium

Lithium is used in the treatment of bipolar disorder and has many side effects. (See Chapter 13 for details.) Lithium use is closely monitored by measuring drug levels in the blood. When the blood levels get too high or if the person becomes symptomatic, then emergent dialysis may be necessary. Here are a few key points concerning lithium overdose:

- ✔ Therapeutic serum lithium levels are 0.8 to 1.2 mmol/L. An absolute indication for dialysis is a level of 3 mmol/L.

- ✔ Initial treatment includes aggressive use of intravenous fluids, preferably normal saline. Volume depletion and dehydration can aggravate lithium toxicity.

- ✔ Lithium has a large volume of distribution, and sometimes multiple dialysis treatments may be needed to remove the excess lithium from the body.

Negating narcotics

Many adults are prescribed narcotics for the treatment of pain. Although narcotics can be effective, they're not without significant side effects. A common side effect from narcotic use is constipation, and significant side effects from narcotic overuse include lethargy, confusion, and somnolence. Older patients can be difficult to arouse.

On examination of a patient, you may notice a decreased respiratory rate and even hypotension. An ABG may show an acute respiratory acidosis. If hypotension or hypoxemia is present, you may see an associated metabolic acidosis.

Treatment involves securing the airway, and if the person experiences significant somnolence, he or she may require intubation and mechanical ventilation. You may prescribe a medication such as naloxone (Narcan) to reverse some of the effects of the narcotic.

If a person has been chronically taking narcotics, the last thing you want to do is completely reverse them with naloxone; otherwise, you'll precipitate acute symptoms of withdrawal. Often, you see small doses given to negate the respiratory depression, and the person is monitored closely.

Narcotics isn't the only medication class that can cause respiratory depression; you also need to be careful with the benzodiazepines. This class includes medications like lorazepam (Ativan) and alprazolam (Xanax). In fact, at least 35 generics are in the class, with multiple brand names for most of them. The treatment for a benzodiazepine overdose isn't naloxone. It's flumazenil (Romazicon).

Recognizing Common Drug Interactions

With the advent of polypharmacy came the danger of significant drug-drug interactions. This section describes the common interactions and what you need to know about them.

Being careful about warfarin (Coumadin)

Nonprofessionals call warfarin (Coumadin) a *blood thinner*. This frequently prescribed anti-coagulant is used to treat many conditions, including atrial fibrillation, mechanical heart valves, and deep venous thrombosis/pulmonary embolism.

Warfarin is hepatically metabolized and can interact with many, many medications that can either increase or decrease PT/INR levels. Close monitoring is essential, as is being aware of possible interactions whenever a patient gets a new medication. Here are some key points about warfarin interactions:

✔ Medications that can increase warfarin levels are enzymatic inhibitors, such as amiodarone (Cordarone), and the macrolide antibiotics, such as clarithromycin (Biaxin). You may see a question concerning the interaction between amiodarone and warfarin, because amiodarone is commonly prescribed for rhythm control of atrial fibrillation.

✔ Anything that affects the metabolism of vitamin K can affect the PT/INR levels. For example, malnutrition or malabsorption can alter bowel flora and increase PT/INR levels. Ingestion of foods containing vitamin K, such as leafy greens, can affect levels as well. Warfarin dosing needs to be adjusted (usually decreased) or even held in some instances until the INR levels begin to normalize.

✔ Vitamin K can be used in the treatment of a high INR, but you need to be careful. It can lower the PT/INR level. Vitamin K can be given orally or subcutaneously. For any acute bleeding episodes, you can and should use fresh frozen plasma (FFP).

 Although one of the treatments for a very high level of warfarin is vitamin K, vitamin K doesn't work in heparin overdose. The treatment for a heparin overdose is protamine sulfate given intravenously.

Assessing the antiarrhythmic interactions

Antiarrythmic medications come in many classes (see Chapter 3 for details), and they have the potential for significant interactions with other medications. Many classes of antiarrhythmics can prolong the QT interval, and some medication interactions increase the likelihood of developing ventricular arrythmias, including the dreaded *torsades de pointes*. Watch for these interactions both for test-taking purposes and especially when taking care of a patient.

For example, enzymatic inhibitors that increase the half-life of quinidine and/or procainamide (Procaine) can increase the risk of prolongation of the QT interval. Any electrolyte abnormalities, especially low potassium and magnesium, can also increase the risk of arrhythmias. Hypomagnesemia can increase the risk of ventricular arrhythmias, especially torsades de pointes.

Having HAART: Interactions with anti-HIV meds

Here we're talking about highly active antiretroviral therapy (HAART). The medications in this drug cocktail have been the mainstay of HIV treatment for years and have improved the lives of many with this condition. Medications used to treat HIV, however, have the potential for so many medication interactions that it boggles the mind. One big interaction that you see in test questions about drug interactions in HIV therapy involves rifampin (Rifadin), which is used in the treatment of tuberculosis. Rifampin can significantly interact with many HIV medications, including zidovudine (AZT), indinavir (Crixivan), and saquinavir (Invirase). It can increase their metabolism and decrease their effectiveness.

One possible side effect of the HIV medication indinavir is kidney stones, which can be difficult to treat.

Watching over transplant medications

A significant drug interaction you're likely to see on the test concerns medications used for solid-organ transplants (for example, a kidney transplant). Rich takes care of several kidney transplant patients, and he has to watch their medications like a hawk. Commonly prescribed medications that you need be aware of include cyclosporine (Neoral or Sandimmune) and tacrolimus (Prograf).

Medication classes that increase the levels of cyclosporine and tacrolimus include macrolide antibiotics such as clarithromycin (Biaxin), antifungal agents like fluconazole (Diflucan), and calcium channel blockers like verapamil (Calan). Like many of the meds listed in this chapter, these transplant medications are closely monitored by a drug level in the blood. If the levels are too high, they can be toxic to the kidney and cause acute kidney failure. They also can suppress the immune system even more than they're supposed to.

Seizing the antiseizure medications

Many commonly prescribed antiseizure medications like phenytoin (Dilantin) are in fact enzymatic inducers and can lower the levels of other medications, including the following:

- Warfarin (Coumadin)
- Transplant medications such as cyclosporine (Neoral) and tacrolimus (Prograf)
- Antifungals like fluconazole (Diflucan)

One major consequence of long-term use of medications like phenytoin and phenobarbital is low vitamin D levels. Vitamin D is metabolized in the liver, and many of these medications, being enzymatic inducers, can hasten the metabolism of the vitamin. In anyone you see who's on phenytoin, check a vitamin D level and supplement as needed.

Probing serotonin

The selective serotonin reuptake inhibitors (SSRIs) are used in treating depression. They're hepatically metabolized, and you need to be aware of the other medications that can interact with them, including blood thinners, especially warfarin. SSRIs can raise warfarin levels.

SSRIs and other nonselective medications, such as bupropion (Wellbutrin) and venlafaxine (Effexor), can interact to affect the reuptake of serotonin. That can lead to *serotonin syndrome,* a potentially life-threatening reaction caused by the release of too much serotonin. An older but important class of medications you should also watch for is the monoamine oxidase (MAO) inhibitors — phenelzine (Nardil) and tranylcypromine (Parnate).

Symptoms of serotonin syndrome include tachycardia, nausea, vomiting, significant agitation, and labile blood pressure. You may also see fevers, muscle spasms, and myoclonus. Treatment consists of hospitalization, intravenous fluids, and the use of benzodiazepines to decrease agitation and muscle spasms/jerking. You can also use meds that block serotonin production, such as cyproheptadine (Periactin).

Looking at neuroleptic malignant syndrome (NMS)

Neuroleptic malignant syndrome can be a side effect of certain psychotropic medications, including haloperidol (Haldol). Although not very common, this syndrome is important to recognize so you won't be led astray. You see NMS in younger people, particularly men. Here are the key points concerning NMS:

- ✔ The person may have significant hyperthermia, labile blood pressure, significant diaphoresis, and a change in mental status.

- ✔ More importantly, the person with NMS becomes rigid. He may have significant muscle damage, and you may see significant rhabdomyolysis with elevated CPK levels. One of the treatments, then, is aggressive volume repletion with normal saline.

- ✔ In addition to stopping the medication that caused NMS, other therapy includes administering the muscle relaxant dantrolene sodium (Dantrium) and using a dopamine agonist such as bromocriptine (Parlodel).

Understanding tyramine reactions

A *tyramine reaction* is potentiated when a person taking a MAO inhibitor eats a food that contains the amino acid tyramine, commonly found in wine, cheese, and about 30 other culinary delights. A person may have a hypertensive crisis, informally known as the *cheese effect,* when the MAO inhibitor and the food mix. Be aware of foods that contain tyramine, and have your patient avoid them if he or she is on a MAO inhibitor. This is one of those syndromes you should know mainly for the test, because in clinical practice, MAO inhibitors aren't prescribed that much anymore.

Being alert to the anticholinergics

Anticholinergic toxicity is a must-know syndrome for you to recognize and treat. Certain medication classes can predispose people to acute anticholinergic syndrome. These classes include antihistamines, antidepressants, certain psychotropic medications, and medications used to treat Parkinson's disease.

The anticholingergic syndrome can affect many organs of the body. It can cause urinary retention, fever, fast heart rate, decreased bowel function (or an ileus), and mydriasis (dilated pupils). The person can also be extremely agitated and may experience hallucinations. The treatment is generally supportive because no specific antidote is available.

A cholinergic reaction, which is the opposite of an anticholinergic reaction, occurs when a lot of acetylcholine is being released. The symptoms include diaphoresis, salivation, and miosis (constricted pupils). These symptoms are the complete opposite of the mydriasis, dry skin, and dry eyes and mouth seen in the anticholinergic syndrome.

You're evaluating a 57-year-old man who presents to your office with complaints of significant lethargy and fatigue. He states that since starting a medication, his mouth is very dry. Which of the following medications is the likely cause of this patient's symptoms?

(A) Amlodipine (Norvasc)

(B) Clonidine (Catapres)

(C) Terazosin (Hytrin)

(D) Lisinopril (Zestril)

(E) Furosemide (Lasix)

The answer is Choice (B). Clonidine (Catapres) works centrally and can cause dry mouth, lethargy, and fatigue. This medication can also cause a withdrawal reaction when stopped abruptly, including tachycardia and hypertension. Another class of medications that can lead to withdrawal is the beta blockers.

Managing the Toxic Ingestions

As the cliché goes, too much of anything is not good. And we might add that even a little of a bad thing is really bad. This rings especially true when you talk about toxic ingestions. Here we're talking mainly about toxic reactions to nonprescription medications. That includes over-the-counter drugs, street drugs, and a few substances that amount to poison. In this section, we review the evaluation and management of common toxic ingestions.

Being aware of acetaminophen overdoses

Millions of people use acetaminophen (Tylenol) for mild to moderate pain relief. Acetaminophen can also be complexed with stronger prescription pain relievers. For example, the commonly prescribed narcotic Percocet is a combination of acetaminophen and oxycodone, and Vicodin is a combination of acetaminophen and hydrocodone.

The maximum recommended dose of acetaminophen is no more than 4 g (4,000 mg) a day, but if liver disease is present, doses less than the maximum may be toxic. Here are the key points about evaluating and managing an acetaminophen overdose:

✔ Measure an acetaminophen level. You also want to order blood work to evaluate liver function and kidney function. Depending on the presentation, you may want to screen for concomitant drug use and/or alcohol use. Usually the person presents with really high elevated liver enzymes. You want to treat early and aggressively to prevent fulminant liver failure.

✔ Treatment depends on the acetaminophen level. For test-taking purposes, simply remember that the treatment for an acetaminophen overdose is intravenous N-acetylcysteine (Mucomyst). The usual loading dose is 140 mg/kg followed by 14 more doses of 70 mg/kg every 4 hours.

Avoiding the aspirin overdose

Acetylsalicylic acid (aspirin) is a very common pain reliever, and people use it for cardiac protection as well. Like acetaminophen, the treatment for a salicylate overdose first depends on checking the salicylate level. Here are the key points concerning salicylate overdose:

✔ Salicylate toxicity can cause a gapped metabolic acidosis and respiratory alkalosis.

✔ Intravenous bicarbonate is necessary to help in the renal excretion of salicylate.

✔ If the salicylate level is greater than 100 mg/dL, then dialysis is recommended.

Treating the toxic alcohols

Ingestion of the toxic alcohols (ethylene glycol, methanol, and isopropyl alcohol) is often a result of a suicide attempt. Prompt recognition and treatment is important, because these ingestions can be fatal and, even when not, often result in permanent organ damage.

Ingesting ethylene glycol, which is present in antifreeze, can damage the body, including the brain and the kidneys. Ingesting methanol (also known as wood alcohol) can be toxic to the eyes and cause blindness. People really do drink this stuff! Here are a few key points:

✔ The initial evaluation for ethylene glycol, methanol, and isopropyl alcohol (rubbing alcohol) is measuring a serum osmolality. All three can cause an osmolar gap. Knowing this info can pay off for you on the PANCE. Here's how to interpret the results:

- For ethylene glycol and methanol, you want to send off a level for each as well. The serum osmolality will be low early on before you begin to see a gapped metabolic acidosis.

- Isopropyl alcohol can show positive serum and urine ketones in the absence of an acidosis.

Remember that ethylene glycol and methanol can cause both an osmolar gap and an anion gap acidosis. Isopropyl alcohol causes an elevated osmolar gap but not an elevated anion gap acidosis. Isopropyl alcohol can cause a lactic acidosis but in and of itself doesn't cause a gapped metabolic acidosis like ethylene glycol and methanol do.

✔ The initial management for ethylene glycol and methanol ingestion consists of intravenous saline, intravenous bicarbonate if an acidosis is present, and 4-methylpyrazole (fomepizole). 4-MP inhibits alcohol dehydrogenase, an enzyme that breaks down and metabolizes ethylene glycol and methanol into their more toxic metabolites.

✔ Indications for emergent dialysis include a high ethylene glycol or methanol level, gapped metabolic acidosis, acute renal failure, and/or a change in mental status.

Always check for other potential toxic ingestions or drug overdoses, including an ethyl alcohol (booze) level and an acetaminophen level. Ethyl alcohol (sometimes called grain alcohol, even if it's made from fruit, vegetables, or honey) is a psychoactive drug. In large doses, it's toxic.

Which of the following is a cause of a metabolic alkalosis?

(A) Salicylates

(B) Methanol

(C) Diuretics

(D) Diabetes

(E) Kidney failure

The answer is Choice (C). Diuretics are a commonly prescribed class of medications known to cause a metabolic alkalosis. The other choices are causes of a gapped metabolic acidosis. To remember these causes, think about the mnemonic MUDPILES (methanol; uremia; DKA [diabetic ketoacidosis]; paraldehyde; INH [isoniazid] or idiopathic; lactic acidosis; ethanol or ethylene glycol; and salicylate).

Messing with methamphetamines

Methamphetamines are stimulants of the central nervous system. Common clinical presentations are tachycardia, hypertension, and an elevated body temperature, especially after an overdose. Here are the important points about a methamphetamine overdose:

✔ Meth can especially affect the heart. Overdoses can cause complete collapse of the entire cardiovascular system, including damage to the heart valves. Methamphetamine users can develop a cardiomyopathy both chronically and after an acute overdose.

✔ The sympathetic overload can affect many organs of the body. You may see neuropsychiatric presentations as well, including severe agitation.

✔ The diagnosis is confirmed by a positive urine drug screen.

✔ Treatment includes aggressive volume replacement, intravenous bicarbonate if needed, and pressor medications to raise the blood pressure if shock is present.

 Never ever give acetaminophen or any antipyretic to a patient with a meth overdose who has a fever. The fever is due to increased activity of the muscles. Treatment for an overdosed patient with a fever includes benzodiazepines, aggressive volume replacement, and paralysis if needed.

Closing in on cocaine overdoses

Like methamphetamine, cocaine is a stimulant, and an overdose can be fatal. One of the major organs of the body that cocaine can affect is the heart. Cocaine is a potent vasoconstrictor, and it can cause a myocardial infarction (MI), a hypertensive crisis, or even a coronary thrombosis. It can actually depress left ventricular function.

People using crack can have lung complications, including allergic reactions and pneumonitis related to the cocaine or other toxic substances that can be mixed in with it.

 Don't give a beta blocker to any patient with a cocaine overdose if he or she has either chest pain or a hypertensive crisis. Both alpha and beta receptors are in the body, and if you use a beta blocker in such a case, you can get significant unopposed alpha blockade. That can lead to vasoconstriction of the alpha receptors, which can cause increased ischemia and actually make the situation worse. Use an agent other than a beta blocker to lower the blood pressure.

Combating carbon monoxide poisoning

Carbon monoxide (CO) is a gas without odor or taste. CO is also super ammunition for a test question. Exposure to gas and kerosene heaters, motor vehicle exhaust fumes, and smoke (think firefighters) — especially in a poorly ventilated area — can cause CO poisoning. If CO ingestion isn't recognized early, it can be fatal.

Exposure to CO can cause changes in mental status, including confusion, lethargy, and forgetfulness. Nausea, vomiting, belly pain, and shortness of breath are likely. Higher levels of CO can induce unconsciousness and death. There may be hypotension. Here are some key points on recognizing and treating CO poisoning:

✔ If you were to measure a pulse oximetry on someone with CO poisoning, the results could be normal, but this is the wrong test. The confirmatory test, which is called a *CO-oximetry,* detects the amount of carboxyhemoglobin in the body. A carboxyhemoglobin level greater than 50 percent can be fatal.

✔ The treatment involves administering oxygen with a well-fitting oxygen mask in order to get rid of the excess CO. To secure the airway, endotracheal intubation may be needed. Depending on the severity of the CO poisoning, the person may need hyperbaric oxygen.

Anyone who smokes already has a low level of carbon monoxide in his or her body — usually 10 percent or less carboxyhemoglobin. This is still too much. Stop smoking, folks!

Practice Pharmacology/Toxicology Questions

These practice questions are similar to the PANCE pharmacology and toxicology questions.

1. Which one of the following is true concerning salicylate intoxication?

   (A) High blood levels cannot be removed by dialysis.

   (B) If a respiratory alkalosis is present, do not administer intravenous bicarbonate.

   (C) Salicylate intoxication causes both a metabolic acidosis and a metabolic alkalosis.

   (D) The recommended treatment is intravenous fluids without dextrose.

   (E) Oil of wintergreen can cause salicylate poisoning.

2. You are evaluating a 35-year-old woman who presents with an acute lithium overdose. Which one of the following statements concerning lithium is true?

   (A) Aggressive diuresis is needed to augment lithium excretion.

   (B) Hypocalcemia can be seen as a side effect of lithium.

   (C) Lithium cannot be removed by dialysis.

   (D) It is recommended that you avoid the use of saline in lithium intoxication.

   (E) You should evaluate thyroid function in anyone taking lithium.

3. Which one of the following is the treatment for a heparin overdose?

   (A) Vitamin K

   (B) Fresh frozen plasma

   (C) Protamine sulfate

   (D) Desmopressin acetate (DDAVP)

   (E) Cryoprecipitate

4. Which one of the following antidotes matches the underlying toxicity?

   (A) Benzodiazepines — naloxone (Narcan)

   (B) Narcotics — flumazenil (Romazicon)

   (C) Ethylene glycol — ethanol (booze)

   (D) Acetaminophen — fomepizole (4-methylpyrazole)

   (E) High carboxyhemoglobin — methylene blue

5. Which one of the following statements concerning digoxin is true?

   (A) Digoxin is used in treating diastolic heart failure.

   (B) Digoxin toxicity is treated with dialysis.

   (C) Digoxin dosing must be increased when kidney disease is present.

   (D) Amiodarone and quinidine can decrease digoxin levels.

   (E) Hypokalemia can exacerbate digoxin toxicity.

6. You are asked to see a 40-year-old man in the emergency room because of fever and altered mental status. He was recently started on fluphenazine (Prolixin). He is agitated and his temperature is 39.4°C (103°F). His blood pressure is 160/100 mmHg. A CPK level is 50,000. What is the most appropriate treatment at this time?

   (A) Urgent hemodialysis

   (B) Intravenous saline alone for the rhabdomyolysis

   (C) Lorazepam (Ativan) for agitation

   (D) Dantrolene

   (E) Cyproheptadine

Answers and Explanations

Use this answer key to score the practice pharmacology/toxicology questions in this chapter. The answer explanations give you some insight into why the correct answer is better than the other choices.

1. **E.** Oil of wintergreen is a topical methyl salicylate that can cause salicylate poisoning. Levels greater than 100 mg/dL and a metabolic acidosis can be indications for dialysis. Even if a respiratory alkalosis is present, intravenous bicarbonate is still recommended to enhance the renal elimination of salicylic acid. Choice (C) is incorrect because salicylate intoxication causes a *respiratory* alkalosis and a metabolic acidosis. And intravenous fluids *with* dextrose are often recommended because even if the serum glucose level is normal, there can be low blood glucose levels in the central nervous system.

2. **E.** Thyroid function tests should be obtained in anyone on lithium. The woman needs intravenous saline to facilitate lithium excretion, so Choice (D) is out. Never use diuretics; in fact, volume depletion and dehydration can increase the risk of lithium toxicity. Other metabolic effects of lithium include hypercalcemia (not hypocalcemia), hypothyroidism, hyperthyroidism, and diabetes insipidus. Lithium can be removed by dialysis.

3. **C.** Use protamine sulfate. Vitamin K and fresh frozen plasma can be used for a warfarin (Coumadin) overdose. Cryoprecipitate is another type of clotting factor, high in vWf and Factor VIII. Desmopressin acetate can be used to treat bleeding in someone with von Willebrand's disease.

4. **C.** Before the use of methylpyrazole (fomepizole), ethanol was used to block the breakdown of ethylene glycol and methanol into their more toxic metabolites. Ethanol has a pretty high affinity for alcohol dehydrogenase, the first enzyme in that metabolic pathway.

   Naloxone (Narcan) is used for an opiate overdose, and flumazenil (Romazicon) is used for a benzodiazepine overdose. N-acetylcysteine is the antidote for acetaminophen overdose, not fomepizole. And there's no match between high carboxyhemoglobin and methylene blue. Sometimes test-writers try to trick you with terminology. An elevated carboxyhemoglobin level means CO poisoning; the treatment is oxygen.

5. **E.** Hypokalemia exacerbates digoxin toxicity. Digoxin is used to treat *systolic* heart failure, not diastolic heart failure. Digoxin is not eliminated by dialysis; its toxicity is treated using Fab antibody fragments. Its dosing is decreased in kidney disease. Both quinidine and amiodarone can increase, not decrease, digoxin levels.

6. **D.** The patient has neuroleptic malignant syndrome (NMS) and likely has muscle rigidity, so give him dantrolene. Pay attention to key words when answering test questions. Certainly if you were seeing this patient clinically, you'd start IV fluids, especially in the setting of rhabomyolysis. Choice (A), urgent hemodialysis, isn't the best answer here. You'd need more information for this choice to be the correct answer. The word *alone* in Choice (B) makes it a wrong answer. Choice (C) isn't correct because the use of a benzodiazepine isn't the most complete answer here. Choice (E) isn't the right answer because cyproheptadine can be used for the treatment of serotonin syndrome, and this is NMS.

Part V
The Brain, Blood, Bugs, Skin, and Glands

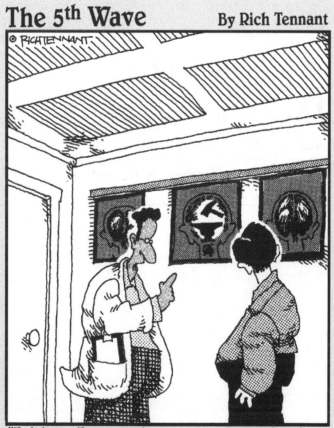

The 5th Wave — By Rich Tennant

"Initially I was going to say your migraines were caused by a hormonal trigger to the hypothalamus. But this X-ray indicates you actually have a tiny hammer striking an anvil in your head."

In this part . . .

Part V covers the endocrine system (Chapter 15), neurology (Chapter 16), dermatology (Chapter 17), hematology and oncology (Chapter 18), and infectious diseases (Chapter 19). These topics won't constitute a big portion of the exam, but they'll be represented.

Chapter 15

Evaluating the Endocrine System

. . . .

In This Chapter

▶ Dealing with diabetes and hypoglycemia

▶ Evaluating calcium and magnesium

▶ Adoring adrenals

▶ Thinking thyroid

▶ Looking at lipids

. . . .

The endocrine system is one of the most fascinating systems of the human body. In other systems, the various components — the brain and nerves, the heart and blood vessels, the bones and connective tissue, and so on — are all connected to each other. But the endocrine system isn't located in one particular area. The system's awesomeness comes from the interactive nature of different organs located in separate parts of the body. For example, the hypothalamus-pituitary-adrenal axis takes you inside the brain, to the base of the brain, and to the top of the kidneys.

The medical conditions in this chapter concern abnormalities of the endocrine system. The endocrine system is Rich's second-favorite body system (the genitourinary system being the first, of course!). We include sections on diabetes as well as conditions that affect the thyroid and adrenal glands. In addition, you find out how to evaluate and manage abnormalities related to calcium and magnesium. Finally, you see how to treat various forms of hyperlipidemia. And don't forget about those pesky practice questions at the end of the chapter.

Dealing with Diabetes and Other Glucose Problems

Diabetes mellitus (DM) is due to abnormal insulin metabolism in the body. In type 1 diabetes mellitus, the pancreas doesn't produce insulin, and in type 2, the body resists the actions of insulin.

In North America, the incidence and prevalence of diabetes mellitus has reached epidemic proportions. Diabetes is a leading cause of kidney disease and dialysis, and it increases the risk of developing coronary artery disease, hyperlipidemia, and peripheral vascular disease. It also increases total body inflammation. You can bet your bottom dollar you'll see questions concerning diabetes mellitus on the PANCE. In this section, we discuss diabetes mellitus and other conditions related to blood glucose levels.

Looking at the shared traits of type 1 and type 2 diabetes

Diabetes mellitus is diagnosed a few different ways:

- ✔ The most common way is registering a fasting blood sugar of > 126 mg/dL two different times.

- ✔ A postprandial (after-eating) glucose level of 200 mg/dL on two occasions is indicative of diabetes.

- ✔ If someone is having symptoms of the three *p*'s — *polyphagia* (eating a lot), *polydipsia* (drinking a lot), and *polyuria* (voiding a lot) — diabetes is likely present.

Both type 1 and type 2 diabetes mellitus can affect the eyes (diabetic retinopathy), nerves (diabetic neuropathy), and kidneys (diabetic nephropathy). Here are some key points about these conditions:

- ✔ **Retinopathy:** Because of the risk of retinopathy, a person with diabetes should see an ophthalmologist annually. Tight blood sugar control is important in reducing ophthalmologic risk.

- ✔ **Nephropathy:** Diabetic nephropathy is the leading cause of kidney disease in this country (as Rich, a kidney doctor, can attest). It's also the leading reason people with kidney disease need dialysis. About a third of people with type 1 diabetes go on to develop kidney disease; only about 10 percent of people with type 2 diabetes develop kidney disease. (See Chapter 10 for more information about diabetic nephropathy.)

- ✔ **Neuropathy:** The neuropathy that diabetes causes can be debilitating. It's typically a peripheral neuropathy, usually in a stocking-glove distribution. The condition can be so bad that it affects the person's ability to walk and even drive a car, especially if he or she has no sensation of the feet touching the pedals.

Diabetic neuropathy is much more than a peripheral neuropathy; neuropathies can affect other areas of the body. Autonomic neuropathy related to diabetes can be difficult to treat. Basically, the sitting or supine blood pressure is high but drops big time when the person stands up.

Diabetic gastroparesis is also a significant problem with both types of diabetes. Problems with gastric and intestinal motility can lead to malnutrition as well as problems with labile blood sugars, due to the inconsistent digestion of carbohydrates.

Missing insulin: Reviewing type 1 diabetes

In *type 1 diabetes mellitus,* the beta cells of the pancreas don't produce insulin. Experts think that the failure of the beta cells to produce insulin may be an autoimmune phenomenon, perhaps stimulated by a viral process. Either way, the person needs insulin. Because type 1 diabetes is a failure of the body to make insulin, it's diagnosed at a very young age.

When you think about the initial presentation of someone with type 1 diabetes, remember the three *p*'s: polyphagia, polydipsia, and polyuria. Despite all the eating and drinking, though, the person keeps losing weight. Without insulin, the body is in a catabolic state.

Here are the general points concerning type 1 diabetes:

✔ The beta cells of the pancreas are not making insulin. Insulin levels are low, and the levels of the hormone *glucagon* (made by the gamma cells of the pancreas) are very high.

✔ In addition to adhering to an insulin regimen, someone with type 1 diabetes needs to follow their blood glucose levels closely. Patients are often asked to keep a blood glucose diary and bring it with them during their clinic visits. You may ask a patient to check either preprandial or postprandial glucose levels.

✔ Following a diabetic diet is important. Understanding how to count carbohydrates is also important, especially for people adjusting an insulin regimen. In general, roughly half of the diet should contain complex carbohydrates, and about a quarter of the diet should come from fat. The remaining quarter should be protein, although you may need to restrict protein if proteinuria or kidney disease is present.

✔ A glycosylated hemoglobin (or Hgb A1c) is a test that measures how "sweet" the blood has been over the past 3 months. It's been used to monitor compliance with an insulin or medication regimen, although some guidelines have proposed that the A1c also be used to diagnose diabetes. The goal Hgb A1c level is < 6.5 percent.

✔ Treatment of type 1 diabetes is the administration of insulin, because the person's pancreas isn't secreting insulin. Many different insulin regimens are out there, and many seek to mimic what the insulin does (or would do) physiologically. In people without type 1 diabetes, insulin is continually being secreted (given in a continuous pulse dose), and the secretion increases during a carbohydrate meal.

Weighing in on type 2 diabetes

Type 2 diabetes mellitus is due to the body's resistance to the actions of insulin. The pancreas is secreting insulin, but because of insulin resistance, the insulin can't get into the cells to do its job. Experts think that in addition to the insulin resistance, the beta cells of the pancreas just wear out — the workload of pumping out insulin and trying to lower the blood glucose levels is too much, and they can't keep up.

The most common reason for insulin resistance is obesity. Unlike type 1 diabetes, type 2 diabetes is typically found in middle-aged or older adults, but with the current obesity epidemic in the United States, you see younger people being diagnosed with type 2 diabetes.

Metabolic syndrome isn't diabetes per se, but it clearly increases the risk of developing type 2 diabetes. You'll no doubt see a question about this in some form or fashion. *Metabolic syndrome* has several components: impaired fasting glucose, large waist circumference, hypertriglyceridemia (high triglycerides) with low cholesterol, and elevated blood pressure. Any three of these components are enough to diagnose metabolic syndrome.

The long and short of it: Combined insulin action

When Rich was in medical school, using neutral protamine Hagedorn (NPH) insulin and regular insulin dosing was all the rage. Diabetes management has come a long way since then. One popular dosing regimen is using long-acting insulin glargine (Lantus) with short-acting insulins such as insulin lispro (Humalog). This way, the body always has background insulin with short-acting insulin, if needed.

There are other combination types of insulin with both long- and short-acting insulins together. One very cool advance is the insulin pump, which allows for the tonic secretion of insulin. The regimen can be personalized to the needs of each person.

Managing type 2 diabetes with diet and exercise

Diet and exercise are crucial in managing type 2 diabetes. Because obesity is so closely connected with type 2 diabetes, weight loss is essential. In many cases, not only does weight loss allow you to decrease the medications a person takes, but it also helps normalize the blood sugar by lowering the insulin resistance. And not only are you decreasing insulin resistance, but you're also helping to preserve beta cell function.

Understanding medication classes for type 2 diabetes

Be aware of the different medication classes that you can use to treat diabetes mellitus type 2. One of the most commonly prescribed medications is the biguanide metformin, originally sold as Glucophage. This substance helps the peripheral utilization of glucose and also decreases *gluconeogenesis* (the liver's production of glucose). Some people think that this medication helps with weight loss as well. Because of its mechanism of action, biguanide is low-risk for causing hypoglycemia. One main potential side effect of metformin — diarrhea — is GI-related.

Look at the patient's kidney function before you prescribe metformin. If the serum creatinine is greater than 1.5 mg/dL for men or 1.4 mg/dL for women, don't use this medication, because it may cause lactic acidosis. For anyone who may be at risk for lactic acidosis (that is, people with congestive heart failure, liver disease, or peripheral vascular disease), use metformin with caution.

The PANCE may also ask you about key characteristics and potential side effects of other diabetes medication classes:

- **Sulfonylureas:** Many clinicians still prescribe the oral sulfonylureas, which work on the beta cells to stimulate insulin secretion. This medication class has many examples, including glimeperide (Amaryl) and glipizide (Glucotrol). Unlike metformin, the sulfonylureas can predispose a person to hypoglycemia.

   Some of the first-generation class of sulfonylureas, such as chlorpropamide (Diabenese), had the propensity for causing hyponatremia. A patient shouldn't drink any booze with these medications because he or she can get violently ill afterward with a disulfuram-like reaction. The second-generation class of sulfonylureas, including glimepiride (Amaryl), is more commonly prescribed.

- **Meglitinides:** This group of medications increases the pancreatic secretion of insulin by acting on the beta cells of the pancreas. An example is repaglinide (Prandin). It's shorter acting and can be used by a person with kidney disease.

- **Alpha-glucosidase inhibitors:** This class of medications slows down carbohydrate absorption in the GI tract. An example of a medication in this class is acarbose (Precose). Many of its side effects, such as flatus, are GI-related.

- **Thiazolidinediones (TZDs):** TZDs such as pioglitazone (Actos) have received a lot of attention. Side effects for this class can include weight gain, especially fluid retention. Watch liver function tests like a hawk as well. Don't give this med to anyone diagnosed with congestive heart failure or liver disease.

- **Dipeptidyl peptidase-4 (DPP-4) inhibitors:** These meds, such as sitagliptin (Januvia), constitute a newer class of medications approved by the U.S. Food and Drug Administration (FDA) in 2006. To understand how this medication works, think of putting elements of the sulfonylureas and the biguanides together: DPP-4 inhibitors increase beta cell production of insulin and decrease hepatic gluconeogenesis. Because of its dual mechanism of action, the risk for hypoglycemia is significant when someone uses a DPP-4 inhibitor with another diabetes medication. There's also a major risk of pancreatitis with this medication.

- **Exenatide (Byetta):** Exenatide works on the glucagon-like-receptor 1 (GLP-1) by increasing the beta cell secretion of insulin while also inhibiting secretion of glucagon. It's administered as a subcutaneous injection. You should never give this med to someone with type 1 diabetes. Many of the potential side effects are GI-related, including nausea, vomiting, and diarrhea. This medication can also cause significant weight loss.

Sometimes, despite all these medications, a person can't get blood sugar levels under control and needs to be treated with insulin. In that situation, the insulin regimen is personalized. Often, the insulin is used in conjunction with the oral medication(s) the person is taking.

For many of the medication classes used to treat type 2 diabetes mellitus, including the biguanides, sulfonylureas, exenatide (Byetta), and insulin, the dosing needs to be reduced or the medication needs to be changed in someone with kidney disease. Kidney disease prolongs the half-life of many of these medications, including insulin.

Which of the following medications needs to be held 48 hours prior to cardiac catheterization and/or angiogram?

(A) Metformin (Glucophage)

(B) Glimepiride (Amaryl)

(C) Acarbose (Precose)

(D) Repaglinide (Prandin)

(E) Exenatide (Byetta)

The answer is Choice (A). Metformin (Glucophage) should be held 48 hours before any interventional procedure where contrast dye is going to be given. Contrast dye can be associated with acute renal failure, which increases the risk of lactic acidosis associated with metformin in the setting of decreased kidney function.

Blasting super-high blood glucose

In people with uncontrolled diabetes mellitus, the blood glucose levels can be super duper high, even ≥ 1,000 mg/dL. High blood sugars due to uncontrolled diabetes mellitus are usually related to either diabetic ketoacidosis (DKA) or hyperosmolar hyperglycemic nonketotic coma (HHNK). These emergency medical conditions require a high level of care, often in the intensive care unit.

On the test, you usually see questions about recognizing and/or managing DKA or HHNK or recognizing the differences between these two critical conditions. We cover each condition in the following sections.

Doubling down on DKA

Diabetic ketoacidosis (DKA) is usually a complication of type 1 diabetes. The person has an insulin deficiency, and without insulin, the body goes into a ketotic, catabolic, acidemic state (with high concentrations of ketone bodies). This condition can be life-threatening.

One way to think about diabetic ketoacidosis is to separate the various components:

- ✔ **Diabetic:** Blood sugar > 250 mg/dL, although it's usually a lot higher
- ✔ **Keto:** Positive serum acetone and positive urine ketones
- ✔ **Acidosis:** Bicarbonate level < 15 mEq/L and a pH < 7.3

Here are some key points concerning diabetic ketoacidosis:

- ✔ Symptoms of diabetic ketoacidosis can be confusion and lethargy, especially at higher blood glucose levels. Another common symptom is abdominal pain.
- ✔ Sometimes the cause of DKA is more than just a missed dose of insulin. Also look for a medical condition that could've put someone into diabetic ketoacidosis. Think of the three *i*'s: infection, inflammation, or infarction.

> ✔ Because diabetic ketoacidosis is commonly seen in type 1 diabetes, which is a state of insulin deficiency, insulin needs to be started with a bolus and followed by continuous infusion to help correct the ketosis and acidosis.
>
> ✔ Someone who has diabetic ketoacidosis needs intravenous fluids, usually intravenous saline with insulin, because the person is likely to be volume depleted.
>
> ✔ Potassium and phosphorous need to be adjusted and replaced during the treatment for diabetic ketoacidosis, because insulin pushes potassium and phosphorous into the cell. This requires frequent monitoring of the blood glucose, potassium, and phosphate levels.

Which of the following is true concerning diabetic ketoacidosis (DKA)?

(A) Management initially consists of normal saline with intravenous insulin.

(B) Hyperglycemia is most commonly due to insulin resistance.

(C) The insulin drip is changed to subcutaneous dosing when the blood sugar normalizes.

(D) Hypophosphatemia can also be seen initially.

(E) Diabetic ketoacidosis never occurs in type 2 diabetes mellitus.

The answer is Choice (A). This question tests how well you understand the nuances of managing DKA. When you first encounter someone with DKA, the management includes initiating an insulin infusion and isotonic saline. This is the opposite of the treatment for HHNK (see the following section).

You can initially see hyperkalemia and hyperphosphatemia (not hypophosphatemia), usually due to an insulin deficiency and hyperglycemia: Insulin isn't present to push potassium and phosphorus into cells (see Chapter 8 for details), and high blood sugars can pull potassium out of cells (an osmotic effect). Concerning Choice (B), diabetic ketoacidosis most often occurs in type 1 diabetes, which is due to an insulin deficiency. Type 2 diabetes is caused by insulin resistance and beta-cell burnout. Choice (C) isn't a true statement because the insulin drip is converted to a subcutaneous insulin regimen when the anion gap normalizes, not when the blood sugar normalizes. This point is critical to remember in diabetic ketoacidosis: It's an anion-gap acidosis. Even if the blood sugar has normalized, usually the intravenous insulin infusion stays until the anion gap is normalized.

Although diabetic ketoacidosis is a state of insulin deficiency and nine times out of ten is seen in type 1 diabetes, the right physiologic stressors (such as severe sepsis) can, on rare occasions, cause diabetic ketoacidosis. So although it's rare, diabetic ketoacidosis can happen in type 2 diabetes.

Pay attention to the wording of the answers. If you see a question that says something "can occur," odds are the answer is true. Does it occur commonly? Probably not. Can it occur sometimes? Probably.

Helping people with HHNK

People usually think of hyperosmolar hyperglycemic nonketotic coma (HHNK) as a complication of uncontrolled type 2 diabetes. You need to look for an underlying cause. What was the stimulus that put the person into this state in the first place? Remember the three *i*'s and apply them here: infection, inflammation, and infarction. Here are some key points concerning HHNK:

> ✔ Blood glucose levels can be high in diabetic ketoacidosis, but they're often higher in HHNK, usually ≥ 500 mg/dL.
>
> ✔ You usually don't see an acidosis with HHNK (unlike diabetic ketoacidosis, in which an acidosis is present).

✔ HHNK happens to older people, whereas diabetic ketoacidosis happens more often to younger people. Commonly, HHNK is seen predominantly in those with type 2 diabetes, whereas diabetic ketoacidosis is seen in those with type I diabetes.

✔ In diabetic ketoacidosis, you think of giving insulin first and then volume. But in HHNK, you think the opposite: Give fluid first (usually normal saline to start), and if that doesn't bring down the blood glucose level, then you think about giving insulin.

Handling blood glucose when it bottoms out: Hypoglycemia

Hypoglycemia can be a significant problem. Realize that hypoglycemia can be more than just a side effect of insulin or medication therapy. Other medical conditions are also related to low blood sugar levels.

The two big types of hypoglycemia you need be aware of are fasting hypoglycemia and postprandial hypoglycemia:

✔ **Fasting:** Causes of fasting hypoglycemia include adrenal insufficiency, liver disease (with decreased hepatic gluconeogenesis as a cause), and even kidney disease. Not only can liver disease be a cause of hypoglycemia, but so can alcohol use. The administration of diabetic medications, including insulin, is also in the differential etiology.

✔ **Postprandial:** If hypoglycemia is detected after a meal (postprandial), think about a problem with the GI tract. Look for gastroparesis, and ask whether the patient has ever had gastric surgery. Look for other potential GI problems, including malabsorption.

Whipple's triad is three signs that can alert the clinician that a person's diaphoresis, tremulousness, and/or shakiness may be due to hypoglycemia. This triad suggests that an insulinoma may be present. Although insulinomas are rare, test-makers like asking about this particular triad on tests. The triad goes like this:

✔ The patient demonstrates diaphoresis, tremulousness, and/or shakiness, alerting the clinician that hypoglycemia may be present.

✔ While the person is having the symptoms, a blood glucose level is checked to verify that hypoglycemia is present *at the same time* as the symptoms.

✔ Normalizing the blood glucose normalizes the person's symptoms.

Discerning Calcium and Magnesium Problems

Understanding the evaluation of abnormal calcium and magnesium levels is rather straightforward. And that's good, because knowing how to treat these electrolyte abnormalities, especially hypercalcemia, is really important. Calcium metabolism, as you find out in this section, is intricately involved with the parathyroid gland. Magnesium is an important co-factor for more than 300 enzymatic reactions in the body. Having labs that are out of whack can affect the heart, increasing the risk of dysrhythmias. In this section, you read about evaluating and managing hypo/hypercalcemia and hypo/hypermagnesemia.

Hampering hypercalcemia

A normal calcium level on reference labs is usually 8.5 to 10.2 mg/dL. Higher levels than this are called *hypercalcemia.* The symptoms of hypercalcemia depend on the calcium level:

✔ At levels of around 11 to 12 mg/dL, common complaints include fatigue, weakness, and constipation.

✔ At levels around 14 to 16 mg/dL, someone may experience changes in mentation, difficulty thinking, and polyuria. There can also be abdominal pain.

Because calcium is a potent vasoconstrictor, very high levels can cause peptic ulcer disease and pancreatitis as well. Hypercalcemia can also be a cause of acute kidney injury (AKI).

You need to correct the calcium level for the albumin level. Otherwise, you could miss a hypercalcemia. For every decrease by 1 mg/dL in the albumin, add 0.8 to the calcium level. This is Rich's easy shortcut for remembering the formula commonly used: (0.8 × normal albumin [assume a level of 4.0 mg/dL] – patient's albumin) + serum calcium level. For example, if the calcium level is 9.0 mg/dL and the albumin level is 3.0 mg/dL, the corrected calcium is 9.8 mg/dL. If you have a question about the calcium level, then check an ionized calcium level.

Looking at causes of hypercalcemia

The two most common causes of hypercalcemia are primary hyperparathyroidism (PHP) and malignancy. Remember the triad of primary hyperparathyroidism:

✔ The calcium level is normal or elevated.

✔ The parathyroid gland value is normal or elevated. (***Note:*** In the setting of hypercalcemia, the intact parathyroid hormone [PTH] level should be depressed, so even a normal level would be abnormal in this situation.)

✔ The 24-hour urinary calcium level is elevated (hypercalciuria).

The most common cause of primary hyperparathyroidism is a parathyroid adenoma, which usually affects one of the parathyroid glands. The initial evaluation, in addition to biochemical testing, can include obtaining an ultrasound of the neck as well as a nuclear scan (termed a *sestamibi*) to get a better look at the parathyroid glands.

The treatment is usually surgical removal of the parathyroid adenoma once identified. Common indications for parathyroid surgery include an elevation in the serum creatinine level, recurrent kidney stones, osteoporosis, and hypercalcemia.

Secondary hyperparathyroidism relates to kidney disease (see Chapter 8). The cause of secondary hyperparathyroidism relates to parathyroid hyperplasia of some or all of the parathyroid glands.

Many of the malignancies that cause hypercalcemia are solid-organ tumors and do so either by directly invading the bone (that is, bone metastasis) or by secreting a parathyroid-like hormone (referred to as the *humoral hypercalcemia of malignancy*). This is why part of the workup for hypercalcemia can involve checking not only an intact PTH level but also a PTH-related peptide (for looking for a solid-organ malignancy that's causing hypercalcemia via the PTH-like hormone).

Examples of common malignancies that can cause hypercalcemia include lung, breast, and prostate cancer. In addition, if a solid-organ malignancy is suspected, a "metastatic workup" is undertaken. It can involve CT scans of the thorax, abdomen, and pelvis; a bone scan; and brain imaging.

Here are a few key points concerning the evaluation of hypercalcemia:

✔ Differential diagnoses for a high calcium level include a plasma cell dyscrasia like multiple myeloma, vitamin D or vitamin A excess, and medications like hydrochlorothiazide, lithium, and theophylline.

✔ Granulomatous diseases such as sarcoidosis (in addition to causing the lung issues we describe in Chapter 4) can also cause hypercalcemia and hypercalciuria. The mechanism of hypercalcemia is increased 1,25-hydroxyvitamin D_3 from the granulomas themselves. Thus, checking a 1,25-hydroxyvitamin D_3 level can be part of the initial lab evaluation for hypercalcemia.

✔ On an ECG, hypercalcemia can cause a shortening of the QT interval.

✔ Milk alkali is a funky cause of hypercalcemia that consists of the triad of ingesting lots of milk, taking a lot of antacids (high in calcium), and having kidney failure or kidney stones. Many patients also have a metabolic alkalosis.

Treating hypercalcemia

Many, if not all, patients who present with hypercalcemia are significantly volume-depleted. The first line of treatment consists of intravenous hydration with normal saline.

Other treatments include the use of furosemide (Lasix) and calcitonin-salmon (Miacalcin). Give this subcutaneously if and only if you first do an intradermal test dose and it's negative. In addition, bisphosphonates can be administered intravenously. In rare instances, if the calcium level is very high (that is, > 20 mg/dL), the patient may need dialysis to remove the calcium.

Loop diuretics such as furosemide (Lasix) can cause hypokalemia and hypomagnesemia. If they are given, electrolyte levels need to be watched closely and replaced. Concerning intravenous hydration, be careful in certain patient populations, such as the elderly and in those with a history of congestive heart failure.

The bisphosphonates administered intravenously, including pamidronate disodium (Aredia) and zoledronic acid (Zometa), both have the potential to cause acute kidney failure. If kidney disease is present, the doses may have to be reduced or delayed until the kidney function is better. And if the GFR is < 30 mL/min, these medications should not be given.

Which one of the following represents symptoms and/or complications of hypercalcemia?

(A) Diarrhea

(B) Psychoses

(C) Gallstones

(D) Hypertension

(E) Proteinuria

The answer is Choice (D). Hypercalcemia is a vasoconstrictor and can cause hypertension. Choice (A) is out because high calcium levels tend to cause constipation, not diarrhea. Very high calcium levels can cause an encephalopathy and lethargy, not a psychosis (B). Hypercalcemia is associated with kidney stones, not gallstones, so Choice (C) is incorrect. Hypercalcemia does not cause proteinuria, Choice (E).

Getting down with hypocalcemia

Hypocalcemia, usually defined as a corrected calcium level < 8.5 mg/dL, is relatively uncommon. However, you should be aware of some key points about hypocalcemia:

- ✔ If the corrected calcium level is low, first check a magnesium level (see the earlier section "Hampering hypercalcemia" for details on the corrected calcium level). A very low magnesium level (usually ≤ 1.4 mg/dL) can cause hypocalcemia.

- ✔ Your initial workup includes checking vitamin D levels, phosphorous, magnesium, and an intact PTH level.

  The patterns of the calcium and phosphorus levels can clue you in on what may be going on:

  - If both the corrected calcium and phosphorous levels are low, think vitamin D deficiency. Recall that vitamin D is responsible for the absorption of calcium and phosphorous from the small intestine.

  - If the phosphorous levels are high and the corrected calcium levels are low, think renal failure.

- ✔ Checking an ECG is important. Look for prolongation of the QT interval.

Reviewing hypomagnesemia

Hypomagnesemia is defined as a magnesium level of < 1.6 mg/dL. Very low magnesium levels can contribute to both low potassium and low calcium levels. Like hypocalcemia, low magnesium levels can cause QT interval prolongation on the ECG.

The most common cause of hypomagnesemia is renal losses, usually from medications like diuretics, amphotericin B, and cisplatin. (These last two medications also can cause kidney failure; see Chapter 10.)

GI losses like those found in certain malabsorption syndromes and inflammatory bowel disease (IBD) can also cause hypomagnesemia.

Therapy consists of either oral magnesium replacement such as magnesium oxide or intravenous replacement with magnesium sulfate. You need to watch some of the oral magnesium replacements because they can cause diarrhea.

Helping hypermagnesemia

The kidney is the main organ of excretion for magnesium, and normally your kidney is pretty good at getting rid of it. Thus, the primary cause of hypermagnesemia is excessive magnesium intake in the setting of kidney failure. Therapies to help with the renal excretion of magnesium include intravenous fluids, high dose furosemide (Lasix), and, when needed, dialysis.

Pursuing Those Pesky Adrenals

The adrenal gland is important physiologically. It's responsible for the production of cortisol, aldosterone, and the sex hormones as well. You don't want to miss an abnormally functioning adrenal gland, either in clinical practice or on the PANCE. Two clinical syndromes we discuss in this section are adrenal insufficiency and Cushing's syndrome.

The *hypothalamus-pituitary-adrenal axis* is a mini endocrine system that's well-connected. When you evaluate test questions on problems that affect any of these three organs, first think about how a dysfunction in one organ affects the others in the system.

Awakening lazy adrenals

With adrenal insufficiency, first figure out whether you're dealing with primary or secondary adrenal insufficiency:

- ✔ **Primary:** Primary adrenal insufficiency (PAI), also known as Addison's disease, refers to a problem with the adrenal gland itself. There are abnormalities related to both cortisol and aldosterone secretion.

- ✔ **Secondary:** Secondary adrenal insufficiency refers to a problem with the pituitary gland (it's unable to secrete ACTH), affecting the adrenal gland's ability to secrete cortisol. Unlike with primary adrenal insufficiency, aldosterone production stays intact in secondary adrenal insufficiency. This is a key point to remember for questions on adrenal insufficiency.

Although there can be several etiologies of primary adrenal insufficiency, the biggest cause is an autoimmune adrenalitis that can destroy the adrenal gland. Other causes include malignancy and other infiltrative conditions and certain infectious processes.

Waterhouse-Friderichsen syndrome (WFS) is hemorrhage of the adrenal glands secondary to meningococcemia. This infection is very bad and is usually caused by *Neisseria meningitidis.* The infection is a systemic problem and can be fatal if not recognized early — we're talking shock and the potential for developing disseminated intravascular coagulation (DIC).

Here are the key points about primary adrenal insufficiency:

- ✔ Early symptoms are nonspecific and can include just fatigue, weakness, and weight loss. As the condition worsens, orthostatic symptoms can occur, with a drop in blood pressure upon standing.

- ✔ Classic findings include hyperpigmentation along the skin creases and decreased hair in the axillary and pubic areas.

- ✔ An abnormal blood work lab includes hyponatremia, hyperkalemia, and anemia. Eosinophilia may be present as well.

  Note that hyponatremia and hyperkalemia are present in primary adrenal insufficiency, not secondary adrenal insufficiency. This happens because aldosterone, whose job is the retention of sodium and the excretion of potassium, is low to nonexistent in primary adrenal insufficiency but is present in secondary adrenal insufficiency.

- ✔ A suggestive diagnostic test is a low morning cortisol of < 5 mg/dL. The confirmatory test is the cosyntropin (ACTH) stimulation test. In response to ACTH, the cortisol level should increase by 8 to 10 points in 60 minutes. If primary adrenal insufficiency is present, then a cosyntropin stimulation test will get little or no response.

- ✔ The treatment is usually oral steroid replacement, usually in divided doses totaling 5 to 7.5 mg/day. If a person is deficient in aldosterone, then synthetic fludrocortisone acetate (Florinef) can be given.

An *Addisonian crisis* is a medical emergency and requires prompt recognition and treatment. In this situation, a significant body stressor (such as an infection) stresses out an already-underfunctioning adrenal gland. The gland can't make enough cortisol to deal with the body stressor. The key is the administration of intravenous steroids, in addition to volume repletion, and pressor medications if needed to help maintain blood pressure. A search for and treatment of the underlying cause, such as infection, is vital. If you suspect an Addisonian crisis, don't wait for a cortisol level to come back before treating the condition. The intravenous steroids can be life-saving in this situation.

Confronting Cushing's syndrome

Cushing's syndrome represents an excess secretion of cortisol. First, establish that the person hasn't been taking steroids (for example, for the treatment of a connective tissue disease), because steroids cause similar symptoms. Then the key is figuring out what's causing the Cushing's syndrome.

Symptoms of excess cortisol secretion from any cause include the classic moon face, buffalo hump, abdominal striae, and hypertension. People with Cushing's may also have muscle weakness in the proximal muscles. You also see weight gain and centripetal obesity with Cushing's syndrome. Metabolic syndrome or hyperglycemia, as well as edema, can also be present.

Cushing's syndrome is diagnosed either by an elevated 24-hour urinary free cortisol test or via a *low-dose dexamethasone suppression test.* Normally, after administering 1 mg of dexamethasone at midnight, you see inhibition of cortisol secretion by the adrenal gland, as evidenced by a very low cortisol level in the morning. But in Cushing's syndrome, the morning cortisol isn't suppressed.

Did you know that for Cushing's syndrome, you can "check it in the spit"? In addition to urinary and blood tests, you can check the saliva for evidence of Cushing's syndrome. The cortisol levels of saliva are usually low at night but can be elevated in people with Cushing's syndrome.

After one of these tests confirms that someone has Cushing's syndrome, you need to ask, "Where in the body is the excess cortisol being secreted from?" *Cushing's disease* represents excess ACTH secretion from the pituitary gland. But Cushing's disease is just one cause of Cushing's syndrome; other causes include a tumor in the adrenal gland or paraneoplastic ACTH secretion from a primary lung malignancy.

Here are key points about Cushing's syndrome:

- ✔ MRI is the test of choice to diagnose a pituitary adenoma.

- ✔ Imaging the adrenals, usually with a CT scan, is important in looking for an adrenal tumor. If you find an adrenal or pituitary tumor, surgical removal is recommended.

- ✔ Ectopic ACTH production secondary to a lung cancer can be associated with significant hypokalemia and a metabolic alkalosis.

You are evaluating a 25-year-old woman who has been transferred to the ICU secondary to profound hypotension. Her blood pressure is 75/40 mmHg with a pulse of 120 beats per minute. Her monitor shows she is in a normal sinus rhythm. Despite intravenous fluids and pressor medications, her blood pressure remains low. You suspect adrenal insufficiency. What is your next step?

(A) Check a stat random cortisol level.

(B) Do a 24-hour urinary free cortisol.

(C) Do an ACTH stimulation test.

(D) Do a low-dose dexamethasone suppression test.

(E) Give hydrocortisone 100 mg intravenously stat.

The answer is Choice (E). This patient is likely having an Addisonian crisis. Give intravenous steroids in this situation. Choices (B) and (D) are part of the initial workup for Cushing's syndrome. And you wouldn't do an ACTH stimulation test on someone who is in shock.

Thinking about the Thyroid

The thyroid is a vital organ. One of its big responsibilities is regulating the basal metabolic rate. If your thyroid gland becomes lethargic, you may have problems with weight gain and extreme fatigue. If your thyroid is overactive, you may have oodles and oodles of energy and lose weight. Hyperthyroidism can cause undue stress on your body, particularly your heart. Hyperthyroidism is in fact a risk factor for the development of atrial fibrillation. In this section, we look at three conditions: hypothyroidism, hyperthyroidism, and thyroid cancer.

Helping hypothyroidism

Hypothyroidism refers to a thyroid that's underactive. Here are four possible causes:

- *Hashimoto's thyroiditis* is an autoimmune condition. It's the most common cause of hypothyroidism, and it mainly affects women around their 30s.

- *DiGeorge syndrome* (DGS) is a hereditary cause of hypothyroidism. The syndrome causes not only thyroid and parathyroid problems but also heart problems, developmental delays, and hypocalcemia. A person with DiGeorge syndrome may also have a cleft palate problem.

- If you see a question on the PANCE about non-autoimmune causes of hypothyroidism, look for an answer that includes prior neck surgery, usually from prior thyroid or parathyroid surgery.

- Commonly prescribed medications that can cause hypothyroidism include amiodarone (Cordarone) and lithium (Lithobid).

Note that if someone's on steroids, secretion of thyroid-stimulating hormone (TSH) can decrease. For someone in the critical care unit, the medication dopamine can also lower TSH secretion. The key is to recheck thyroid function tests when the patient is off these medications.

The symptoms of hypothyroidism often depend on how underactive the thyroid gland is. They can include hoarseness, profound weakness and fatigue, weight gain, cold intolerance, constipation, and amenorrhea, as well as depression. In fact, part of the initial workup of depression includes screening for hypothyroidism.

Hypothyroidism can cause pain in the muscles (a proximal type of myopathy). Physical examination can reveal loss of the eyebrows (the lateral aspect), and a neck exam can reveal a goiter. There can be bradycardia and elevated blood pressure. Examination of the deep tendon reflexes (especially the Achilles reflex) can show a delayed relaxation response.

There's a close relationship among the hypothalamus, pituitary gland, and thyroid glands. The hypothalamus secretes thyroid releasing hormone (TRH), which stimulates the pituitary to make thyroid stimulating hormone (TSH), which finally stimulates the thyroid to make thyroxine (T4). Continue to follow the logic here:

- Primary hypothyroidism (a problem of the thyroid) is characterized by a low free T4 and an elevated TSH.

- Secondary hypothyroidism (a problem with the pituitary) is characterized by a low TSH and a low free T4.

- Tertiary hypothyroidism, which is not common clinically, is caused when the hypothalamus doesn't make TRH.

The treatment for hypothyroidism is oral thyroid replacement. The usual treatment is levo-thyroxine (Synthroid). After beginning this medication, it's customary to wait about 6 weeks before doing a follow-up TSH level.

An emergent medical condition resulting from long-standing untreated hypothyroidism is *myxedema coma*. This condition is characterized by extreme lethargy (sometimes even to the point of being comatose), confusion, and hypothermia. There's often significant total body edema. On blood work, hyponatremia may be present. Lab values often show a very elevated TSH level. The treatment is usually thyroid replacement, most often given intravenously. Intravenous steroids are often given first before the thyroid replacement.

Which of the following is characteristic of Hashimoto's thyroiditis?

(A) Serum high T4 and low TSH

(B) The presence of antimicrosomal antibodies

(C) Association with atrial fibrillaton

(D) No association with other autoimmune conditions

(E) Treatment includes radioactive iodine

The answer is Choice (B). Choice (A) is incorrect because it lists the characteristic findings in someone with primary hyperthyroidism, and hyperthyroidism is associated with atrial fibrillation, Choice (C). Both hypothyroidism and hyperthyroidism are associated with other autoimmune conditions. And as for Choice (E), radioactive iodine is used in the treatment of hyperthyroidism, namely Graves' disease, which we cover next.

Handling hyperthyroidism

Hyperthyroidism refers to an overactive thyroid gland. Hyperthyroidism has many causes, but the most common is Graves' disease. Like Hashimoto's thyroiditis (for hypothyroidism; see the preceding section), Graves' disease is an autoimmune condition that usually affects young women. In Graves' disease, the body forms antibodies that have an extremely high affinity for the TSH receptor (TSHR), the place on the thyroid that TSH would normally bind to.

Other causes of hyperthyroidism are easy to remember because they begin with the letter *t*. The two "toxic" causes are *toxic adenomas* and *toxic multinodular goiter* (TMG). These are common etiologies of hyperthyroidism, not as prevalent as Graves' disease but in second place in the developed world. Toxic adenomas are benign nodules that actively take up radioactive iodine on thyroid testing — the adenoma is the only area that's active for the iodine uptake. With toxic multinodular goiter, you may see multiple areas of active iodine uptake. Thyroid nodules may not be present.

Signs and symptoms of hyperthyroidism

The classic triad of Graves' disease includes goiter, pretibial myxedema, and exopthalmos. *Exophthalmos* is significant swelling of the eye tissues that can cause the eyeball to protrude. (Think of Bart Simpson with his big eyeballs.) In many cases of Graves' disease, though, there's milder ophthalmic involvement.

Other signs and symptoms can include high blood pressure with a widened pulse pressure, tachycardia, intolerance to heat, fever, diaphoresis, hyperdefecation, palpitations, tremor, increased reflexes, and moist skin (as opposed to the dry skin seen in hypothyroidism). Other behavioral abnormalities can include psychotic behavior and delirium.

If hyperthyroidism remains undiagnosed and unchecked, long-term sequelae include the development of atrial fibrillation, high calcium levels, and osteoporosis.

Older people can have a condition called *apathetic hyperthyroidism.* They have none of the symptoms we mention earlier, but they can present with atrial fibrillation. "Apathetic" here does not mean that they don't care about their atrial fibrillation.

Labs showing hyperthyroidism include a high free T4 and a low TSH level. The T3 level is often elevated.

Treating hyperthyroidism

The treatment of hyperthyroidism is multifaceted. It involves treating not only the thyroid gland itself but also the peripheral manifestations of thyroid disease. One important medication class is the beta blocker, the most common of which is propranolol (Inderal). It inhibits the peripheral conversion of T4 to T3, and because it's lipophilic, it can cross the blood-brain barrier. It's good for helping not only high blood pressure and tachycardia but also tremor and other symptoms.

Thyroid-specific medications such as propylthiouracil (PTU) and methimazole (Tapazole) are used as well. Significant side effects of methimazole include hepatitis, drug-induced lupus-like syndrome, and negative effects on the bone marrow. These include thrombocytopenia, anemia, and agranulocytosis. Propylthiouracil, like methimazole, carries a risk of bone marrow suppression and liver problems. It increases the risk of developing significant autoimmune problems such as vasculitis and glomerulonephritis.

Two other options for hyperthyroidism are radioactive iodine-131 ablation and surgery. Radioactive iodine is the more customary therapy because it's a permanent therapy. One side effect is the development of hypothyroidism over time; thyroid replacement therapy is often needed.

Radioactive iodine-131 (I131) ablation shouldn't be used in pregnancy, nor should methimazole (Tapazole), which can cause fetal harm. Because methimazole has been found in breast milk, nursing mothers shouldn't use methimazole, either. Opt for propylthiouracil if you're taking care of a pregnant woman.

Surgery is less common because of its increased risk. Because the vagus nerve (recurrent laryngeal nerve branch) runs along this area, hoarseness related to injury to this nerve can be a complication of surgery.

Thyroid storm (thyrotoxicosis) is a potentially fatal condition if not recognized. The affected person can present with high fevers, very high blood pressure, tachycardia, and psychotic and/or profound diaphoresis. The symptoms are the opposite those of a myxedema coma. The treatments include using beta blockers for managing the peripheral symptoms and either propylthiouracil or methimazole to decrease the synthesis of thyroid hormone. Intravenous steroids can be administered as well. Close hemodynamic support and monitoring is essential.

Identifying the similarities between Hashimoto's and Graves'

When you prepare for test questions about the thyroid, don't just compare and contrast causes of the differences between hypothyroidism and hyperthyroidism. Noting some similarities is also useful.

Three amigos of thyroiditis

Besides Hashimoto's thyroiditis and Graves' disease, another cause of abnormal thyroid function (again, most commonly seen in women) is *subacute thyroiditis*. The three different types of subacute thyroiditis are the painless one (lymphocytic thyroiditis), the painful one (de Quervain thyroiditis), and postpartum thyroiditis. What's unique about all three of these is that they typically follow the same clinical course: They can present with hyperthyroid symptoms and then become hypothyroid, and all can return to normal afterward. Many times these conditions are self-limiting.

The painless condition can sometimes be difficult to distinguish from Graves' disease on initial presentation and is thought to be an autoimmune process. The painful one is thought to be more viral in nature. Sometimes prednisone can be given for the painful thyroiditis. The postpartum variant can occur up to 6 months after delivery and can persist for several months afterward.

Hashimoto's thyroiditis (the most common cause of hypothyroidism) and Graves' disease (the most common cause of hyperthyroidism) are both autoimmune diseases. Both occur primarily in younger women (usually in their 30s), and both of these conditions can include a goiter. There are also links to other autoimmune diseases, such as diabetes mellitus and adrenal insufficiency. Hashimoto's thyroiditis and Graves' disease are so different, yet they have so much in common.

Both Hashimoto's thyroiditis and Graves' disease also have measurable antibody levels. Two antibodies that you can order to help confirm the diagnosis of Hashimoto's thyroiditis are antimicrosomal antibodies and antibodies to thyroid peroxidase. In Graves' disease, you can see antithyroglobulin antibodies as well as circulating antibodies to the TSH receptor site.

Throttling thyroid cancer

As with thyroid disease in general, thyroid cancer affects women more often than men. The most common clinical presentation is a thyroid nodule. Other symptoms can include hoarseness and difficulty swallowing. Ask about any prior radiation exposure, especially to the neck area. The only way to determine which type of cancer you're dealing with is via a fine needle biopsy.

The thyroid is located in the anterior mediastinum. Differential diagnoses of anterior mediastinal masses include four *t*'s — thyroid masses, teratomas, terrible lymphomas, and thymomas.

Here are the types of thyroid cancer you may need to know for the PANCE:

- **Papillary thyroid cancer:** This is the most common cause of thyroid malignancy. It accounts for about 75 percent of all thyroid cancer and is usually insidious in onset. Papillary cancer spreads via the lymph nodes. This malignancy isn't usually considered to be very aggressive, and surgical intervention with total thyroidectomy can be done, depending on the size of the nodule.

- **Follicular cancer:** Follicular cancer accounts for about 10 percent of thyroid malignancies. Whereas papillary cancer spreads via the lymph nodes, follicular cancer spreads via the blood (hematogenously). The treatment is surgery.

- **Medullary thyroid cancer (MTC):** Medullary thyroid cancer is uncommon, accounting for only 2 to 5 percent of all cases of thyroid cancer. There are two points concerning medullary cancer worth mentioning:

  - Medullary thyroid cancer can have high levels of calcitonin, made by the parafollicular cells (C-cells).

- Medullary thyroid cancer can be part of several endocrine disorders, including the multiple endocrine neoplasia (MEN) complex of syndromes. It's associated with both MEN 2A and MEN 2B. Look for the presence of a pheochromocytoma and problems with the parathyroid (usually hyperparathyroidism).

Medullary thyroid cancer is a fairly aggressive cancer, and surgery is the treatment of choice. Calcitonin levels can be followed to monitor recurrence of disease.

✔ **Anaplastic thyroid cancer:** This form of cancer is rare (less than 1 percent of all thyroid cancers) and is very, very aggressive, with a very high mortality rate: The ten-year survival rate is 14 percent. The workup includes a fine needle biopsy, thyroid function tests, calcitonin and thyroglobulin levels, and imaging for metastatic disease.

✔ **Lymphomas:** Lymphomas represent only a small percentage of causes of thyroid malignancies.

Looking Over Lipids

Any person who goes to see a healthcare provider gets a lipid panel done as part of a comprehensive workup. Most lipid panels show levels for high-density lipoprotein (HDL), low-density lipoprotein (LDL), triglyceride (TG), and total cholesterol. Author Barry loves reading his own labs, because the computer printout shows the normal range and flags any results that are out of range.

Understanding HDL, LDL, triglyceride, and cholesterol levels is important because of their link with coronary artery disease and association with other conditions like diabetes mellitus:

✔ Diabetes mellitus can be associated with high triglycerides and low HDL levels.

✔ Hypothyroidism, obesity, sedentary lifestyle, and metabolic syndrome all increase the risk of developing hyperlipidemia.

✔ High LDL levels, low HDL levels, and high triglycerides are associated with an increased risk of coronary artery disease.

Very high triglyceride levels (usually > 1,000 mg/dL) and extremely high cholesterol levels are risk factors not only for heart disease but also for pancreatitis.

With newer medical guidelines, just screening for total cholesterol and triglycerides is a no-no. HDL and LDL need to be included.

Blaming relatives for some forms of hyperlipidemia

Become familiar with some of the hereditary forms of hyperlipidemia, because they could appear on the PANCE:

✔ *Familial hypercholesterolemia* (FH) is a hereditary condition in which the affected person can have super-high cholesterol and LDL levels. This condition is thought to be due to a mutation of the LDL receptor (LDLR) gene. FH is inherited in an autosomal dominant fashion, and this disorder has both homozygous and heterozygous forms. People with the homozygous form don't survive long as adults.

✔ In *familial dysbetalipoproteinemia,* not only are there increased total cholesterol, LDL, and triglyceride levels, but there are also low HDL levels. Experts think that this condition is due to a defect with apolipoprotein E's role in catabolism of lipids.

> ✔ *Familial hypertriglyceridemia* causes (you guessed it) high triglycerides.
>
> ✔ *Familial combined hyperlipidemia* is just that: Elevated total cholesterol and triglycerides.

Familial hypercholesterolemia and other familial conditions can present with xanthomas, which represent lipid deposition in joints or in tendons. There may be *xanthelasmas,* which are deposits along the eyelids. You see these deposits only with very high cholesterol levels.

Treating hyperlipidemia

Certainly, diet and lifestyle changes, including exercising and stopping smoking, are very important in improving lipid health. A diet low in saturated fat and high in fiber can help lower cholesterol. Diet and lifestyle changes can also lower LDL and triglyceride levels and raise HDL levels. Sometimes, though, that may not be enough, and medication is necessary.

The statins, including atorvastatin (Lipitor) and simvastatin (Zocor), are commonly prescribed for the treatment of hyperlipidemia. Side effects of these medications include liver problems and myopathy. Some people have reported problems with memory.

A common class of medication used to treat *hypertriglyceridemia* (high triglycerides) is the *fibrate* class. Derivatives include fenofibrate (Tricor). With this med, you need to watch liver enzymes closely. If a patient is on both a statin and fenofibrate, his or her risk of hepatotoxicity increases. Omega-3 (fish oil) has also been used in the treatment of hypertriglyceridemias.

Low HDL levels can be treated with nicotinic acid (niacin). However, liver enzymes may be affected. A common side effect of nicotinic acid is flushing, so to reduce the risk, sometimes aspirin is prescribed before the person takes the medication.

Bile acid sequestrants work in the intestine but have different modes of action. Ezetimibe (Zetia) inhibits the absorption of cholesterol in the intestine. *Bile acid resins* like cholestyramine (Questran) and colestipol (Colestid) function as bile acid binders in the intestine.

Practice Endocrine System Questions

These practice questions are similar to the PANCE endocrinology questions.

1. Which of the following can be used in the evaluation of Addison's disease?

   (A) 24-hour urinary free cortisol

   (B) Low-dose dexamethasone suppression test

   (C) High-dose dexamethasone suppression test

   (D) Morning cortisol level

   (E) MRI of the brain

2. You are seeing a 50-year-old man who has been treated with a diuretic for hypertension and edema. You do routine lab work and discover a potassium level of 3.4 mg/dL and a calcium level of 10.8 mg/dL. Which medication is this patient likely taking?

   (A) Furosemide (Lasix)

   (B) Acetazolamide (Diamox)

   (C) Chlorthalidone (Hygroton)

   (D) Amiloride (Midamor)

   (E) Aldactone (Spironolactone)

3. You are evaluating a 35-year-old man with no significant past medical problems. You obtained a lipid panel, and it shows an LDL level of 130 mg/dL. Based on National Cholesterol Education Program (NCEP) guidelines, which of the following would you recommend?

   (A) Recommend lifestyle and dietary changes and then reevaluate.

   (B) Begin ezetimibe (Zetia).

   (C) Initiate treatment with atorvastatin (Lipitor).

   (D) Begin ezetimibe (Zetia) in addition to lifestyle and dietary intervention.

   (E) Initiate treatment with atorvastatin (Lipitor) in addition to lifestyle and dietary interventions.

4. Which of the following would be on indication for surgical treatment of hyperparathyroidism?

   (A) Development of recurrent kidney stones

   (B) A normal DEXA (also called DXA) scan

   (C) Elevation in the serum sodium level

   (D) Hypophosphatemia

   (E) Persistently low calcium level

5. A 35-year-old woman with a history of manic depression presents to the clinic with excessive thirst. She doesn't remember her medication list but recalls one was abruptly stopped. She also states she is urinating a lot more than usual. Her vitals, including blood pressure, are stable. You order some lab work, and the sodium level is 141 mEq/L, the creatinine level is 1.2 mg/dL, the blood glucose level is 100 mg/dL, and the calcium level is 9.5 mg/dL. Which test would you order next?

   (A) Urinalysis to look for glucosuria

   (B) Morning (a.m.) cortisol to screen for adrenal insufficiency

   (C) Chemistry panel

   (D) Urine osmolality

   (E) Serum osmolality

6. You are seeing a 68-year-old man with type 2 diabetes in your office. His last Hgb A1c, done one month ago, was 9.2. In the last three weeks, you made some adjustments in his medication. Which test could you order to see whether there has been any change in his condition?

   (A) Repeat glycosylated hemoglobin (Hgb A1c)

   (B) Sequential postprandial glucose monitoring

   (C) Oral glucose tolerance test

   (D) Albumin/creatinine ratio

   (E) Glycated serum fructosamine (GSP) level

Answers and Explanations

Use this answer key to score the practice endocrine system questions from the preceding section. The answer explanations give you some insight into why the correct answer is better than the other choices.

1. **D.** A morning (a.m.) cortisol level is used in evaluating adrenal insufficiency and hyponatremia. All the other tests listed are used in evaluating Cushing's syndrome. You use an MRI of the brain to evaluate for Cushing's disease (not the same as Cushing's syndrome) secondary to a pituitary adenoma.

2. **C.** Choices (D) and (E) are potassium-sparing diuretics and would cause hyperkalemia. Although Choices (A), (B), and (C) all can cause hypokalemia, only Choice (C) can cause hypercalcemia, because it's a thiazide diuretic. Choice (B) is a carbonic anhydrase inhibitor and can cause hypokalemia and a metabolic acidosis.

3. **A.** He has no significant risk factors, so his goal LDL is < 160. He requires only lifestyle intervention and dietary modification. If a person has known coronary artery disease and one additional risk factor, the goal should be < 130. If someone has coronary artery disease, congestive heart failure, or diabetes mellitus, you strive to get the LDL level below 100 mg/dL.

4. **A.** None of the choices except Choice (A) are indications for parathyroidectomy. Recurrent kidney stones, bone disease (including osteoporosis), hypercalcemia, and worsening renal insufficiency are indications for surgery. Low phosphorous levels, although they may accompany hyperparathyroidism, are not in and of themselves indications for surgery. An elevation in the serum calcium level, not the serum sodium level, would be considered an indication for surgery if the elevation were persistent.

5. **D.** For this question, you need to be able to pick up the clues. The first sentence tells you a lot. The woman has a history of manic depression, is polydipsic, and is polyuric. The serum glucose is normal, so her polyuria is not due to an osmotic diuresis from diabetes. Her calcium level is normal, so polyuria is not from a high calcium level causing a nephrogenic diabetes insipidus. She likely had been on lithium and has a nephrogenic diabetes insipidus from this. You'd obtain a urine osmolality to see whether the urine is dilute.

   With diabetes insipidus, whether it be central or nephrogenic, you expect a dilute urine with a urine osmolality < 100 mOsm/kg. Common causes of nephrogenic diabetes insipidus include hypercalcemia, hypokalemia, and medications like lithium (Eskalith). There's typically low urine osmolality. *Central diabetes insipidus* refers to a problem in the posterior pituitary, where ADH is stored. Causes can include trauma, surgery, or infiltrative conditions.

6. **E.** You want to check the serum fructosamine level. The Hgb A1c reflects changes in blood sugars over 3 months, whereas the fructosamine level, Choice (E), can reflect changes over the past few weeks. The oral glucose tolerance test is not routinely used but is a method of diagnosing type 2 diabetes mellitus and gestational diabetes. This person has already been diagnosed with diabetes, and he doesn't need to be retested. We're also pretty confident that he isn't pregnant, either. There's no such test as sequential postprandial glucose monitoring, although it's recommended that both pre- and postprandial blood glucose levels be monitored in diabetes. Albumin/creatinine ratio testing should be done at least yearly in someone diagnosed with diabetes mellitus.

Chapter 16

Keeping Neurology in Mind

- -

- -

*T*he neurologic system comprises both the central nervous system (CNS) and the peripheral nervous system (PNS). This chapter covers many important subject areas you see on the PANCE/PANRE, including headaches, seizures, movement disorders, delirium, and the cerebrovascular accident (CVA). Don't lose your nerve!

Changes in Mental Status: When It's Not Okay to Change Your Mind

Changes in mental status can occur quickly or over a long period of time. Sometimes changes in mental status are reversible, such as when they occur because of a medication or temporary medical condition. In other cases, all you and the patient's family can do is try to mitigate the inevitable decline as best you can. In this section, we point out some of the medications and conditions that can cause a change in mental status, and then we describe dementia, which is irreversible.

Tracing an altered status to meds or medical conditions

For the PANCE, you should be aware of conditions and medications that can cause a change in mental status. They're a common reason for admission to the hospital.

Common medications that can cause a change in mental status, especially in older people, include antipsychotics, anticholinergics, and benzodiazepines. Medication overdoses do it, too.

Common conditions that can cause a change in mental status include hypoglycemia, electrolyte abnormalities (such as hypernatremia and hyponatremia), infection (including urinary tract infections, pneumonia, and bacteremia), hypotension with resultant lowered cerebral perfusion, and volume depletion.

Note that trauma, especially falls in the elderly and motor vehicle accidents, can also be a cause of brain injury with a change in mentation. In those situations, obtaining a CT scan of the head is vital to evaluate for possible bleeding, including a subdural hematoma.

When reading a test question concerning a change in mental status, look for the underlying etiology of the person's confusion. There will be a reason.

Dealing with dementia

Dementia essentially refers to brain degeneration, and it's irreversible. It's a significant problem, especially in the older population. Alzheimer's is on the rise, and with the epidemic of obesity, diabetes, and hypertension, you'll see more and more cases of vascular dementia. This section describes the various forms of dementia from a PANCE and clinical perspective.

Different types of dementia can affect different areas of the brain. For example, in a clinical scenario where an older person is behaving like an infant (for example, sucking his thumb and displaying infant-like reflexes), think of a dementia affecting the frontal lobe. When the frontal lobe is affected, the person loses all inhibitions. An example of a frontal lobe type of dementia is Pick's disease.

Distinguishing dementia from delirium and pseudodementia

On the PANCE, expect to see a question in which a person, usually an older person, is admitted with a change in mental status. You'll have to determine whether you're dealing with delirium or dementia. The answer depends on a couple of factors:

- **Time frame:** Although dementia is a process that occurs over a long period of time (months to years), delirium usually occurs over the course of a few days. For example, a urinary tract infection, pneumonia, or volume depletion can cause a change in mental status acutely over the period of a few days, if not faster, and cause delirium. Medications can cause delirium big time.

- **Types of change:** Delirium can be associated with changes in thinking and perception. The affected person can be hyperactive or completely lethargic. Sometimes the behavior patterns can change in a single day. The key concerning the management of delirium is in looking for an underlying cause.

  Dementia, on the other hand, is a serious loss of mental faculties, which can include cognition, memory, attention, perception, language, problem-solving, and interpersonal skills.

Don't confuse dementia with pseudodementia, which commonly afflicts older individuals. In *pseudodementia,* the person appears to be demented but typically is just extremely depressed. The difference is in how the person answers your questions. In the person with pseudodementia, the cognition and perception are generally intact. The demented person answers questions strangely and may not even pay attention to what you're asking.

Understanding Alzheimer's dementia

Alzheimer's dementia (commonly called *Alzheimer's disease*) is by far the most common form of dementia. It likely accounts for more than half of all the cases of dementia. The typical scenario is an older person who initially experiences worsening problems with memory, especially short-term memory. Over time, the affected person begins to have other problems, including confusion, labile mood (mood swings), and trouble with speaking. The person can become isolated and unable over time to perform activities of daily living (ADL). This condition can be extremely difficult for caregivers and for family members, who often are the caregivers.

The symptoms usually present in individuals in their mid-60s; however, Alzheimer's dementia can be early onset as well.

Here are four key points about Alzheimer's dementia:

- ✔ If you were to look under the microscope, you would see that beta amyloid plaques and neurofibrillary tangles are present in the brain of someone with Alzheimer's. It's postulated that the plaques and the tangles inhibit and destroy the function of the nerve cells somehow. This destruction may be the cause of the dementia symptoms.

- ✔ The diagnosis is made from having a high clinical suspicion of the dementia plus exclusion of other, reversible causes of dementia. Imaging studies such as an MRI and a PET scan can help in the diagnosis.

- ✔ Medications may prevent worsening of the disease. Examples are donepezil (Aricept), which is an anticholinesterase inhibitor, and memantine (Namenda), which is a glutamate receptor antagonist.

- ✔ In the later stages of Alzheimer's dementia, regular caregiving becomes impossible for family members and significant others because the person requires 24-hour care. The person often needs to be placed in a supervised care facility.

Recognizing vascular dementia

Vascular dementia, or *multi-infarct dementia,* is the most common type of dementia after Alzheimer's. Although Alzheimer's dementia is more common in women, vascular dementia is more common in men.

Risk factors for vascular dementia include hypertension, diabetes, and long-standing vascular disease. Atherosclerosis, inflammation, small vessel disease, and infarctions all likely play a role in the development of vascular dementia. Atrial fibrillation can also be a risk factor, usually due to multiple embolic infarcts. All these processes are damaging to the blood vessels and affect the circulation in the brain. These blood vessels have been damaged over time. Here are a couple of key points about vascular dementia:

- ✔ Loss of abilities can occur in steps as the small vessels in the brain (the *lacunae*) are affected (a *lacunar infarct*). Therefore, this type of dementia is considered a stepwise dementia.

- ✔ Treatment of risk factors can delay vascular dementia. This means controlling blood pressure, regulating blood glucose levels, decreasing factors of inflammation, and watching cholesterol levels.

Many medical conditions, especially B_{12} and folic acid deficiencies, can cause dementia if left untreated for a long period of time. Syphilis can also be a cause of dementia. Myxedema, which results from long-standing uncontrolled hypothyroidism, can also present with a dementia-like picture.

Note that in a small percentage of people, vascular dementia and Alzheimer's dementia can co-exist. This can be very difficult to diagnose and to manage.

Learning about Lewy body dementia

Lewy body dementia, which combines many of the features of Alzheimer's dementia with Parkinson's disease, is the third most common type of dementia. It's caused by Lewy bodies, which you find in the neurons of people affected by this syndrome. The main symptoms of this type of dementia include significant changes in the level of alertness throughout the day. Hallucinations, especially visual hallucinations, can also be present. Lewy body dementia has a motor component as well; motor symptoms can resemble Parkinson's disease (read about Parkinson's in the next section).

The treatment of Lewy body dementia involves treatments utilized for both Alzheimer's dementia and Parkinson's disease. Medications such as donepezil (Aricept), which is an anticholinesterase inhibitor, and a glutamate receptor antagonist such as memantine (Namenda) are used for some of the dementia symptoms of this condition. Anti-Parkinson's medications are used to help treat the motor symptoms.

Reviewing Movement Disorders

Different types of neurologic conditions can present with different types of problems. Some disorders, such as the peripheral neuropathies, present with a sensory type of neuropathy. You can read about them later. The disorders in this section concern problems with motor function. For PANCE purposes, the four fundamental types of movement disorders are essential tremors, Parkinson's disease, Huntington's disease, and cerebral palsy.

Stressing over essential tremors

Stop shaking! This topic's easy! An *essential tremor* (kinetic tremor) is a tremor of the arm or arms, worsened with movement or any type of stressor, such as emotional stress. The essential tremor doesn't occur all the time. Note that although an essential tremor typically involves an extremity, it can also involve other body areas, including the head. In a test question, an intermittent tremor brought on by a stressor is the key.

Here are three points about the essential tremor:

✔ These tremors don't occur at rest; they're usually absent during sleep.

✔ One effective treatment is a beta blocker, particularly propranolol (Inderal). Propranolol is lipophilic and can penetrate the blood-brain barrier.

✔ An essential tremor doesn't mean that the person has Parkinson's disease. Both conditions are progressive and degenerative, but Parkinson's has a more precise etiology and slightly different symptoms.

Blaming brain chemistry for Parkinson's disease

Parkinson's disease (called the "shaking palsy" in 1817) is a progressive and degenerative disorder characterized by a deficiency of dopamine. Clinical manifestations include the four so-called cardinal signs: bradykinesia, pill-rolling tremor, rigidity (including lead-pipe rigidity and cogwheel rigidity), and postural instability. Parkinson's usually presents in someone who's middle aged.

Here are some key points concerning Parkinson's disease:

✔ It's caused by a deficiency of dopamine production by the substantia nigra in the brain. The exact cause of the death of dopamine-generating cells isn't known.

✔ Significant muscle rigidity and ambulatory dysfunction, including a shuffling gait, can be present.

✔ Parkinson's disease can be associated with other conditions, some of which can affect the integrity of the autonomic nervous system — think multiple system atrophy.

✔ The person may have a failure to thrive, and cognition problems can develop.

Treating Parkinson's is pharmacologic. One of the big medications used is carbidopa/levodopa (Sinemet). The body changes levodopa into a synthetic dopamine. The carbidopa stops some of the metabolism of the levodopa, so the patient can receive a smaller dose.

Another medication for treating Parkinson's is amantadine (Symmetrel), which was once used to treat influenza A. It's no longer recommend for treating influenza B, and both the A and B viruses are now resistant to amantadine, but for Parkinson's, this med can reduce some of the symptoms. It may be used as monotherapy in early stage Parkinson's, but it's often used in combination with carbidopa/levodopa. It may work as an antagonist of the NMDA (N-methyl-D-aspartate) type glutamate receptor, which increases dopamine release and blocks reuptake of dopamine. It can help especially with bradykinesia.

Pramipexole (Mirapex), which is a dopamine agonist, can help with the tremors and dyskinesias of Parkinson's. It can cause sleepiness.

For another important class of medications used in the treatment of Parkinson's disease, look at the following example question.

Which class of medications is used in treating Parkinson's disease?

(A) Antipsychotics

(B) Antidiarrheals

(C) Anticholinergics

(D) Steroids

(E) Plasmapheresis

The correct answer is Choice (C). Dopamine and acetylcholine normally exist in the brain in equal amounts, and the medications used in treating Parkinson's disease can upset this balance, hence the worsening symptoms. Anticholinergics are used to help with the symptoms of Parkinson's and to maintain a healthy balance between dopamine and acetylcholine. As for the other choices, antipsychotics would make Parkinson's worse, because antipsychotics antagonize dopamine. Antidiarrheals are used in treating diarrhea. Steroids are used in treating a multiple sclerosis exacerbation, and plasmapheresis is used in treating Guillain-Barré syndrome, a myasthenic crisis, and certain forms of vasculitis.

Chorea: Getting a handle on Huntington's disease

Huntington's disease is a genetic disorder that's inherited in an autosomal dominant manner, resulting in trinucleotide CAG repeats. It's characterized by *choreiform movements,* which are involuntary, irregular movements of the arms. The arms make it look like the person is dancing. In addition to chorea, Huntington's can be associated with dystonia. *Dystonia* is an involuntary movement characterized by muscle spasm. Huntington's disease is associated with an increased mortality — the average lifespan in young adulthood is about 15 to 20 years after the onset of symptoms.

Here are some key points concerning Huntington's disease:

- ✔ This condition affects the brain and can cause confusion, psychosis, and dementia. It's associated with a host of cognitive and psychiatric symptoms. A main symptom is depression, which may have an *organic* cause deriving from the effect of Huntington's disease on the brain.

- ✔ In people with Huntington's, a leading cause of mortality is infectious, usually aspiration pneumonia. Huntington's is also associated with cardiomyopathy, which is the second leading cause of mortality.

- ✔ Huntington's has no cure. The treatment is supportive with medications used to help the symptoms. Medications include antipsychotics and antidepressants.

Besides Huntington's chorea, another condition that can cause choreiform movements is Sydenham's chorea (St. Vitus' Dance), which is associated with rheumatic fever.

Understanding cerebral palsy

Cerebral palsy is a condition that commonly affects motor function. Cerebral palsy comes in various types, and the most common type causes spastic movements. Like multiple sclerosis (MS), which we cover later in "Looking for the right signals in multiple sclerosis," cerebral palsy is an upper motor neuron lesion.

Note that cerebral palsy can present with a variety of symptoms, from problems with balance to spastic movements, involuntary gesturing, and significant ambulatory dysfunction. Treatment is based on the predominant presenting symptoms.

Getting the Upper Hand on Peripheral Nerve Problems

Many disorders can affect the integrity of the peripheral nerves. In this section, we pick two likely candidates for PANCE questions: peripheral neuropathy and complex regional pain syndrome (CRPS).

Managing peripheral neuropathies

One of the best examples of a peripheral neuropathy is *diabetic neuropathy,* a polyneuropathy that affects the hands and feet in a glove-stocking distribution. A peripheral neuropathy sometimes affects just one nerve (a *mononeuropathy*), as in carpal tunnel syndrome, which affects the median nerve. A neuropathy can also affect multiple nerves, as in vasculitis or a connective tissue disease like systemic lupus erythematosus (see Chapter 6 for details on lupus).

Peripheral neuropathies can be debilitating. Common presenting symptoms include sensory symptoms (including numbness, tingling, and paresthesias) and motor symptoms (including weakness).

The treatment of the peripheral neuropathy depends on the underlying cause. Look at the following examples:

- ✔ The treatment for diabetic neuropathy is prevention with intensive blood glucose control. Medications such as gabapentin (Neurontin), duloxetine (Cymbalta), and the tricyclic antidepressants can help with the pain.

- ✔ The treatment for peripheral neuropathy secondary to B_{12} and folic acid deficiency is replacement. B_{12} deficiency can cause subacute combined degeneration, which is a loss of vibration and proprioception.

- ✔ Amyloidosis can cause a peripheral polyneuropathy, an autonomic neuropathy, or a restrictive cardiomyopathy. The treatment is chemotherapy.

- ✔ Exposure to heavy metals, including lead, can cause a peripheral neuropathy. The treatment for this involves intravenous chelation.

- ✔ HIV can cause many kinds of neuropathy. The treatment includes the use of some of the medications you read about in this section in addition to treatment directed against the HIV.

 Another example of a peripheral neuropathy is an *autonomic neuropathy,* which involves a blunting of the sympathetic nervous system. The most common cause of this is diabetes mellitus. With an autonomic neuropathy, there's usually orthostatic hypotension but without a corresponding increase in heart rate.

Relieving the intensity of complex regional pain syndrome

Complex regional pain syndrome (CRPS), formerly known as *reflex sympathetic dystrophy* (RSD), can be a very debilitating condition. An extremity is often in extreme pain after some inciting event, usually a significant trauma. The thought is that after inciting event, the person has an exaggerated inflammatory response, which worsens the pain. Another thought is that the person has a heightened sympathetic tone. The nerve is affected, either directly or indirectly, as a result of the injury.

The affected extremity is red, warm, and painful to touch. Complex regional pain syndrome involves nerve damage, which can affect the muscles and even the bone. On a radiograph or bone scan, the bone can have the look of osteoporosis.

Here are key points about complex regional pain syndrome:

- ✔ The pain is out of proportion to the injury that caused it *(allodynia)*.
- ✔ The affected person's extremity is very sensitive *(hyperalgesia)*.
- ✔ The pain and paresthesias can worsen over weeks to months.
- ✔ The person may have a low blood flow and labile temperatures over the affected limb.
- ✔ The muscles of that extremity can atrophy.

Treatment is based on trying to help with pain, and that may decrease sympathetic tone or even stimulate the nerves. If this condition is diagnosed too late, it may not be reversible.

Identifying Brain Infections

The two big nervous-system infection types you need to be aware of are meningitis and encephalitis. These conditions can be fatal if not quickly recognized and treated. Not knowing about them for the PANCE can be fatal in another way.

Covering meningitis

Meningitis is an inflammation of the membrane that blankets the spinal cord and brain. Meningitis comes in two types: bacterial and aseptic. The two conditions have similar presentations, but the similarities end there.

Bacterial meningitis

Bacterial meningitis is fatal unless it's quickly diagnosed and treated. Symptoms of bacterial meningitis include fever, headache, photophobia, and neck pain. On physical examination, you can see nuchal rigidity, Kernig's sign, and Brudziński's sign.

The key in diagnosis lies in the cerebrospinal fluid (CSF) total protein count. With bacterial meningitis, you see a high protein count, low glucose level, and leukocytosis with a neutrophilic predominance. The person also has an increased opening pressure.

Common causes of bacterial meningitis include *Streptococcus pneumoniae*, group B strep, and *Neisseria meningitidis*. You commonly see group B strep as a cause of meningitis in neonates. *Listeria monocytogenes* is a cause of meningitis in infants, the immunocompromised, and the elderly.

The treatment for bacterial meningitis involves antibiotics, including vancomycin and ceftri-axone (Rocephin). For someone with *Listeria monocytogenes,* the treatment is ampicillin. In addition, dexamethasone (Decadron) is used in conjunction with antibiotics to treat bacterial meningitis.

Aseptic meningitis

Unlike bacterial meningitis, aseptic meningitis isn't usually fatal. The symptoms can mimic those of bacterial meningitis, but aseptic meningitis isn't as severe. Causes of aseptic meningitis can be viral or secondary related to medications such as NSAIDs. Concerning the cerebrospinal fluid count, you usually see normal or near normal protein and glucose levels. The treatment is supportive.

Cryptococcal meningitis, caused by the yeast *Cryptococcus neoformans,* can occur in anyone, but it has a predilection for someone who is immunocompromised. For example, in someone with HIV, you may see this infection when the CD4 count is less than 200. The treatment includes strong antifungal medications, including intravenous amphotericin B (Fungilin). Another cause of meningitis is cancer, so it's called (get ready) *carcinomatous meningitis.*

You're evaluating a 65-year-old man who presents with a fever and a severe headache. His mental status is intact. On exam, his Kernig's and Brudziński's signs are positive. You obtain a lumbar puncture, which shows a cerebrospinal fluid glucose of 30 mg/dL and protein levels of 600 mg/dL. The cerebrospinal fluid opening pressure is increased. Which one of the following would you use for treatment?

(A) Acyclovir (Zovirax)

(B) Fluconazole (Diflucan)

(C) Ceftriaxone (Rocephin)

(D) Indomethacin (Indocin)

(E) Phenytoin (Dilantin)

The correct answer is Choice (C), ceftriaxone, because the cerebrospinal fluid findings indicate bacterial meningitis. Choice (A), acyclovir, is used in treating herpes simplex encephalitis. Choice (B), fluconazole, is used in the treatment of a fungal meningitis. Choice (D), indomethacin, isn't indicated here and in fact would be a cause of aseptic meningitis. Choice (E), phenytoin, isn't indicated because the patient hasn't had any seizure activity (although encephalitis can present with seizures, especially if the temporal lobe is affected).

When clinically treating someone with bacterial meningitis, vancomycin (Vancocin) is given in addition to ceftriaxone (Rocephin). In an older patient, or in someone in whom *Listeria* is suspected, ampicillin (Polycillin) is also added.

Getting into encephalitis

Encephalitis is a nasty, nasty inflammatory and infectious process of the brain. Like meningitis, it can be fatal if not quickly diagnosed and treated. Common presenting symptoms of encephalitis include a change in mental status that can worsen quickly, fever, neck pain, and neuropsychiatric symptoms.

The most common causes of encephalitis are viral and vector-associated (for example, West Nile virus). Another viral form of encephalitis you should be familiar with is *herpes simplex encephalitis* (HSE), sometimes called *herpesviral encephalitis.* Here are a few key points about herpes simplex encephalitis:

✔ The diagnosis can be confirmed by lumbar puncture and brain imaging. The MRI can show abnormalities in the temporal lobe.

✔ The treatment for herpes simplex encephalitis is intravenous acyclovir (Zovirax).

✔ Herpes simplex encephalitis is actually a meningoencephalitis. A change in mental status and seizure-like activity confirm the presence of accompanying encephalitis.

Handling Headaches

Headaches are a common reason people visit a healthcare provider, and at their worst, headaches can be debilitating. For PANCE purposes, we bring up migraine headaches, tension headaches, and cluster headaches.

Managing migraines

Migraine headaches are probably one of the most common forms of headache. Any migraine sufferer will tell you that these headaches are the worst. Migraines tend to affect the frontal and temporal parts of the head. Common presenting symptoms (aside from hurting like hell) include photophobia and phonophobia. Picture the person lying quietly in a dark room with an acute migraine headache. The acute phase can sometimes last for 48 to 72 hours before dissipating. Migraine headaches are diagnosed from their clinical presentation.

Sometimes migraines occur spontaneously without warning, and sometimes they're accompanied by an *aura,* a perceptual preview of coming attractions. People may experience visual auras (the scintillating scotoma, for example) or other auras, including certain sounds and smells. One risk factor for migraine headaches is a positive family history.

Treating migraines involves a two-pronged approach: acute treatment to stop the migraines and medications that attempt to prevent the migraines in the first place (that is, *migraine prophylaxis*). Various medication classes are used to treat an acute migraine headache. Two common examples are the ergotamine derivatives and the triptans. Medications used to prevent migraines include beta blockers such as propranolol (Inderal) and calcium channel blockers.

Easing tension headaches

We live in a world of stress. Stress and tension can manifest in many ways, including headaches. Tension headaches, unlike migraine headaches, occur more in the back of the head. The tension headache is a steady ache that won't go away. It's often described as pressure, squeezing, or a vise-like headache. The acute headache can be treated with NSAIDs; ibuprofen is a common med. Muscle relaxants such as cyclobenzaprine (Flexeril) can also be used. Other modalities include exercise and stress management.

Clustering headaches

The cluster headache, also known as the *suicide headache* because the pain is so severe, occurs predominantly in middle-aged men. The cluster headache usually presents as an acute lancinating pain behind the eye. It can be debilitating. The headaches often occur in cycles that become predictable. A person can experience several headaches each day for as little as a week to as long as several months. These headache episodes are separated by pain-free intervals of time. Note that the duration of these pain-free intervals can vary from person to person. Other symptoms can include ptosis and increased eye tearing. The treatment can include 100 percent oxygen and steroids.

Losing Consciousness

Passing out is never a good thing. When you're evaluating a test question involving someone who has lost consciousness, you often need to figure out whether the person had a syncopal episode or a seizure. We cover both here.

Fainting: Recovering from syncope

Syncope (fainting) is a condition in which a person loses consciousness and will recover, often spontaneously, without any kind of assistance. One of the most common flavors of syncope is vasovagal syncope, brought to you by the vagus nerve.

Here are some key points concerning the evaluation and management of syncope:

✔ Some causes of syncope are heart-related. Examples include cardiac arrhythmias, including ventricular arrhythmias, bradyarrhythmias, and conduction disturbance, such as heart block. Structural problems of the heart, including aortic stenosis and hypertrophic cardiomyopathy, can also cause syncope.

✔ Syncope can have neurologic causes. An example is orthostatic hypotension caused by an autonomic neuropathy. Refer to Chapter 3 for details on orthostatic hypotension.

✔ Another cause of syncope is idiopathic, meaning that the cause isn't readily apparent.

Sorting out seizure types and treatments

Seizures are a completely different animal from fainting. *Seizures* refer to an abnormal electrical activity in the brain. For PANCE purposes, you should be familiar with the types of seizures and some of the medications used to treat them:

✔ **Partial simple seizures:** The person doesn't lose consciousness.

✔ **Partial complex seizures:** The affected person loses consciousness.

✔ **Absence seizure:** The person experiences an alteration in consciousness for only a few seconds. The patient may seem like he or she is daydreaming.

✔ **Tonic-clonic seizure:** The person loses consciousness with loss of postural tone and generalized myoclonic/convulsive activity.

Laboratory abnormalities that you can see during a patient's acute seizure include lactic acidosis and rhabdomyolysis, especially after a tonic-clonic seizure.

Risk factors for seizures include stress, sleep deprivation, alcoholism, and electrolyte abnormalities such as hyponatremia, hypocalcemia, and hypomagnesemia. Many medications, including the fluoroquinolones, can lower the seizure threshold.

Here are some key points about treating a seizure:

✔ Phenytoin (Dilantin), especially in the water-soluble form, fosphenytoin, is often given during an acute seizure. This is one of the most common medications used in the treatment of an acute seizure. Phenytoin can be associated with gingival hyperplasia and osteoporosis. Too high of a phenytoin level can cause symptoms of toxicity, including nausea, confusion, tremors, and nystagmus, so drug levels are followed.

✔ Phenobarbital (Solfoton) can also be used in the treatment of an acute seizure. Clinically it's prescribed when phenytoin can't be used or isn't tolerated. Phenobarbital is also used in conjunction with phenytoin. Like phenytoin, phenobarbital is followed with blood levels. Side effects include sedation and neurological effects, including ataxia and nystagmus.

✔ The benzodiazepines are used in treating an acute seizure. Examples include diazepam (Valium) and midazolam (Versed).

✔ The next three medications are commonly prescribed antiseizure medications that are often added as needed after the person has been treated acutely. Be aware of the side effects of these medications:

  • Lamotrigine (Lamictal) can be associated with a skin rash. Note that this medication can also be used for the treatment of bipolar disorder.

  • Valproic acid (Depakote) can be associated with elevated liver function tests and pancreatitis. This medication is followed by drug levels.

  • Carbamazepine (Tegretol) can cause hyponatremia and leukopenia as side effects. This medication is followed by drug levels.

After a seizure, especially if the person has lost consciousness, the person will be in a postictal state. If a test question asks you for signs that a seizure has occurred, remember the postictal state as well as tongue biting, extensor plantar response (Babinski sign) in the immediate postictal response, loss of bowel function, and loss of bladder function.

Status epilepticus is a continuous abnormal electrical activity of the brain — one that doesn't stop and is refractory to treatment. This is a life-threatening condition. To be technical, it's seizure activity that continues for a half hour or more. The evaluation is comprehensive and can involve brain imaging, a lumbar puncture to rule out an infection, and lab work (for example, glucose level and arterial blood gas). Review the person's medications to look for changes in existing antiseizure drugs or for a new med that may lower the levels of antiseizure medication or lower the seizure threshold. Changes in medication levels are especially significant in someone with a history of epilepsy. The first-line of treatment is usually benzodiazepines.

Todd's paralysis, also known as *Todd's paresis,* is temporary weakness in a body part (focal weakness) occurring after a seizure. Symptoms can take up to 2 days to subside.

Viewing the Brain's Vascular System

In the field of neurology, be aware of the vascular system. When the arteries in the brain get messed up, bad things can happen. Arteries can be blocked, they can rupture, and they can bleed. That's plenty for any brain! This section describes the cerebrovascular accident and bleeding disorders that can occur in the brain.

Identifying and preventing the transient ischemic attack

Welcome to the world of the mini-stroke, the *transient ischemic attack*. Picture this: A 60-year-old man comes to your office for an urgent visit, demanding to be seen. He states he was sitting home reading when he noticed vision in his left eye "became dark." He says it's as if "someone pulled a window shade over my left eye." It lasted for a few minutes but then suddenly went away. He denies feeling weak in any one area of the body or talking funny. What happened? This person had one version of a transient ischemic attack (TIA).

The changes to the man's eye are termed *amaurosis fugax* (Latin for "fleeting darkening"), which is the acute onset of blindness in one eye. Another common scenario suggesting a transient ischemic attack is the person who presents to the emergency room with weakness on one side of her face and "arms and legs that went away." Another common scenario is the person who, according to the family, starts to talk funny. This usually refers to an acute episode of aphasia that occurs and then resolves.

What do these transient ischemic attack variants have in common? They occur and then spontaneously resolve. By definition, the symptoms of a transient ischemic attack don't persist for more than 24 hours. If they do, you then need to think about something else — the ever-popular stroke, for example.

Think of a transient ischemic attack as analogous to an angina episode of the heart. The person has a short period of ischemia to the affected artery in the brain that spontaneously resolves. Given the quick timeframe, you're usually dealing with an embolic phenomenon.

Here are some other key points concerning the transient ischemic attack:

✔ The risk factors include hypertension, diabetes mellitus, tobacco use, hyperlipidemia, chronic inflammation, and peripheral vascular disease present elsewhere.

✔ Part of the initial evaluation involves a carotid ultrasound to evaluate the patency of the carotid arteries and an echocardiogram to evaluate for a possible embolic source.

✔ Other studies can include a magnetic resonance angiography (MRA) and/or angiogram.

✔ The treatment involves the use of antiplatelet agents, including aspirin, and clopidogrel (Plavix). Also, identifying and reducing the risk factors is essential.

Stroke: Treating the brain attack

A *brain attack* isn't an incursion of zombies. We're referring to an acute *cerebrovascular accident* (CVA), commonly called a stroke. If a transient ischemic attack is like an anginal episode, then an acute stroke is like an acute heart attack. Both require immediate intervention for survival and a good outcome.

The transient ischemic attack sufferer usually recovers spontaneously, but the stroke sufferer doesn't. The time course in treating a stroke is especially important.

Looking at types of stroke

Strokes may be ischemic or hemorrhagic (we cover the hemorrhagic stroke later in "Treating the bleeding brain"). Furthermore, the acute ischemic stroke may be embolic or thrombotic:

✔ **Embolic strokes:** These strokes most commonly occur in the setting of a heart issue, such as underlying atrial fibrillation — as if the heart problem weren't bad enough. Another possible cause of an embolic stroke is infective endocarditis with valvular vegetation (see Chapter 3). In someone with a very low ejection fraction or a very hypokinetic left ventricle, a ventricular thrombus can be present. Of course, this increases the risk of an embolic stroke.

✔ **Thrombotic strokes:** A thrombotic stroke most commonly occurs in the setting of significant atherosclerosis. The carotid arteries are most commonly affected. Other risk factors for a thrombotic stroke include vasculitis and/or the presence of a hypercoagulable state.

Examining stroke symptoms

Stroke symptoms depend on the area of the brain affected. In a hospital setting and on the PANCE, you'll likely deal with the acute ischemic embolic presentation — someone who presents with a weakness of the right arm and right leg, with or without *aphasia* (impairment of language ability).

Stroke symptoms aren't always a right arm/right leg thing. When the presentation is different, you must have some idea of the vascular territory involved:

✔ A stroke involving the right anterior cerebral artery produces weakness in the left leg compared to the left arm. There are sensory disturbances as well.

✔ A stroke involving the right middle cerebral artery produces weakness in the left arm compared to the left leg. Understand that a stroke affecting this area of the brain is a biggie because it affects the blood supply to more than 60 percent of the anterior circulation of the brain. Additional symptoms can include aphasia and increased reflexes.

Hypoglycemia is an example of a disease that mimics a stroke. In someone who has a history of a prior cerebrovascular accident, if the blood sugar is low, the patient can present like he or she is having an acute stroke. Normalize the blood glucose level, and the symptoms go away.

Treating acute stroke

For the PANCE, be very, very familiar with the time course in treating an acute ischemic stroke. We're specifically talking about the use of *thrombolytics,* also known as clot-busters. Here are some key points about treating an acute ischemic stroke:

✔ The time course for treating an acute ischemic stroke is within 4½ hours from the onset of symptoms (or from the last time the person was observed to be normal), especially when you're considering thrombolysis. If the time is more than 4½ hours, for testing purposes, no thrombolytics can be used.

✔ If the time course of the acute stroke is within the 4½-hour window, then you first need to make sure that hemorrhagic stroke isn't present (see the next section). A CT scan of the brain without contrast is a really good and quick way to check for hemorrhagic stroke.

✔ Before giving thrombolytics, you have to ask certain questions because of contraindications to using thrombolytics. Contraindications include any bleeding, the use of blood thinners like warfarin (Coumadin), significant thrombocytopenia, and any recent traumatic events or surgeries.

In anyone presenting with hypertensive urgency and an acute stroke, be careful not to lower the blood pressure too quickly. Maintain the cerebral perfusion pressure (CPP) by keeping a higher mean arterial pressure (MAP).

Treating the bleeding brain

The major types of bleeding in the brain you have to know about are the hemorrhagic stroke, the hematomas (epidural and subdural), and the subarachnoid hemorrhage:

- ✔ **Hemorrhagic stroke:** A hemorrhagic stroke is usually a consequence of uncontrolled high blood pressure. It starts in a small area and can extend over a larger area. The most common areas of the brain affected are the putamen and the pons. Street drugs that really raise the blood pressure, like cocaine, also increase the risk of an intracerebral hemorrhage.

- ✔ **Hematoma:** As the Greeks said, a *hematoma* is a "body of blood." An *epidural hematoma* is bleeding between the dura mater and the skull. A *subdural hematoma* is between the dura mater and the arachnoid mater.

- ✔ **Subarachnoid hemorrhage:** The real mother of them all is the *subarachnoid hemorrhage* (SAH), bleeding between the arachnoid mater and pia mater. The death rate is 40 to 50 percent. One major etiology of this bleed is an aneurysmal rupture. In all cases, trauma is the most likely cause of subarachnoid hemorrhage.

Here's a classic clinical scenario you're likely to see on the PANCE: A person comes into the ER or the doctor's office with the worst headache of his or her life. The onset of the headache is very, very quick. It's the notorious *thunderclap headache,* which can mean subarachnoid hemorrhage big time.

With a hemorrhagic stroke, a CT scan of the head is pretty reliable for diagnosing an intracerebral bleed. With the subarachnoid hemorrhage, although the CT of the head is pretty reliable, it's not always so. If you have a high clinical suspicion that a subarachnoid hemorrhage has occurred and the CT scan of the head is negative, the affected person needs a lumbar puncture (LP) — if xanthochromia is present, then it's a pretty good indicator that the person has a subarachnoid hemorrhage.

You're evaluating a man who presents with a change in mental status. On admission, he has a blood pressure of 260/150 mmHg. He is diffusely encephalopathic. From what you're able to discern, there are no focal deficits. A CT scan of the head doesn't demonstrate a bleed. After he spends two days in the ICU, his blood pressure is 170/110 mmHg, and his mental status has improved. What's the likely cause of his original change in mental status?

(A) Hypoglycemia

(B) Hypertensive encephalopathy

(C) Transient ischemic attack

(D) Hemorrhagic bleed

(E) Seizure

The correct answer is Choice (B). This man's mentation improved when the blood pressure dropped, so his change in mental status was caused by hypertensive encephalopathy. (See the earlier section "Tracing an altered status to meds or medical conditions" for info on changes in mental status.) No information indicates hypoglycemia, Choice (A). He had no areas of focal weakness, so Choice (C), transient ischemic attack, is out. The CT scan of the head didn't show any areas of focal bleeding, so Choice (D), hemorrhagic bleed, is out. There was no evidence of any seizure-like activity, so Choice (E) isn't right.

Reviewing Other Neurological Disorders

We're not done yet. You need to know about other neurologic disorders for the PANCE. Among them are myasthenia gravis, multiple sclerosis, Guillain-Barré syndrome, and Tourette's syndrome.

Losing power: Mulling over myasthenia

Picture a scenario in which a person says he or she becomes weaker as the day wears on. The person feels better when sitting down and resting, but the symptoms return after the next period of activity. The person may notice worsening vision problems, including double vision as well as drooping of the eyelids. When you see a scenario like this, you need to think about myasthenia gravis (MG).

Myasthenia gravis is an autoimmune condition in which the most profound clinical symptom is muscular weakness. If you remember the anatomy of a skeletal muscle, recall how important the neuromuscular junction is for transmission of nerve impulses across the synaptic membrane. Acetylcholine is an important neurotransmitter, especially in regard to motor function. What happens in myasthenia gravis? Antibodies are formed against the postsynaptic receptor that acetylcholine binds to. This is the main reason for the profound weakness.

Here are the key clinical points about myasthenia gravis:

✔ The main presenting symptoms grow worse as the day goes on. The eyes are the main organs affected, but many other skeletal muscles can be affected as well. The person may have problems with talking, chewing, and in the most severe form, breathing.

✔ You can order a blood test to look for antibodies to the acetylcholine receptor. It's diagnostic in many cases. However, after that, you still need further testing.

✔ The gold standard test for establishing a diagnosis of myasthenia gravis is the Tensilon test. Tensilon is a brand name for edrophonium chloride, which works to prevent the breakdown of acetylcholine at the neuromuscular junction. If the person has myasthenia gravis, edrophonium chloride causes him or her to get better for a little while because there's more acetylcholine around. The test also differentiates myasthenia gravis from cholinergic crisis.

Note that additional studies are used in the diagnosis of myasthenia gravis, including electromyography (EMG) testing.

✔ Because myasthenia gravis is an autoimmune condition, it's associated with other autoimmune conditions, including rheumatologic conditions and diabetes mellitus.

 Myasthenia gravis is associated big time with a *thymoma,* an uncommon but nasty tumor of the thymus. The thymoma is an anterior mediastinal mass, and you can usually find it on a CT scan of the thorax, although it can be suggested on a chest radiograph.

The treatment of myasthenia gravis is multidimensional. If a thymoma is present, its removal is certainly recommended. Cholinesterase inhibitors, such as pyridostigmine bromide (Mestinon), are used to help with symptoms. Other medications, such as prednisone or immunosuppressive agents, can also be used. Plasmapheresis is used primarily during a myasthenic crisis.

The PANCE may ask you to differentiate myasthenia gravis from Lambert-Eaton syndrome (also known as Lambert-Eaton *myasthenic* syndrome). Lambert-Eaton is a paraneoplastic syndrome usually associated with a lung malignancy. It's autoimmune in origin and somewhat rare. With Lambert-Eaton, the symptoms get better as the day goes on, which is the opposite of myasthenia gravis.

Treating Guillain-Barré syndrome

Guillain-Barré (acute inflammatory demyelinating polyneuropathy) is a syndrome you must spot quickly. Otherwise, the affected person can die of respiratory failure. (No pressure in this job, right?) The most common presentation of Guillain-Barré syndrome is an ascending neuropathy, starting at the lower extremities and spreading upward. The first symptoms of Guillain-Barré can be weakness or paresthesias in the lower extremities. The acute respiratory failure part comes in when the neuropathy affects the lungs. Respiratory failure is due to respiratory muscle paralysis. The person needs to be intubated to protect the airway.

People with Guillain-Barré usually require ICU-level care. The vital capacity is an objective measurement used clinically to see whether acute respiratory failure is imminent and therefore whether intubation is necessary.

Here are three key points about Guillain-Barré syndrome:

- ✔ The trigger is thought to have an infectious etiology, such as an upper respiratory infection or gastroenteritis.
- ✔ The time course of Guillain-Barré can vary from a few hours to several days.
- ✔ The treatment is supportive and may also include plasmapheresis or intravenous immunoglobulin (IVIG).

Looking for the right signals in multiple sclerosis

Multiple sclerosis (MS) is a demyelinating disorder characterized by a problem in nerve signaling. Multiple sclerosis involves significant damage to the myelin sheath. When this happens, nerves in the brain and the spinal cord don't communicate well. Like myasthenia gravis, multiple sclerosis is thought to be autoimmune in nature.

The clinical presentation of multiple sclerosis can be varied. You're dealing with many different neurologic areas. Symptoms can include weakness in the extremities, paresthesias, and/or problems with ambulation. Because multiple sclerosis affects the upper motor neurons, it can cause muscle spasticity. For the PANCE, consider one of the most common presenting symptoms to be optic neuritis, which can present with eye pain, diplopia, and/or vision loss.

Concerning the eye, multiple sclerosis affects the medial longitudinal fasciculus (MLF). This structure connects cranial nerves III, IV, and VI. With multiple sclerosis, you see a Marcus Gunn pupil (relative afferent pupillary defect), which roughly equates to less constriction during a swinging flashlight test.

Here are some key points about multiple sclerosis:

- ✔ Women are affected more than men, and the median age is in the 30s.
- ✔ Multiple sclerosis has four subtypes, the most common of which is the relapsing-remitting subtype.

✔ The diagnosis can be confirmed through an MRI of the brain with gadolinium, showing enhancement in the periventricular white matter.

✔ If a lumbar puncture is done in addition to an MRI, you can test the cerebrospinal fluid for the presence of IgG oligoclonal bands.

Treatment involves treating both the acute attack and the chronic condition. During an acute multiple sclerosis flare, steroids are commonly used to decrease the severity of the symptoms and to calm the inflammation. Chronically, interferon has been used, although it's not without side effects, including flu-like symptoms and depression. Monoclonal antibodies have also been used in treating common multiple sclerosis.

Understanding Tourette's syndrome

Tourette's syndrome is a genetic condition characterized by tic-like movements and/or utterances. The affected person doesn't have control over these movements. Many times, they occur in the facial area and manifest as uncontrolled blinking and constant word repetition. People associate Tourette's with yelling curse words, but that form of Tourette's doesn't occur a lot.

Here are three key points concerning Tourette's syndrome:

✔ The diagnosis is a clinical one, usually based on symptoms and strong family history.

✔ Tourette's often doesn't occur alone. It can be accompanied by disorders such as attention deficit disorder and obsessive compulsive disorder.

✔ The treatment often involves medication, including the antipsychotics and some antidepressants. The treatment Rich has seen a lot clinically is pimozide (Orap), a dopamine-receptor blocker.

Concussions: Bruising the brain

Watch any football game, and you may see one of the players, especially the quarterback, taken off the field with a concussion. The concussion is a form of brain trauma. With a concussion, the brain moves quickly in a way it's not supposed to.

In school, you hear about coup and contrecoup mediated brain injury, both of which likely play a role in the damage due to a concussion. The *coup* refers to the part of the brain that's directly affected by the brain trauma; the *contrecoup* refers to the opposite part of the brain that's affected after a trauma.

Initially, the person with the concussion may lose consciousness. Symptoms of a concussion can include headache, visual problems, photosensitivity, and/or balance problems. The affected person can also be lethargic and slow to respond to commands or questions. Brain scanning is often done to rule out a head bleed.

Repeated concussions can have long-term ramifications, including dementia and neurological damage. After an acute concussion, a person may still be affected weeks or even months later: In *post-concussive syndrome,* the person can be emotionally labile, have intermittent headaches, and/or have trouble in school because of difficulty concentrating for any length of time (this is not ADD). He or she may also complain of lightheadedness. The treatment is usually supportive, and in many cases, these symptoms resolve with time and rest.

Practice Neurology Questions

These practice questions are similar to the PANCE neurology questions.

1. You're evaluating a 50-year-old man who presents with a headache. He says that he notices that before his headaches, like now, he sees "funny squiggly things." He asks if you can turn off the light as you come into the room, because the bright light is "driving him nuts." Which one of the following would you give to help with his headache?

   (A) Oxygen

   (B) Cyclobenzaprine (Flexeril)

   (C) Lisinopril (Zestril)

   (D) Terazosin (Hytrin)

   (E) Ergotamine and caffeine (Cafergot)

2. In which one of the following disorders would you see choreiform movements?

   (A) Parkinson's disease

   (B) Rheumatic fever

   (C) Complex regional pain syndrome

   (D) Multiple sclerosis

   (E) Tourette's syndrome

3. Which one of the following signs is associated with meningitis?

   (A) Applebee's sign

   (B) Kernig's sign

   (C) Tinel's sign

   (D) Trousseau's sign

   (E) Homans' sign

4. You're evaluating a 45-year-old woman with a history of a solid organ transplant. She's on immunosuppression and presents with a fever and a change in mental status. She isn't arousable and has become very lethargic. There's a question as to whether she had a seizure at home. An MRI showed hemorrhagic changes and increased enhancement in the temporal lobe. Which one of the following does she need at this point?

   (A) Intravenous methylprednisolone (Medrol)

   (B) Plasmapheresis

   (C) Intravenous azithromycin (Zithromax)

   (D) Intravenous acyclovir (Zovirax)

   (E) Oral amoxicillin (Trimox)

5. Which one of the following would be used in treating a peripheral neuropathy secondary to heavy metal toxicity?

   (A) Chelation

   (B) Dialysis

   (C) Electromyography

   (D) A good colonic

   (E) B_{12} supplementation

6. Which of the following could be seen with the chronic use of phenytoin (Dilantin)?

   (A) Leukocytosis

   (B) Increased liver function levels

   (C) Hyponatremia

   (D) Hypovitaminosis D

   (E) Hypercalcemia

Answers and Explanations

Use this answer key to score the practice neurology questions from the preceding section. The answer explanations give you some insight into why the correct answer is better than the other choices.

1. **E.** This person has symptoms consistent with a migraine headache and the visual disturbances described are likely scotomas (and an aura). Choice (E), ergotamine and caffeine, is used in treating an acute migraine. Choice (A), oxygen, is one treatment for cluster headaches. Choice (B), cyclobenzaprine, is a muscle relaxer used for treating tension headaches. Choice (C), lisinopril, is used first-line to treat hypertension as well as proteinuria and albuminuria secondary to diabetes. Choice (D), terazosin, is used for hypertension as well as for benign prostatic hyperplasia.
2. **B.** With rheumatic fever, you may see subsequent Sydenham's chorea. With Parkinson's, Choice (A), you see bradykinesia, muscle rigidity, and a pill-rolling tremor. Choice (C), complex regional pain syndrome, is associated with pain, usually in an extremity with bone changes and usually after a significant trauma. Choice (D), multiple sclerosis, is an upper motor neuron lesion, so it's associated with spasticity. Choice (E), Tourette's, is associated with tic-like movements, especially facial and verbal tics.
3. **B.** Kernig's sign (knee/leg extension) is a test for meningitis. Choice (A) isn't really a clinical sign; it's a sign that Rich is hungry and really wants to go out to eat. Choice (C), Tinel's sign, is associated with carpal tunnel syndrome. Choice (D), Trousseau's sign, is associated with two things: hypocalcemia and a migratory thrombophlebitis, usually associated with pancreatic cancer. Choice (E), Homans' sign, is associated with a deep venous thrombosis.
4. **D.** This woman has encephalitis, namely herpes encephalitis, and you're going to give intravenous acyclovir. Look at the question setup: The patient is immunosuppressed, presents with a fever, and has had a change in mental status. You see the characteristic finding in hemorrhage of the temporal lobe. Choice (A), methylprednisolone, is given for a multiple sclerosis exacerbation. Choice (B), plasmapheresis, is given to treat myasthenia gravis and Guillain-Barré syndrome. Choice (C), azithromycin, is one of the treatments for community-acquired pneumonia, and Choice (E), amoxicillin, is used for treating otitis media or bacterial sinusitis.
5. **A.** Heavy metal toxicity can present with a peripheral neuropathy. The treatment is chelation therapy, because these metals are in the tissues and can't be removed by dialysis, Choice (B). Choice (C), electromyography (EMG), is used to evaluate and diagnose a peripheral neuropathy. Pretty much anyone can benefit from a good colonic, Choice (D), but the colonic won't treat the problem at hand. Vitamin B_{12} supplementation, Choice (E), helps only with B_{12} deficiency.
6. **D.** Phenytoin (Dilantin) is associated with low vitamin D levels because the drug increases the metabolism of the liver and can deplete the vitamin D levels quickly. This can lead to osteoporosis. Choice (A), leukocytosis, is associated with lithium. You can see Choice (B), increased liver function levels, with valproic acid (Depakote). You can see Choice (C), hyponatremia, with carbamazepine (Tegretol). Concerning Choice (E), phenytoin isn't associated with hypercalcemia.

Chapter 17

Touching on Dermatology

・・

In This Chapter

▶ Mastering malignancies of the skin

▶ Examining the eczematous eruptions

▶ Treating skin infections

▶ Looking at pigmentation, bumps, sores, scales, and rashes

▶ Inspecting bug and spider bites

▶ Understanding skin and hair loss

・・

Welcome to the wonderful world of dermatology. From rashes to eczema and from bacterial infections to viral exanthems, you read about the skin in this chapter. There are few thrills greater than diseases of the skin.

In this chapter, we describe the appearance of many skin conditions, but that's not the same as viewing a rash or lesion on the body. To get a better idea of what many of these conditions look like, check out the slideshow on the CD that accompanies this book. In the slideshow, you can view color photos of many of the skin diseases we mention here and read brief descriptions of them. *Note:* If you're using a digital version of this book, go to http://booksupport.wiley.com for access to the additional content.

Mastering Skin Malignancies

Skin cancer is a common finding, and it's usually identified by a person's primary care provider. The four cutaneous malignancies you should know about for the PANCE/PANRE are Kaposi's sarcoma, basal cell carcinoma, squamous cell cancer, and melanoma.

Keeping up with Kaposi's sarcoma

Kaposi's sarcoma is a purplish maculopapular rash on the extremities and mucous membranes of the body. It's associated with immunosuppression, especially HIV. This cancer can improve with the treatment of the immunosuppression. The treatment is otherwise multifactorial, involving chemotherapy, radiation, and surgery, if needed.

Intervening with basal cell carcinoma

Basal cell carcinoma is the most common skin malignancy in the United States. It isn't considered a cancer because it doesn't spread to other organs in the same way that most cancer does. Nevertheless, basal cell carcinoma usually requires surgical intervention because it can be an eyesore and can become disfiguring when it gets too large, especially when it affects the facial area.

The lesion is diagnosed by a biopsy. Basal cell carcinoma is more likely to occur in the fair-skinned person who spends a lot of time in the sun (the risk factors are similar for squamous cell carcinoma and malignant melanoma — see the next two sections). About 70 percent of basal cell carcinomas occur in sun-exposed areas of the skin. Treatments can include surgery, topical chemotherapy, and radiation.

Seeing squamous cell carcinoma

Whereas basal cell carcinoma is a benign condition, squamous cell carcinoma (SCC) is a bad malignancy. You usually see it in someone who has had long-term daily sun overexposure or exposure to ultraviolet light. Older adults, especially people who are fair-skinned, are more at risk for developing this condition. It commonly occurs on the face and ears, although you can find it on the extremities and other parts of the body.

As with any skin lesion, an increase in size is a sign of a malignancy. In addition, the surface is often flaky or scaly in nature, with a reddish center. The diagnosis is made by a skin biopsy. Treatment can include surgical excision of the lesion as well as radiation. If you find evidence of metastatic spread, then the affected person may need chemotherapy.

Here are two other points concerning squamous cell carcinoma:

✔ Bowen's disease is a premalignant skin condition, also referred to as *squamous cell carcinoma in situ.*

✔ A small percentage of actinic keratosis cases can develop into squamous cell carcinoma. You read about actinic keratosis later in "Horny growths: Examining keratosis lesions."

Battling malignant melanoma

Melanoma is a very aggressive form of skin cancer. The other skin cancers, including basal cell and squamous cell cancer, are referred to as *nonmelanoma skin cancers.* The risk factors for developing melanoma include being fair-skinned, having had excessive exposure to ultraviolet radiation, and being older in age. The person may have a family history of melanoma as well.

One of the main tools you can use in evaluating melanoma is the alphabetic classification system — A, B, C, D, and E:

✔ **Asymmetry:** If one side of the lesion is different from the other, the odds are higher that you're dealing with melanoma.

✔ **Borders:** Are the borders of the lesion regular or irregular? Are they smooth or spiculated? The more irregular they are, the greater the likelihood that you're dealing with a malignancy.

✔ **Colors:** The melanoma may have more than one color.

✔ **Diameter:** The larger the lesion, the greater the risk that it's melanoma. A skin lesion of > 9–10 mm is usually felt to be more suspicious for melanoma.

✔ **Evolution:** Changes over time in terms of appearance and size can signal a melanoma.

Note that this classification scheme doesn't apply to nodular melanoma, which is the most dangerous form of melanoma. There are several types of melanoma. The most common type of melanoma is superficial spreading melanoma. Lentigo maligna melanoma, which tends to develop very slowly, can be found in the facial area.

If melanoma is likely, an excisional skin biopsy is done; a shave biopsy isn't sufficient for diagnosis. The Breslow scale is one way to tell the depth of invasion.

The treatment depends on the staging. Note that melanoma, like squamous cell carcinoma, has the ability to metastasize. Treatment can involve surgery and/or chemotherapy. Medications that boost the immune system, such as interferon, have been used in treating widely metastatic melanoma.

Inflammation: Examining Eczematous Eruptions

Eczema and dermatitis refer to anything that causes skin inflammation, and the causes are many. *Dermatitis* is a nonspecific term that refers to skin inflammation. *Eczema,* a type of dermatitis, has some characteristic skin findings — the skin can be flaky, itchy, scaly, and red. Sometimes scratching can make it redder. Unfortunately, there's no magic cure.

The gold standard of treatment is searching for the underlying cause and using topical steroids or antipruritic agents (desoximetasone, sold as Topicort Emollient Cream) as needed. Questions you're likely to ask someone who has eczema are along the lines of "Any new allergies?" (for allergy-mediated or atopic eczema) and "Any new shampoos or new detergents you haven't used before?" (for a contact type of dermatitis).

For the purposes of the PANCE, be familiar with two types of eczema:

- **Dyshidrosis:** In this type of dermatitis, skin lesions occur on the palmar surface of the hands and the plantar aspect of the feet. You see these scaly lesions along the digits as well.

- **Lichen simplex chronicus:** If you scratch an eczematous lesion long enough and often enough, you can cause changes consistent with lichen simplex chronicus (LSC, also known as *neurodermatitis*). The underlying pathology is somewhat of a mystery. Is there an inflammatory component? An allergic component? How about both?

   You see lichen simplex chronicus a little more commonly in people with contact dermatitis. A hallmark of lichen simplex chronicus is the "itchy fits," episodes of intense itching. The treatment of this is topical steroids. If the person scratches so much that the skin becomes infected, then you may need to prescribe a topical antibiotic.

You're examining a 35-year-old woman who presents with a scaly, eczematous rash on her elbows and thighs. She was just told she has an intolerance to gluten. Which one of the following conditions are you likely dealing with?

(A) Dyshidrosis

(B) Lyme disease

(C) Acne vulgaris

(D) Dermatitis herpetiformis

(E) Cellulitis

The correct answer is Choice (D), dermatitis herpetiformis. Given the popularity and prevalence of celiac disease (gluten sensitivity-mediated disease), you should be familiar with the close association between celiac disease and dermatitis herpetiformis, a type of eczema. Choice (A), dyshidrosis, is a type of eczema with a different distribution; if dyshidrosis were the answer, the question would mention "pruritic, deep-seated, tapioca-like vesicles." Choice (B), Lyme disease, is characterized by the bull's-eye rash (erythema migrans). Choice (C), acne vulgaris, is the typical acne you fretted over as a teenager. It has a predilection for the facial area and is associated with *Propionibacterium acnes.* Choice (E), cellulitis, is a maculopapular erythematous lesion on the lower extremities. It's caused by a bacterial infection, usually a *Staph* or *Strep* species.

Surveying Skin Infections

For the PANCE, you need to be familiar with various types of skin infections. From bacterial infections to viral infections to cutaneous fungal infections, you read about them in this section. You'll see many of these conditions clinically.

Treating bacterial infections

Most skin infections are caused by *Strep* or *Staph* bacteria and can be treated with antibiotics. We cover several of those conditions here.

Different types of infections can affect different layers of the skin. The first layers are the epidermis and the dermis. Following them is the subcutaneous layer and then the hypodermis, which technically isn't part of the skin. Below are the fascia and muscle layers.

Calling on cellulitis

Cellulitis is a very common bacterial skin infection that you've probably encountered in your clinical rotations. It can involve the skin and the subcutaneous tissues. For cellulitis to occur, the person has to have some break in the integrity of the skin (for example, a scratch or dry skin that's cracking), allowing normal skin flora to penetrate. A classic clinical presentation is a lower-extremity cellulitis in someone who's obese, with corresponding venous insufficiency. Diabetes may be present.

Risk factors for cellulitis include a lowered immune system (for example, diabetes, atherosclerosis, and vascular disease). Presenting symptoms can include a fever, and a leukocytosis may or may not be present. The area affected may also have some degree of adenopathy (for example, inguinal adenopathy for a cellulitis affecting the leg). The most common offending organisms are *Staph* and *Strep* species.

Antibiotics can be oral or intravenous, depending on how much the cellulitis has spread. Penicillins and cephalosporins are commonly used. Examples include the first-generation cephalosporins cephalexin (Keflex) and cefazolin (Ancef).

When someone comes to the hospital with a cellulitis, a black magic marker should be used to mark the edge of the cellulitis on admission. With the administration of intravenous antibiotics, the cellulitis should get better and not spread beyond the marker line.

Containing superficial infections

Erysipelas is a skin infection that doesn't go as deep as cellulitis can. It's actually superficial edematous cellulitis, characterized by raised borders, that is tender to palpation. It's usually caused by group A beta-hemolytic *Streptococci.* The spectrum of antibiotics used to treat erysipelas is the same as with cellulitis, namely penicillins and cephalosporins. Macrolide antibiotics can also be used.

Impetigo is another superficial skin infection also caused by *Strep* or *Staph* species. Rather than being maculopapular, it's a more vesicular/crusting type of "honeycomb" or "honeycrusted" lesion. It can look like dried pie crust. A classic area where impetigo can appear is underneath the nose.

Impetigo caused by *Strep* has been implicated as a cause of post-streptococcal glomerulonephritis, in addition to streptococcal pharyngitis (strep throat).

Candida and Dermatophyte: Fending off fungi

Candida is a fungus you can read about in the infectious diseases chapter (Chapter 19) and in the gastrointestinal chapter (Chapter 5), among others. *Candida* can also affect the skin; the medical name for this condition is *cutaneous candidiasis.* The most common clinical presentation is a skin rash that occurs in the intertriginous areas (under the skin folds) of someone who is massively obese or of a woman with pendulous breasts.

Take a dark, moist place, and you have the right setup for *Candida* infection. For example, diaper rash is in some cases actually a *Candida* infection. In addition to maintaining good hygienic practices, you can treat cutaneous candidiasis with topical antifungals such as ketoconazole (Nizoral). They can be creams or powders. Clinically, for skin folds, powder is probably better. It's also good for diaper rash.

Dermatophyte infections refer to superficial fungal infections that can affect the skin, hair, and nails. The fungus is often named for the site of the infection. Here's a quick rundown of some of these dermatophyte infections:

- **Tinea pedis (athlete's foot):** The most common place to get athlete's foot is between the toes, especially the third, fourth, and fifth toes. In addition to good foot hygiene, the treatment is a topical antifungal ointment. Because athlete's foot causes such a break in skin integrity, there's a risk of a bacterial superinfection.

  Fungus doesn't travel alone. If you're looking at a foot and see tinea pedis, check the nail beds as well to make sure that you aren't dealing with an *onychomycosis,* a fungal infection of the nails on the skin and hand. Onychomycosis is treated with one of two specific agents: terbinafine hydrochloride (Lamisil) or itraconazole (Sporanox). An onychomycosis can take months to heal; it's often treated for 4 to 6 months. Be aware of the side effects of these medications, including increased liver function tests.

- **Tinea corporis (ringworm):** This is a common form of fungal infection that occurs on the upper and lower extremities. The skin lesion is usually circular. You see a thick and scaly circular border with central clearing. If you see this description on the PANCE, think about tinea corporis.

- **Tinea capitis:** This condition, which is one of the most common superficial skin infections in children, affects the scalp.

You're examining an 18-year-old male athlete who presents with itching around the groin area that's been occurring for a couple of days. He denies being sexually active and denies any penile discharge. On examination, you see what looks like red patches around the groin area that are an angry red. Which condition does he most likely have?

(A) Contact dermatitis

(B) Tinea cruris

(C) Gonococcal infection

(D) Tinea corporis

(E) Eczema

The correct answer is Choice (B). This athlete, who likely wears an athletic supporter, has *tinea cruris,* also known as "jock itch" or "crotch rot." With Choice (A), contact dermatitis, you'd expect a larger skin area, such as the arm or torso, to be affected. This man isn't sexually active, making Choice (C), gonococcal infection, less likely. Choice (D), tinea corporis, is a type of dermatophyte infection that occurs on the arms and legs. Choice (E), eczema, is similar to contact dermatitis in presentation.

Putting a pox on viruses

You read a lot about viral diseases and their associated skin manifestations in other chapters, particularly the infectious disease chapter (Chapter 19). Here are a couple of other items not covered in those chapters:

- **Molluscum contagiosum:** This skin condition is caused by the pox virus. The skin lesions first begin looking like a run-of-the-mill papular rash; they then transform into what looks like clear pearls that are umbilicated in the center. They usually occur in the genital area in adults; in children they most commonly occur on exposed skin sites. This condition is transmitted by skin contact (that is, touching an item that someone who has the condition has already touched).

  Unlike herpes simplex virus, molluscum contagiosum shouldn't cause pain. These skin lesions often need to be surgically removed because there isn't a topical or medicinal treatment for them.

- **Verrucae (plantar warts):** These firm, calloused lesions on the plantar surface of the foot are caused by the human papillomavirus. They can cause pain when walking. The subtypes that cause plantar warts differ from the subtypes that cause condyloma acuminata (genital warts). Plantar warts can be transmitted from one person to another. They often resolve without treatment, although treatment can involve the use of topical salicylate derivatives or surgical removal.

Looking at Pigmentation, Bumps, and Sores

This section covers other skin conditions that are excellent fodder for test questions on the PANCE. Some of these conditions involve intensive examination of people's armpits and groin areas. (This is one reason Rich became a kidney specialist and not a dermatologist.) Other conditions involve discoloration of the skin. And then you've got bumps on and under the skin.

Spotting pigmentation problems

You can read about adrenal insufficiency, a medical condition that can cause hyperpigmentation, in Chapter 15. In this section, you read about other skin pigmentation problems you can expect to see on PANCE.

Analyzing acanthosis nigricans

Acanthosis nigricans is a velvety black hyperpigmentation of the skin that can occur under the axillary area, under inguinal areas, and in crevices and folds in other parts of the body. Causes are many. Three big causes of acanthosis nigricans are paraneoplastic phenomenon, Cushing's syndrome, and diabetes. When you see acanthosis nigricans, the key is to look for and treat the underlying cause.

Spotting melasma

Melasma is a skin condition you often see in young women, particularly those who are pregnant or are taking estrogen/progesterone supplementation. Melasma has been called the "mask of pregnancy." The cause of this skin condition isn't known, but melasma is characterized by a macular discoloration of the facial area. This is usually a clinical diagnosis. The treatment is supportive.

Visiting vitiligo

If melasma is a problem of pigmentation of the skin, especially the face, then *vitiligo* is just the opposite. Here, you're dealing with an autoimmune condition that causes portions of the skin, especially the extremities, not to be pigmented. Vitiligo can be associated with other autoimmune conditions. The treatment is steroids or photodynamic therapy.

Facing acne

With just the switch of a letter, you go from talking about a dermatological condition to a supermarket chain that Rich's mom used to shop at when he was a kid. Acne (not Acme) comes in two basic flavors for the test: acne rosacea and acne vulgaris.

Nothing rosy about acne rosacea

Acne rosacea is a maculopapular rash on the face and cheeks that can turn the affected area bright red. It's more common in young to middle-aged females. Common presenting symptoms include a reddened face, especially the cheeks and nasolabial fold. The nose can be red, and the affected skin can burn and itch. In severe cases, you may see *rhinophyma,* which is skin thickening associated with irregular contours occurring on the nose. In addition to papular lesions, you can see small, dilated blood vessels called *telangiectasias.*

The cause of rosacea is unknown, although it can be triggered by the extremes of weather and also by certain foods and chemicals, such as caffeine. The initial treatment is usually the combination of a topical metronidazole such as metronidazole gel (MetroGel) in addition to an oral doxycycline (Vibramycin).

The lesion of rosacea is sometimes confused with the butterfly macular rash of systemic lupus erythematosis. The big difference is that lupus spares the nasolabial fold. For info on lupus, see Chapter 6.

No picking on acne vulgaris

Acne vulgaris (common acne) can make the affected person use vulgar language. Acne vulgaris is the acne that everyone's familiar with. It's characterized by many types of skin lesions on the face. From pimples to papules to lumps to bumps, it's all there.

Acne vulgaris is actually a disease of the pilosebaceous follicles. Factors involved in this condition include thickening of the follicles, increased production of an oily substance (*sebum*) by the sebaceous glands, and increased inflammation. A very high-sugar diet and some dairy products can cause an acne flare.

The treatment is good hygiene. Avoid pimple picking, which can only lead to scarring. Medications for treating acne are topical and oral. For really bad flares, antibiotics include doxycycline (Vibramycin) or the macrolides. Retinoic acid derivatives (Tretinoin) can be prescribed in topical form. In addition, benzoyl peroxide (Basiron) is commonly prescribed for mild to moderate acne. Not only is this medication in PANCE questions, but it's also in the infomercials Rich has seen at 3:00 a.m.

Isotretinoin (Amnesteem), a prescription medication used to treat acne, has some side effects that you need to be aware of. They include photosensitivity and alopecia as well as inflammatory bowel disease and elevated liver function tests. Isotretinoin is highly teratogenic (category X). Although isotretinoin is a commonly prescribed drug, its significant side effect profile requires prescribers to undergo special training before treating a patient.

Horny growths: Examining keratosis lesions

You need to be aware of two types of keratosis lesions (horny growths):

✔ **Actinic keratosis:** This skin lesion is caused by excessive exposure to the sun or UV light. It can take many years to develop. Unlike squamous cell carcinoma, actinic keratosis isn't a malignancy, although a small percentage of the lesions can develop into squamous cell carcinoma over time.

Some of the most common areas to find actinic keratosis are the face and hands. The risk factors are the same as the ones for squamous cell carcinoma: long-term daily sun overexposure or exposure to ultraviolet light. Older adults, especially people who are fairskinned, are more at risk for developing this condition. The nature of the lesion is similar to squamous cell carcinoma in that it's scaly. You can make the diagnosis of actinic keratosis by skin biopsy, and the treatment can include topical creams like imiquimod (Aldara).

✔ **Seborrheic keratosis:** This condition is neither cancerous nor precancerous. It's a benign lesion that occurs on many areas of the body, including the face and back. The lesions are multicolored, raised, and papular, classically described as "stuck on" in appearance.

Seborrheic keratosis is associated with Leser-Trélat syndrome, a paraneoplastic sign that colon cancer may be present. The skin condition is also associated with Parkinson's disease. Seborrheic keratosis is usually treated with topical therapy to try to reduce the size of the lesions.

Papules and scales: Putting up with papulosquamous diseases

A group of *papulosquamous* skin conditions have characteristic findings and are associated with other medical conditions. You predominantly see papular (smooth, elevated skin) lesions that are also scaly in appearance. With this type of lesion, you can see *plaques,* which are a bunch of these papular/scaly lesions coming together.

Loathing lichen planus

Lichen planus is a skin condition that can also affect mucous membranes, specifically the oral area, including the tongue. These lesions are well-described by the 5 *p's:* well-defined pruritic, planar, purple, polygonal papules. On occasion, the oral lesions may ulcerate and become painful. The cause of the lesions isn't known, although lichen planus is associated with hepatitis C. The treatment often involves immunosuppressive medications, including prednisone, both topical and systemic.

Dr. Snyder's dermatology rules

Rich is an internist and kidney specialist, and he's seen his share of rashes. He's gleaned four rules of dermatology from his years of training. These are his general rules for dealing with a rash of any kind:

✔ If the skin is dry, moisten it.

✔ If the skin is moist, dry it out.

✔ If the skin lesion is unknown, get it biopsied. It will be called "inflammatory" or "atypical."

✔ You can use topical oral steroids and a topical fungal cream together. They work most of the time and make you look smart. If the condition is an inflammatory process, the steroids help. If it's a fungus, the antifungal helps.

Identifying the patchwork of pityriasis rosea

Pityriasis rosea can produce a "Christmas tree" appearance on someone's back. On exam, this seasonal rash manifests as papular lesions that are scaly in appearance. In addition to the Christmas tree pattern, be familiar with the herald patch that can be the precursor of other rashes on the skin. The treatment is usually conservative, involving topical anti-inflammatories and antipruritic medications as needed.

Scaling back on psoriasis

Oh, the heartbreak of psoriasis! Actually, it's a skin break. *Psoriasis* is an inflammatory lesion of the skin, characterized by silver-white scaly lesions that can occur all over the body, particularly on extensor surfaces. The cause is unknown. Here are some key points concerning psoriasis:

- ✔ Auspitz's sign is bleeding that occurs after scraping a psoriatic scale. It can also occur with just a minor scrape of skin affected by psoriasis.

- ✔ When psoriasis affects the nail beds, you can see an "oil spot lesion." This is due to the accumulation of cellular debris and schmutz under the nail. The treatment can involve topical steroid injections and/or other oral immunosuppressive agents, including cyclosporine (Neoral).

- ✔ Psoriasis can be associated with psoriatic arthritis. For this form of arthritis, the PANCE may ask about the appearance of "sausage digits" (dactylitis) on the fingers.

- ✔ Psoriasis can be associated with a bacterial infection. *Guttate psoriasis* is a form of psoriasis that can occur about 3 to 4 weeks after a group A beta hemolytic strep infection. You see guttate psoriasis more commonly in children than in adults. The cause is unknown, but treatment can involve the use of steroids, either topical or oral.

- ✔ Phototherapy has been used in the treatment of psoriasis. Immunosupressive therapies, including biologic-based agents, have also been used. The use of tar is a time-honored modality for treating psoriasis, although newer (and less messy) treatment options have reduced its popularity. The precise mechanism of action of tar is unknown; it has an apparent antiproliferative effect.

Blistering bullous pemphigoid

Bullous pemphigoid (BP) is a dermatologic disorder in which large blisters are on the body, usually on the extremities and on the truncal areas. They can itch, especially early on, and they almost resemble an urticarial-type process. Later, they form bullae/blistering lesions. Experts think the condition is autoimmune in nature. The treatment depends on the severity of the bullous pemphigoid. In minor cases, you can use doxycycline (Vibramycin). In more severe cases, immunosuppressive medication may be necessary. Usually a biopsy is required to confirm the diagnosis.

Sweating over hidradenitis

Hidradenitis suppurativa, which can affect the axillary and groin areas, is a clogging of the sweat glands, causing infection. Ask someone with hidradenitis to show you his or her armpits, and you'll likely see small, pus-filled, cyst-like structures that over time can become scarred. The treatment is varied. It includes identifying and alleviating risk factors (losing weight), using antibiotics, and maybe using immunosuppressive agents.

Leaving lipomas alone

A *lipoma* is a benign fatty growth that's freely movable and painless. You can find it anywhere, but it's often in the extremities. The basic advice is to leave lipomas alone because they're benign. When lipomas affect movement or the nerve of a particular area, they're usually removed surgically.

Eliminating hives

Urticaria (hives) is a skin condition usually triggered by some sort of allergic condition. You can see a coalescing area of small, erythematous lumps that can itch a lot. They're raised and can resemble a wheal. Think of a wheal like the wheal you had under your skin after you received a purified protein derivative (PPD) test, which you had to do as a medical professional. Unlike the wheals made by the PPD, the wheals of urticaria are smaller, and there can be a lot of them.

Urticaria has many causes: allergy-mediated, stress, and medication-induced. The treatment is identifying and eliminating the offending cause. Contributors can include the use of antihistamines (Benadryl comes to mind). Steroids, either topical or oral, can also be used.

Dermatographia is a type of physical hives or physical urticaria. Here, the skin becomes acutely red and inflamed when the skin is either rubbed or touched. The cause is not known. Stress may play a role. In *pressure hives,* the pressure of touching the skin itself can invoke an urticarial reaction. In most cases, physical urticaria resolves on its own over time. Antihistamines are also needed.

Pilonidal cyst: Looking at the buttocks

A *pilonidal cyst* is an abscess or hair-filled collection of fluid located at the sacral/coccyx area, although these abscesses can occur anywhere in the body. The most common initial presenting symptom is pain. They can hurt like the dickens. The usual treatment is incision and drainage (I&D).

Bedsores: Scanning the sacrum to detect decubitus ulcers

In a hospital rotation, you've likely been exposed to the sacrum, a major body area where *decubitus ulcers* (also known as *bedsores* or *pressure sores*) occur. The pressure sore/ulcer is an injury to the skin on a dependent area. The sacrum is especially affected because it's a large bony prominence and most people lie in bed on their backs.

The most common clinical presentation is an older patient who is nonambulatory, usually bedridden. This person often has some degree of underlying dementia. He or she may not be able to move or may even be unable to ask to be moved; this may be secondary to advanced dementia or a history of a cerebrovascular accident (stroke), where the person can't verbalize or vocalize his or her wishes. Risk factors include a history of paralysis or significant ambulatory dysfunction.

When someone comes into a hospital (especially a person with bacteremia or a change in mental status), look at the backside — especially the sacrum — to examine for pressure ulcers. You may need to take a picture of the area and put it in the hospital record to demonstrate that the pressure ulcer didn't occur in the hospital. In addition to measuring the diameter of the skin lesion, pay attention to the depth of the pressure ulcer. For PANCE purposes, be aware of the stages of pressure ulcers:

- ✔ **Stage I:** You see a little erythema over the affected area and no evidence of skin breakdown.
- ✔ **Stage II:** You can see the other layers of the skin affected. There's a break in the integrity of the skin, but it isn't deep.
- ✔ **Stage III:** The injury to the skin has gone beyond the skin layers and now affects the subcutaneous fascia.
- ✔ **Stage IV:** You can see the bone in the setting of a *sacral decubitus*. You also need to worry about a possible osteomyelitis.

Prevention of pressure ulcers includes promoting ambulation and turning people (or changing their positions) every 2 hours or so in bed, especially when they're sleeping. The active management of a pressure sore includes constant monitoring for signs of infection, including wound weeping, angry-looking erythema, and skin necrosis. In addition, surgical debridement or intravenous systemic antibiotics may be necessary.

Inspecting the Body for Insects and Arachnids

It's not nice to be bitten by insects or spiders — especially spiders. Rich saw the movie *Arachnophobia* and didn't sleep for a month. In this section, you read about lice, scabies, and spider bites.

Lice aren't so nice

Lice (singular *louse*) are insects, and they can be anywhere on the body, especially the head. When Rich was in grade school, he remembers the school nurse checking the kids for head lice. This affliction is spread from person to person. It's not a vector-associated disease like Lyme disease or Rocky Mountain spotted fever. Just the same, it's extremely contagious. Risk factors include spending time in places where people are in close quarters and have poor hygiene. Outbreaks have occasionally occurred in schools and nursing homes, although nursing home outbreaks of lice are very uncommon.

Head lice attach to the hair follicles, often at the nape and behind the ears. They do bite and can leave small, red welts on the scalp. They lay their eggs, or *nits,* in the hair about ¼ inch from the scalp. They are very hard to get rid of.

The treatment is meticulous hygiene and a medication called permethrin (Elimite). Clothes and bedding have to laundered, too, often repeatedly in very hot water, to kill the eggs. For head lice, you want to comb the hair with a very fine comb every few days when it's wet. Doing so helps break up the eggs. Medicated shampoos are often used as well.

Anyone who may have come in contact with someone with head lice needs to change his or her clothes and launder them with hot water at the very least, because lice can be on the clothes.

Treating the mite-y scabies

Scabies (the seven-year itch) is a skin condition that, like lice, is transmitted from person to person. Scabies is transmitted by the mite *Sarcoptes scabiei* (the "itch mite"). Outbreaks have occurred in nursing homes and schools, where individuals are in a lot of close contact.

On examination, look for evidence of the mite that has burrowed under the skin. You may see small pustular and papular lesions or what looks like tracks made in the skin. You can find them on the extremities, especially in the interdigital areas of the fingers and toes. Treatments include lindane, permethrin, and the antiparasite medication ivermectin (Stromectol). People in contact with the affected person should also receive treatment.

Sorting out spider bites

Spider bites can look like insect bites and stings. The more dangerous spider bites are often necrotic, which can cause confusion. For the most part, spider bites in the United States are deadly only if they're from a black widow or brown recluse spider. You need to have a high index of suspicion that your patient was in fact bitten by one of these deadly spiders:

- ✔ Brown recluse spider bites may occur when cleaning out storage areas, leaf debris, or wood piles, or the patient may not recall when he or she was bitten. Within 24 hours after the bite, the area surrounding the bite site typically turns a reddish-blue color and may develop a blister. Necrosis follows.

- ✔ Black widow spider bites cause pain at the envenomation site, nausea, vomiting, and abdominal rigidity, along with other neurological effects.

Treatment of a bite from the black widow or brown recluse includes cleaning the area with soap and water. If the bite is on an extremity, the person should elevate the arm or leg and tie a tourniquet above the bitten area to prevent the venom from spreading. Getting the person to an emergency room pronto is mandatory. Talking with a toxicology expert is important. The affected person needs antivenin.

Remaining Sensitive to the Loss of Skin or Hair

In this section, you read about some very serious and potentially life-threatening stuff: skin conditions where you can lose the outer layer, the epidermis of the skin. This section includes desquamating diseases, burns, and a very nonfatal skin condition, alopecia.

Losing the top layer of skin: Desquamating diseases

Desquamation is the loss or shedding of the outermost layers of the skin. Causes of desquamation include Stevens-Johnson syndrome, toxic epidermal necrolysis (TEN, or Lyell's syndrome), erythema multiforme, and burns.

You never forget Stevens-Johnson syndrome and toxic epidermal necrolysis once you see them. With both conditions, the epidermis, the outermost layer of the skin, is completely destroyed. Toxic epidermal necrolysis is a more severe disease than Stevens-Johnson syndrome, although they're both life-threatening. The causes of both conditions are many, including hypersensitivity reactions to medications, rheumatologic conditions, and HIV. Medication use is often cited as a major cause of toxic epidermal necrolysis.

The treatment is, in many ways, similar to burn treatment. It includes aggressive fluid resuscitation, nutrition, and electrolyte replacement. Antibiotic and intravenous steroids may be used. One big medication used in the treatment of toxic epidermal necrolysis is gamma globulin. The goal is to modulate the immune response.

Erythema multiforme is a desquamating disorder with multiple causes, including medications, viruses, and rheumatologic causes. This condition is thought to recur because it may be related to an allergen-mediated immune phenomenon. The minor form of erythema multiforme just consists of macular papular lesions. The major form is desquamation, along with papules. You see involvement of the mucous membranes. There's a strong association between erythema multiforme and the herpes simplex virus.

Assessing and staging burns

Burns are a very serious skin condition. For the PANCE, you should be aware of the staging of burns — first, second, and third degree. The key to understanding staging is to review the skin layers:

- ✔ **First degree:** These burns are very, very superficial. Stick your hand on a hot stove for a split second, and you usually get a local, superficial redness. You may also get a first-degree burn from lying in the sun too long.

- ✔ **Second degree:** These burns go a little deeper than first degree burns. Note that a burn that first appears to be a first degree burn can become a second degree burn over time. A person who touched a hot stove may have initially had erythema on the affected area; now you can begin to see blisters, which are a hallmark of a second degree burn.

- ✔ **Third degree:** These burns mean the loss of the first two layers of the skin. In addition to skin, vascular structures and nerves can be injured as well.

In addition to knowing the degrees of burns, you need to know how much of the body is burned. Medical professionals often use the *rule of nines* in second and third degree burns to assess how much of the body is damaged.

Treating burns comprises aggressive hydration, electrolyte replacement, and nutrition. Antibiotics are also needed. When the skin layers are lost, the affected person can lose tons of fluid and electrolytes and be prone to infection. People with major burns (second or third degree) are often treated at a burn center.

Alopecia: Where did the hair go?

When you see someone without any hair or eyebrows, think about alopecia. *Alopecia* means loss of hair, but like ice cream, it comes in several flavors. Here are the three types, based on location of the hair loss:

- ✔ **Alopecia areata:** Hair is on the head but with patches of baldness.
- ✔ **Alopecia totalis:** No hair is on the head.
- ✔ **Alopecia universalis:** The person has no hair anywhere.

Normal male pattern baldness is referred to as *androgenic alopecia*.

Experts think alopecia is a type of autoimmune process. Right now, there's no accepted cure for this condition. Minoxidil (Rogaine) may slow the loss of hair.

Practice Dermatology Questions

These practice questions are similar to the PANCE dermatology questions.

1. Which one of the following can develop into squamous cell carcinoma over time?

   (A) Onychomycosis

   (B) Actinic keratosis

   (C) Seborrheic keratosis

   (D) Psoriasis

   (E) Impetigo

2. You're evaluating a 25-year-old woman who presents with a rash on her face. She states she may be having a reaction to some food that she ate, but she isn't sure. The rash is reddened and macular on both cheeks, and there is no sparing of the nasolabial fold. Which one of the following would you order at this point?

   (A) ANA and complement levels

   (B) Oral prednisone

   (C) Oral doxycycline (Vibramycin)

   (D) Oral amoxicillin (Trimox)

   (E) Rheumatoid factor

3. You're evaluating a 44-year-old man who presents with a new rash. He takes off his shirt and raises his arms to show you. In the left axillary area, you see a new hyper-pigmented, macular rash. Which one of the following medical conditions could be associated with this skin lesion?

   (A) Diabetes mellitus

   (B) Hypertension

   (C) Benign prostatic hyperplasia

   (D) Kidney stones

   (E) Hepatitis B

4. Which one of the following represents a manifestation of measles?

   (A) Coronary artery disease

   (B) Koplik spots

   (C) Pneumonitis

   (D) Slapped-cheek appearance

   (E) Impetigo

5. Which one of the following is true concerning the evaluation and management of lipomas?

   (A) They are usually painful and tender on examination.

   (B) They are usually associated with a malignant condition.

   (C) They can usually be watched without surgical intervention.

   (D) They usually require surgical removal to prevent further complications.

   (E) They are associated with diabetes mellitus.

6. Which of the following is the likely etiology of a paronychia?

   (A) A fungal infection

   (B) A viral infection

   (C) An autoimmune reaction

   (D) A prescribed medication

   (E) A bacterial infection

Answers and Explanations

Use this answer key to score the practice dermatology questions from the preceding section. The answer explanations give you some insight into why the correct answer is better than the other choices.

1. **B.** Actinic keratosis is a skin lesion that can develop into squamous cell carcinoma of the skin. This happens less than 10 percent of the time. Choice (A), onychomycosis, is a fungal infection of the nails. Choice (C), seborrheic keratosis, is a keratinized type of skin lesion that's benign, but it's associated with colon cancer (Leser-Trélat sign). Psoriasis, Choice (D), can be associated with the HLA-B27 antigen, which increases the risk of developing psoriatic arthritis. Choice (E), impetigo, is caused by a bacterium, namely *Staph* or *Strep*. When caused by *Strep*, it increases the risk of developing post-streptococcal glomerulonephritis.

2. **C.** This woman has acne rosacea. One big clue in the question is the statement "no sparing of the nasolabial fold." If you see sparing of the nasolabial fold, then you're dealing with the malar (butterfly) rash of lupus. The treatment of acne rosacea is oral doxycycline (Vibramycin) or a topical metronidazole (Flagyl). Choice (A), ANA and complement levels, would be a serological workup for systemic lupus erythematosis. Oral prednisone, Choice (B), is for Bell's palsy or for temporal arteritis. Choice (D), oral amoxicillin (Trimox), is a first-line choice for acute bacterial sinusitis, impetigo, and otitis media. Choice (E), rheumatoid factor, is part of the evaluation for rheumatoid arthritis and other rheumatologic conditions.

3. **A.** This lesion is acanthosis nigricans. It's associated with diabetes mellitus and can be a paraneoplastic phenomenon associated with certain cancers. You don't see it with the other conditions listed (hypertension, benign prostatic hyperplasia, kidney stones, and hepatitis B).

4. **B.** Measles can cause Koplik spots. Concerning Choice (A), coronary artery involvement can be a complication of Kawasaki disease. Measles is not associated with a pneumonitis, Choice (C). A slapped-cheek appearance, Choice (D), is associated with erythema infectiosum, or fifth disease. Streptococcal and staphylococcal infections are common causes of impetigo, Choice (E).

5. **C.** A lipoma is a benign fatty tumor; it's painless and freely movable and usually can be watched without surgical intervention. There's no direct association between lipomas and diabetes mellitus.

6. **E.** A paronychia, an infection around the nail, is usually caused by bacteria. It usually requires incision and drainage (I&D) of the affected area as well as oral antibiotics. Onychomycosis is a fungal infection of the nail, Choice (A). Herpetic whitlow is a viral cause of nail infection, Choice (B), usually seen in healthcare workers. Choices (C) and (D), an autoimmune reaction and prescription drugs, aren't thought to be causes of paronychia.

Chapter 18

Handling Hematology and Oncology

. . . .

In This Chapter

▶ Examining anemias

▶ Understanding myeloproliferatives

▶ Understanding thrombocytopenia

▶ Sorting out coagulation disorders and clotting problems

▶ Examining leukemia, lymphoma, and other blood-related malignancies

. . . .

*A*nemia is one of the most common conditions you'll encounter, not only on examinations but over the course of your clinical career. Co-author Rich is a nephrologist, and he sees a lot of anemia. Anemia has many causes, and knowing how to evaluate and treat the many kinds of anemia is important — especially for doing well on the PANCE.

This chapter covers several important hematology topics, including diagnosing and managing anemias and evaluating abnormalities of both platelet count and function.

In addition, we discuss malignant conditions of the blood, bone, and bone marrow, including lymphomas and leukemias. We cover the solid organ cancers, including lung cancer and prostate cancer, in their respective anatomic chapters.

Analyzing Anemia

Anemia is defined as a condition in which the body has a reduced quantity of red blood cells. It is often recognized by a low hemoglobin and hematocrit in the lab work. Many types of anemia exist, and they have a multitude of causes.

In this section, you review vital points concerning diagnosing and managing anemia. One key approach to anemia questions is to know what the patient's *mean corpuscular volume* (MCV) means. The MCV can help you think about the cause of the anemia and how to evaluate for it.

The MCV is a measure of the average size of red blood cells. If you look at any lab report, a normal reference range for the MCV is about 80–99 femtoliters (fL). A *microcytic anemia* has an MCV below normal, a *normocytic anemia* has an MCV in a normal range, and a *macrocytic anemia* has an MCV above normal.

In this section, you review anemias based on their MCVs, starting with the microcytic anemias. You also read about aplastic anemia, hemolytic anemia, and the hereditary anemias.

Mastering the microcytic anemias

Microcytic anemias are characterized by a low MCV, usually < 79 fL. The main microcytic anemias on the PANCE are iron-deficiency anemia, anemia of chronic disease, thalassemia, and lead poisoning. The key to answering these questions is to recognize the laboratory patterns of each type of anemia.

Iron-deficiency anemia

Iron-deficiency anemia is the most common type of microcytic anemia. Here are the main causes of this kind of anemia:

- ✔ **Bleeding in the gastrointestinal (GI) tract, usually from the colon:** This is the primary cause of iron-deficiency anemia. If a test question asks about new onset iron-deficiency anemia in an older adult, the test of choice is a colonoscopy to check for bleeding. In this case, you first need to rule out colon cancer. Besides a colonic malignancy, other causes of bleeding from the lower GI tract can include diverticulosis and angiodysplasia. Refer to Chapter 5 for causes of GI bleeding.

- ✔ **Malabsorption in the GI tract:** Recall that iron is absorbed in the small intestine. If you see a test question in which a person has iron deficiency and no cause of bleeding can be identified, think malabsorption. The most common cause of malabsorption is *celiac disease* (sensitivity to gluten). For other causes, see Chapter 5.

You need to order four labs to assess for iron deficiency: *iron, transferrin, transferrin saturation* (TSAT for short), and *ferritin*. In iron-deficiency anemia, the *ferritin level,* which is a measure of storage iron, is low, and so is the TSAT. The transferrin level is high because the body wants to pick up as much iron from the circulation as possible.

Picture transferrin as a vacuum that wants to suck up all the circulating iron, no matter how little is available. The transferrin is saturated with the circulating iron. That is why the transferrin level is high and the TSAT is low in iron-deficient states. The ferritin represents storage iron and is low in states of iron deficiency.

Iron can be replaced two ways, either orally or intravenously. Ferrous sulfate is a commonly used oral iron replacement. Giving vitamin C at the same time as oral iron can increase the amount of iron absorbed in the intestine.

You started a patient on iron replacement for iron-deficiency anemia. Which of the following labs is initially used to monitor response to therapy?

(A) Ferritin level

(B) Repeat transferrin level

(C) Reticulocyte count

(D) Homocysteine level

(E) Haptoglobin level

The answer is Choice (C). A *reticulocyte* is an immature red blood cell. In iron-deficiency anemia, the reticulocyte count is initially low. Within 1 week, you should begin to see an increase in the reticulocyte count as the iron is replaced. You need to do blood work for several weeks' time to check the ferritin and transferrin levels, because it takes that long to see a response. Homocysteine levels are used in evaluating macrocytic anemias, particularly folate deficiency. The haptoglobin level is used in evaluating hemolytic anemias.

Which of the following is a cause of a microcytic anemia?

(A) Alcoholism

(B) Hypothyroidism

(C) Chronic liver disease

(D) Hemolysis

(E) Bleeding duodenal ulcer

The answer is Choice (E). The bleeding from a duodenal ulcer would cause an iron-deficiency anemia, which is a microcytic anemia. Choices (A) through (D) represent causes of macrocytic anemias. Alcoholism can be a cause of many types of nutritional deficiencies, including B_{12} and folic acid. Hypothyroidism can be a cause of a macrocytic anemia (and normocytic anemia as well). Chronic liver disease and hemolysis are other causes of macrocytic anemia that you should be aware of.

Anemia of chronic disease

Anemia of chronic disease is also called *anemia of inflammation*. It's a common cause of anemia, especially in older adults who have many complex medical conditions. You can see anemia with many inflammatory states, especially the connective tissue diseases and cancer. You also see this type of anemia with chronic infections, such as osteomyelitis.

Test questions about this kind of anemia usually include clues such as references to some long-standing disease, chronic infection, or inflammatory condition. For example, the question may mention a newly discovered anemia in someone with rheumatoid arthritis (RA). Rheumatoid arthritis, a chronic inflammatory process, can certainly have an anemia of inflammation or chronic disease associated with it.

One key to differentiating anemia of chronic disease from iron-deficiency anemia (see the preceding section) is the pattern of the iron studies:

Type of Anemia	Ferritin Level	Transferrin Level	TSAT Level
Iron-deficiency anemia	Low	High	Low
Anemia of chronic disease	High	Low	Low

Ferritin is not only a measure of iron stores in the body but also a marker of inflammation, so it makes sense that a high ferritin level is a sign of anemia of chronic disease. Ferritin can be elevated in inflammatory states (such as cancer) or connective tissue disease (such as rheumatoid arthritis or systemic lupus erythematosus). In medical conditions like Still's disease, it can even be > 3,000 ng/mL.

Thalassemia

Thalassemia is a type of microcytic anemia that's important to recognize because the test always includes a question or two about it. Thalassemia is very common in people of African or Mediterranean descent.

You may recall that hemoglobin is made of two different types of protein: beta globin (HBB) and alpha globin (HBA). *Thalassemia* is a hereditary condition concerning a problem in the gene that makes one of these two proteins, leading to anemia. If a gene that makes beta globin is affected, then you have *beta thalassemia*. If a gene that makes alpha globin is affected, then you can have *alpha thalassemia*.

The thalassemia can be either a major problem (thalassemia major) or a minor problem (thalassemia minor). Both beta globin and alpha globin can have their own major and minor problems. Therefore, you can see a beta thalassemia major and minor and an alpha thalassemia major and minor.

If someone has thalassemia major, he or she inherited the problem gene from both parents. If someone has thalassemia minor, the problem gene came from only one parent. Two types of beta thalassemia and four types of alpha thalassemia exist because two genes code for beta globin, and four genes code for alpha globin.

Here are a couple of key points concerning the thalassemias:

- ✔ **Beta thalassemia minor (beta thalassemia trait):** The affected person can have a microcytosis but with a very mild anemia. You'll see target cells on a peripheral smear.

- ✔ **Beta thalassemia major:** The person can be severely affected as a child. He or she can develop a hemolytic anemia, problems with growth, and congestive heart failure because the anemia causes a high output state. Patients can also develop a very large liver and spleen, which for many can be fatal at a young age. Those who survive are often transfusion dependent and can develop problems with iron overload in their twenties and thirties.

There are four basic alpha thalassemias. They can range in severity from being asymptomatic (clinical carriers) to being fatal in utero (hydrops fetalis). Alpha thalassemia minor is a lot like beta thalassemia minor in its presentation: mild microcytosis.

You can confirm the diagnosis of thalassemia with a hemoglobin electrophoresis.

Lead poisoning

Lead poisoning (lead toxicity) is a condition you commonly see in young children exposed to lead. This exposure occurs especially in people who live in older homes that contain lead paint. Lead gets into the body when people eat it or inhale small particles into the lungs. It causes anemia, primarily by inhibiting the synthesis of heme.

Here are two key points concerning lead poisoning and anemia:

- ✔ On a peripheral smear, you can see basophilic stippling.

- ✔ Ferritin and iron levels can be normal.

The lead level and the presenting symptoms of lead exposure and lead poisoning differ. Low level exposures can cause anemia, peripheral neuropathy, and kidney disease. Lead poisoning can affect nerve function big time. The symptoms of lead poisoning include neurologic symptoms such as confusion, seizures, and coma at very high levels. Abdominal symptoms include pain and vomiting. Poisoning usually occurs at levels from 80–120 mcg/dL, which are toxic.

The treatment for lead poisoning is chelation, depending on the presenting symptoms and the lead level.

Vitamin deficiencies: Mastering macrocytic anemias

Macrocytic anemias are associated with a large MCV, usually > 100 fL. The two most common causes are vitamin B_{12} and folate (folic acid) deficiencies.

In addition to being macrocytic anemias, vitamin B_{12} and folic acid deficiencies are both *megaloblastic anemias*. Therefore, you see hypersegmented neutrophils on a peripheral blood smear.

Vitamin B_{12} deficiency

B_{12} deficiency can affect the blood, nerve function, and yes, even bowel function. This cause of anemia is easy to test for and easier to treat.

Following are some points on the causes of anemia due to B_{12} deficiency:

- B_{12} is found in meat, and the Western animal-based diet is built around meat, so unless someone's a vegan, being B_{12} deficient due to diet is very hard.

- Common causes of B_{12} deficiency include malabsorption syndromes (such as celiac sprue or tropical sprue), any prior intestinal surgeries (including gastric bypass and other stomach surgeries), inflammatory bowel disease (IBD), *Diphyllobothrium latum* infection, pancreatic insufficiency, and pernicious anemia. *Pernicious anemia* is caused by a lack of intrinsic factor, usually due to an autoimmune condition in which the body forms antibodies against the gastric parietal cells and can destroy them.

- Any type of *bacterial overgrowth syndrome* in the bowel can cause malabsorption of key nutrients, including B_{12}. You can see this with any process that can affect bowel integrity (for example, diverticulosis or colonic stricture) or bowel motility (diabetes mellitus is the most common example).

Here are some high-yield points concerning the symptoms, testing, and treatment of B_{12} deficiency:

- Signs of B_{12} deficiency include weakness, diarrhea or constipation, weight loss, and feeling just awful. The deficiency can also affect the nervous system and cause numbness and tingling of the hands and feet because of its effect on the peripheral nerves. It can cause *subacute combined degeneration* (SACD), which concerns a diminishing of the positional and vibratory senses. SACD is caused by a degeneration of the lateral and posterior columns of the spinal cord. B_{12} deficiency can also be a cause of dementia.

- You can diagnose B_{12} deficiency with a simple blood test, namely a B_{12} level. A normal level is > 300 pg/mL.

- You may have a suspicion that someone with low-level normal levels of B_{12} has B_{12} deficiency. In that situation, you'd order a *methylmalonic acid* level and *homocysteine* level. In B_{12} deficiency, both of these would be elevated, whereas only homocysteine would be elevated in folic acid deficiency.

- To assess for pernicious anemia as a cause of B_{12} deficiency, you'd order *antiparietal cell antibodies* and *anti-intrinsic factor antibodies* lab tests. Treatment with steroids may help, although this practice isn't common.

- No one does a Schilling test anymore. These tests are cumbersome and a pain to do.

- Treatment for B_{12} deficiency is B_{12} supplementation. Intramuscular injections of B_{12} can be given, usually once a week. These injections can transition to once a month or oral supplementation. B_{12} can be given sublingually (under the tongue) as well.

Folic acid deficiency

You commonly see folic acid deficiency along with B_{12} deficiency. Common causes of folic acid deficiency include the malabsorption syndromes, including celiac disease (celiac sprue) and tropical sprue.

Here are the high-yield tips concerning folic acid deficiency:

✔ A simple blood test can help you assess for folic acid deficiency.

✔ Pregnant women need to take prenatal vitamins fortified with folic acid to prevent birth defects, including *spina bifida*.

✔ Folic acid deficiency can be caused by malabsorption, excessive alcohol intake, and certain medications, such as methotrexate used for the treatment of rheumatoid arthritis or phenytoin sodium (Dilantin) and other seizure medications. Another common medication that causes folic acid deficiency is zidovudine (AZT), which is used in the treatment of HIV.

✔ The treatment is folic acid supplementation. Supplements are usually given orally in doses of 400 mcg to 1,000 mcg (1 mg) daily. Because folic acid can be found in leafy greens, eating veggies is also important.

In addition to B_{12} and folic acid deficiencies, other causes of macrocytic anemias include alcoholism, hypothyroidism, chronic liver disease, and hemolysis.

Narrowing in on normocytic anemias

How about anemias with a normal MCV (76–100 fL)? In these anemias, the hemoglobin is low. They include the following:

✔ Anemia secondary to kidney disease (the kidney produces little or no erythropoietin)

✔ Anemia of chronic disease (it can be either normocytic or microcytic — see the earlier section "Mastering the microcytic anemias" for details on this anemia)

✔ Myelophthisic anemia (anemia secondary to cancer, fibrosis, or granulomatous process that has spread to the bone marrow)

Be aware of this short list in case you're asked on the test.

Ameliorating aplastic anemia

Aplastic anemia is a disorder in which the bone marrow no longer produces red blood cells. The person is also *pancytopenic* because the bone marrow doesn't make platelets or white blood cells, either. In a person with aplastic anemia, the CBC shows pancytopenia and a low reticulocyte count. On presentation, the person is usually normocytic but occasionally has a large MCV (yet another cause of a macrocytic anemia).

Known causes of aplastic anemia include viruses (including hepatitis, Epstein-Barr, HIV, and parvovirus B19), medications (including antibiotics, chloramphenicol, NSAIDs, anti-seizure medications, and chemotherapy), toxin exposure (including heavy metals such as mercury), and autoimmune diseases. There can also be congenital causes of this condition. However, in many cases, the etiology of aplastic anemia isn't clear.

One particular medical condition that's closely associated with aplastic anemia is *paroxysmal nocturnal hemoglobinuria,* or PNH. It's characterized by a hemolytic anemia and venous thrombosis. The bone marrow isn't doing its job, and you see low white cell and low platelet counts on a CBC. People diagnosed with paroxysmal nocturnal hemoglobinuria are at risk of developing aplastic anemia later in life. Given the strong connection between the two conditions, people with aplastic anemia are often screened for PNH.

The treatments for aplastic anemia can include a stem cell transplant and/or immunosuppressive therapy through drugs such as cyclosporine (Neoral). Immunosuppressive medication is used especially if the cause of the aplastic anemia is likely autoimmune in nature. Often the person requires blood and platelet transfusions.

Harping on hemolysis: The destruction of red blood cells

Normal red blood cells live for about 3 to 4 months. *Hemolysis* is the destruction of red blood cells in the circulation way before their life span is over. Hemolysis has many causes; one easy way to think about those causes is whether you're dealing with extravascular hemolysis or intravascular hemolysis:

- ✔ **Extravascular hemolysis:** This hemolysis occurs primarily in the reticuloendothelial system (RES). The reticuloendothelial system is the part of the immune system consisting of cells whose job is to engulf and remove defective blood cells from the circulation. The liver's Kupffer cells and the spleen are main parts of the reticuloendothelial system.

  Common causes of extravascular hemolysis include autoimmune hemolytic anemia and hereditary disorders.

- ✔ **Intravascular hemolysis:** Intravascular hemolysis is the destruction of red blood cells occurring *intravascularly,* or within the circulation. Common causes include microangiopathic processes (such as hemolytic uremic syndrome, or HUS; thrombotic thrombocytopenic purpura, or TTP; or disseminated intravascular coagulation, or DIC), medications, hereditary conditions, tumor lysis syndrome (TLS), and autoimmune diseases.

For the PANCE, you need to be familiar with the laboratory evaluation of hemolysis. Table 18-1 shows how the lab results for intravascular and extravascular hemolysis compare.

Table 18-1	Lab Evaluation for Hemolysis	
Lab Test	*Intravascular Hemolysis*	*Extravascular Hemolysis*
LDH test	Lactate dehydrogenase (LDH), reticulocyte count, and total bilirubin (with an elevated unconjugated portion) are increased.	LDH and haptoglobin are normal. No hemoglobin is released into the circulation because the abnormal cell contents are all completely engulfed by the reticuloendothelial system.
Peripheral smear	You see *schistocytes,* or helmet cells, especially if there's a microangiopathic process.	You see spherocytes (sphere-shaped cells).
Urine dip	The urine dips positive for blood but doesn't show any red cells (positive for hemoglobinuria). See Chapter 10 for details.	The urine dips negative for blood (no hemoglobinuria).

Handling hereditary anemias

The PANCE may ask you about two basic hereditary causes of anemias: glucose-6-phosphate dehydrogenase (G6PD) deficiency and sickle cell anemia.

G6PD deficiency

G6PD deficiency is a hereditary condition in which the body is unable to produce enough glucose-6-phosphate dehydrogenase. It affects millions of people throughout the world, especially African-American males and people of Mediterranean descent.

Most kids with G6PD deficiency have no symptoms until their bodies are exposed to certain triggers or oxidative stresses. For the PANCE, be aware of the triggers: sulfa antibiotics, bacterial and viral illnesses, and medications used in the treatment of malaria, including primaquine phosphate (Primaquine) and dapsone.

Here's how to recognize G6PD deficiency:

- ✔ The diagnosis is based on a high clinical suspicion; tests can evaluate the degree of enzymatic activity, but they can also yield false-negative results.

- ✔ You can see Heinz bodies on a peripheral smear.

Treatment consists of removing the offending trigger and transfusing as needed.

Sickle cell disease

Sickle cell disease causes the body to make blood cells that are "sickle shaped" in times of physical stress. Examples can include low-oxygen states, such as hypoxemia and pneumonia, as well as infection and dehydration. Sickle cell disease primarily affects people of African descent but can also affect people of Indian and Mediterranean heritage.

If you have *sickle cell trait,* you're a carrier — you've inherited one gene for sickle hemoglobin and one normal gene, so you won't develop any of the symptoms of sickle cell disease. People who have the sickle cell trait need to undergo genetic counseling to be aware of their risk of passing the sickle gene on to their children.

Here are some aspects of sickle cell disease to be aware of:

- ✔ Sickle cell anemia is characterized by painful sickle cell crises, persistent anemia, and damage to organs of the body, including the heart, lungs, kidneys, and bones. Bone infarctions and avascular necrosis are long-term bone sequelae of sickle cell disease.

- ✔ Sickle cell crisis can include vaso-occlusive crisis, aplastic crisis, sequestration crisis, and hemolytic crisis. An episode can last 5 to 7 days.

  Sickle cell crisis is a life-threatening medical condition. Common precipitants include infection, any pulmonary process that causes hypoxemia, and volume-depleted states such as diarrhea. It can affect the lungs (acute chest syndrome), kidneys (kidney infarction), and bones (bone infarction). The treatment consists of oxygen, aggressive hydration, pain management, and folic acid supplementation. Exchange transfusions may also be needed.

- ✔ Sickle cell disease comes in different types, including hemoglobin sickle cell disease. Hemoglobin electrophoresis can confirm the type of sickle cell.

- ✔ People with sickle cell disease need chronic folic acid supplementation.

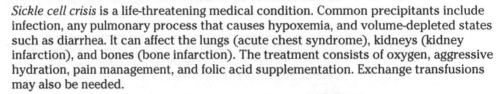

✔ People who have sickle cell disease are at risk for recurrent infections, especially from encapsulated organisms, because of problems with opsonization. Therefore, people who have sickle cell disease need to keep up-to-date with immunizations, specifically the pneumococcal vaccine. Because of recurrent bone infarctions, these patients are also at risk for osteomyelitis.

In a patient with sickle cell disease, which of the following bacterial agents is a common cause of osteomyelitis?

(A) *Staphylococcus*

(B) *Shigella*

(C) *E. coli*

(D) *Salmonella*

(E) *Streptococcus*

The answer is Choice (D). People with sickle cell disease and *Salmonella* are very susceptible to bone infections. Of the other choices, *Staph* and *Strep* are also Gram-positive organisms that can cause osteomyelitis.

Probing Polycythemia Vera: The Opposite of Anemia

Polycythemia vera is a myeloproliferative disorder (MPD). *Myeloproliferative disorders* are diseases of the bone marrow that involve increased cell turnover. There are different types of myeloproliferative disorders, but for the PANCE, we focus on polycythemia vera.

Polycythemia is the exact opposite of anemia — too many red blood cells are being produced. You commonly see polycythemia in both men and women over the age of 60. Here are some key points concerning *polycythemia vera* (PV):

✔ Clinical presentation includes vision problems and headaches. After a hot shower, a person with polycythemia may feel intense itching (yet another reason to take a cold shower!).

✔ Physical examination can show high blood pressure and splenomegaly.

✔ The CBC clues you in to a possible diagnosis with an elevated hemoglobin and hematocrit. You make the diagnosis by determining red cell mass. Some patients can also have a high platelet count (thrombocytosis) as well.

✔ The treatments include phlebotomy to keep the hematocrit lower, as well as hydroxyurea or anagrelide as needed. It's also recommended that the patient take an antiplatelet agent such as aspirin to minimize the risk of stroke, coronary events, and other clotting events.

The second type of polycythemia is called *secondary polycythemia,* meaning that something in the body, usually lack of oxygen, or hypoxemia, is driving erythropoietin production. Examples of this include COPD and cyanotic heart disease. Remember that renal cell carcinoma and polycystic kidney disease can have a secondary polycythemia as well through increased production of erythropoietin.

The third type of polycythemia is called *relative polycythemia*. It refers to a state when the hemoglobin and hematocrit levels are elevated because of extreme volume depletion and/or dehydration. The hemoglobin and hematocrit levels normalize with IV hydration.

Getting the Lowdown on Platelets: Testing for Thrombocytopenia

Thrombocytopenia is defined as a platelet count of < 150,000. For test-taking purposes, the primary causes of low platelets are idiopathic thrombocytopenic purpura (ITP), thrombotic thrombocytopenic purpura (TTP), and disseminated intravascular coagulation (DIC). We discuss all three conditions as well as the complicating factor of splenomegaly in this section.

When you read a test question about thrombocytopenia, ask yourself the following questions:

- ✔ Is this a problem of platelet production, or is something destroying the platelets?
- ✔ Are only the platelets low, or are the other cell lines (Hgb/HCT and white cell count [WBC]) affected as well? If all three lines are affected, then you know you're dealing with pancytopenia and that the bone marrow is completely unresponsive.

Looking for ITP: Platelet production problems

Idiopathic thrombocytopenic purpura (ITP) is a common cause of low platelets. Only the platelets are affected. The affected person usually has a normal WBC and Hgb/HCT.

When you think about ITP, differentiate between two types: one found in adults and one found in children. Here are the fundamental points about *chronic ITP,* the adult form of ITP:

- ✔ Adults with ITP usually have a chronically low platelet count with a mean platelet count around 50,000.
- ✔ People with chronic ITP do not have a large spleen, and petechiae may be present.
- ✔ Chronic ITP is more common in women than in men; it can coexist with other connective tissue diseases or autoimmune syndromes.
- ✔ The first line of treatment is prednisone. If this doesn't work, other treatments, including intravenous immune globulin (IVIG), are utilized. If other therapies don't work, splenectomy is a last resort. Because chronic ITP is a platelet-production problem, a person with ITP can receive transfusions as needed.

ITP in children is a different animal. Here are the key points about ITP in children:

- ✔ It has an abrupt onset compared to the adult condition.
- ✔ ITP in children is usually caused by a viral illness. Contrast this with ITP in adults, where you should think autoimmune process.
- ✔ The childhood form often gets better on its own, although in some cases prednisone may be needed.
- ✔ Expect petechiae and purpura to be present, much moreso than in chronic ITP seen in adults.

Homing in on heparin-induced thrombocytopenia (HIT)

Just about everyone you see in the hospital gets heparin, either subcutaneously for DVT prophylaxis or intravenously as part of the treatment for a myocardial infarction or pulmonary embolism. Heparin is a medication that can cause the platelet count to drop. Recognize that there are actually two different types of *heparin-induced thrombocytopenia* (HIT).

- ✔ **Type I:** Type I occurs 24 to 48 hours after exposure to heparin. The platelet counts will normalize, and the heparin doesn't need to be stopped. This reaction isn't immune mediated.

- ✔ **Type II:** Type II can occur about 5 to 10 days after exposure to heparin. This is the biggie, mediated by the immune system, and it can be life-threatening. Even though heparin is an anticoagulant, in this situation it can cause the blood to clot! Blood clots can form in the arteries or veins. The treatment for Type II HIT is to *discontinue* the heparin.

Dealing with disseminated intravascular coagulation (DIC)

Disseminated intravascular coagulation (or DIC for short) is a syndrome that causes the platelets to be chewed up. Patients who have DIC are really sick — you usually find them in the intensive care unit. DIC has many causes, including sepsis, malignancy, and obstetrical complications. Here are the key points on DIC:

- ✔ The lab values are vital in diagnosing DIC: low platelets, low fibrinogen levels, elevated levels of D-dimer, and a prolonged prothrombin time (PT). The prothrombin time and its derived measures of prothrombin ratio (PR) and international normalized ratio (INR) are measures of the extrinsic pathway of coagulation.

- ✔ A small percentage of the time, a hemolytic anemia can be present.

- ✔ The treatment depends on what's occurring: If there's bleeding, you need to administer fresh frozen plasma (FFP) or cryoprecipitate to replace fibrinogen. If the patient is clotting, then you may need to start heparin.

- ✔ Presenting signs include bleeding from mucous membranes, digital ischemia, and gangrene.

Testing for thrombotic thrombocytopenic purpura (TTP)

Thrombotic thrombocytopenic purpura (TTP) is a systemic process where, as in disseminated intravascular coagulation (DIC), the platelets are chewed up. Common causes include medications, malignancy, and pregnancy. Here are some key points on TTP:

- ✔ TTP is closely associated with a pentad: hemolytic anemia, thrombocytopenia, kidney failure, fever, and change in mental status. Note that not all five criteria need to be present; hemolytic anemia and low platelets can be enough to make the diagnosis if other laboratory parameters fit.

✔ Key labs are an elevated LDH level and a peripheral smear that shows schistocytes (helmet cells). You can also see an increased bilirubin and reticulocyte level.

✔ The gold standard of treatment is plasmapheresis. If this isn't an option on a test question, then look for transfusion with fresh frozen plasma (FFP). It's the next-best choice.

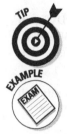

The INR and fibrinogen are normal in TTP, whereas in DIC, the fibrinogen is low and INR is high. This is a key differentiating point between the two conditions that you need to know for the test.

Which of the following medical conditions does not match its corresponding treatment?

(A) Idiopathic thrombocytopenic purpura — steroids

(B) Thrombotic thrombocytopenic purpura — fresh frozen plasma infusion

(C) Heparin-induced thrombocytopenia — protamine sulfate

(D) Disseminated intravascular coagulation — fresh frozen plasma infusion

(E) Idiopathic thrombocytopenic purpura — splenectomy

The answer is Choice (C). The treatment of HIT (Type II) is discontinuation of heparin. Protamine sulfate is used in the treatment of a heparin coagulopathy, in which the blood is too thin. All the other answers are correct.

When looking at this question, you could be fooled because protamine is associated with heparin, but it isn't for this particular question. Remember to take a couple of seconds to see what the question is really asking. You may have considered Choice (B); remember that although the gold standard of TTP treatment is plasmapheresis, fresh frozen plasma can also be used. Fresh frozen plasma can be used in the treatment of DIC as well.

Helping kids with hemolytic uremic syndrome

Hemolytic uremic syndrome (HUS) is like TTP (see the preceding section) but is usually found in children. Hemolytic uremic syndrome is rare in adults. The most common cause is Gram-negative sepsis, commonly caused by infection with *E. coli* 0157:H7. Other bacterial agents (such as *Salmonella*) and viral agents can cause hemolytic uremic syndrome as well. Here are the key points:

✔ As with TTP, you may see the pentad (hemolytic anemia, thrombocytopenia, kidney failure, fever, and change in mental status). However, mental status changes may be more significant in TTP, whereas kidney failure is more common in hemolytic uremic syndrome.

✔ You don't do plasma exchange in children with hemolytic uremic syndrome; the treatment is conservative and involves treating the underlying infection.

Sequestering platelets in the spleen

Remember that your spleen sequesters about one-third of your platelets at any one time. If splenomegaly is present, more platelets can be held in the spleen. A very common cause of splenomegaly is liver disease. Liver disease can cause cirrhosis with resulting portal hypertension and splenomegaly. On a CBC, you see both a lower white cell count and thrombocytopenia because of the splenomegaly. Another cause of splenomegaly is a malignancy, such as leukemia.

Confronting Coagulation Disorders

On the PANCE, some blood-related questions concern coagulation problems and their evaluation and management. This section focuses on platelets' coagulation and factor disorders.

Many things can affect platelets' ability to stick together. Medications, including antiplatelet agents, hinder clotting. Commonly prescribed medications like aspirin, antiplatelet agents like ticlopidine (Ticlid), clopidogrel (Plavix), and nonsteroidals like ibuprofen (Motrin) also can affect platelet clotting.

One major medical condition that can affect how platelets work is *uremia*. The uremic toxins in advanced kidney disease can affect the ability of platelets to clump. In that case, the treatment is dialysis.

The administration of clotting factors depends on which coagulation problem you're dealing with. *Fresh frozen plasma* (FFP) is part of the blood that's frozen and kept after a blood transfusion; it contains all the coagulation factors. Compared to FFP, *cryoprecipitate* (which is also frozen) contains Factor VIII, fibrinogen, vWF, and Factor XIII.

Viewing von Willebrand disease: Mucous membrane bleeding

Von Willebrand disease (vWD) is an extremely common hereditary coagulation disorder that's characterized by mucous membrane bleeding. It's inherited in an autosomal dominant fashion. There are several different types of von Willebrand disease, but for the purposes of the test, concern yourself only with Type I. Here are the key points about this condition:

- Clinical presentations can include minor or major bleeding. Minor cases include excessive bleeding after a trauma or dental surgery. Major bleeding includes recurrent nosebleeds (epistaxis), GI bleeding, and bleeding from the GU tract.

- Important labs include an abnormal bleeding time, reduced plasma von Willebrand's factor (vWF) levels, and low Factor VIII activity levels. Understand that physiologically, von Willebrand disease is linked to Factor III. This link comes up again in regard to hemophilia A (see the next section).

- Treatments involve giving Factor VIII concentrates or desmopressin. This can raise the vWF level; however, these treatments are indicated only for certain forms of vWF.

Handling hemophilia

Hemophilia comes in various types, but for test-taking purposes, focus on hemophilia A. Hemophilia A, the most common type, is an X-linked inherited disease. Here are some key points about hemophilia A:

- One can have significant bleeding into almost any body cavity; common places include the joints (hemarthroses), the head, the gastrointestinal tract, and the genitourinary tract (hematuria). If not treated, bleeding can persist from days to weeks.

- ✔ Hemophilia A causes significant bleeding due to a deficiency in Factor VIII, so to diagnose hemophilia A, you need to order a specific assay for Factor VIII. Labwise, the PTT level is prolonged.

- ✔ Do not use any antiplatelet agents.

- ✔ The gold standard is transfusion with Factor VIII concentrate that is purified to reduce the incidence of infection.

Christmas disease (hemophilia B) is important to differentiate from other causes of hemophilia because the treatment differs. Christmas disease involves a deficiency of Factor IX. Clinically, Factor IX deficiency can present in a similar way to Factor VIII, so make sure you know which factor deficiency you're dealing with. To diagnose hemophilia B, you order a specific assay for Factor IX. The treatment involves administering a purified or recombinant Factor IX concentrate.

Concentrates of Factor VIII and Factor IX can cause activation of the clotting cascade and promote a clotting problem. An alternative solution is to give fresh frozen plasma to the person with hemophilia who is unable to receive the Factor concentrates.

Kicking it with vitamin K: The clotting pathway

Vitamin K is a fat-soluble vitamin that's important in the clotting pathway. Working in the medical field, we've come across patients on warfarin (Coumadin) whose PT/INR levels (which measure the extrinsic pathway of coagulation) were scary high. If you recall, warfarin works on a vitamin K–dependent pathway.

Here are some key points concerning vitamin K deficiencies:

- ✔ Common causes of low vitamin K levels include advanced liver disease, antibiotics, poor nutrition, and malabsorptive processes.

- ✔ The PT/INR is elevated in people with vitamin K deficiency.

- ✔ Coagulation and vitamin K synthesis can be significantly compromised in a cirrhotic liver. If liver disease is advanced, the liver enzymes can be normal because not enough functioning hepatic cells are left to increase the liver enzymes.

- ✔ Vitamin K can be given orally or subcutaneously. Vitamin K supplements may not be effective in liver disease because the liver may not be able to process the vitamin K.

Clamoring Over Clotting Problems

In this section, we deal with problems involving too much clotting. These problems are often associated with a hypercoagulable or thrombophilic state. Medical conditions that predispose someone to a hypercoagulable state are often abnormalities in one or more aspects of Virchow's triad: *venous stasis, hypercoagulable state,* and/or *endothelial dysfunction.* (For information on this triad, see Chapter 22.)

Here are the key points on evaluating someone with a clotting problem or suspected thrombophilic disorder:

✔ Look at the family history for a history of clotting. Family history is important in trying to figure out which particular problem you're dealing with.

✔ The key testing clues for deep venous thrombosis (DVT) are a long plane trip or car trip, ambulatory dysfunction, and a history of immobilization. These issues are related to the problems of venous stasis that increase the risk of developing a deep venous thrombosis.

✔ Many causes of hypercoagulable state can cause deep venous thrombosis. A few can also cause arterial thromboses, including antiphospholipid antibody syndrome and Factor V Leiden mutation (homozygous).

Reviewing some hereditary causes

Here are several hereditary causes of a hypercoagulable state:

✔ Factor V Leiden mutation is the most common hereditary cause of thrombophilia in the world. It can be homozygous or heterozygous. It's caused by a genetic mutation that prevents Factor V from being broken down by Protein C.

✔ Prothrombin G mutation is a gene defect for prothrombin. It increases the risk of clots.

Other causes of a hypercoagulable state include deficiencies in antithrombin III, Protein C, and Protein S. You establish the deficiencies by measuring specific factor levels.

When an acute thrombosis develops, the standard treatment is intravenous heparin and then warfarin (Coumadin). This treatment has two caveats:

✔ Heparin works by potentiating antithrombin III, so higher levels of heparin may be needed if someone has antithrombin III deficiency

✔ In patients with Protein C and S deficiencies, the use of warfarin may actually raise the pro-clotting effect. Before you initiate warfarin, the affected person should be fully anti-coagulated on heparin.

For many hereditary causes, after a deep venous thrombosis has been diagnosed, the treatment for thrombophilia is lifelong anticoagulation.

Evaluating some acquired causes of thrombophilia

You should be aware of two acquired causes of thrombophilia: malignancy and the anti-phospholipid antibody syndrome.

Malignancies related to solid organ cancers, particularly pancreatic cancer, can increase the risk of forming a deep venous thrombosis. The treatment is usually lifelong anticoagulation and treatment of the underlying cancer.

Antiphospholipid antibody syndrome (APS) is an acquired coagulation disorder that can present with thrombocytopenia, venous (or arterial) thromboses, and spontaneous abortions, usually in the second trimester. In addition to the clinical history, lab tests that can confirm antiphospholipid antibody syndrome include a lupus anticoagulant and anticardiolipin antibody. The treatment is anticoagulation.

Which of the following statements concerning the use of warfarin (Coumadin) is true?

(A) It works by increasing the activity of vitamin K.

(B) It is used for chronic anticoagulation for medical conditions such as deep venous thrombosis and atrial fibrillation.

(C) A rare side effect is bone necrosis.

(D) It is used for anticoagulation acutely in the setting of a myocardial infarction.

(E) It can be given during pregnancy.

The answer is Choice (B). Warfarin antagonizes the activity of vitamin K. It causes warfarin-induced skin necrosis, not bone necrosis. Because warfarin does not inhibit platelet aggregation, warfarin isn't used in the acute treatment of a myocardial infarction. Heparin and other antiplatelet agents are used. And it can't be given during pregnancy.

Understanding Hematologic Malignancies

In this section, you read about the various hematologic malignancies. They include multiple myeloma, amyloidosis, leukemia, and lymphoma. They can occur together, or they can occur separately. They can also affect multiple organs of the body, a big one being the kidney. Co-author Rich sees a lot of these conditions in his clinical practice.

Mastering multiple myeloma

Multiple myeloma (MM) is referred to as a *plasma cell dyscrasia*. It's cancer of the plasma cell (the memory cell), and it most frequently affects older adults. This condition can be deadly. Here are the key points concerning multiple myeloma:

- ✔ Clinical presentation includes back pain and weight loss. Initial presentation can be a fracture after a fall that reveals a cancer (pathologic fracture).

- ✔ Initial lab abnormalities suggestive of multiple myeloma include anemia, kidney failure, hypercalcemia, an increased total protein level, and an elevated sedimentation rate.

- ✔ Screening tests for multiple myeloma include a serum and protein electrophoresis (SPEP and UPEP) to look for this paraprotein. You're looking for a monoclonal spike (or M spike) on the SPEP. Other parts of the initial examination are a serum-free light chain assay and serum immunoelectrophoresis. Bence Jones proteins (light chains of immunoglobulin) are found in the urine.

  The diagnosis of multiple myeloma is made by the degree of the M spike seen on the SPEP. As people get older, they can become carriers of this paraprotein without having features of multiple myeloma. This condition is called *monoclonal gammopathy of undetermined significance* (MGUS).

- ✔ You make the confirmatory diagnosis by bone marrow biopsy, looking for more than 10 percent plasma cells in the bone marrow.

- ✔ Other testing includes a skeletal survey, looking for lytic lesions.

- ✔ The treatment is chemotherapy, which can include melphalan and steroids like prednisone or dexamethasone. Thalidomide has been used, as well as newer agents like bortezomib, which is a monoclonal antibody.

If you see a question asking for a radiologic study to search for multiple myeloma, the answer is *not* bone scan or MRI. The skeletal survey using radiographs is preferred for this diagnosis. Remember that multiple myeloma is only *osteolytic,* not *osteoblastic.* If you're asked about staging for a solid organ cancer with osteoblastic activity (such as prostate or breast cancer), *then* the answer would be bone scan.

Asking about amyloidosis

A condition closely related to multiple myeloma is *amyloidosis.* It's an abnormal, toxic, inflammatory protein that can deposit in places that it shouldn't and cause some major damage. Approximately 10 percent of people diagnosed with multiple myeloma can have coexistent amyloidosis, although amyloidosis can exist on its own. We're referring here to *primary amyloidosis* — there can be several different types of amyloidosis. Here are some key facts concerning primary amyloidosis:

✔ Amyloidosis can affect multiple organs in the body, including the nerves (peripheral neuropathy), the heart (cardiac amyloidosis), and the kidneys (renal failure and proteinuria).

✔ You can make the diagnosis by doing an abdominal-wall fat pad biopsy. If needed, you can biopsy a specific organ (for example, the kidney if kidney disease is present). A positive Congo red stain under polarized light is diagnostic for amyloidosis.

✔ The treatment for amyloidosis is chemotherapy.

 Know that when amyloidosis affects the kidney, proteinuria and kidney failure occur. Multiple myeloma can also affect the kidney in a number of ways, including myeloma cast nephropathy and light chain disease, which can also cause proteinuria. Both multiple myeloma and amyloidosis can cause the kidneys to appear enlarged on kidney ultrasound.

Looking at the leukemias

Leukemias are high levels of abnormal white cells that overwhelm and overtake the bone marrow. They can also invade and take over other organs. For PANCE purposes, be familiar with four types of leukemias — two acute leukemias and two chronic leukemias. The acutes are acute myeloid leukemia (AML) and acute lymphocytic leukemia (ALL). The chronic forms are chronic myelogenous leukemia (CML) and chronic lymphocytic leukemia (CLL).

 Try to pick up on key points that differentiate the leukemias from each other. For example, Auer rods (needle-shaped, lysosomal-like material within the cytoplasm of the leukemic cell) are a key finding in AML, and the Philadelphia chromosome is important for diagnosing CML. This type of hematologic minutiae is high yield for test questions.

Evaluating acute lymphocytic leukemia

Acute lymphocytic leukemia (ALL) is a condition primarily of childhood and young adulthood, although it can also occur in older adults. The cell line affected in ALL is the lymphoblast, whereas acute myeloid leukemia (AML) affects the myeloblast. Here are some key points concerning ALL:

✔ Risk factors of acquiring ALL include having Down syndrome and perhaps radiation exposure. The risk due to other toxic exposures is uncertain.

✔ Clinical presentation can include type B constitutional symptoms, including fevers, chills, drenching night sweats, and weight loss as well as easy bleeding and bruising.

✔ On physical examination, lymphadenopathy and hepatosplenomegaly can be present.

✔ Initial labs can show a significant leukocytosis with blasts. Anemia and thrombocytopenia can be present.

✔ In someone with ALL, do a chest radiograph to make sure that there's no mediastinal mass.

✔ Treatments include chemotherapy and bone marrow transplant.

People with ALL can test positive for terminal deoxynucleotidyl transferase (TDD). Common acute lymphoblastic leukemia antigen (CALLA) is expressed by most types of lymphoblastic leukemias. You may see either of these on the PANCE.

Reviewing acute myeloid leukemia

Acute myeloid leukemia (AML) is a very bad disease that can present either insidiously or abruptly. Different types of AML exist. One classification system, the French-American-British (FAB), has seven different types of AML.

Having a high clinical suspicion is the key to recognizing leukemia. Here are the key points you need to know about AML:

✔ Risk factors include a history of benzene exposure.

✔ Chromosomal aberrations such as Down syndrome and Klinefelter's syndrome increase the risk of developing AML. Anti-cancer medications also can increase the risk of developing AML.

✔ Clinical presentation can include bruising and bleeding and type B constitutional symptoms, including fever, weight loss, and overwhelming fatigue.

✔ On physical examination, lymphadenopathy, petechiae, and splenomegaly can be present. A small percentage of people present with retinal bleeding.

✔ Initial labs can show a significant leukocytosis with blasts or leukopenia. Anemia and thrombocytopenia can be profound.

✔ The treatment is high-dose chemotherapy.

On a bone marrow aspirate of someone with AML, you can see Auer rods. You see Auer rods in certain forms of myelodysplasia as well.

When treating leukemias or high-grade lymphomas with chemotherapy, a potential complication is tumor lysis syndrome (TLS). Before giving chemo, give prophylaxis with intravenous fluids with bicarbonate to alkalinize the urine (with the goal of getting urine pH above 6.5) and with allopurinol to reduce hyperuricemia. In a condition called *spontaneous tumor lysis syndrome,* TLS occurs in the absence of chemotherapy.

How about a medication side effect that can be high yield on the PANCE? *Retinoic acid syndrome* is a reaction to the medication tretinoin, which is used to treat a form of AML called *acute promyelocytic leukemia.* It's high yield for tests because it can cause a unique syndrome that presents with an ARDS-like (acute respiratory distress syndrome) picture, including hypoxemia and opacification of both lung fields. The treatment is supportive and intravenous steroids. Other immunosuppressive medications may be given.

Clarifying chronic lymphocytic leukemia (CLL)

Chronic lymphocytic leukemia (CLL) is the most common type of leukemia you'll encounter. You usually see CLL in the older population. The first indication of CLL is often an abnormality of blood work, specifically an elevated white count with a significant lymphocytosis. Here are the main points about CLL concerning the Rai staging of classification for CLL:

✔ **Stage 0:** You see an isolated lymphocytosis.

✔ **Stage I:** Lymphadenopathy is present.

✔ **Stage II:** You see splenomegaly.

✔ **Stage III:** Anemia is present.

✔ **Stage IV:** You see thrombocytopenia.

CLL often follows an indolent course, although it does have the potential for malignant transformation. Usually chemotherapy is indicated for Stage II or above unless significant adenopathy is present.

The preferred treatment for CLL is now imatinib (Gleevec). Other treatment options include a bone marrow transplant.

Considering chronic myelogenous leukemia (CML)

Chronic myelogenous leukemia (CML), also known as *chronic myeloid leukemia,* peaks in incidence for people in their mid 40s. Testing for the Philadelphia chromosome, which is a translocation between chromosomes 9 and 22, is highly indicative that CML may be present. Philadelphia chromosome is associated with a BCR/ABL fusion protein.

✔ Risk factors of CML include smoking and perhaps high doses of radiation.

✔ Clinical presentation can include type B constitutional symptoms, fatigue, and abdominal discomfort because of a large spleen. If the platelet or white cell counts are high enough, people can have related problems, including strokes, visual problems, lung problems, and heart problems (including MIs).

✔ On physical examination, lymphadenopathy and splenomegaly can be present. Sometimes you can detect hepatomegaly on physical examination as well.

✔ The lab pattern of CML is leukocytosis, thrombocytosis, high B_{12} levels, high uric acid levels, high LDH levels, and low leukocyte alkaline phosphatase.

✔ The only CML treatment that has any shot at a cure is stem cell transplantation. Sometimes the medication imatinib (Gleevec) is used to help manage the disease process.

Identifying hairy cell leukemia (HCL)

In a subtype of leukemia called *hairy cell leukemia* (HCL), blood cells actually look like hair when seen under a microscope. This condition has nothing to do with the hairiness of the individual. HCL is a disorder of B cells. The patient can have pancytopenia, and yes, splenomegaly. The treatment is 2-chlorodeoxyadenosine (2CDA).

Examining the lymphomas

The lymphomas are malignancies that affect the lymphatic system. The two major groups of lymphoma that you should be familiar with are Hodgkin's disease and non-Hodgkin's lymphoma.

Harping on Hodgkin's disease

Hodgkin's disease (HD) is a type of lymphoma that affects young people, usually in the mid-teen years, but it also occurs in people into their late 40s. HD involves a unique type of cell called the Reed-Sternberg cell. It's a huge cell that has a multilobed nucleus. The Reed-Sternberg cell is crucial in the diagnosis of Hodgkin's disease.

Look at the key points about Hodgkin's disease:

✔ Clinical presentation can include lymphadenopathy, often along the cervical nodes. The adenopathy is usually painless. Type B symptoms and/or pruritus may be present.

✔ In addition to lymphadenopathy, physical examination can reveal hepatosplenomegaly.

✔ Staging is really important because Hodgkin's disease is very curable in the early stages. CT scans are the key to staging this disease. Depending on the stage at the time of diagnosis, radiation and/or chemotherapy may be used.

The Ann Arbor staging system and the REAL/WHO staging system are two systems for staging Hodgkin's lymphoma.

Narrowing in on non-Hodgkin's lymphoma

Lymphomas that don't contain the Reed-Sternberg cell are referred to as non-Hodgkin's lymphomas (NHL). A lymph node biopsy is very important in NHL.

Although staging of NHL is important for diagnosis, perhaps even more important is the *grade* of the lymphoma. Non-Hodgkin's lymphoma has three different grades: low, intermediate, and high.

✔ **Low grade:** Examples of low-grade lymphomas include follicular lymphoma, mantle cell lymphoma, and mucosa-associated lymphoid tissue lymphoma (MALToma or MALT lymphoma).

✔ **Intermediate grade:** An example of an intermediate-grade lymphoma is diffuse large cell lymphoma.

✔ **High grade:** Examples of high-grade lymphomas include lymphoblastic lymphoma and Burkitt's lymphoma.

Here are some key points on NHL:

✔ Important connections link HIV, Sjögren's syndrome, and NHL.

✔ Especially with high-grade lymphoma, LDH levels are important markers of disease activity (for example, the degree of cell turnover).

✔ Richter's syndrome is a rare condition in which the CLL transforms into a high-grade lymphoma. The diagnosis is made by a lymph node biopsy.

✔ The treatment regimen can include radiation, chemotherapy, and/or bone marrow transplant, depending on the type of lymphoma you're dealing with.

MALTomas that affect the gastric area are caused by *Helicobacter pylori,* a Gram-negative bacterium (see Chapter 5). The treatment consists of using a proton pump inhibitor and antibiotics. This regimen has a pretty decent cure rate, although close follow-up is needed.

Practice Hematology and Oncology Questions

These practice questions give you a sense of what to expect of PANCE hematology and oncology questions. They also address important subject areas you need to be familiar with, without regard to the test.

1. You're evaluating a 43-year-old man who presents to the ER with an abnormal complete blood count (CBC). The white blood cell count is 6.3 mg/dL, the hemoglobin is 7.4 mg/dL, and the platelet count is 40 mg/dL. You order a peripheral smear, and there are schistocytes. The LDH level is 2,500. Plasmapheresis isn't available at your hospital facility. What would be your next immediate step?

   (A) Platelet transfusion

   (B) Intravenous steroids

   (C) Intravenous immunoglobulin (IVIG)

   (D) Fresh frozen plasma (FFP) transfusion

   (E) Splenectomy

2. Which of the following is an example of a macrocytic anemia?

   (A) Anemia of kidney disease

   (B) Chronic liver disease

   (C) Myelophthisic anemia

   (D) Multiple myeloma

   (E) Pure red cell aplasia

3. You're evaluating a patient with anemia. During the course of your examination, you note that the patient has a positive monoclonal spike on a serum protein electrophoresis. You're not sure of the significance of this. Which one of the following tests would you order next?

   (A) CT scan of thorax, abdomen, and pelvis

   (B) Nuclear medicine bone scan

   (C) A radiographic skeletal survey

   (D) MRI spine survey with gadolinium

   (E) CT scan of the spine with intravenous contrast

4. What is the most common cause of a hypercoagulable state?

   (A) Prothrombin gene mutation

   (B) Factor V Leiden mutation

   (C) Nephrotic syndrome

   (D) Antiphospholipid antibody syndrome

   (E) Antithrombin III deficiency

5. You are evaluating a 23-year-old woman who presents with recurrent epistaxis. She also experiences some bleeding from her gums when she brushes her teeth. Other past medical history is unremarkable, and the patient denies taking any medications, including NSAIDs. On examination, there is no splenomegaly. The CBC shows a WBC of 7.4 mg/dL, hemoglobin of 11.3 mg/dL, and a platelet count of 220,000. What would be your next step?

   (A) Obtain an abdominal ultrasound to be sure splenomegaly is not present.

   (B) Order a bone marrow biopsy.

   (C) Test for von Willebrand disease.

   (D) Obtain stat creatinine to evaluate kidney function.

   (E) Send peripheral blood for flow stat creatinine.

6. Which one of the following tumor markers and its association is correct?

   (A) CA125 — breast cancer

   (B) CA19-9 — ovarian cancer

   (C) Alpha-fetoprotein — hepatocellular carcinoma (HCC)

   (D) Prostate-specific antigen (PSA) — testicular cancer

   (E) Carcinoembryonic antigen (CEA) level — prostate cancer

Answers and Explanations

1. **D.** This patient has thrombotic thrombocytopenic purpura (TTP), so you would transfuse fresh frozen plasma. Platelet transfusions are good in the treatment of idiopathic thrombocytopenic purpura (ITP) but not TTP. Steroids and splenectomy are treatments for ITP. Some clinicians also use intravenous immunoglobulin in the treatment of ITP.

2. **B.** Chronic liver disease is associated with a macrocytic anemia. All the other choices are associated with a normocytic, normochromic anemia. *Pure red cell aplasia* is an autoimmune process in which antibodies are produced against erythropoietin. This causes a hypoproliferative bone marrow concerning the production of red blood cells, but the patient has normal leukocytes and platelets.

3. **C.** You suspect that the patient has multiple myeloma based on the initial positive monoclonal spike on the serum protein electrophoresis, but the patient may have a monoclonal gammopathy of unknown significance (MGUS). You'd order a skeletal radiographic survey to look for lytic lesions. Choice (A) isn't right because a CT scan of the thorax, abdomen, and pelvis is used for staging many solid organ cancers as well as lymphomas. A bone scan is good only when you're looking for bone metastasis concerning solid organ cancers that have osteoblastic activity. You wouldn't expect to see multiple myeloma, which is predominantly a lytic process. An MRI, Choice (D), or CT scan, Choice (E), with their respective contrasts, wouldn't be indicated at this time.

4. **B.** The most common cause of a hypercoagulable state is a Factor V Leiden mutation. Patients can be homozygous or heterozygous for this mutation. The other choices are causes of a hypercoagulable state but are not as common as Factor V Leiden mutation. Antithrombin III deficiency is a common cause of clotting in younger people, as are Protein C and Protein S deficiencies.

5. **C.** The patient has recurrent problems with mucosal bleeding, which suggests a problem with platelet function. Her platelet count is normal, which should suggest a qualitative platelet problem. Although kidney disease, Choice (D), could cause qualitative platelet function, there are usually other issues present (anemia, uremic symptoms, and so forth). The other answers are not applicable to this problem. Flow cytometry, Choice (E), is sometimes ordered by a hematologist for evaluation of malignancy. A bone marrow biopsy, Choice (B), is not indicated, and Choice (A), an abdominal ultrasound, doesn't make sense. You would test for von Willebrand disease.

6. **C.** Alpha-fetoprotein is associated with hepatocellular carcinoma (HCC). The other choices don't represent the correct tumor markers with their corresponding cancers. CA19-9 is associated with breast cancer, and CA125 is associated with ovarian cancer. CEA is a tumor marker associated with colon cancer. PSA is associated with prostate cancer, not testicular cancer.

Chapter 19

Dealing with Bugs and Drugs: Infectious Diseases

- -

In This Chapter

▶ Sorting out spirochetes and other bacteria

▶ Finding fungal infections

▶ Looking at HIV and other viruses

▶ Getting rid of worms and other parasites

- -

We're surrounded by bugs known as *microorganisms.* They're all around us. Beneficial organisms give us beer, wine, cheese, bread, and compost. The rest go straight to our bodies and wreak havoc. (The exception is the intestinal flora; the intestine is full of beneficial bacteria that contribute to keeping your body in balance and maintaining health.)

On the PANCE/PANRE, you need to know about some of these nasty organisms, their effects, and the drugs used to treat them. Don't get bugged!

Keeping Spirochetes and Rocky Mountain Spotted Fever from Spiraling Out of Control

The spirochete-related diseases can be debilitating and disabling to the max if they aren't detected early. The spirochetes are Gram-negative bacteria that are responsible for conditions such as syphilis and Lyme disease, which you read about in this section. We also discuss Rocky Mountain spotted fever (RMSF), which is caused by a Gram-negative coccobacillus, not a spirochete. Its clinical presentation and mode of transmission are very similar to Lyme disease.

Ticking off key points on Rocky Mountain spotted fever

Rocky Mountain spotted fever (RMSF) is a tick-borne illness that can be fatal if it isn't recognized and promptly treated. It's caused by the bacterium *Rickettsia rickettsii*. Historically, it was found in and around the Rocky Mountains, but today you can find it all across the United States. It's particularly prevalent in the Southeast.

The initial symptoms can include high fever, nausea, anorexia, and vomiting. This combination can be confusing to the clinician because you can attribute these generalized symptoms to a number of illnesses. The classic triad for Rocky Mountain spotted fever is fever, rash, and headache. These symptoms can occur anywhere from 3 to 14 days after the initial tick bite. Note that geographic location, season, and history of a tick bite should be significant factors in making your diagnosis.

The big tipoff that someone has Rocky Mountain spotted fever is the classic skin rash. Look for a maculopapular rash on the palms and soles. It can also spread to (or initially be found on) the distal extremities, including the ankles and wrists. However, in many cases, the rash isn't even present.

Here are three key points concerning Rocky Mountain spotted fever:

- ✔ The fever associated with this condition isn't a sissy fever. People with Rocky Mountain spotted fever are toxic and sick, with fevers on the order of 38.9–39.4°C (102–103°F).

- ✔ This illness can affect multiple organ systems and can cause acute respiratory distress syndrome (ARDS), acute renal failure (ARF), elevated liver enzymes, and low platelets, to name but a few.

- ✔ The treatment is doxycycline (Vibramycin). It's usually given for 10 to 14 days. Be aware that a side effect of this medication is photosensitivity.

Hitting the bull's-eye with Lyme disease

Lyme disease is similar to Rocky Mountain spotted fever (see the preceding section) in three ways: Lyme disease is a tick-borne illness, it has a characteristic skin rash (which isn't always present), and it's treated with doxycycline (Vibramycin); however, treatment for Lyme disease lasts 21 days, not 10 to 14.

Lyme disease is transmitted by the deer tick (genus *Ixodes*), and the bacterium mainly responsible is *Borrelia burgdorferi*. Lyme disease can affect multiple body areas, and the presentations can be confusing because Lyme disease is a great mimicker of other medical conditions, including rheumatologic conditions. Here are three key points about Lyme disease:

- ✔ The characteristic skin rash is called *erythema migrans*. It looks like a bull's-eye, and it usually appears on an extremity, although it can appear anywhere. The time course to presentation of the rash can vary. It can occur a few days after the tick bite, or it may not present itself for a few weeks. Again, this characteristic skin rash isn't always present.

- ✔ Lyme disease can do a lot more than just cause a skin rash. It can affect the heart, the joints, and the central nervous system. One big clinical manifestation you need to be aware of is Lyme-induced meningitis.

- ✔ Lyme disease can cause a *Lyme carditis*. The most common clinical presentation of Lyme carditis is second- or third-degree heart block in a person with no cardiac risk factors. The person usually needs emergent cardiac pacing (that is, a transcutaneous or transvenous pacemaker) as well as intravenous ceftriaxone (Rocephin) for treatment, not just oral doxycycline (Vibramycin). This is a very high-yield testing point.

The laboratory evaluation of Lyme disease is based on two tests: the enzyme-linked immunosorbent assay (ELISA) and the western blot. Both must be positive to confirm a diagnosis of Lyme disease. They may be negative early in the course of the disease, so they need to be clinically repeated, especially if you have a high clinical suspicion that Lyme disease is present.

Lyme disease has been implicated in chronic fatigue and fibromyalgia syndrome (FMS) as an inciting factor of a persistent systemic inflammatory response. Fibromyalgia syndrome can be debilitating.

Lyme disease can be a presenting cause of acute monoarticular arthritis; however, if someone in a test question has acute monoarticular arthritis, start thinking of differential diagnoses. Besides Lyme disease, other causes include gonorrhea, gout, pseudogout, and a septic joint (see Chapter 6 for info on joint conditions). Lyme disease can also be a cause of Bell's palsy. What else would be in your differential diagnosis for Bell's palsy? Herpes zoster (Ramsay Hunt syndrome), sarcoidosis, or idiopathic origin.

Knowing the progression of syphilis

Syphilis, an STD, is caused by the bacterium *Treponema pallidum*. Syphilis occurs in several stages: primary, secondary, and tertiary. If you treat it early, you can usually prevent progression to the next stage. Think about the clinical aspects of syphilis as they pertain to each stage of the disease:

- ✔ **Primary syphilis:** The initial manifestation of syphilis is the painless lesion known as the *chancre.* It can present within 1 week or as late as 3 months after exposure. The lesion is maculopapular, usually located in the penile region in males and the cervical region in females. The treatment is one dose of benzathine penicillin administered intramuscularly.

- ✔ **Secondary syphilis:** If untreated, primary syphilis can progress to a secondary syphilis. The main clinical manifestation is a rash that can affect the hands and feet as well as the upper and lower extremities. Symptoms include *condyloma latum,* which are grapelike clusters of warts that can present in various places. Reddish papules all over the body are a possibility, too.

- ✔ **Tertiary syphilis:** Tertiary syphilis, also called *neurosyphilis,* can cause dementia, which may be an initial presentation. We counted another 18 symptoms, too, including blindness, depression, and seizures. The treatment for tertiary syphilis is intravenous penicillin, given over several weeks.

The initial lab test used to screen for syphilis is the rapid plasma reagent (RPR). If it's positive, then a Venereal Disease Research Laboratory (VDRL) test is often ordered next. The best confirmatory test for syphilis is the fluorescent treponemal antibody absorption test (FTA-Abs). This test can stay positive for a lifetime — it doesn't wane with treatment.

For test-taking purposes, don't confuse two different conditions. A *chancre* is associated with primary syphilis, whereas *chancroid* is associated with *Haemophilus ducreyi.* *Condyloma latum* is associated with secondary syphilis, whereas *condyloma acuminata* is associated with the human papillomavirus (HPV; see Chapter 9).

Be aware of other neurologic manifestations of syphilis. One that you may be tested on is *Tabes dorsalis,* which affects the dorsal columns of the spinal cord; vibration and sensation can be affected.

You're evaluating a 65-year-old man who is being treated for a bacterial infection. He complains of shortness of breath and shaking chills. On physical examination, his temperature is 37.8°C (100°F), pulse is 100 beats per minute, and his blood pressure is 90/60 mmHg. He says that these symptoms occurred a few hours after taking the prescribed antibiotic. What's the most likely cause of this man's symptoms?

(A) Resistant syphilitic infection

(B) Untreated *Gonococcus*

(C) Immunosuppression with HIV

(D) Jarisch-Herxheimer reaction

(E) Complicated urinary tract infection (UTI)

The correct answer is Choice (D). Sometimes after you initiate treatment for bacterial infection, the person begins to feel worse before he or she feels better. In this case, the released contents of the dead bacteria begin to stimulate the immune system acutely, causing the *Jarisch-Herxheimer reaction.* The Jarisch-Herxheimer reaction is associated with syphilis, but you can see it with other bacterial infections as well.

Having a resistant syphilitic infection, Choice (A), is rare. Nothing in the question suggests that Choice (B), *Gonococcus,* or Choice (C), immunosuppression, is present. Also, the question offers no suggestion that the man has a urinary tract infection, Choice (E), because no symptoms of urgency or dysuria are present.

Beating Bacterial Infections

Many bacterial infections exist, but for the PANCE, there are seven biggies. Bacterial causes of diarrhea, especially food poisoning, can make someone deathly ill. Rheumatic fever isn't commonly seen, but tests ask about it a lot. In this section, you read about diarrhea, rheumatic fever, botulism, and other bacterial infections.

Causes of diarrhea: When what goes in comes out too fast

For most people, diarrhea is merely inconvenient. But for people in the developing world, especially children, it's a leading cause of death. The three big causes of diarrhea are cholera, shigella, and salmonella.

Cholera

Cholera is caused by *Vibrio cholerae,* which is introduced when a person eats or drinks food or water contaminated by the feces of an infected person. You see cholera mainly in Africa and Third World countries. Cholera can cause a profuse secretory diarrhea (rice water stools), and the affected person can lose massive amounts of fluid. The person is at risk of significant dehydration if the fluid isn't aggressively repleted. The treatment for dehydration includes aggressive oral and/or intravenous rehydration. Cholera is treated with tetracycline derivatives or macrolide antibiotics.

Shigella

Shigella (bacillary dysentery) is a bacterium that can cause an infectious colitis. This bacterium has several subtypes, though for this book, we're talking about *Shigella flexneri* (although *S. dysenteriae* is pretty terrible, too). It can be transmitted by eating food or drinking water that's contaminated.

One of the main presenting symptoms of shigella is bloody diarrhea. Anyone who has contact with infected stool (for example, healthcare workers) can acquire shigella. The best advice to practitioner and patient: Wash your hands!

Children are especially at high risk of acquiring shigella. In children, in addition to bloody diarrhea, an initial presenting symptom can be seizures. Without adequate volume repletion, dehydration and electrolyte abnormalities can occur.

Shigella diarrhea is usually a self-limited disease that runs its course in about 7 to 10 days in immunocompetent individuals. Antibiotics are used in moderate to severe cases. Penicillin and fluoroquinolones have also been used.

E. coli O157:H7 is a cause of hemolytic-uremic syndrome (HUS) (see Chapter 18 for details). The Shiga toxin that can be seen in some cases of shigellosis can also cause hemolytic-uremic syndrome.

Salmonellosis

Salmonellosis (popularly "salmonella") is caused by *Salmonella enterica,* a bacterium that can produce an infectious diarrhea or an infectious colitis. Symptoms of nausea, vomiting, and diarrhea can develop as soon as a few hours after infection, or they can take as long as 3 days to develop. *Salmonella enterica* has several subtypes (in particular, *Salmonella enterica enterica*). People can acquire this bacterium through infected food, such as infected meat and eggs that aren't properly cooked.

In the United States, you see periodic high-profile outbreaks of salmonella, with, for example, millions of pounds of ground turkey or beef being recalled. The salmonellosis peanut-butter outbreak of 2009 sickened about 691 people in 46 states and resulted in 9 deaths! Salmonellosis is far more serious than just being a case of the runs.

Here are some key points about salmonellosis:

✔ Symptoms of salmonellosis can be gastrointestinal upset and/or a flu-like illness. An initial presentation can be bloody diarrhea.

✔ Antibiotic treatment is given only in moderate to advanced cases of salmonella. Many experts think that early antibiotic treatment may actually prolong the illness. Sulfa drugs and fluoroquinolones are often used.

In someone with sickle cell anemia, salmonella can be a common cause of osteomyelitis, a condition we cover in Chapter 6. This is a very high-yield topic.

Rheumatic fever: Reviewing a rare disease

An older adult may tell you that he or she has a history of rheumatic fever, which is a reaction to a bacterial infection caused by a beta hemolytic Group A streptococcus *(Streptococcus pyogenes)* infection. It usually affects the heart about 3 weeks after pharyngitis or a skin infection, and it's a leading cause of mitral stenosis.

Rheumatic fever is diagnosed by the Jones criteria, which consists of major and minor criteria:

✔ **Major criteria:** The major Jones criteria are Sydenham's chorea, carditis, polyarticular joint inflammation, subcutaneous nodules, and a characteristic skin rash, erythema marginatum. The carditis can be myocarditis or pericarditis.

Don't confuse the Jones criterion erythema marginatum with *erythema migrans,* which is the skin rash associated with Lyme disease. *Erythema marginatum* can be found on the upper and lower extremities and is macular or papular. It can coalesce to form a ring shape. The edges can be flat or raised, and over time, there can be central clearing. This rash appears in about 15 percent of people with rheumatic fever.

✔ **Minor criteria:** The minor Jones criteria can include fever, joint pain, an elevated white cell count on a CBC, laboratory evidence of inflammation (including a high sed rate), and signs of conduction block on a ECG. (See Chapter 3 for ECG images.)

If you have one minor criterion and two of the major criteria in the setting of a recent *Strep* infection, you have your diagnosis of rheumatic fever.

Rheumatic fever as a new diagnosis is rare these days, because many *Strep* infections are caught and treated early. The initial treatments consist of antibiotics, including penicillin, as well as medications to reduce inflammation. Sometimes prednisone is given.

Botulism: An illness patients can avoid

Botulism is caused by *Clostridium botulinum*. The clinical scenario is eating something from a damaged can or from an improperly home-canned product, either a vegetable or a meat product, and getting sick. Within several hours (and up to a day afterwards), nasty symptoms can develop, including vision problems and gastrointestinal upset. The really bad symptoms include paralysis and respiratory failure. That's approximately equal to death. Other symptoms can include problems with talking or swallowing food — these symptoms represent the body's muscles becoming paralyzed because of the botulinum toxin. The paralysis is so bad that the affected person needs to be put on a ventilator. The treatment is the administration of antitoxin.

In addition to acquiring botulism from eating contaminated canned food, someone can acquire botulism from an infected wound.

Tetanus: Getting the lowdown on lockjaw

Tetanus, also known as *lockjaw,* is caused by the bacterium *Clostridium tetani,* which is found in the soil. It usually gets into a body through some kind of injury, such as by stepping on a rusty nail.

The bacteria make a toxin that can produce significant muscle spasms, which begin in the jaw and spread. The muscle spasms can become more intense, so strong that they can actually cause a tear in the muscle. Muscle rigidity increases. The person can have difficulty swallowing. Sometimes a person can present with seizures.

The treatment for tetanus is antibiotics, usually penicillin or metronidazole (Flagyl). If you see a PANCE question about treating tetanus and one of the answer choices is metronidazole, pick it. Benzodiazepines can help relax the muscles. The most important treatment for tetanus is the administration of immunoglobulin.

A question that you may see on the PANCE is whether or when a person needs a tetanus shot. Be aware of some of the newer recommendations:

- ✔ If someone hasn't been vaccinated before, he or she needs to have a tetanus, pertussis, and diphtheria (TPD) vaccination, with a tetanus booster to be given every 10 years after that.

- ✔ The DTaP (diphtheria, tetanus, and acellular pertussis) vaccination is given to children five times: at ages 2 months, 4 months, 6 months, 15 to 18 months, and 4 to 6 years.

- ✔ The Tdap is the booster shot, given to adolescents and adults (ages 11 to 64). It confers immunity to tetanus, diphtheria, and pertussis. People should get this shot every 10 years.

Diphtheria: A disease on the decline

Diphtheria is a condition you may have heard your grandparents or great-grandparents talk about when they discussed their childhoods. Before immunization, it was a common cause of death. The United States had an estimated 100,000 to 200,000 cases in the 1920s. In the period from 2000 to 2007, there were only 3 cases! Not being vaccinated is a serious risk factor for acquiring diphtheria. ("Two, four, six, eight! It always pays to vaccinate!")

Diptheria is caused by *Corynebacterium diphtheriae*. The initial symptoms of diphtheria can resemble a common upper respiratory tract infection or pharyngitis. Then they can turn nasty. Here are some key points to remember about diphtheria:

✔ Diphtheria infection can cause the formation of a gray pseudomembrane on the pharynx of the affected person.

✔ The significant adenopathy caused by diphtheria can give the sufferer a bull-neck appearance.

✔ Diphtheria can be a cause of myocarditis.

✔ The treatment is the use of erythromycin (Emycin) or penicillin that is given intramuscularly. A specific diphtheria antitoxin is used when significant symptoms, such as a pseudomembrane, develop.

Figuring Out the Fungus among Us

The fungal infections in this chapter can be serious, causing bacteremia as well as affecting specific organs, including the lung. Some of the organisms are opportunistic infections and can wreak havoc in someone with a weaker immune system. For the PANCE, you should be aware of four different fungal conditions: pneumocystis, histoplasmosis, cryptococcosis, and candidiasis. You see several of these with increasing prevalence with an advanced HIV infection. (For information on superficial fungal infections, flip to Chapter 17, where we discuss dermatology.)

Knowing pneumocystis

Pneumocystis jirovecii (formerly known as *Pneumocystis carinii*) is an infection in the lung, usually in people who are immunosuppressed. A common clinical test scenario involves someone who's a solid organ transplant patient or who has advanced HIV and presents with shortness of breath.

Here are some key points concerning *Pneumocystis jirovecii*:

✔ It's often seen in an HIV patient with a CD4 count of 250 or less.

✔ A chest radiograph can show diffuse bilateral infiltrates. This pneumonia can be very destructive.

✔ This pneumonia can be characterized by an elevated LDH level.

✔ The initial treatment of choice is intravenous trimethoprim/sulfamethoxazole (Bactrim). If the patient has a sulfa allergy, the next treatment of choice is pentamidine.

✔ If you encounter a test question in which the person is hypoxemic with a very low pO_2 and low oxygen saturation, he or she needs intravenous steroids in addition to the trimethoprim/sulfamethoxazole.

Digging into histoplasmosis

Histoplasmosis is also known as *Ohio Valley disease* or *cave disease*. It mainly affects the lungs. If a test question mentions that the patient lives (or has lived) in the Ohio River Valley or near the Mississippi River, start thinking about histoplasmosis. The person presents with shortness of breath and may have a cough or flu-like symptoms.

Histoplasmosis is caused by *Histoplasma capsulatum,* a fungus that's found in soil that contains infected bird or bat feces. Here are some key points about histoplasmosis:

- ✔ Histoplasmosis primarily affects the lung. The chest radiograph can show a "bullet-like" appearance.

- ✔ Histoplasmosis can affect areas other than the lungs, producing bone and joint infections and pericarditis.

- ✔ The person can be put on oral itraconazole if he or she is an outpatient. If the person is admitted to the hospital, he or she is put on amphotericin B.

Sticking your neck out to diagnose cryptococcus

Cryptococcus infection is caused by the fungus *Cryptococcus neoformans.* A common clinical scenario involves someone with a headache with fever and nuchal rigidity. For PANCE purposes, be aware that *Cryptococcus* can cause a severe form of meningitis, especially in people who are immunosuppressed. The treatment is amphotericin B initially and then an oral fluconazole (Diflucan).

Which one of the following is an adverse effect associated with amphotericin B?

(A) Heart failure

(B) Liver failure

(C) Bone marrow toxicity

(D) Kidney failure

(E) Lung fibrosis

The correct answer is Choice (D). In someone who's being treated with amphotericin B, the main side effect is kidney disease. In addition, the drug can cause low potassium and low magnesium. Anyone on amphotericin B needs to be treated with intravenous saline to reduce the risk of kidney disease.

Correcting candidiasis

Candidiasis is a fungal infection produced mainly by *Candida albicans,* although there are many species of *Candida.* This not-so-friendly fungus pops up in Chapters 5, 9, and 17. In someone with uncontrolled diabetes, the first manifestation can be recurrent fungal or yeast infections. People who are immunosuppressed can have *Candida* esophagitis. And this fungus is one of three big causes of vaginitis. It looks wretched on the tongue or skin.

In addition to diabetes and immunosuppression (think HIV here as well), another risk factor is overuse of antibiotics. Antibiotics can really disrupt bowel flora and promote candidal overgrowth. Total parenteral nutrition (TPN) can also increase the risk of getting a fungal infection.

For *Candida* vulvovaginitis, the recommended treatment is one dose of fluconazole (Diflucan) 150 mg or a topical miconazole cream (Monistat) applied twice a day. For *Candida*-induced esophagitis, the recommended treatment is intravenous fluconazole (Diflucan).

Viewing the Viral Syndromes

There are many viral syndromes that you not only need to know about but likely have been exposed to during your life and medical career. Thank the stars for immunity! In this section, you read about those viral syndromes, some of which we touch on in other chapters in this book.

Contemplating cytomegalovirus

Cytomegalovirus (CMV) is one of those viruses that can affect a lot of organs. From the liver to the eye to the intestine, it can cause much badness, to use professional medical terminology. Here are some key points about cytomegalovirus-related infection:

- Cytomegalovirus infections are commonly seen in people with a suppressed immune system. Classic examples include people who've received solid organ transplants, those on chemotherapy, and people with HIV.

- When cytomegalovirus affects the eyes, it can cause a chorioretinitis, which can result in vision loss. You see this condition in very advanced HIV infection.

- Although cytomegalovirus can occur anywhere along the gastrointestinal tract (see Chapter 5), common clinical manifestations include cytomegalovirus esophagitis and cytomegalovirus colitis.

- Cytomegalovirus can affect the liver and cause cytomegalovirus-induced hepatitis, usually a transaminitis.

- You can diagnose either by culturing the affected tissue or by measuring antibody levels in blood. A common test for antibodies is the enzyme-linked immunosorbent assay (ELISA).

- Under a microscope, you can see inclusion bodies in white blood cells that are definitive for cytomegalovirus.

Treating cytomegalovirus involves medications such as ganciclovir (Cytovene) and valganciclovir (Valcyte). These meds are usually first-line. When these two can't be used, you can use foscarnet. The main side effect of ganciclovir is neutropenia, and one of the main side effects of foscarnet is hypocalcemia.

Minimizing herpes recurrences

You've likely heard the joke concerning the difference between love and herpes: "Herpes is forever." Once you have it, you have it. The goal is to prevent recurrent exacerbations.

There are two herpes simplex viruses:

- HSV-1 is a common cause of mouth ulcers, gingival infections, and pharyngitis. HSV-1 is usually transmitted via kissing.

- HSV-2 is a cause of genital herpes. The key is in looking for herpetic lesions in the mouth or in the genital area.

Medical professionals used to simplify the diagnosis by assuming that HSV-1 occurred above the waist and HSV-2 occurred below the waist. However, sexual behaviors determine the spread of the virus, and either type can be found in each of these areas and can cause symptoms there.

The treatment for herpes simplex virus is similar to treatment for varicella (see the next section). Commonly prescribed medications include acyclovir (Zovirax) and famciclovir (Famvir). There are distinct regimens for acute outbreaks and for reduction of transmission to partners.

With some of these infectious diseases, be aware of the histologic findings that can be in a question. With herpes simplex virus, you're looking for a Tzanck smear showing large cells with multiple nuclei. With cytomegalovirus, you can see inclusion bodies that have an "owl's-eye" appearance. With human papillomavirus (see Chapter 9), you can see koilocytes on a Pap smear.

Identifying varicella's painful lesions

You may see the scenario of an older person who presents with pain in an extremity or along the trunk. The pain follows a dermatomal distribution. On examination, you see skin lesions that can be in various stages: Many are vesicular, and many of them may be crusted over. In addition, the person may have early lesions that are macular in nature. The bottom line is that you remember the vesicular lesions in a dermatomal pattern that can hurt like the dickens in an older person. That's varicella-zoster virus (VZV), also known as *shingles,* in a nutshell.

Here are a few key points concerning varicella:

- ✔ It occurs very commonly in older adults because they have lowered immune systems. It can also occur in anyone who is immunocompromised.

- ✔ The lesions typically occur in a dermatomal distribution because the virus can stay dormant in nerve cells for a long time and recur when the immune defenses are lowered.

- ✔ People who are affected with varicella are given acyclovir (Zovirax) or a derivative thereof. To be most effective, this med usually needs to be given within 24 hours of when the rash began.

- ✔ People over the age of 60 should get a varicella vaccination, which is just one injection.

- ✔ In children, varicella-zoster is a cause of chicken pox. The clinical presentation is similar to that of shingles (that is, vesicular skin lesions in a dermatomal distribution). If the child received the varicella vaccine, he or she can still get chicken pox, but it's a milder form. The antiviral medications typically given to adults with shingles aren't typically given to children unless their immune systems aren't intact or they have significant underlying lung disease.

Be aware that significant nerve pain can occur with varicella, often after the acute flare is over. This is called *post-herpetic neuralgia,* and it can be debilitating. Medications used to treat this pain can include the tricyclic antidepressants, gabapentin (Neurontin), and topical capsaicin (Zostrix).

Knowing what Epstein-Barr leads to

Epstein-Barr virus (EBV) is the cause of mononucleosis, and infectious mononucleosis is a cause of viral pharyngitis, with posterior cervical adenopathy, exudative pharyngitis, and atypical lymphocytes later in the course of the disease. With mono, you also see splenomegaly, which also occurs in other EBV-related diseases. With severe Epstein-Barr virus, you can also see an autoimmune hemolytic anemia and a thrombocytopenia.

Epstein-Barr virus isn't a cause of just mono. It can also cause hepatitis, which is characterized by elevated liver enzymes. Epstein-Barr virus has been implicated in certain malignancies and lymphoproliferative disorders, including Burkitt's lymphoma, because high viral titers have been found in patients. In people who have undergone solid organ transplants, Epstein-Barr virus has been linked to a lymphoma that can occur post-transplant.

Titers of the virus can be ordered (look for an IgM titer, not so much an IgG, because everyone walking around likely has antibodies to Epstein-Barr virus). A monospot test can be ordered early on in the disease process. The treatment for Epstein-Barr virus is supportive.

Keeping up with kids' viruses

All the viruses in this section affect children, especially if they haven't been immunized. Although adults can acquire these viruses, for the PANCE, think of them as causing childhood diseases.

- ✔ **Measles:** Measles is a highly contagious viral syndrome characterized by certain clinical findings. Like all viral syndromes, initial symptoms include fever, cough, and upper respiratory tract infection symptoms. The fever usually lasts 3 to 4 days. In addition, the child has a diffuse rash that's maculopapular in nature. Measles is transmitted via respiratory droplets.

  One of the hallmarks of measles is the presence of *Koplik spots,* which are white lesions found in the mouth, often before measles begins.

- ✔ **Mumps:** Mumps can be summed up by the -itises: parotitis, orchitis, and sometimes pancreatitis. The most common clinical finding is significant parotitis. As with measles, the child can also have a fever and a skin rash. Like measles, mumps is transmitted via respiratory droplets. An infected person is able to transmit the virus for at least 1 week after acquiring the disease.

- ✔ **Rubella:** Rubella is another virus transmitted by respiratory droplets. Also known as German measles, it's also associated with a skin rash. The rash is erythematous and papular.

  Be aware that rubella can be transmitted from mother to fetus, leading to *congenital rubella syndrome.* It can cause multiple birth defects and can affect the heart and brain, among other body organs.

  The MMR (measles, mumps, and rubella) inoculation that children get between 12 and 15 months of age confers immunity to measles, mumps, and rubella. Because of the MMR vaccine, rubella is now a very uncommon illness.

- ✔ **Erythema infectiosum:** Erythema infectiosum, which is caused by parvovirus B19, is also called *fifth disease.* The classic physical finding for this condition is a characteristic skin rash on the cheeks, lending a "slapped-cheek" appearance. The rash has often been described as "lace-like." The child also has maculopapular appearance on the arms and legs.

- ✔ **Roseola:** Roseola, also known as *sixth disease,* is a viral infection that affects infants, generally from 4 to 12 months of age. Roseola is caused by human herpes virus 6 (HHV-6B). Initially, the child has flu-like symptoms. In addition, he or she may have conjunctivitis and high fevers. After about 2 to 3 days, the child develops a characteristic skin rash that begins on the chest and spreads over the body to include the upper and lower extremities. In addition to the rash, one big characteristic is that the affected child looks relatively nontoxic despite the high fevers. Roseola is usually self-resolving after a few days.

Why do we have a fifth and a sixth disease? They're part of the historical classification of childhood rashes: 1) measles, 2) scarlet fever, 3) rubella, 4) Duke's disease, 5) fifth disease (erythema infectiosum), and 6) sixth disease (roseola).

Which one of the following is associated with parvovirus B19?

(A) Asymmetric polyarthritis

(B) Diarrhea

(C) Hemolytic anemia

(D) Kidney failure

(E) Lung fibrosis

The correct answer is Choice (A). For PANCE purposes, parvovirus B19 can do three things: It can cause erythema infectiosum, it can cause asymmetric polyarthritis in young women, and it can cause aplastic anemia in someone diagnosed with sickle cell anemia.

Handling HIV

For the PANCE, you should be familiar with some general stuff concerning HIV, specific infections related to HIV, and side effects of certain medications. HIV is such a big topic that we gave it its own section separate from the other viral syndromes.

HIV stands for *human immunodeficiency virus.* Risk factors for acquiring HIV include high-risk sexual behavior (unprotected sex) and drug abuse, especially intravenous use with dirty needles. Coming into contact with contaminated blood from someone with HIV is also a cause, which is a special concern for healthcare workers.

Almost right after someone is infected, he or she may experience an *acute syndrome* related to the HIV infection. It can cause typical flu-like symptoms, with gastrointestinal upset, sore throat, fever, muscle aches, and joint pains. You may also see neuropathy and a skin rash.

Testing for HIV includes an initial enzyme-linked immunosorbent assay (ELISA), followed by the confirmatory western blot. The big issue with HIV is establishing how well the immune system is functioning, which you do by ordering a CD4 count and a plasma HIV RNA level.

The lower the CD4 count, the higher the risk of acquiring certain infections. HIV also involves an acquired deficiency of T cells, which are important for conferring cellular immunity.

The treatment, which is a science in and of itself, has transformed the lives of millions of people. It involves using different categories of medications, including protease inhibitors, reverse transcriptase inhibitors, and others. Here are four high-yield items about HIV meds you should know for the test:

- ✔ Zidovudine (AZT) causes a macrocytic anemia. You can see a mean corpuscular volume (MCV) > 100 in someone on this medication. Folate replacement may be needed.

- ✔ Didanosine (DDI, brand name Videx) causes pancreatitis.

- ✔ Tenofovir disoproxil fumarate (TDF, brand name Viread) causes acute kidney failure.

- ✔ Indinavir (Crixivan) causes kidney stones.

Some PANCE questions concern infections, especially at the lower CD4 counts. These infections include toxoplasmosis and atypical mycobacterial infections. They're rampant in the HIV population, and the majority of test questions about infections are likely to involve underlying HIV. Here are some key points related to infections:

✔ A normal CD4 count is ≥ 500 cells. The risk for many opportunistic infections occurs when the CD4 count falls below 250. A CD4 count of < 200 is considered diagnostic for AIDS.

✔ Remember the four *c*'s, which you can see in advanced HIV: *Candida*, *Cryptococcus*, *Cryptosporidium*, and *CMV* (cytomegalovirus). *Cryptosporidium* is a cause of infectious diarrhea in someone with advanced HIV. You can read about the other three conditions in the earlier sections on fungal and viral infections.

✔ Toxoplasmosis is caused by a parasite. Cats are actually the ones primarily infected, because *Toxoplasma gondii* shows up in their feces. Someone who deals with cats and doesn't wash his or her hands can become infected. In someone with HIV, the infections are potentially fatal. This parasite can cause encephalitis. On a CT scan of the head with contrast, toxoplasmosis has been described as a "ring-enhancing lesion." The treatment for toxoplasmosis is a combination of pyrimethamine (Daraprim) and sulfadiazine (Lantrisul).

In someone with a low CD4 count, trimethoprim/sulfamethoxazole (Bactrim) is used for pneumocystis and toxoplasmosis prophylaxis.

Tuberculosis and atypical mycobacterial disease are more prevalent in the HIV population. We discuss tuberculosis at length in Chapter 4. Concerning atypical mycobacterial infections, the big one to be familiar with is the *Mycobacterium avium* complex (MAC). You can see this infection in advanced HIV, with CD4 counts < 50. The most glaring presenting symptom of a MAC attack is significant adenopathy. It can disseminate and can cause gastrointestinal problems, including ulcers and diarrhea. It can also cause joint and muscle infections.

Treatments can include macrolide antibiotics, rifabutin, and the fluoroquinolones. Rifabutin and clarithromycin (Biaxin) seem to be the more popular meds asked about in test questions.

Looking at Parasites That Worm Their Way In

You don't want to be called a parasite any more than you want to have one. Recall that *parasitism* is a nonmutual relationship in which the parasite benefits at the expense of the host. In this section, you read about malaria, pinworms, and helminths (flukes, tapeworms, roundworms, and the like).

Meeting malaria

Someone contracts malaria after being bitten by an infected mosquito. These mosquitoes usually live in Asia, Africa, and South America and are carrying an infectious bug from the genus *Plasmodium* — technically, a eukaryotic protist.

When these little parasitic creatures get into the bloodstream, they can stay dormant in the liver for a while, and then they wreak havoc. They can affect multiple body systems, including the liver, blood cells, and kidney.

Signs and symptoms of malaria can include gastrointestinal upset, fever, icterus, hematochezia, myopathy, and even seizures. Labs can confirm the presence of a hemolytic anemia. You may see hepatosplenomegaly on physical examination or on imaging studies.

With malaria, you need to order a special malarial peripheral blood smear called a *thick and thin blood smear.* On this smear, you're looking for the presence of parasites. This test can be repeated, and repeating the test is necessary if the initial smears are negative and you have a high clinical suspicion of malaria.

Medications such as chloroquine, the antibiotic doxycycline (Vibramycin), and atovaquone are frequently used together because of the high incidence of resistance to treatment. The atovaquone/proguanil combination (Malarone) can be used for malaria prophylaxis as well. If a patient is planning travel to areas where malaria is endemic, remind him or her to check the CDC's travelers' health website (www.cdc.gov/travel/).

Make sure you know the type of malaria you're dealing with. The *Plasmodium* genus contains 200 known species, and at least 11 of them love humans. The most common species are *Plasmodium falciparum* and *Plasmodium vivax. Plasmodium falciparum* is the most deadly, with the highest rate of fatalities compared to the other forms.

Eliminating pinworms

The most common pinworm is the *Enterobius vermicularis.* You can eliminate pinworms by eliminating them, but that doesn't eliminate them. Is this a Buddhist kōan? Nope.

Pinworms are parasites that you acquire by eating them. The pinworm replicates in the gastrointestinal system. Then the pinworm lays its eggs in the anal region, where the person eliminates. From there, with the action of wiping or cleaning the anus, the eggs get on the hands and can spread to anything the person touches. This usually happens with children, who may be careless about wiping — and washing — after a bowel movement. Diagnosis may be confirmed by visual inspection of the pinworms around the anus or a cellophane tape test in an attempt to identify the ovum or parasites.

The medication used to treat pinworms, albendazole (Albenza), eliminates them. It often needs to be administered for several months because there's a high risk of reinfection, even when you're treating this condition with medication. Hygiene, washing hands in particular, is very important in preventing reinfection. In addition, clothes should be washed frequently.

Facing creepy, crawly helminths

Helminths (parasitic worms) fall into four groups: monogeneans, cestodes (tapeworms), nematodes (roundworms), and trematodes (flukes). The trematodes include *Necator americanus* (hookworm) and parasites in the genus *Schistosoma,* which cause snail fever and other conditions.

Depending on the type of helminth you're dealing with, symptoms can include liver failure, biliary problems, and intestinal issues. The tapeworm can cause malabsorption and other intestinal problems.

Only certain medications can be used to treat helminth infections. Examples are albendazole (Albenza) and mebendazole (Vermox).

Practice Infectious Disease Questions

These practice questions are similar to the PANCE infectious disease questions.

1. You're evaluating a 35-year-old man who presents with arthritis, fever, urethritis, and conjunctivitis. This has been occurring a few days. He states that about a week ago, he came down with what felt like a viral bug that went away. What is the likely cause of this person's symptoms?

   (A) *Enterobius vermicularis*

   (B) *Plasmodium falciparum*

   (C) Schistosomiasis

   (D) *Shigella flexneri*

   (E) Rotavirus

2. Which one of the following would be used to treat tetanus?

   (A) Fluconazole (Diflucan)

   (B) Prednisone (Deltasone)

   (C) Metronidazole (Flagyl)

   (D) Doxycycline (Vibramycin)

   (E) Azithromycin (Zithromax)

3. You're evaluating a 55-year-old man with advanced HIV who presents with significant diarrhea. He has a CD4 count of 100. What is the likely cause of his diarrhea?

   (A) *Cryptosporidium*

   (B) *Cryptococcus*

   (C) Norwalk virus (norovirus)

   (D) *Giardia*

   (E) *Salmonella*

4. Which one of the following is a criterion for rheumatic fever?

   (A) Erythema migrans

   (B) Erythema nodosum

   (C) Leukopenia

   (D) Erythema marginatum

   (E) Meningitis

5. Which of the following is recommended for treating a *Chlamydia trachomatis* infection?

   (A) Metronidazole (Flagyl)

   (B) Diflucan (Fluconazole)

   (C) Azithromycin (Zithromax)

   (D) Gentamicin

   (E) Amoxicillin (Trimox)

6. Which one of the following is recommended for treating Rocky Mountain spotted fever?

   (A) Metronidazole (Flagyl)

   (B) Doxycycline (Vibramycin)

   (C) Azithromycin (Zithromax)

   (D) Diflucan (Fluconazole)

   (E) Amoxicillin (Trimox)

Answers and Explanations

Use this answer key to score the practice infectious disease questions from the preceding section. The answer explanations give you some insight into why the correct answer is better than the other choices.

1. **D.** This man has reactive arthritis, or Reiter's syndrome, likely caused by *Shigella flexneri*. Reiter's is a reactive illness that occurs after being infected by *Shigella*. Choices (A) and (C), *Enterobius vermicularis* and schistosomiasis, are parasitic diseases that would present with ongoing intestinal symptoms. Choice (B), *Plasmodium falciparum*, is one of the most common causes of malaria; it causes flu-like symptoms and icterus. Rotavirus, Choice (E), is a common cause of diarrhea in children.

2. **C.** Choice (C), metronidazole, is the treatment of choice for tetanus. Choices (A) and (B), fluconazole and prednisone, are an antifungal and a steroid, respectively. They aren't used in the treatment of tetanus, which is caused by a bacteria, *Clostridium tetani*. Choice (D), doxycycline, is used in treating Lyme disease. Choice (E), azithromycin, is used in treating community-acquired pneumonia.

3. **A.** This person likely has a *Cryptosporidium* protozoan in him. This parasite is the most common cause of diarrhea you'd expect, given his HIV status and the fact that his CD4 count is less than 200. Choice (B), *Cryptococcus*, is a cause of meningitis. Choice (C), norovirus, is a common viral cause of diarrhea in children. Don't forget norovirus outbreaks on cruise ships, too. Choice (D), *Giardia*, is a protozoan parasite that can cause diarrhea; it's usually related to infected well water. Choice (E), *Salmonella*, is a bacterial cause of diarrhea.

4. **D.** Erythema marginatum, a characteristic skin rash, is a criterion for rheumatic fever. Choice (A), erythema migrans, is seen with Lyme disease. Choice (B), erythema nodosum, occurs with sarcoidosis and other rheumatologic diseases. Choice (C), leukopenia, isn't a criterion for rheumatic fever; leukocytosis, not leukopenia, is a minor criterion. Meningitis, Choice (E), isn't a criterion for rheumatic fever, either.

5. **C.** There are two treatments for *Chlamydia* infection: One is giving one dose of azithromycin, and the other is 7 days' worth of doxycycline twice a day.

6. **B.** The treatment for Rocky Mountain spotted fever is doxycycline.

Part VI
Tackling a PANCE Practice Test

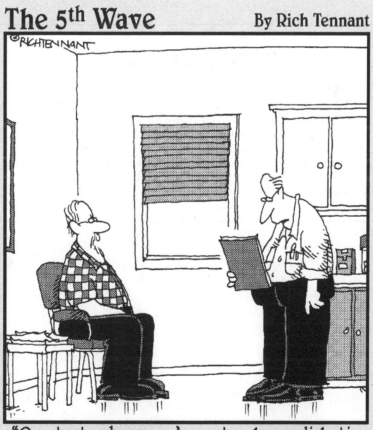

The 5th Wave   By Rich Tennant

"Our tests show you're not only prediabetic,
you're also preeminent, predictable,
and precocious."

In this part . . .

The practice questions in the various chapters are important, but are you ready for a full practice test? Chapter 20 has a complete 300-question practice PANCE, and Chapter 21 explains the correct answers. When you're ready for even more practice, you can take the three digital PANCEs and digital PANRE that came with this book.

Chapter 20

PANCE Practice Test

*T*est preparation books have practice tests, and this book is no exception. This chapter contains a complete PANCE practice test. It has five blocks of 60 questions each. The idea is to approach this test as you would the real PANCE exam. Try to simulate as many exam conditions as you can by following these guidelines:

- ✔ Find a quiet place, such as a library or an isolated room in your home, to take the test. A bustling coffee shop won't work for this exercise.

- ✔ Don't use any study aids, including references, notes, or a calculator. Use nothing but a pencil.

- ✔ You have 60 minutes to complete each block. If you finish a block early, you may go on to another.

- ✔ If you want to truly imitate the real test, take all the blocks in a row. You may take any portion of the allotted 45 minutes for breaks between blocks.

- ✔ Don't eat or drink anything during the practice test, because that won't be allowed on the real test. You can use your break time to eat and answer nature's calls. Do not consult a reference or make any cell calls during your breaks.

Here are some handy test-taking tips:

- ✔ Try to answer the questions in the order they appear, without skipping any. You can pass on an answer and come back to it, but we think that's dangerous. You may have too little time near the end of the hour to return to skipped questions.

- ✔ Yes, you can change answers, but only in the block you're currently working on. No going back to previous blocks or jumping ahead to the next one. That's the way it works during the real PANCE.

- ✔ If you finish the block before the 60 minutes are up, recheck your answers. If you've opted to skip some questions, go back and answer them.

- ✔ Try not to look at the answer explanations (found in Chapter 21) until you've completed the entire block. We won't ask you to complete the entire test (unless you really want to imitate the real test experience), because that would mean a five-hour delay before you started checking.

The answers to the five blocks in this chapter are in Chapter 21.

This book provides three additional digital PANCE practice tests and one additional digital PANRE practice test. You can find these tests on the CD that accompanies this book. If you are using a digital or enhanced digital version of this book, go to http://booksupport.wiley.com to access the additional content.

Answer Sheet for PANCE Practice Test

Block 1

1 Ⓐ Ⓑ Ⓒ Ⓓ Ⓔ	21 Ⓐ Ⓑ Ⓒ Ⓓ Ⓔ	41 Ⓐ Ⓑ Ⓒ Ⓓ Ⓔ
2 Ⓐ Ⓑ Ⓒ Ⓓ Ⓔ	22 Ⓐ Ⓑ Ⓒ Ⓓ Ⓔ	42 Ⓐ Ⓑ Ⓒ Ⓓ Ⓔ
3 Ⓐ Ⓑ Ⓒ Ⓓ Ⓔ	23 Ⓐ Ⓑ Ⓒ Ⓓ Ⓔ	43 Ⓐ Ⓑ Ⓒ Ⓓ Ⓔ
4 Ⓐ Ⓑ Ⓒ Ⓓ Ⓔ	24 Ⓐ Ⓑ Ⓒ Ⓓ Ⓔ	44 Ⓐ Ⓑ Ⓒ Ⓓ Ⓔ
5 Ⓐ Ⓑ Ⓒ Ⓓ Ⓔ	25 Ⓐ Ⓑ Ⓒ Ⓓ Ⓔ	45 Ⓐ Ⓑ Ⓒ Ⓓ Ⓔ
6 Ⓐ Ⓑ Ⓒ Ⓓ Ⓔ	26 Ⓐ Ⓑ Ⓒ Ⓓ Ⓔ	46 Ⓐ Ⓑ Ⓒ Ⓓ Ⓔ
7 Ⓐ Ⓑ Ⓒ Ⓓ Ⓔ	27 Ⓐ Ⓑ Ⓒ Ⓓ Ⓔ	47 Ⓐ Ⓑ Ⓒ Ⓓ Ⓔ
8 Ⓐ Ⓑ Ⓒ Ⓓ Ⓔ	28 Ⓐ Ⓑ Ⓒ Ⓓ Ⓔ	48 Ⓐ Ⓑ Ⓒ Ⓓ Ⓔ
9 Ⓐ Ⓑ Ⓒ Ⓓ Ⓔ	29 Ⓐ Ⓑ Ⓒ Ⓓ Ⓔ	49 Ⓐ Ⓑ Ⓒ Ⓓ Ⓔ
10 Ⓐ Ⓑ Ⓒ Ⓓ Ⓔ	30 Ⓐ Ⓑ Ⓒ Ⓓ Ⓔ	50 Ⓐ Ⓑ Ⓒ Ⓓ Ⓔ
11 Ⓐ Ⓑ Ⓒ Ⓓ Ⓔ	31 Ⓐ Ⓑ Ⓒ Ⓓ Ⓔ	51 Ⓐ Ⓑ Ⓒ Ⓓ Ⓔ
12 Ⓐ Ⓑ Ⓒ Ⓓ Ⓔ	32 Ⓐ Ⓑ Ⓒ Ⓓ Ⓔ	52 Ⓐ Ⓑ Ⓒ Ⓓ Ⓔ
13 Ⓐ Ⓑ Ⓒ Ⓓ Ⓔ	33 Ⓐ Ⓑ Ⓒ Ⓓ Ⓔ	53 Ⓐ Ⓑ Ⓒ Ⓓ Ⓔ
14 Ⓐ Ⓑ Ⓒ Ⓓ Ⓔ	34 Ⓐ Ⓑ Ⓒ Ⓓ Ⓔ	54 Ⓐ Ⓑ Ⓒ Ⓓ Ⓔ
15 Ⓐ Ⓑ Ⓒ Ⓓ Ⓔ	35 Ⓐ Ⓑ Ⓒ Ⓓ Ⓔ	55 Ⓐ Ⓑ Ⓒ Ⓓ Ⓔ
16 Ⓐ Ⓑ Ⓒ Ⓓ Ⓔ	36 Ⓐ Ⓑ Ⓒ Ⓓ Ⓔ	56 Ⓐ Ⓑ Ⓒ Ⓓ Ⓔ
17 Ⓐ Ⓑ Ⓒ Ⓓ Ⓔ	37 Ⓐ Ⓑ Ⓒ Ⓓ Ⓔ	57 Ⓐ Ⓑ Ⓒ Ⓓ Ⓔ
18 Ⓐ Ⓑ Ⓒ Ⓓ Ⓔ	38 Ⓐ Ⓑ Ⓒ Ⓓ Ⓔ	58 Ⓐ Ⓑ Ⓒ Ⓓ Ⓔ
19 Ⓐ Ⓑ Ⓒ Ⓓ Ⓔ	39 Ⓐ Ⓑ Ⓒ Ⓓ Ⓔ	59 Ⓐ Ⓑ Ⓒ Ⓓ Ⓔ
20 Ⓐ Ⓑ Ⓒ Ⓓ Ⓔ	40 Ⓐ Ⓑ Ⓒ Ⓓ Ⓔ	60 Ⓐ Ⓑ Ⓒ Ⓓ Ⓔ

Block 2

1 Ⓐ Ⓑ Ⓒ Ⓓ Ⓔ	21 Ⓐ Ⓑ Ⓒ Ⓓ Ⓔ	41 Ⓐ Ⓑ Ⓒ Ⓓ Ⓔ
2 Ⓐ Ⓑ Ⓒ Ⓓ Ⓔ	22 Ⓐ Ⓑ Ⓒ Ⓓ Ⓔ	42 Ⓐ Ⓑ Ⓒ Ⓓ Ⓔ
3 Ⓐ Ⓑ Ⓒ Ⓓ Ⓔ	23 Ⓐ Ⓑ Ⓒ Ⓓ Ⓔ	43 Ⓐ Ⓑ Ⓒ Ⓓ Ⓔ
4 Ⓐ Ⓑ Ⓒ Ⓓ Ⓔ	24 Ⓐ Ⓑ Ⓒ Ⓓ Ⓔ	44 Ⓐ Ⓑ Ⓒ Ⓓ Ⓔ
5 Ⓐ Ⓑ Ⓒ Ⓓ Ⓔ	25 Ⓐ Ⓑ Ⓒ Ⓓ Ⓔ	45 Ⓐ Ⓑ Ⓒ Ⓓ Ⓔ
6 Ⓐ Ⓑ Ⓒ Ⓓ Ⓔ	26 Ⓐ Ⓑ Ⓒ Ⓓ Ⓔ	46 Ⓐ Ⓑ Ⓒ Ⓓ Ⓔ
7 Ⓐ Ⓑ Ⓒ Ⓓ Ⓔ	27 Ⓐ Ⓑ Ⓒ Ⓓ Ⓔ	47 Ⓐ Ⓑ Ⓒ Ⓓ Ⓔ
8 Ⓐ Ⓑ Ⓒ Ⓓ Ⓔ	28 Ⓐ Ⓑ Ⓒ Ⓓ Ⓔ	48 Ⓐ Ⓑ Ⓒ Ⓓ Ⓔ
9 Ⓐ Ⓑ Ⓒ Ⓓ Ⓔ	29 Ⓐ Ⓑ Ⓒ Ⓓ Ⓔ	49 Ⓐ Ⓑ Ⓒ Ⓓ Ⓔ
10 Ⓐ Ⓑ Ⓒ Ⓓ Ⓔ	30 Ⓐ Ⓑ Ⓒ Ⓓ Ⓔ	50 Ⓐ Ⓑ Ⓒ Ⓓ Ⓔ
11 Ⓐ Ⓑ Ⓒ Ⓓ Ⓔ	31 Ⓐ Ⓑ Ⓒ Ⓓ Ⓔ	51 Ⓐ Ⓑ Ⓒ Ⓓ Ⓔ
12 Ⓐ Ⓑ Ⓒ Ⓓ Ⓔ	32 Ⓐ Ⓑ Ⓒ Ⓓ Ⓔ	52 Ⓐ Ⓑ Ⓒ Ⓓ Ⓔ
13 Ⓐ Ⓑ Ⓒ Ⓓ Ⓔ	33 Ⓐ Ⓑ Ⓒ Ⓓ Ⓔ	53 Ⓐ Ⓑ Ⓒ Ⓓ Ⓔ
14 Ⓐ Ⓑ Ⓒ Ⓓ Ⓔ	34 Ⓐ Ⓑ Ⓒ Ⓓ Ⓔ	54 Ⓐ Ⓑ Ⓒ Ⓓ Ⓔ
15 Ⓐ Ⓑ Ⓒ Ⓓ Ⓔ	35 Ⓐ Ⓑ Ⓒ Ⓓ Ⓔ	55 Ⓐ Ⓑ Ⓒ Ⓓ Ⓔ
16 Ⓐ Ⓑ Ⓒ Ⓓ Ⓔ	36 Ⓐ Ⓑ Ⓒ Ⓓ Ⓔ	56 Ⓐ Ⓑ Ⓒ Ⓓ Ⓔ
17 Ⓐ Ⓑ Ⓒ Ⓓ Ⓔ	37 Ⓐ Ⓑ Ⓒ Ⓓ Ⓔ	57 Ⓐ Ⓑ Ⓒ Ⓓ Ⓔ
18 Ⓐ Ⓑ Ⓒ Ⓓ Ⓔ	38 Ⓐ Ⓑ Ⓒ Ⓓ Ⓔ	58 Ⓐ Ⓑ Ⓒ Ⓓ Ⓔ
19 Ⓐ Ⓑ Ⓒ Ⓓ Ⓔ	39 Ⓐ Ⓑ Ⓒ Ⓓ Ⓔ	59 Ⓐ Ⓑ Ⓒ Ⓓ Ⓔ
20 Ⓐ Ⓑ Ⓒ Ⓓ Ⓔ	40 Ⓐ Ⓑ Ⓒ Ⓓ Ⓔ	60 Ⓐ Ⓑ Ⓒ Ⓓ Ⓔ

Block 3

1 Ⓐ Ⓑ Ⓒ Ⓓ Ⓔ	21 Ⓐ Ⓑ Ⓒ Ⓓ Ⓔ	41 Ⓐ Ⓑ Ⓒ Ⓓ Ⓔ
2 Ⓐ Ⓑ Ⓒ Ⓓ Ⓔ	22 Ⓐ Ⓑ Ⓒ Ⓓ Ⓔ	42 Ⓐ Ⓑ Ⓒ Ⓓ Ⓔ
3 Ⓐ Ⓑ Ⓒ Ⓓ Ⓔ	23 Ⓐ Ⓑ Ⓒ Ⓓ Ⓔ	43 Ⓐ Ⓑ Ⓒ Ⓓ Ⓔ
4 Ⓐ Ⓑ Ⓒ Ⓓ Ⓔ	24 Ⓐ Ⓑ Ⓒ Ⓓ Ⓔ	44 Ⓐ Ⓑ Ⓒ Ⓓ Ⓔ
5 Ⓐ Ⓑ Ⓒ Ⓓ Ⓔ	25 Ⓐ Ⓑ Ⓒ Ⓓ Ⓔ	45 Ⓐ Ⓑ Ⓒ Ⓓ Ⓔ
6 Ⓐ Ⓑ Ⓒ Ⓓ Ⓔ	26 Ⓐ Ⓑ Ⓒ Ⓓ Ⓔ	46 Ⓐ Ⓑ Ⓒ Ⓓ Ⓔ
7 Ⓐ Ⓑ Ⓒ Ⓓ Ⓔ	27 Ⓐ Ⓑ Ⓒ Ⓓ Ⓔ	47 Ⓐ Ⓑ Ⓒ Ⓓ Ⓔ
8 Ⓐ Ⓑ Ⓒ Ⓓ Ⓔ	28 Ⓐ Ⓑ Ⓒ Ⓓ Ⓔ	48 Ⓐ Ⓑ Ⓒ Ⓓ Ⓔ
9 Ⓐ Ⓑ Ⓒ Ⓓ Ⓔ	29 Ⓐ Ⓑ Ⓒ Ⓓ Ⓔ	49 Ⓐ Ⓑ Ⓒ Ⓓ Ⓔ
10 Ⓐ Ⓑ Ⓒ Ⓓ Ⓔ	30 Ⓐ Ⓑ Ⓒ Ⓓ Ⓔ	50 Ⓐ Ⓑ Ⓒ Ⓓ Ⓔ
11 Ⓐ Ⓑ Ⓒ Ⓓ Ⓔ	31 Ⓐ Ⓑ Ⓒ Ⓓ Ⓔ	51 Ⓐ Ⓑ Ⓒ Ⓓ Ⓔ
12 Ⓐ Ⓑ Ⓒ Ⓓ Ⓔ	32 Ⓐ Ⓑ Ⓒ Ⓓ Ⓔ	52 Ⓐ Ⓑ Ⓒ Ⓓ Ⓔ
13 Ⓐ Ⓑ Ⓒ Ⓓ Ⓔ	33 Ⓐ Ⓑ Ⓒ Ⓓ Ⓔ	53 Ⓐ Ⓑ Ⓒ Ⓓ Ⓔ
14 Ⓐ Ⓑ Ⓒ Ⓓ Ⓔ	34 Ⓐ Ⓑ Ⓒ Ⓓ Ⓔ	54 Ⓐ Ⓑ Ⓒ Ⓓ Ⓔ
15 Ⓐ Ⓑ Ⓒ Ⓓ Ⓔ	35 Ⓐ Ⓑ Ⓒ Ⓓ Ⓔ	55 Ⓐ Ⓑ Ⓒ Ⓓ Ⓔ
16 Ⓐ Ⓑ Ⓒ Ⓓ Ⓔ	36 Ⓐ Ⓑ Ⓒ Ⓓ Ⓔ	56 Ⓐ Ⓑ Ⓒ Ⓓ Ⓔ
17 Ⓐ Ⓑ Ⓒ Ⓓ Ⓔ	37 Ⓐ Ⓑ Ⓒ Ⓓ Ⓔ	57 Ⓐ Ⓑ Ⓒ Ⓓ Ⓔ
18 Ⓐ Ⓑ Ⓒ Ⓓ Ⓔ	38 Ⓐ Ⓑ Ⓒ Ⓓ Ⓔ	58 Ⓐ Ⓑ Ⓒ Ⓓ Ⓔ
19 Ⓐ Ⓑ Ⓒ Ⓓ Ⓔ	39 Ⓐ Ⓑ Ⓒ Ⓓ Ⓔ	59 Ⓐ Ⓑ Ⓒ Ⓓ Ⓔ
20 Ⓐ Ⓑ Ⓒ Ⓓ Ⓔ	40 Ⓐ Ⓑ Ⓒ Ⓓ Ⓔ	60 Ⓐ Ⓑ Ⓒ Ⓓ Ⓔ

Block 4

1 Ⓐ Ⓑ Ⓒ Ⓓ Ⓔ	21 Ⓐ Ⓑ Ⓒ Ⓓ Ⓔ	41 Ⓐ Ⓑ Ⓒ Ⓓ Ⓔ
2 Ⓐ Ⓑ Ⓒ Ⓓ Ⓔ	22 Ⓐ Ⓑ Ⓒ Ⓓ Ⓔ	42 Ⓐ Ⓑ Ⓒ Ⓓ Ⓔ
3 Ⓐ Ⓑ Ⓒ Ⓓ Ⓔ	23 Ⓐ Ⓑ Ⓒ Ⓓ Ⓔ	43 Ⓐ Ⓑ Ⓒ Ⓓ Ⓔ
4 Ⓐ Ⓑ Ⓒ Ⓓ Ⓔ	24 Ⓐ Ⓑ Ⓒ Ⓓ Ⓔ	44 Ⓐ Ⓑ Ⓒ Ⓓ Ⓔ
5 Ⓐ Ⓑ Ⓒ Ⓓ Ⓔ	25 Ⓐ Ⓑ Ⓒ Ⓓ Ⓔ	45 Ⓐ Ⓑ Ⓒ Ⓓ Ⓔ
6 Ⓐ Ⓑ Ⓒ Ⓓ Ⓔ	26 Ⓐ Ⓑ Ⓒ Ⓓ Ⓔ	46 Ⓐ Ⓑ Ⓒ Ⓓ Ⓔ
7 Ⓐ Ⓑ Ⓒ Ⓓ Ⓔ	27 Ⓐ Ⓑ Ⓒ Ⓓ Ⓔ	47 Ⓐ Ⓑ Ⓒ Ⓓ Ⓔ
8 Ⓐ Ⓑ Ⓒ Ⓓ Ⓔ	28 Ⓐ Ⓑ Ⓒ Ⓓ Ⓔ	48 Ⓐ Ⓑ Ⓒ Ⓓ Ⓔ
9 Ⓐ Ⓑ Ⓒ Ⓓ Ⓔ	29 Ⓐ Ⓑ Ⓒ Ⓓ Ⓔ	49 Ⓐ Ⓑ Ⓒ Ⓓ Ⓔ
10 Ⓐ Ⓑ Ⓒ Ⓓ Ⓔ	30 Ⓐ Ⓑ Ⓒ Ⓓ Ⓔ	50 Ⓐ Ⓑ Ⓒ Ⓓ Ⓔ
11 Ⓐ Ⓑ Ⓒ Ⓓ Ⓔ	31 Ⓐ Ⓑ Ⓒ Ⓓ Ⓔ	51 Ⓐ Ⓑ Ⓒ Ⓓ Ⓔ
12 Ⓐ Ⓑ Ⓒ Ⓓ Ⓔ	32 Ⓐ Ⓑ Ⓒ Ⓓ Ⓔ	52 Ⓐ Ⓑ Ⓒ Ⓓ Ⓔ
13 Ⓐ Ⓑ Ⓒ Ⓓ Ⓔ	33 Ⓐ Ⓑ Ⓒ Ⓓ Ⓔ	53 Ⓐ Ⓑ Ⓒ Ⓓ Ⓔ
14 Ⓐ Ⓑ Ⓒ Ⓓ Ⓔ	34 Ⓐ Ⓑ Ⓒ Ⓓ Ⓔ	54 Ⓐ Ⓑ Ⓒ Ⓓ Ⓔ
15 Ⓐ Ⓑ Ⓒ Ⓓ Ⓔ	35 Ⓐ Ⓑ Ⓒ Ⓓ Ⓔ	55 Ⓐ Ⓑ Ⓒ Ⓓ Ⓔ
16 Ⓐ Ⓑ Ⓒ Ⓓ Ⓔ	36 Ⓐ Ⓑ Ⓒ Ⓓ Ⓔ	56 Ⓐ Ⓑ Ⓒ Ⓓ Ⓔ
17 Ⓐ Ⓑ Ⓒ Ⓓ Ⓔ	37 Ⓐ Ⓑ Ⓒ Ⓓ Ⓔ	57 Ⓐ Ⓑ Ⓒ Ⓓ Ⓔ
18 Ⓐ Ⓑ Ⓒ Ⓓ Ⓔ	38 Ⓐ Ⓑ Ⓒ Ⓓ Ⓔ	58 Ⓐ Ⓑ Ⓒ Ⓓ Ⓔ
19 Ⓐ Ⓑ Ⓒ Ⓓ Ⓔ	39 Ⓐ Ⓑ Ⓒ Ⓓ Ⓔ	59 Ⓐ Ⓑ Ⓒ Ⓓ Ⓔ
20 Ⓐ Ⓑ Ⓒ Ⓓ Ⓔ	40 Ⓐ Ⓑ Ⓒ Ⓓ Ⓔ	60 Ⓐ Ⓑ Ⓒ Ⓓ Ⓔ

Block 5

1 Ⓐ Ⓑ Ⓒ Ⓓ Ⓔ	21 Ⓐ Ⓑ Ⓒ Ⓓ Ⓔ	41 Ⓐ Ⓑ Ⓒ Ⓓ Ⓔ
2 Ⓐ Ⓑ Ⓒ Ⓓ Ⓔ	22 Ⓐ Ⓑ Ⓒ Ⓓ Ⓔ	42 Ⓐ Ⓑ Ⓒ Ⓓ Ⓔ
3 Ⓐ Ⓑ Ⓒ Ⓓ Ⓔ	23 Ⓐ Ⓑ Ⓒ Ⓓ Ⓔ	43 Ⓐ Ⓑ Ⓒ Ⓓ Ⓔ
4 Ⓐ Ⓑ Ⓒ Ⓓ Ⓔ	24 Ⓐ Ⓑ Ⓒ Ⓓ Ⓔ	44 Ⓐ Ⓑ Ⓒ Ⓓ Ⓔ
5 Ⓐ Ⓑ Ⓒ Ⓓ Ⓔ	25 Ⓐ Ⓑ Ⓒ Ⓓ Ⓔ	45 Ⓐ Ⓑ Ⓒ Ⓓ Ⓔ
6 Ⓐ Ⓑ Ⓒ Ⓓ Ⓔ	26 Ⓐ Ⓑ Ⓒ Ⓓ Ⓔ	46 Ⓐ Ⓑ Ⓒ Ⓓ Ⓔ
7 Ⓐ Ⓑ Ⓒ Ⓓ Ⓔ	27 Ⓐ Ⓑ Ⓒ Ⓓ Ⓔ	47 Ⓐ Ⓑ Ⓒ Ⓓ Ⓔ
8 Ⓐ Ⓑ Ⓒ Ⓓ Ⓔ	28 Ⓐ Ⓑ Ⓒ Ⓓ Ⓔ	48 Ⓐ Ⓑ Ⓒ Ⓓ Ⓔ
9 Ⓐ Ⓑ Ⓒ Ⓓ Ⓔ	29 Ⓐ Ⓑ Ⓒ Ⓓ Ⓔ	49 Ⓐ Ⓑ Ⓒ Ⓓ Ⓔ
10 Ⓐ Ⓑ Ⓒ Ⓓ Ⓔ	30 Ⓐ Ⓑ Ⓒ Ⓓ Ⓔ	50 Ⓐ Ⓑ Ⓒ Ⓓ Ⓔ
11 Ⓐ Ⓑ Ⓒ Ⓓ Ⓔ	31 Ⓐ Ⓑ Ⓒ Ⓓ Ⓔ	51 Ⓐ Ⓑ Ⓒ Ⓓ Ⓔ
12 Ⓐ Ⓑ Ⓒ Ⓓ Ⓔ	32 Ⓐ Ⓑ Ⓒ Ⓓ Ⓔ	52 Ⓐ Ⓑ Ⓒ Ⓓ Ⓔ
13 Ⓐ Ⓑ Ⓒ Ⓓ Ⓔ	33 Ⓐ Ⓑ Ⓒ Ⓓ Ⓔ	53 Ⓐ Ⓑ Ⓒ Ⓓ Ⓔ
14 Ⓐ Ⓑ Ⓒ Ⓓ Ⓔ	34 Ⓐ Ⓑ Ⓒ Ⓓ Ⓔ	54 Ⓐ Ⓑ Ⓒ Ⓓ Ⓔ
15 Ⓐ Ⓑ Ⓒ Ⓓ Ⓔ	35 Ⓐ Ⓑ Ⓒ Ⓓ Ⓔ	55 Ⓐ Ⓑ Ⓒ Ⓓ Ⓔ
16 Ⓐ Ⓑ Ⓒ Ⓓ Ⓔ	36 Ⓐ Ⓑ Ⓒ Ⓓ Ⓔ	56 Ⓐ Ⓑ Ⓒ Ⓓ Ⓔ
17 Ⓐ Ⓑ Ⓒ Ⓓ Ⓔ	37 Ⓐ Ⓑ Ⓒ Ⓓ Ⓔ	57 Ⓐ Ⓑ Ⓒ Ⓓ Ⓔ
18 Ⓐ Ⓑ Ⓒ Ⓓ Ⓔ	38 Ⓐ Ⓑ Ⓒ Ⓓ Ⓔ	58 Ⓐ Ⓑ Ⓒ Ⓓ Ⓔ
19 Ⓐ Ⓑ Ⓒ Ⓓ Ⓔ	39 Ⓐ Ⓑ Ⓒ Ⓓ Ⓔ	59 Ⓐ Ⓑ Ⓒ Ⓓ Ⓔ
20 Ⓐ Ⓑ Ⓒ Ⓓ Ⓔ	40 Ⓐ Ⓑ Ⓒ Ⓓ Ⓔ	60 Ⓐ Ⓑ Ⓒ Ⓓ Ⓔ

Block 1

Time: 60 minutes for 60 questions

Directions: Choose the *best* answer to each question. Mark the corresponding oval on the answer sheet.

1. Which of the following is true concerning nephrotic syndrome?

   (A) Hematuria is an aspect of nephrotic syndrome.

   (B) Proteinuria of 2 grams or less is diagnostic for nephrotic syndrome.

   (C) Common causes of nephrotic syndrome include hypertension and obstructive uropathy.

   (D) Anemia needs to be present for nephrotic syndrome to be considered.

   (E) A high cholesterol level is usually seen in nephrotic syndrome.

2. Which of the following is the recommended treatment for Torsades de Pointes?

   (A) Intravenous (IV) steroids

   (B) IV metoprolol (Lopressor)

   (C) IV diltiazem (Cardizem)

   (D) IV magnesium

   (E) IV digoxin (Lanoxin)

3. Which of the following medications has been demonstrated to reduce mortality in patients with systolic congestive heart failure (CHF)?

   (A) Digoxin (Lanoxin)

   (B) Terazosin (Hytrin)

   (C) Lisinopril (Zestril)

   (D) Diltiazem (Cardizem)

   (E) Hydrochlorothiazide, or HCTZ (Microzide)

4. Which of the following is a common side effect of calcium channel blockers?

   (A) Hypokalemia

   (B) Hypomagnesemia

   (C) Diarrhea

   (D) Edema

   (E) Cough

5. A 77-year-old man with a history of gastrointestinal (GI) bleeding and gait instability — with a history of falls — is admitted to the hospital with sudden onset of shortness of breath. A ventilation/perfusion (V/Q) scan shows high probability for a pulmonary embolism (PE). What's your next step in management?

   (A) Administer a heparin bolus, infuse heparin, and then start warfarin (Coumadin).

   (B) Infuse heparin only, and then start warfarin (Coumadin).

   (C) Obtain CT angiography to confirm PE.

   (D) Have inferior vena cava (IVC) filter placed.

   (E) Give subcutaneous enoxaparin (Lovenox) injections.

6. A 20-year-old woman presents to the ER in May complaining of a rash and fever. She lives near the woods in North Carolina but is unsure whether she was bitten by a tick. She feels nauseous and "aches all over." Physical exam shows a temperature of 38.3°C (101°F) and a petechial rash over her ankles and the palms of her hands. Which of the following would be your next step in management?

   (A) Advise her that this condition is viral; discharge her with a follow-up with her doctor.

   (B) Order intravenous (IV) ceftriaxone (Rocephin) and admit her to the hospital.

   (C) Give her a prescription for azithromycin (Zithromax) and send her home.

   (D) Administer doxycycline (Doxy-Caps) and admit her to the hospital.

   (E) Obtain a stat creatine phosphokinase (CPK) level.

Go on to next page

7. Which of the following is a paraneoplastic phenomenon associated with lung cancer?

    (A) Hypocalcemia

    (B) Hypernatremia

    (C) Ectopic ACTH secretion

    (D) Hyperkalemia

    (E) Polycythemia

8. What is the test of choice to diagnose an aortic dissection?

    (A) Chest radiograph

    (B) Transthoracic echocardiogram (TTE)

    (C) MRI of the chest with contrast

    (D) CT scan of the thorax with contrast

    (E) PET scan of the chest

9. You are evaluating a 43-year-old man for anemia. Labs show he has a hemoglobin of 7.6 mg/dL and a mean corpuscular volume (MCV) of 102. A peripheral smear demonstrates hypersegmented neutrophils. What is the likely cause of the patient's anemia?

    (A) Hypothyroidism

    (B) Liver disease

    (C) Myelodysplasia

    (D) Vitamin B_{12} deficiency

    (E) Hemolytic anemia

10. Which of the following maneuvers can be used to diagnose vertigo?

    (A) Phalen's maneuver

    (B) Tensilon test

    (C) Epley maneuver

    (D) Dix-Hallpike maneuver

    (E) Tilt table test

11. A 65-year-old man presents with shortness of breath. A chest radiograph demonstrates a large right pleural effusion. A thoracentesis is done and shows a pleural fluid LDH of 300 and a protein of 23. A corresponding serum LDH is 443. Which of the following would be a cause of this person's effusion?

    (A) Pneumonia

    (B) Systolic congestive heart failure (CHF)

    (C) Diastolic CHF

    (D) Liver disease

    (E) Kidney failure

12. Which of the following would you prescribe for the treatment of septic arthritis?

    (A) Physical therapy

    (B) Intra-articular steroid injection

    (C) Oral colchicine

    (D) Intravenous (IV) vancomycin (Vancocin)

    (E) Oral doxycycline (Vibramycin)

13. Which of the following is used in the treatment of an autonomic neuropathy?

    (A) Metoprolol (Lopressor)

    (B) Prednisone

    (C) Midodrine (ProAmatine)

    (D) Antibiotics

    (E) Intravenous (IV) fluids

14. You are evaluating a 28-year-old woman with gestational hypertension. Which of the following medications is contraindicated in this patient?

    (A) Hydralazine (Apresoline)

    (B) Methyldopa (Aldomet)

    (C) Labetalol (Trandate)

    (D) Lisinopril (Zestril)

    (E) Amlodipine (Norvasc)

Go on to next page

15. In addition to excessive alcohol use, what is the most common cause of hepatitis in the United States today?

    (A) Autoimmune disease

    (B) Viral hepatitis

    (C) Nonalcoholic steatohepatitis (NASH)

    (D) Statin use

    (E) Celiac disease

16. In acute appendicitis, what is the name of the test by which palpation of the left lower quadrant elicits pain at McBurney's point?

    (A) Psoas sign

    (B) Obturator sign

    (C) Rovsing's sign

    (D) Murphy's sign

    (E) Blumberg's sign

17. A 40-year-old man who's hospitalized with a change in mental status has periods of complete lucidity followed by periods of confusion. He is afebrile and shows no neck rigidity. He is given thiamine intravenously without any change in his condition. His blood glucose level is normal. What's your next immediate step in management?

    (A) Give additional intravenous (IV) thiamine.

    (B) Perform a lumbar puncture (LP).

    (C) Obtain blood and urine cultures.

    (D) Get a noncontrast CT scan of the head.

    (E) Get a stat chest radiograph.

18. Which of the following medications is the treatment of choice for bacterial vaginosis (BV)?

    (A) Fluconazole (Diflucan)

    (B) Azithromycin (Zithromax)

    (C) Metronidazole (Flagyl)

    (D) Ceftriaxone (Rocephin)

    (E) Doxycycline (Vibramycin)

19. Which of the following antibody tests would most likely be positive in systemic lupus erythematosus (SLE)?

    (A) Anti-Smith antibody

    (B) Anti-SSA antibody

    (C) Anti-ribonucleoprotein (RNP) antibody

    (D) HLA-B27

    (E) Anti-mitochondrial antibody (AMA)

20. Which of the following is associated with heart block and meningitis?

    (A) Gout

    (B) Septic joint

    (C) Lyme disease

    (D) Pseudogout

    (E) Still's disease

21. Which of the following is a common metabolic abnormality in both the tricyclic antidepressants and selective serotonin reuptake inhibitors (SSRIs)?

    (A) Hyponatremia

    (B) Hypercalcemia

    (C) Hypokalemia

    (D) Hyperglycemia

    (E) Hypothyroidism

22. A 21-year-old woman presents with hypotension and weakness. She is hemodynamically stable at the moment. An AM cortisol is equivocal at 13. What is your next diagnostic step?

    (A) 24-hour urinary free cortisol

    (B) Low-dose dexamethasone suppression test

    (C) High-dose dexamethasone suppression test

    (D) Cosyntropin stimulation test

    (E) Metyrapone test

Go on to next page

23. In someone with Addison's disease, a sudden drop in blood pressure that does not improve with intravenous (IV) fluids requires which of the following interventions?

    (A) Give another fluid bolus.

    (B) Start IV phenylephrine.

    (C) Get a stat cardiac echocardiogram.

    (D) Obtain cultures and start antibiotics.

    (E) Administer IV hydrocortisone.

24. Which of the following is a cause of high-output heart failure?

    (A) Polycythemia

    (B) Hypothyroidism

    (C) Paget's disease of bone

    (D) Vitamin D deficiency

    (E) Vitamin B_{12} deficiency

25. Which of the following is a potential complication of ulcerative colitis but not of Crohn's disease?

    (A) Bowel obstruction

    (B) Colonic strictures

    (C) Anal fistulas

    (D) Sclerosing cholangitis

    (E) Colon carcinoma

26. A 5-year-old child presents with significant edema. The urinalysis shows 3+ protein but no blood. The serum albumin is 2.3 mg/dL. A 24-hour urine protein is 4.5 grams. What is the most likely cause of proteinuria in this young child?

    (A) Membranous nephropathy

    (B) Focal segmental glomerulosclerosis

    (C) Minimal change disease

    (D) Benign orthostatic proteinuria

    (E) IgA nephropathy

27. Osteomyelitis in a patient with sickle cell anemia is usually due to which of the following organisms?

    (A) *Staphylococcus aureus*

    (B) *Alpha-hemolytic streptococcus*

    (C) *Enterococcus faecalis*

    (D) *Salmonella enteritidis*

    (E) *Candida albicans*

28. A 46-year-old man is admitted to the hospital with a change in mental status. Labs show a hemoglobin of 7.6 mg/dL and a platelet count of 42. A peripheral blood smear shows schistocytes. What's the next step in treatment?

    (A) Platelet transfusion

    (B) Intravenous (IV) steroids

    (C) Emergent splenectomy

    (D) Plasmapheresis

    (E) Intravenous gamma globulin (IVIG)

29. A 4-year-old has a temperature of 38.9°C (102°F), left-sided cervical adenopathy, and a reddened tongue. You also notice that his hands and feet are red and that he has a rash on his chest. What's the most likely diagnosis?

    (A) Measles

    (B) Syphilis

    (C) Kawasaki disease

    (D) Mononucleosis

    (E) Fifth disease

30. Which of the following organs does not produce alkaline phosphatase?

    (A) Intestine

    (B) Liver

    (C) Bone

    (D) Placenta

    (E) Lung

31. An 80-year-old man presents with shortness of breath. He has a history of rheumatic heart disease. On physical exam he has jugular venous distention (JVD) and an absent S1. His chest radiograph demonstrates pulmonary edema. An electrocardiogram (ECG) shows a short PR interval. What's the most likely diagnosis?

    (A) Aortic stenosis

    (B) Mitral regurgitation

    (C) Aortic regurgitation

    (D) Mitral stenosis

    (E) Pulmonic stenosis

Go on to next page

32. An 87-year-old nursing home resident presents with a temperature of 38.3°C (101°F), shortness of breath, and a cough productive of brown sputum. On oral examination he has dry mucous membranes. Initial chest radiograph is negative. Which of the following organisms is the likely cause of the patient's pneumonia?

    (A) *Legionella pneumophilia*

    (B) *Pseudomonas aeruginosa*

    (C) *Streptococcus viridans*

    (D) *Chlamydia pneumonia*

    (E) *Candida albicans*

33. On physical examination of a patient you notice pigmented areas in the neck and axilla. What is this condition referred to as?

    (A) Acanthosis nigricans

    (B) Hemochromatosis

    (C) Adrenal insufficiency

    (D) Tinea capitis

    (E) Purpura

34. You're evaluating a 22-year-old woman for amenorrhea. A urine β-hCG test is negative. Which of the following tests would be ordered next as a further work-up?

    (A) Serum cortisol level

    (B) Thyroid-stimulating hormone (TSH) level

    (C) Estrogen level

    (D) Repeat serum β-hCG

    (E) Complete blood count (CBC)

35. You're evaluating a 56-year-old man for hypercalcemia. What's the most common cause of hypercalcemia?

    (A) Multiple myeloma

    (B) Sarcoidosis

    (C) Hyperparathyroidism

    (D) Hypomagnesemia

    (E) Milk-alkali syndrome

36. An 11-year-old boy presents with a chronic cough. His mother states the cough has been ongoing for several months. It is a productive, foul-smelling cough. In addition, he states that his stool "floats" and that this has been occurring for quite a while. On physical examination you notice testicular atrophy. What test would you order next?

    (A) Sweat chloride test

    (B) Alpha-1 antitrypsin level

    (C) Angiotensin converting enzyme (ACE) level

    (D) Urinary pneumococcal antigen

    (E) Mantoux test

37. You're evaluating a 70-year-old man who presents with weakness. He has atrial fibrillation and is on warfarin (Coumadin). He has no history of diarrhea or weight loss. His stool is negative for occult blood. Labs show a hemoglobin of 6.0 mg/dL. His PT/INR is 5.5. His serum LDH and haptoglobin are normal. He has no history of fall or trauma. What is your likely diagnosis?

    (A) Gastrointestinal (GI) bleeding

    (B) Hemolysis

    (C) Malabsorption syndrome

    (D) Retroperitoneal bleed

    (E) Hemothorax

38. You're evaluating a 70-year-old man who has not been feeling well. He's been feeling more tired over the last few months. Per his wife, "he sleeps all day." He also has a decreased appetite and says that his wife's cooking is awful. When asked why, he states, "everything she cooks tastes like metal." In addition to asking this gentleman to apologize to his distraught wife, what would you order first?

    (A) Thyroid-stimulating hormone (TSH) level

    (B) Hepatic function panel

    (C) Serum blood urea nitrogen (BUN) and creatinine level

    (D) Complete blood count (CBC)

    (E) Vitamin B$_{12}$ level

Go on to next page

39. The triad of miosis, ptosis, and anhidrosis is seen with which malignancy?

    (A) Colon

    (B) Esophageal

    (C) Breast

    (D) Prostate

    (E) Lung

40. You're evaluating a 75-year-old man with worsening confusion. His daughter states he has had a significant decline over the past few months. Which of the following would be part of your initial evaluation?

    (A) Vitamin B_{12} level

    (B) Phosphorous

    (C) Potassium level

    (D) 24-hour urinary free cortisol

    (E) Vitamin D level

41. A 36-year-old man with a history of seizure disorder presents with a new onset rash. He states that he was started on a new medication for his seizure disorder, but he doesn't remember which one. On exam you see a diffuse maculopapular rash. The man is afebrile, looks well, and has no other symptoms. Which medication is responsible for the rash?

    (A) Phenytoin (Dilantin)

    (B) Lamotrigine (Lamictal)

    (C) Phenobarbital (Solfoton)

    (D) Valium (Diazepam)

    (E) Carbamazepine (Tegretol)

42. A 63-year-old man with a history of hypertension and diabetes mellitus presents with angina. When you see the patient in the ER, he is having chest pain. His blood pressure is 132/50 mmHg, and an electrocardiogram (ECG) shows ST depression in leads V1, V2, and V3. Initial troponin is less than 0.05. What's your initial step in management?

    (A) Give sublingual nitroglycerin and start intravenous (IV) heparin.

    (B) Consult cardiology for emergent cardiac catheterization.

    (C) Order a thallium stress test.

    (D) Order a stat cardiac echocardiogram.

    (E) Obtain stat chest radiograph.

43. What is the goal Protime (PT/INR) for a patient with atrial fibrillation?

    (A) 1.0 to 1.5

    (B) 1.5 to 2.0

    (C) 2.0 to 2.5

    (D) 2.5 to 3.0

    (E) 2.0 to 3.0

44. You are evaluating a 25-year-old man with a history of diarrhea who presents with weakness. He denies any bloody stools. He has had a 10-pound weight loss over the past six months. He has no family history of colon cancer. You also note pale conjunctivas, and his stool for occult blood is negative. Labs show a hemoglobin of 9.0 mg/dL, a mean corpuscular volume (MCV) of 84. His ferritin is 11 mg/dL, and a vitamin B_{12} level is 100. The serum calcium is 6.8 mg/dL when corrected for his albumin. What's your next step in management?

    (A) Order a bone marrow biopsy.

    (B) Order a colonoscopy.

    (C) Order a tissue transglutaminase antibody test.

    (D) Start vitamin B_{12} injections.

    (E) Administer intravenous (IV) iron.

45. What's the imaging study of choice to evaluate for avascular necrosis?

    (A) Radiograph of hips

    (B) PET scan

    (C) MRI

    (D) CT scan with contrast

    (E) Bone scan

46. A 35-year-old man presents with pain in his right hand. He states that he has been having pain in his thumb. The pain is reproduced when he wraps his fingers around his thumb to form a fist and the fist is bent toward the pinky finger. What's the most likely cause of his pain?

    (A) Ganglion cyst

    (B) Carpal tunnel syndrome

    (C) Dupuytren's tenosynovitis

    (D) Colles' fracture

    (E) Scaphoid fracture

Go on to next page

47. You are evaluating a 46-year-old obese man who's experiencing a chronic cough. The cough only occurs at night. He denies any seasonal allergies. What's your next step in management?

    (A) Prescribe a nasal steroid.

    (B) Advise the patient to avoid eating after dinner.

    (C) Order a methacholine challenge test.

    (D) Order a Z-pack.

    (E) Order saline nasal spray.

48. Which of the following symptoms is commonly associated with Ménière's disease?

    (A) Headache

    (B) Anosmia

    (C) Vertigo

    (D) Early satiety

    (E) Decreased vision

49. Which of the following statements is true concerning the epithelium of the esophagus?

    (A) It has squamous epithelium at the proximal end and columnar epithelium near the GE junction.

    (B) It has columnar epithelium at the proximal end and squamous epithelium near the GE junction.

    (C) It is entirely lined by squamous epithelium.

    (D) It is lined by cuboidal epithelium.

    (E) It is lined by columnar epithelium.

50. Which of the following infusions would you order for the treatment of rhabdomyolysis?

    (A) An infusion of D5W

    (B) A furosemide (Lasix) infusion

    (C) Intravenous (IV) half-normal saline at 80 mL/hr

    (D) IV normal saline at 125 mL/hr

    (E) A bicarbonate infusion

51. A 35-year-old woman presents with a cough. She does not have a history of smoking or any significant occupational exposures. A chest radiograph shows a lung mass. What is the likely cause of her cancer?

    (A) Adenocarcinoma

    (B) Small-cell carcinoma

    (C) Squamous-cell carcinoma

    (D) Bronchoalveolar carcinoma

    (E) Large-cell carcinoma

52. Which of the following is a side effect of quetiapine (Seroquel)?

    (A) Hypoglycemia

    (B) Weight gain

    (C) Hypothyroidism

    (D) Agranulocytosis

    (E) Hyponatremia

53. A 3-year-old boy presents with pain in the right lower quadrant (RLQ). He has a recent history of rectal bleeding. What's the most likely diagnosis?

    (A) Acute appendicitis

    (B) Meckel's diverticulum

    (C) Diverticulitis

    (D) Regional enteritis

    (E) Pyloric stenosis

54. You're evaluating a 65-year-old man with systolic heart failure. Which of the following would you prescribe for treating this condition?

    (A) Lisinopril (Zestril)

    (B) Hydrochlorothiazide, or HCTZ (Microzide)

    (C) Terazosin (Hytrin)

    (D) Clonidine (Catapres)

    (E) Diltiazem (Cardizem)

Go on to next page

55. Which of the following would you do for the treatment of prehypertension in a patient who is otherwise healthy?

    (A) Start on lisinopril (Zestril).

    (B) Start on amlodipine (Norvasc).

    (C) The patient does not need any interventions at this time.

    (D) Recommend dietary interventions and lifestyle modification.

    (E) Start on hydrochlorothiazide, or HCTZ (Microzide).

56. Which of the following is a feature of rheumatoid arthritis (RA)?

    (A) High blood pressure

    (B) Elevated pulmonary pressures

    (C) Sclerodactyly

    (D) Subcutaneous nodules

    (E) Heartburn

57. You are evaluating a 15-year-old boy who's experiencing knee pain. He is an athlete on the high school track team. The pain gets worse after he runs or jumps. On physical examination he yelps in pain when you try to straighten the leg out. You notice a lump on the lower leg below the knee that is very tender when you touch it. What's the most likely cause of this young man's knee pain?

    (A) Chondromalacia

    (B) Osgood-Schlatter disease

    (C) Stress fracture

    (D) Quadriceps tear

    (E) Sciatica

58. Which of the following concerning iron replacement is true?

    (A) The most common complaint with oral iron therapy is diarrhea.

    (B) The reticulocyte count can be used to assess the bone marrow response to iron therapy.

    (C) The addition of vitamin D can increase the absorption of oral iron.

    (D) Oral iron should never be given separately from other medications.

    (E) Iron can be given subcutaneously for replacement if needed.

59. Which of the following is a cause of sensorineural hearing loss?

    (A) Ménière's disease

    (B) Otitis media

    (C) Tympanic membrane rupture

    (D) Otosclerosis

    (E) Cerumen impaction

60. You are evaluating a 75-year-old woman diagnosed with *Clostridium difficile* colitis. Which of the following medications would be effective in treating this condition?

    (A) Clindamycin (Cleocin)

    (B) Oral vancomycin (Vancocin)

    (C) Amoxicillin (Amoxil)

    (D) Doxycycline (Doryx)

    (E) Intravenous (IV) vancomycin

STOP DO NOT TURN THE PAGE UNTIL TOLD TO DO SO.
DO NOT RETURN TO A PREVIOUS TEST.

Block 2

> **Time:** 60 minutes for 60 questions
>
> **Directions:** Choose the *best* answer to each question. Mark the corresponding oval on the answer sheet.

1. Which statement is correct concerning an S2?

    (A) It represents ventricular volume overload.

    (B) It is always heard in a patient with atrial fibrillation.

    (C) It represents closure of the aortic and pulmonic valves.

    (D) It represents atrial contraction into a noncompliant ventricle.

    (E) It represents the closure of the mitral and tricuspid valves.

2. You're seeing a 17-year-old girl with a history of asthma. She states that she usually has an attack only once a week, if that. She feels fine otherwise and has no history of seasonal allergies. What classification of asthma would best describe her condition?

    (A) Mild persistent asthma

    (B) Intermittent

    (C) Moderately persistent

    (D) Severely persistent

    (E) Exercise induced

3. Which of the following is true concerning diabetes mellitus (DM)?

    (A) Type I DM is characterized by insulin resistance.

    (B) Type I DM usually occurs at an older age compared to type II.

    (C) C-peptide levels can only be measured in type I DM.

    (D) Metformin (Glucophage) can be used in type I DM.

    (E) Hypertriglyceridemia can be found in uncontrolled DM.

4. You're treating a 65-year-old man for painless rectal bleeding. A barium swallow demonstrates an apple-core deformity. What is the most likely cause of his rectal bleeding?

    (A) Diverticulosis

    (B) Arteriovenous malformation (AVM)

    (C) Colonic malignancy

    (D) Chronic constipation

    (E) Ulcerative colitis

5. You're performing a school physical on a 20-year-old man and notice a heart murmur that increases in response to the Valsalva maneuver. You ask the patient to make a fist with his left hand, and this action decreases the loudness of the murmur. What condition do you suspect that the patient has?

    (A) Coarctation of the aorta

    (B) Eisenmenger syndrome

    (C) Hypertrophic cardiomyopathy

    (D) Atrial septal defect

    (E) Tetralogy of Fallot

6. You're evaluating a 35-year-old man with a history of human immunodeficiency virus (HIV) who presents with shortness of breath. A chest radiograph demonstrates extensive bilateral infiltrates. His CD4 count is 150. What would you treat this patient with?

    (A) Trimethoprim/sulfamethoxazole (Bactrim)

    (B) Metronidazole (Flagyl)

    (C) Azithromycin (Zithromax)

    (D) Cefepime (Maxipime)

    (E) Ciprofloxacin (Cipro)

Go on to next page

7. Which of the following would you prescribe for the treatment of histoplasmosis?

   (A) Isoniazid (Tubizid)

   (B) Prednisone (Deltasone)

   (C) Ciprofloxacin (Cipro)

   (D) Itraconazole (Sporanox)

   (E) Trimethoprim/sulfamethoxazole (Bactrim)

8. You're evaluating a 2-year-old child who presents to the clinic with bright red cheeks. His mother states his only other symptoms were a runny nose and mild cough. You check his records and see that he is up to date on all of his immunizations. On exam you notice a maculopapular rash that extends to his arms, chest, and legs. What is the most likely cause of this child's rash?

   (A) Measles

   (B) Parvovirus B19

   (C) *Streptococcus*

   (D) Respiratory syncytial virus (RSV)

   (E) Rhinovirus

9. Which of the following represents the most common cause of acute bronchitis?

   (A) Fungal

   (B) Viral

   (C) Gram-positive organisms

   (D) Anaerobic organisms

   (E) Gram-negative organisms

10. Which of the following symptoms correlate with the highest mortality in aortic stenosis?

    (A) Syncope

    (B) Angina

    (C) Dyspnea

    (D) Palpitations

    (E) Leg swelling

11. A 45-year-old man presents with several episodes of flushing, palpitations, and blood pressure that is "all over the place." On examination you hear a murmur. You suspect carcinoid syndrome. What would you order as your next step?

    (A) 24-hour urinary 5-hydroxyindoleacetic acid (5-HIAA) level

    (B) Serum serotonin level

    (C) Plasma aldosterone level

    (D) 24-hour urinary metanephrines

    (E) 24-hour urinary free cortisol

12. You're evaluating a 35-year-old obese woman for headache and blurry vision. On fundoscopic examination you notice a swollen optic disc in both eyes as well as a significant blurring of the disc margins. A CT scan of the head is normal, and her blood pressure is 146/86 mmHg. What is the likely cause of the headache and blurry vision in this patient?

    (A) Ischemic stroke

    (B) Malignant hypertension

    (C) Intracranial bleed

    (D) Encephalitis

    (E) Pseudotumor cerebri (PTC)

13. Which of the following medications is used in the treatment of glaucoma?

    (A) Amphotericin B (Amphotec)

    (B) Furosemide (Lasix)

    (C) Gentamicin (Garamycin)

    (D) Trimethoprim/sulfamethoxazole (Bactrim, Septra)

    (E) Acetazolamide (Diamox)

Go on to next page

14. You're evaluating a 40-year-old woman who presents with a palpable thyroid mass. She states that over the past few months she has had weight gain and constipation and has missed cycles. On exam her blood pressure is 148/90 mmHg. You also find a delayed Achilles reflex. What is the most likely diagnosis?

    (A) Graves' disease

    (B) Hashimoto's thyroiditis

    (C) Papillary thyroid cancer

    (D) Toxic adenoma

    (E) Pituitary microadenoma

15. You are evaluating a 26-year-old woman who complains of hematemesis. She has a history of bulimia. She has no history of alcoholism, excessive nonsteroidal anti-inflammatory drug (NSAID) use, or laxative abuse. What's the most likely cause of the hematemesis?

    (A) Esophageal varices

    (B) Duodenal ulcer

    (C) Mallory-Weiss tear

    (D) Gastroesophageal reflux disease (GERD)

    (E) Barrett's esophagus

16. In someone diagnosed with bulimia, which of the following would be found on physical examination?

    (A) Moist mucous membranes

    (B) Skin hyperpigmentation

    (C) Parotid gland hypertrophy

    (D) Macular rash

    (E) Buffalo hump

17. Which of the following medications can cause edema and hypokalemia as a significant side effect?

    (A) Midodrine (ProAmatine)

    (B) Terazosin (Hytrin)

    (C) Fludrocortisone (Florinef)

    (D) Furosemide (Lasix)

    (E) Spironolactone (Aldactone)

18. Which of the following is a common cause of adult respiratory distress syndrome (ARDS)?

    (A) Congestive heart failure (CHF)

    (B) Pulmonary embolism (PE)

    (C) Aortic stenosis

    (D) Pancreatitis

    (E) Anemia

19. You are seeing a 16-year-old boy for hematuria. He had a sore throat 1 week ago and has now developed gross hematuria. His urinalysis is positive for 3+ blood and 2+ protein. His creatinine is 1.6 mg/dL. Which of the following is a likely cause of the young man's kidney failure?

    (A) Hypertension

    (B) IgA nephropathy

    (C) Henoch-Schonlein purpura

    (D) Minimal change disease

    (E) Diabetic nephropathy

20. You're evaluating a 50-year-old man with a sore left toe. He denies any trauma but states he eats a lot of meat and drinks alcohol quite frequently. What would you expect to see on a synovial fluid analysis?

    (A) Synovial fluid white cell count greater than 100,000 with a left shift

    (B) No inflammatory cells in white cell count

    (C) Positively birefringent, rhomboid-shaped crystals

    (D) Needle-shaped crystals with negative birefringence under polarized light

    (E) Elevated eosinophil count in synovial fluid

Go on to next page

21. You're seeing a 30-year-old man who presents with jerking movements of his arms and legs. You notice that when looking at you, he turns his whole head rather than shifting his eyes. He is concerned because his father also had a history of jerking-like movements. You find out his father passed away at a relatively young age. What is the most likely diagnosis?

    (A) Sydenham chorea

    (B) Huntington's disease

    (C) Parkinson's disease

    (D) Cerebral palsy

    (E) Multiple sclerosis (MS)

22. What rhythm is shown on the strip provided?

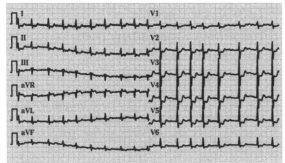

    (A) Atrial fibrillation

    (B) Atrial flutter

    (C) Multifocal atrial tachycardia

    (D) Wolf-Parkinson-White syndrome

    (E) Sinus tachycardia

23. What medical condition can be a cause of atrial fibrillation, particularly in the elderly?

    (A) Hypokalemia

    (B) Chronic obstructive pulmonary disease (COPD)

    (C) Hyperthyroidism

    (D) Obesity

    (E) Polycythemia

24. Which of the following is a cause of pseudogout?

    (A) Steroid use

    (B) Diabetes mellitus

    (C) Wilson's disease

    (D) Hyperthyroidism

    (E) Hyperparathyroidism

25. You're evaluating a 67-year-old woman in the hospital who has been diagnosed with *Clostridium difficile* colitis. She complains of worsening abdominal pain. Her abdomen is very distended, is diffusely tender to palpation, and presents decreased bowel sounds. A radiograph shows a dilated colon. What is the condition she is suffering from?

    (A) Abdominal perforation

    (B) Toxic megacolon

    (C) Ulcerative proctitis

    (D) Large bowel obstruction

    (E) Diverticulitis

26. Which of the following would be indicated in the treatment of an acute asthma exacerbation?

    (A) Urine eosinophils

    (B) Neck radiograph

    (C) Methacholine challenge

    (D) Intravenous (IV) antibiotics

    (E) IV steroids

27. You're on call and asked to see a young man who suddenly becomes short of breath. He is tachypneic with a respiratory rate of 30. His blood pressure has decreased to 76/44 mmHg. You don't hear breath sounds at all on the left lung. You notice that the trachea is deviated to the left. What is the likely diagnosis?

    (A) Pulmonary embolism (PE)

    (B) Pulmonary infarction

    (C) Tension pneumothorax

    (D) Left ventricular failure

    (E) Asthma exacerbation

Go on to next page

28. What emergent step would you take when managing a patient with a tension pneumothorax?

    (A) Heparinization

    (B) Stat cardiac echocardiogram

    (C) Chest tube placement

    (D) Intravenous (IV) methylprednisolone (Solu-Medrol)

    (E) Needle decompression

29. You're assessing a 25-year-old man who presents with acute onset of sharp pain in the perineal area. He is toxic-looking and has a temperature of 38.9°C (102°F). Urinalysis demonstrates greater than 50 WBC/HPF. What's your next step in management?

    (A) Perform a prostatic massage to ascertain an adequate sample.

    (B) Place a Foley catheter to obtain an early and midstream sample.

    (C) Obtain a prostatic ultrasound to look for benign prostatic hyperplasia (BPH).

    (D) Perform a digital rectal examination to evaluate for prostatic abscess.

    (E) Avoid any invasive procedure at this time.

30. You're seeing a 50-year-old woman who presents with pain in her arms. She states that the pain is in her shoulders and bicep area; she gets so sore it can be difficult to move her arms. Her creatine phosphokinase (CPK) level is normal but the erythrocyte sedimentation rate (ESR) is 80. What is your likely diagnosis?

    (A) Polymyositis

    (B) Polymyalgia rheumatica (PMR)

    (C) Fibromyalgia

    (D) Polyarteritis nodosa

    (E) Systemic lupus erythematosus (SLE)

31. You're seeing a 4-year-old child whose mother states he has been taking swimming classes. On exam you notice that both eyes are red with a significant discharge. What is the most likely cause of the conjunctivitis?

    (A) Virus

    (B) *Staphylococcus aureus*

    (C) Fungus

    (D) Streptococcus

    (E) *Escherichia coli*

32. Which of the following cardiac anomalies is associated with a fixed split S2 on auscultation?

    (A) Atrial septal defect

    (B) Ventricular septal defect

    (C) Hypertrophic cardiomyopathy

    (D) Patent ductus arteriosus

    (E) Tetralogy of Fallot

33. You are evaluating an 87-year-old man admitted for shortness of breath. On exam he appears toxic, with a temperature of 38.3°C (101°F). You detect a foul odor from his mouth. You notice poor dentition with black and decaying teeth. On lung exam you notice decreased breath sounds at the right lung base. Which of the following do you need to think about as a significant cause of his symptoms?

    (A) Gram-negative rods

    (B) Anaerobic bacteria

    (C) Gram-positive cocci in clusters

    (D) Fungus

    (E) Virus

34. What is one of the most common causes of external otitis in a diabetic patient?

    (A) *Candida albicans*

    (B) *Haemophilus influenzae*

    (C) *Moraxella catarrhalis*

    (D) *Pseudomonas aeruginosa*

    (E) Adenovirus

Go on to next page

35. Which of the following types of thyroid carcinoma has the worst prognosis?

    (A) Papillary

    (B) Follicular

    (C) Medullary

    (D) Anaplastic

    (E) Squamous-cell

36. Which of the following medications would you recommend for the treatment of essential tremor?

    (A) Sertraline (Zoloft)

    (B) Alprazolam (Xanax)

    (C) Carbidopa (Sinemet)

    (D) Propanolol (Inderal)

    (E) Phenytoin (Dilantin)

37. You are evaluating a 35-year-old man of Mediterranean decent who presents with fatigue and weakness. He recently completed a course of trimethoprim/sulfamethoxazole (Bactrim). His hemoglobin is 8.5 mg/dL. A prior hemoglobin level was 13. What's the most likely cause of his anemia?

    (A) Sickle cell disease

    (B) Glucose 6-phosphatase deficiency (G6PD)

    (C) Hereditary spherocytosis

    (D) Autoimmune hemolysis

    (E) Thalassemia

38. You're evaluating a 66-year-old man with abnormal liver function tests (LFTs). His alanine aminotransferase (ALT) level is 500 and his aspartate aminotransferase (AST) level is 340. A right upper quadrant (RUQ) ultrasound demonstrates a large liver mass. The patient has a history of a blood transfusion 20 years ago. What is the most likely cause of this patient's liver mass?

    (A) Hepatitis A

    (B) Hemochromatosis

    (C) Hepatitis C

    (D) Primary biliary cirrhosis

    (E) Epstein-Barr virus

39. You're evaluating an 87-year-old nursing home resident who presents with itching all over. The patient has multiple excoriations on her arms and abdomen from scratching. You notice what look like pencil marks on her arms. You call the nursing home and find out that other residents on her floor have had the same complaints. In addition to washing the bed linens and cleaning the floor and furniture, what else should the treatment include?

    (A) Oral amoxicillin to be taken for a ten-day course

    (B) Hospitalization for intravenous (IV) antibiotics

    (C) Permethrin cream to be applied all over the body

    (D) Antifungal soap and shampoo

    (E) IV amphotericin B

40. Which of the following is true concerning kidney stones?

    (A) The most common cause of kidney stones is uric acid.

    (B) Calcium-based stones are unable to be seen on an abdominal radiograph.

    (C) Struvite stones are hereditary.

    (D) The initial treatment of kidney stones includes the use of loop diuretics.

    (E) Treatment of a uric acid stone includes a low-purine diet and alkalinization of the urine.

41. You're evaluating a 45-year-old woman who presents with a rash. She states that her backyard is near the woods. On examination you see what looks like a bull's-eye rash on her left arm. What is the medical name for this rash?

    (A) Erythema multiforme

    (B) Erythema chronicum migrans

    (C) Erythema marginatum

    (D) Erythema infectiosum

    (E) Erythema nodosum

Go on to next page

42. You're evaluating a patient who complains of numbness and paresthesias. She states she just had neck surgery. On exam, you tap her left cheek at the level of the jaw and notice twitching of the facial muscles on the same side that you tapped. What's the electrolyte abnormality?

    (A) Hypercalcemia

    (B) Hyponatremia

    (C) Hyperkalemia

    (D) Hypokalemia

    (E) Hypocalcemia

43. You're performing a school physical exam on an 11-year-old child. You note a 45° curve in the child's thoracic spine by scoliometer. The curve is confirmed by a spinal radiograph. What's your next step in management?

    (A) Follow up in three months.

    (B) Obtain spinal radiographs at six-month intervals to assess progression.

    (C) Provide a referral to an orthopedic surgeon for further evaluation.

    (D) Follow up in one year.

    (E) Provide a referral to neurosurgery for epidural pain injection.

44. Which of the following is not a manifestation of pellagra?

    (A) Obstipation

    (B) Skin rash

    (C) Dementia

    (D) Peripheral neuropathy

    (E) Cardiomyopathy

45. You're evaluating a 13-year-old boy who presents with aching all over. He states that this aching has been occurring for a few weeks. He says it takes more time in the morning to "loosen up" than before. He has been complaining of "feeling hot." On examination, his temperature is 38.1°C (100.5°F). You notice swelling in his knees, ankles, and hands. On abdominal examination, you notice hepatosplenomegaly. His rheumatoid factor is negative. What's the most likely diagnosis?

    (A) Lyme disease

    (B) Sarcoidosis

    (C) Still's disease

    (D) Systemic lupus erythematosus (SLE)

    (E) Rheumatic fever

46. You're evaluating a 40-year-old woman in the ER who presents with progressive weakness. She states she recently had a sore throat and "swollen glands." She says that yesterday her legs felt heavy and that she noticed numbness and tingling in her legs. Today she has trouble walking and moving her arms. What's the most likely diagnosis?

    (A) Multiple sclerosis (MS)

    (B) Parkinson's disease

    (C) Polymyositis

    (D) Addison's disease

    (E) Guillain-Barré syndrome

47. Which of the following is a recommended treatment for Parkinson's disease?

    (A) Intravenous (IV) steroids

    (B) Interferon

    (C) Plasmapheresis

    (D) Carbidopa/Levodopa (Sinemet)

    (E) Cyclophosphamide (Cytoxan)

48. Which of the following is an example of a mood disorder?

    (A) Paranoia

    (B) Mania

    (C) Catatonia

    (D) Agoraphobia

    (E) Anhedonia

Go on to next page

49. Which type of schizophrenia would be associated with the belief that you or your significant other are in physical danger or are being followed?

    (A) Paranoid

    (B) Manic

    (C) Catatonic

    (D) Undifferentiated

    (E) Disorganized

50. Which of the following is a risk factor for endometriosis?

    (A) Pelvic inflammatory disease (PID)

    (B) Multiparity

    (C) Late menarche

    (D) Amenorrhea

    (E) Endometrial cancer

51. You are evaluating a 30-year-old woman who is complaining of abdominal pain. Three days prior the patient had a placement of an intrauterine device (IUD). She has a fever of 38.9°C (102°F). She denies back pain and urinary symptoms. What's the most likely diagnosis?

    (A) Cystitis

    (B) Vaginitis

    (C) Pyelonephritis

    (D) Endometritis

    (E) Colitis

52. What's the test of choice to evaluate for infectious endocarditis?

    (A) Transthoracic echocardiogram (TTE)

    (B) Transesophageal echocardiogram (TEE)

    (C) CT scan of the chest with intravenous (IV) contrast

    (D) MRI of the heart with gadolinium

    (E) Blood cultures

53. You're seeing a 65-year-old man with a history of shortness of breath. He has a positive smoking history, and he states that he gets short of breath a few months out of the year where he "coughs his head off" but then symptoms seem to subside. This has been going on for a few years. You note that he has a short, stocky build. His pulse oximetry on room air is 95%. What's the most likely diagnosis?

    (A) Emphysema

    (B) Acute epiglottitis

    (C) Interstitial pulmonary fibrosis

    (D) Chronic bronchitis

    (E) Alpha-1 antitrypsin deficiency

54. You're seeing a 25-year-old man who states he feels "empty inside." You know that his parents divorced when he was young and that he lived in foster care for much of his life. You note that last week when the two of you talked he "liked you a lot." Now he "hates your guts." You notice what look like razor marks on his wrist. What type of personality disorder are you most likely dealing with?

    (A) Avoidant

    (B) Paranoid

    (C) Borderline

    (D) Schizotypal

    (E) Antisocial

55. You're evaluating a 55-year-old man with a history of cirrhosis who presents with hematemesis. His hemoglobin is 7.5 mg/dL, and his blood pressure is 94/50 mmHg. A Protime (PT/INR) is 5.6. In addition to transfusing packed red blood cells to correct his coagulopathy, what else would you administer?

    (A) Oral vitamin K

    (B) Subcutaneous vitamin K

    (C) Fresh frozen plasma (FFP)

    (D) Intravenous (IV) desmopressin (DDAVP)

    (E) IV factor VIII

Go on to next page

56. You're evaluating an 87-year-old woman admitted to the hospital three days ago because of pneumonia. She was coherent, alert, and oriented on admission. You were called by the nurse because the patient is now incoherent, trying to jump out of bed, and talking to people who are not in the room. This behavior is most consistent with which of the following psychiatric conditions?

    (A) Dementia

    (B) Delirium

    (C) Dysthymia

    (D) Pseudodementia

    (E) Mania

57. Which of the following syndromes is characterized by right ventricular hypertrophy, overriding aorta, outflow obstruction of the right ventricle, and a subaortic septal defect?

    (A) Tetralogy of Fallot

    (B) Hypoplastic left heart syndrome

    (C) Hypertrophic cardiomyopathy

    (D) Williams syndrome

    (E) Pulmonary atresia

58. Which of the following is not associated with reactive arthritis?

    (A) Arthritis

    (B) Conjunctivitis

    (C) Urethritis

    (D) Dermatitis

    (E) Alopecia

59. You are evaluating a 30-year-old man who tried to commit suicide by overdosing on aspirin. On examination, he is tachypneic. His pH is 7.18 and his salicylate level is 100. In addition to hemodynamic support and starting intravenous (IV) bicarbonate, what's your next immediate step?

    (A) Administer IV fluids with dextrose.

    (B) Administer IV N-acetylcysteine (Mucomyst).

    (C) Administer 4-methylpyrazole (Fomepizole).

    (D) Administer flumazenil (Romazicon).

    (E) Contact the on-call nephrologist regarding dialysis.

60. Which of the following medications would you prescribe to treat the condition shown in the photo?

    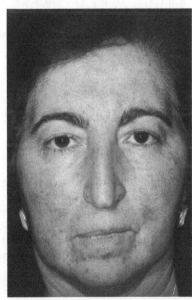

    (A) Topical clotrimazole and betamethasone (Lotrisone)

    (B) Topical metronidazole (Flagyl)

    (C) Oral cephalexin (Keflex)

    (D) Vitamin D derivatives

    (E) Oral clindamycin (Cleocin)

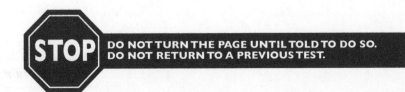

STOP DO NOT TURN THE PAGE UNTIL TOLD TO DO SO. DO NOT RETURN TO A PREVIOUS TEST.

Block 3

Time: 60 minutes for 60 questions

Directions: Choose the *best* answer to each question. Mark the corresponding oval on the answer sheet.

1. You're asked to see a 60-year-old man with hypotension and no detectable pulse. What is the name of the rhythm shown here?

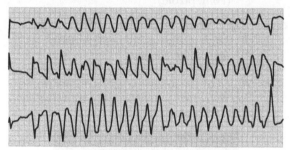

   (A) Ventricular fibrillation

   (B) Torsades de pointes

   (C) Wolff-Parkinson-White syndrome

   (D) Atrial fibrillation

   (E) Multifocal atrial tachycardia

2. A 35-year-old woman presents to the ER with a headache. Her blood pressure is 160/100 mmHg. Physical examination shows no abdominal or femoral bruit. Labs show a Cr of 1.0 mg/dL and potassium of 2.3 mg/dL. What is the most likely cause of her hypertension?

   (A) Pheochromocytoma

   (B) Carcinoid syndrome

   (C) Renal artery stenosis (RAS)

   (D) Hyperaldosteronism

   (E) Hyperthyroidism

3. You're evaluating a 60-year-old man who has had progressive shortness of breath over the past few months. He has a smoking history. On examination you hear rales in both lungs. A chest radiograph demonstrates a reticular nodular pattern. You send the patient for pulmonary function tests (PFTs), which show a restrictive defect and decreased diffusion capacity. What's the most likely cause of his shortness of breath?

   (A) Emphysema

   (B) Chronic bronchitis

   (C) Bronchiectasis

   (D) Asthma

   (E) Interstitial pulmonary fibrosis (IPF)

4. You're evaluating a 35-year-old woman with abdominal pain. She states that she has had trouble with her bowels for years. She says she notices she has diarrhea during the day but her stools are "more formed, more normal at night." She doesn't sleep well and complains of having pain all over. The stool is negative for blood. Stool leukocytes and all other stool studies are negative. She has no family history of cancer. She denies any weight loss. What's your next step?

   (A) Obtain an urgent colonoscopy.

   (B) Recheck stool for fecal occult blood.

   (C) Start a proton pump inhibitor (PPI).

   (D) Emphasize stress management and relaxation techniques.

   (E) Encourage a dairy-free diet.

Go on to next page

5. Which of the following is true concerning rheumatoid arthritis (RA)?

   (A) It is an asymmetric polyarthritis.

   (B) It is more common in women than in men.

   (C) It cannot be diagnosed as a cause of arthritis if the rheumatoid factor is negative.

   (D) One commonly prescribed treatment is sulfasalazine (Azulfidine).

   (E) Radiographic findings can demonstrate chondrocalcinosis.

6. You're evaluating a 67-year-old woman who complains of dizziness that began a few days ago. She states that she had a cold a couple of weeks ago and is slowly recovering from it. She says that she's fine when she sits up, but she notices that when she lies down on her side she feels that the room is spinning. She states that her hearing is fine and denies any ringing in the ears. What's the most likely cause of this person's symptoms?

   (A) Orthostatic hypotension

   (B) Ménière's disease

   (C) Acoustic neuroma

   (D) Labrynthitis

   (E) Cholesteatoma

7. Galactorrhea is caused by an elevation of which of the following?

   (A) Thyroid-stimulating hormone (TSH)

   (B) Estrogen

   (C) Prolactin

   (D) Progesterone

   (E) Dopamine

8. Which of the following is a syndrome that is characterized by physical symptoms that have no apparent organic cause?

   (A) Somatoform disorder

   (B) Schizoaffective disorder

   (C) Bipolar disorder

   (D) Cyclothymia

   (E) Avoidant personality disorder

9. You're evaluating a 17-year-old girl who says she urinates a lot. She's constantly thirsty and drinks lots of water. Despite eating "like a horse" she is still losing weight. She denies any drug use. What test would you order?

   (A) Beta-hCG level

   (B) Serum blood glucose level

   (C) Thyroid-stimulating hormone (TSH) level

   (D) AM cortisol level

   (E) Urine drug screen

10. Which of the following medications can be prescribed effectively for both influenza A and B?

    (A) Amantadine (Symmetrel)

    (B) Acyclovir (Cyclovir)

    (C) Amoxicillin-clavulanic acid (Augmentin)

    (D) Oseltamivir (Tamiflu)

    (E) Doxycycline (Doryx)

11. You're evaluating a 24-year-old woman for a microcytic anemia with a mean corpuscular volume (MCV) of 76. Her iron studies are normal. She has no evidence of any lead exposure and no history of any chronic infections or long-standing medical conditions. What test would you order next?

    (A) Glycosylated hemoglobin

    (B) Reticulocyte count

    (C) Bone marrow biopsy

    (D) Hemoglobin electrophoresis

    (E) Thyroid-stimulating hormone (TSH) level

12. Which of the following statements concerning seminoma is true?

    (A) It is usually found in older men.

    (B) It overall has a very grave prognosis.

    (C) It is mainly treated with chemotherapy and surgery.

    (D) It is an example of a germ cell tumor.

    (E) Tumor markers include an elevated alpha-fetoprotein level.

Go on to next page

13. What condition is this photo consistent with?

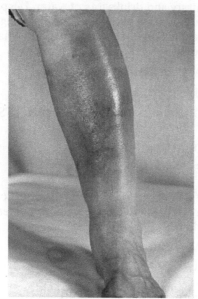

(A) Cellulitis

(B) Vasculitis

(C) Necrotizing fasciitis

(D) Dry gangrene

(E) Erythema migrans

14. You are evaluating an 87-year-old man for worsening confusion. His family states that over the last few months he has become more and more forgetful. He has a history of diabetes, coronary artery disease (CAD), and atrial fibrillation. He had a stent placed in the lower extremity a few years ago secondary to claudication. What's the most likely cause of his dementia?

(A) Alzheimer's disease

(B) Microvascular disease

(C) Vitamin B_{12} deficiency

(D) Hypothyroidism

(E) Neurosyphilis

15. Which electrocardiogram (ECG) findings would be consistent with acute pericarditis?

(A) ST elevation in leads V1, V2, V3, and V4

(B) Diffuse ST segment elevation and PR segment depression

(C) ST elevation in leads V1 through V6 and PR interval prolongation

(D) Diffuse ST segment depression and PR interval prolongation

(E) ST elevation V1–V5 with reciprocal depression in leads II, III, and aVF

16. Which of the following signs would you see in someone with cirrhosis?

(A) Jugular venous distention (JVD)

(B) Kussmaul's sign

(C) Pulsus paradoxus

(D) Shifting dullness

(E) Pulsus alternans

17. Which of the following medications would be used to treat an anaerobic infection?

(A) Levofloxacin (Levaquin)

(B) Ceftriaxone (Rocephin)

(C) Azithromycin (Zithromax)

(D) Erythryomycin (E-Mycin)

(E) Metronidazole (Flagyl)

18. You're evaluating an 87-year-old woman who presents with left lower quadrant (LLQ) abdominal pain and fever. These symptoms occurred after dinner; suddenly she was doubled over in pain. She states she has had three prior attacks like this before, all in the same area. You order a CT scan, which confirms your suspicion. In addition to making the patient NPO and starting intravenous (IV) fluids, which of the following medications would you prescribe?

(A) Ceftriaxone (Rocephin) and azithromycin (Zithromax)

(B) Fluconazole (Diflucan) and clarithromycin (Biaxin)

(C) Vancomycin (Vancocin) and fluconazole (Diflucan)

(D) Ciprofloxacin (Cipro) and metronidazole (Flagyl)

(E) Cephalexin (Keflex) and fluconazole (Diflucan)

Go on to next page

19. Which of the following is the recommended treatment for cauda equina syndrome?

    (A) Recommend neurosurgical evaluation for possible decompressive surgery.

    (B) Check a lumbar spine radiograph and prescribe tramadol (Ultram) for pain.

    (C) Obtain a CT scan of the spine in the next 72 hours.

    (D) Obtain an MRI of the spine in the next 72 hours.

    (E) Obtain an orthopedic consultation for steroid injection.

20. Which of the following medications is indicated for raising HDL levels?

    (A) Atorvastatin (Lipitor)

    (B) Fenofibrate (Tricor)

    (C) Niacin (Niaspan)

    (D) Cholestyramine (Questran)

    (E) Ezetemibe (Zetia)

21. You're evaluating a 16-year-old boy for high blood pressure. He says that he's been having pain in both of his legs while running and that he has to sit down for the pain to subside. On examination you notice the blood pressure in his right arm is 168/116 mmHg, and in the left arm it is 170/104 mmHg. In the lower extremities, you can barely feel a pulse; it is audible by Doppler. What medical condition are you most likely dealing with?

    (A) Fibromuscular dysplasia

    (B) Marfan syndrome

    (C) Hyperaldosteronism

    (D) Coarctation of the aorta

    (E) Pheochromocytoma

22. You are evaluating a 74-year-old man who presents with shortness of breath. He is hypoxemic and his pulse oximetry is 82% on room air. You obtain a chest radiograph. The results look like those shown in the figure. Which of the following treatments would be used to treat this condition?

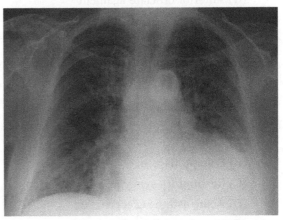

    (A) Intravenous (IV) saline

    (B) IV nitroglycerin

    (C) IV heparin

    (D) IV ceftriaxone (Rocephin)

    (E) IV methylprednisolone (Solumedrol)

23. You're seeing a 40-year-old man who went camping with his friends for the weekend. He admits to drinking from the nearby lake. One week later he develops acute onset of abdominal pain and diarrhea. He says that some of his friends have developed similar symptoms. What is the most likely cause of his diarrhea?

    (A) _Giardia lamblia_

    (B) _Shigella_

    (C) _Salmonella_

    (D) _Cryptosporidium_

    (E) _Campylobacter jejuni_

Go on to next page ⟶

24. For which structure is the Lachman test used to evaluate injury?

 (A) Medial meniscus

 (B) Medial collateral ligament

 (C) Illiotibial band

 (D) Anterior cruciate ligament

 (E) Posterior cruciate ligament

25. You're asked to emergently see a 3-year-old who presents with shortness of breath and drooling. On examination you hear stridor and notice the child is leaning forward on the examination table in order to breathe. What is the emergent condition?

 (A) Croup

 (B) Epiglottitis

 (C) Respiratory syncytial viral infection

 (D) Acute asthma exacerbation

 (E) Pertussis (whooping cough)

26. You're seeing a 16-year-old boy with fever and sore throat. On physical exam you note an exudative pharyngitis as well as adenopathy in the posterior cervical nodes. On abdominal examination you note that the patient has a normal spleen size. Which of the following statements concerning the etiology of his pharyngitis is true?

 (A) The cause of his pharyngitis is thought to be mediated by the Epstein-Barr virus.

 (B) The etiology of his pharyngitis can be associated with atypical lymphocytes and low platelets.

 (C) The cause of his pharyngitis is the most common cause of croup.

 (D) The cause of his pharyngitis is the coxsackievirus.

 (E) Amoxicillin (Trimox) can be used to treat his pharyngitis.

27. You're evaluating a young man who had a recent femur fracture after a fall. He works full time at night and sleeps most of the day. He spends little time outdoors because of his job. He also stays away from dairy products because he says they make him gassy. Which of the following vitamins is he likely deficient in?

 (A) Vitamin A

 (B) Vitamin B_6

 (C) Vitamin C

 (D) Vitamin D

 (E) Vitamin K

28. Which of the following electrolyte abnormalities can be seen in someone with primary hyperparathyroisidm?

 (A) Hypokalemia

 (B) Hypophosphatemia

 (C) Hypomagnesemia

 (D) Hyponatremia

 (E) Hypocalcemia

29. You are evaluating a 35-year-old G3P2 with an estimated gestational age (EGA) of 25 weeks. During a routine office visit, you find that her resting blood pressure is 168/90 mmHg. On a visit at 20 weeks EGA, her blood pressure was normal. Urinalysis shows 3+ protein and no blood. You do a 24-hour urine test, which shows 400 mg of protein. Her serum creatinine is 0.7 mg/dL. Which of the following conditions does this woman have?

 (A) Gestational hypertension

 (B) Gestational diabetes

 (C) Preeclampsia

 (D) Glomerulonephritis

 (E) Eclampsia

Go on to next page

30. Which of the following statements is true concerning the diagnosis of fibrocystic breast disease?

    (A) Patients can experience pain in both breasts that is unrelated to the menstrual cycle.

    (B) Complaints include the breasts feeling swollen or full.

    (C) A nipple discharge is not present.

    (D) In some women, fibrocystic breast disease is considered to be a premalignant condition.

    (E) Treatment includes mastectomy and/or lumpectomy and radiation.

31. You're seeing a 75-year-old man who presents with an acute onset of crushing chest pain. His electrocardiogram (ECG), as shown, is an example of which of the following conditions?

    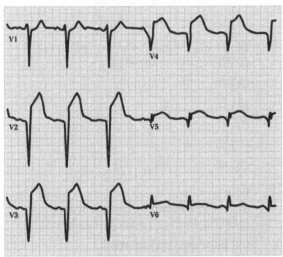

    (A) Inferior wall myocardial infarction (MI)

    (B) Anterior wall MI

    (C) Lateral wall MI

    (D) Posterior wall MI

    (E) Pericarditis

32. What is the standard for treating an ST elevation myocardial infarction (STEMI)?

    (A) Intravenous (IV) heparin and nitroglycerin

    (B) Tissue plasminogen activator (tPA) to be given in the ER

    (C) Clopidogrel (Plavix)

    (D) Emergent cardiac intervention in the catheterization lab

    (E) IV beta blocker

33. What vessel is the primary supplier of blood supply to the left ventricle?

    (A) Left circumflex artery

    (B) Right coronary artery

    (C) Coronary sinus

    (D) Right posterior descending artery

    (E) Left anterior descending artery

34. You're evaluating an older man who has had a change in mental status. His wife states that he fell a few days ago. For the past few days, he has had periods where he is absolutely lucid and clear, but then at other times he is confused. What's the most likely cause of this person's confusion?

    (A) Acute cerebrovascular accident (CVA)

    (B) Subdural hematoma

    (C) Alzheimer's dementia

    (D) Depression

    (E) Meningitis

35. You are evaluating a 70-year-old woman who says that she's embarrassed because her hands shake when she gets really nervous. Her hands shake so badly she can't even use a knife to cut her food. She denies any problems with walking. When she "takes a nip" of alcohol, she notices that her hands stop shaking for a period of time. What does this woman likely suffer from?

    (A) Post-traumatic stress disorder

    (B) Essential tremor

    (C) Parkinson's disease

    (D) Tardive dyskinesia

    (E) Myoclonus

Go on to next page

36. You're interviewing a 45-year-old man with loss of vision. He states that he has trouble seeing out of his right eye and that he's also experiencing severe pain in that eye. On physical examination the left pupil is normal and reactive, but the right pupil is dilated and doesn't constrict in response to light. He has an elevated intraocular pressure. What is the most likely cause of this patient's symptoms?

    (A) Temporal arteritis

    (B) Amaurosis fugax

    (C) Closed-angle glaucoma

    (D) Macular degeneration

    (E) Retinal detachment

37. Optic neuritis is strongly associated with which medical condition?

    (A) Multiple sclerosis (MS)

    (B) Ischemic cerebrovascular accident (CVA)

    (C) Diabetic retinopathy

    (D) Myasthenia gravis

    (E) Orbital cellulitis

38. You're evaluating a 50-year-old woman with abdominal pain. On examination she has a positive Murphy's sign. What's the likely cause of her abdominal pain?

    (A) Hepatitis

    (B) Ischemic colitis

    (C) Cholecystitis

    (D) Diverticulitis

    (E) Regional enteritis

39. Which of the following physical exam signs is associated with pyelonephritis?

    (A) McBurney's point tenderness

    (B) Rovsing's sign

    (C) Costovertebral tenderness

    (D) Psoas sign

    (E) Obturator sign

40. You are evaluating a 5-year-old child who presents with fever and ear pain. On examination you don't see a cone of light reflex. The tympanic membrane is erythematous and hyperemic. The child winces when air is insufflated into the ear canal. What are you likely dealing with?

    (A) Perforated eardrum

    (B) Otitis media

    (C) External otitis

    (D) Mastoiditis

    (E) Acute sinusitis

41. Which of the following is the most common cause of mortality among teenagers?

    (A) Poisoning and toxic ingestions

    (B) Suicide

    (C) Drowning

    (D) Motor vehicle accidents

    (E) Guns and other firearms

42. Obesity is defined as a body mass index (BMI) greater than what?

    (A) 20

    (B) 25

    (C) 30

    (D) 35

    (E) 40

43. Which of the following changes would you expect to find on an electrocardiogram (ECG) in someone with hypocalcemia?

    (A) Shortened QT interval

    (B) Prolonged QT interval

    (C) Prominent U wave

    (D) Diffuse PR interval prolongation

    (E) Widened QRS complex

Go on to next page

44. You're evaluating a 40-year-old woman in the clinic. She complains of a milky, whitish vaginal discharge. During your gynecologic exam you note the appearance of a whitish, cottage-cheese like discharge. What would you prescribe?

    (A) Azithromycin (Zithromax)

    (B) Doxycycline (Vibramycin)

    (C) Ceftriaxone (Rocephin)

    (D) Fluconazole (Diflucan)

    (E) Metronidazole (Flagyl)

45. Which of the following medications can change the color of body secretions to reddish-orange?

    (A) Isoniazid

    (B) Rifampin

    (C) Pyrazinamide

    (D) Myambutol

    (E) Streptomycin

46. What would be the most common cause of meningitis in a 75-year-old woman?

    (A) _Streptococcus pneumoniae_

    (B) _Pneumocystis jiroveci_

    (C) _Haemophilus influenzae_

    (D) _Staphylococcus aureus_

    (E) _Cryptococcus neoformans_

47. You're evaluating a patient with systemic lupus erythematosus (SLE) who was placed on hydroxychloroquine (Plaquenil). What would you recommend that the patient do?

    (A) Have her liver and kidney functions monitored.

    (B) Have a complete blood count (CBC) taken monthly.

    (C) Follow up closely with an ophthalmologist.

    (D) Have an annual audiogram.

    (E) Watch for possible bruising or bleeding.

48. Which of the following symptoms are associated with rheumatoid arthritis (RA)?

    (A) Profound fatigue

    (B) Morning stiffness lasting more than one hour

    (C) Multiple symmetrical tender points

    (D) Inability to get a good night's sleep

    (E) Restless legs syndrome (RLS)

49. You're evaluating a 32-year-old man who was found on the ground after a drug overdose. It's not known how long he was on the ground, but from the history you suspect it may have been several hours. On admission labs you see that his creatinine level is 4.5 mg/dL. His urinalysis is strongly positive for blood, but the microscopic evaluation reveals only 0–2 RBC/HPF. Which of the following is the likely cause of the hematuria and acute renal failure (ARF) in this patient?

    (A) Wegener's granulomatosis

    (B) Acute glomerulonephritis

    (C) Rhabdomyolysis

    (D) Intravascular hemolysis

    (E) Nephrolithiasis

50. What is a major consequence of vitamin B_6 deficiency?

    (A) Decrease in nighttime vision

    (B) Peripheral neuropathy

    (C) Vestibular dysfunction

    (D) Easy bruising

    (E) Brittle bones

Go on to next page ⇨

51. You're evaluating a 35-year-old man who was in a motor vehicle accident, resulting in significant brain trauma and bleeding. He's on a ventilator and is noncommunicative. On his third day of hospitalization, he has a significant urine output and is diuresing almost 3–4 L/day. His serum creatinine is 0.7 mg/dL, and his serum glucose is 88 mg/dL. He's not on any diuretics. What's the most likely cause of his increased urine output?

    (A) Diabetes mellitus

    (B) Diabetes insipidus

    (C) Recovery of acute renal failure (ARF)

    (D) Medication effect

    (E) Osmotic diuresis

52. Which of the following statements concerning digoxin (Lanoxin) is true?

    (A) Its primary effect is on the sinoatrial (SA) node.

    (B) It's used in the treatment of atrial fibrillation.

    (C) It can be removed by hemodialysis.

    (D) It's used in the treatment of diastolic congestive heart failure (CHF).

    (E) The use of this medication increases morbidity.

53. You're evaluating a 45-year-old man who presents with shortness of breath. He reports worsening dyspnea on exertion over the past several months. He states he has worked with glass since he was in his 20s. You order a chest radiograph, which demonstrates eggshell calcifications. What's the medical condition causing his symptoms?

    (A) Silicosis

    (B) Asbestosis

    (C) Coal worker's pneumoconiosis

    (D) Berylliosis

    (E) Interstitial pulmonary fibrosis (IPF)

54. What species of bacterium is most commonly identified as the causative agent of hemolytic uremic syndrome (HUS)?

    (A) *Salmonella*

    (B) *Campylobacter*

    (C) *Shigella*

    (D) *Escherichia coli*

    (E) *Cryptosporidium*

55. What's the cell type associated with Hodgkin's lymphoma?

    (A) Auer rod

    (B) Reed-Sternberg cell

    (C) Atypical lymphocyte

    (D) Target cell

    (E) Schistocyte

56. You're evaluating a 24-year-old vegan who presents with fatigue and weakness. The patient states he has numbness and tingling in his ankles and feet. He also complains of worsening chronic diarrhea for the last few weeks. On exam he has pale conjunctivas, and you notice a swollen, red tongue. What test would you order?

    (A) Folic acid level

    (B) Vitamin B_{12} level

    (C) Thyroid-stimulating hormone (TSH)

    (D) Liver function tests (LFTs)

    (E) Reticulocyte count

57. Which of the following is true concerning metformin (Glucophage)?

    (A) It is associated with weight gain and edema.

    (B) It inhibits carbohydrate absorption in the intestine.

    (C) It increases peripheral utilization of insulin into the tissues.

    (D) It can cause constipation.

    (E) It should be used with caution in anyone with liver disease.

58. What are the deposits of uric acid crystals that can occur on multiple joints referred to?

    (A) Tophi

    (B) Podagra

    (C) Pellagra

    (D) Tender points

    (E) Trigger points

Go on to next page

59. You are evaluating a 35-year-old man who believes he can fly and is bulletproof. What is this is an example of?

    (A) Hallucination

    (B) Delusion

    (C) Somatoform disorder

    (D) Mania

    (E) Paranoid schizophrenia

60. You're evaluating a 23-year-old man who presents to the ER with a blood pressure of 180/110 mmHg and a pulse of 110 beats per minute. Which of the following would you order next?

    (A) Urine drug screen

    (B) Serum sodium and calcium level

    (C) Blood glucose level

    (D) MRI of head

    (E) Salicylate level

STOP DO NOT TURN THE PAGE UNTIL TOLD TO DO SO.
DO NOT RETURN TO A PREVIOUS TEST.

Block 4

Time: 60 minutes for 60 questions

Directions: Choose the *best* answer to each question. Mark the corresponding oval on the answer sheet.

1. Which of the following is true about an S3?

    (A) It represents ventricular volume overload.

    (B) It is always heard in a patient with atrial fibrillation.

    (C) It represents closure of the aortic and pulmonic valves.

    (D) It represents atrial contraction into a noncompliant ventricle.

    (E) It represents closure of the mitral and tricuspid valves.

2. You're evaluating a 46-year-old man for tachycardia. He complains of nausea, vomiting, and abdominal pain for the past three days. You obtain an electrocardiogram (ECG) that demonstrates sinus tachycardia at a rate of 120 beats per minute with no ischemic changes. On physical examination the person has a temperature of 38.9°C (102°F) and a blood pressure of 90/60 mmHg. You also note he has very dry mucous membranes and tenderness to palpation of the abdomen. Which of the following statements is true concerning the treatment of his sinus tachycardia?

    (A) He should be started on intravenous (IV) fluids.

    (B) He should be given IV diuretics.

    (C) He should be given IV metoprolol (Lopressor).

    (D) He should be given IV hydrocortisone (Solu Medrol).

    (E) He needs to have a stress test done.

3. What type of fluids would you prescribe for someone who is volume depleted?

    (A) 0.45% normal saline

    (B) Dextrose 5% in water (D5W)

    (C) Intravenous (IV) fluids with bicarbonate

    (D) Isotonic saline

    (E) Fresh frozen plasma (FFP)

4. You're evaluating a 36-year-old man with a 20-year history of type I diabetes who has nausea and vomiting with most of his meals. He also experiences early satiety. In addition to small, frequent meals, what medication would you prescribe?

    (A) Ranitidine (Zantac)

    (B) Sucralfate (Carafate)

    (C) Metoclopramide (Reglan)

    (D) Pantoprazole (Protonix)

    (E) Cisapride (Propulsid)

5. You're evaluating a 65-year-old man with emphysema. You want to prescribe ipratropium bromide (Atrovent). Which of the following statements is true regarding its mechanism of action?

    (A) It is used to treat bronchiectasis.

    (B) It is not indicated for the treatment of asthma.

    (C) It works as a muscarinic receptor agonist.

    (D) It works synergistically with albuterol to promote better bronchodilatory effects.

    (E) It has predominantly cholinergic side effects.

Go on to next page

6. You're evaluating a 48-year-old man who presents with shortness of breath. He's been living in the Ohio River Valley the last few months. For the past week he has been having a cough and flu-like symptoms. The chest radiograph shows some hilar adenopathy as well as lower lobe infiltrates. What's the most likely diagnosis?

   (A) Tuberculosis

   (B) Aspergillosis

   (C) Sarcoidosis

   (D) Coccidiomycosis

   (E) Histoplasmosis

7. A 65-year-old man with a 30 pack-year smoking history presents with painless gross hematuria. He had worked as a dye maker several years before retirement. He denies any flank pain and has no history of kidney stones. His urinalysis is positive for blood and trace protein. The microscopic evaluation shows 8–10 RBC/HPF. A 24-hour protein is undetectable. What is your next diagnostic test?

   (A) Pursue a kidney biopsy to evaluate for glomerulonephritis.

   (B) Order a CT scan of the abdomen and cystoscopy.

   (C) Obtain a urine culture and start trimethoprim/sulfamethoxazole (Bactrim).

   (D) Check blood creatine phosphokinase (CPK) level.

   (E) Repeat the 24-hour urine protein test.

8. You're evaluating a 67-year-old man who has difficulty swallowing and has been losing weight. He has a smoking history. He denies any cough or hemoptysis. He states he has had a history of heartburn for years. An endoscopy is performed and reveals a mass in the distal part of the esophagus. What's the most likely type of malignancy you're dealing with?

   (A) Adenocarcinoma

   (B) Squamous cell carcinoma

   (C) Transitional cell cancer

   (D) Esophageal dysplasia

   (E) Esophageal lymphoma

9. Most gallstones are cholesterol-based stones. Which of the following is a risk factor for the development of pigment stones?

   (A) Female gender

   (B) Diabetes

   (C) Gastric bypass surgery

   (D) Sickle cell disease

   (E) Obesity

10. Which of the following is histologically necessary for the diagnosis of Barrett's esophagus?

    (A) Peyer's patches

    (B) Goblet cells

    (C) Howell-Jolly bodies

    (D) Epithelial cell hyperplasia

    (E) Keratinized epithelium

11. You are evaluating a 36-year-old man with a sore and tender right shoulder and fever. He has had no trauma and has no prior history of gout or pseudogout. You review the chart and find out that he has positive blood cultures as well as vegetation on his mitral valve. What is the most likely source of pain in his right shoulder?

    (A) Gout

    (B) Pseudogout

    (C) Osteoarthritis

    (D) Lyme disease

    (E) Septic arthritis

12. Which of the following statements is correct concerning an S4?

    (A) An S4 represents the closing of the mitral and tricuspid valves.

    (B) An S4 is always heard in a patient with atrial fibrillation.

    (C) An S4 represents the closing of the aortic and pulmonic valves.

    (D) An S4 represents atrial contraction into a noncompliant ventricle.

    (E) An S4 is always heard after an S3.

Go on to next page

13. Which of the following has a positive effect on bone density?

    (A) Steroid use

    (B) Hydrochlorothiazide, or HCTZ

    (C) Testosterone deficiency

    (D) Heparin

    (E) Phenytoin (Dilantin)

14. You're evaluating a 56-year-old woman who complains of a headache when she eats. You probe further and find out it is actually her jaw that hurts when she eats. She recently went to the dentist who told her she "ground" her teeth at night. On examination, the proximal part of her left jaw is tender when she opens her mouth. Which of the following are you most likely dealing with?

    (A) Temporal arteritis

    (B) Dental cavity

    (C) Temporomandibular joint (TMJ) syndrome

    (D) Cervical disc disease

    (E) Bell's palsy

15. You're seeing a 65-year-old man who fell on his right shoulder several weeks ago. At the time he didn't tell anyone because he was "sick and tired of going to the doctor." Over the past few days, he has noticed problems moving his shoulder. On exam his shoulder seems "stiff." He has a limited range of motion in abduction, adduction, and rotation. What are you most likely dealing with?

    (A) Adhesive capsulitis

    (B) Shoulder dislocation

    (C) Osteoarthritis

    (D) Clavicular fracture

    (E) Gout flare

16. Which of the following is true concerning the diagnosis of dacryocystitis?

    (A) It is an infection of the conjunctiva.

    (B) The etiology is due to obstruction of the lacrimal sac.

    (C) The infection is considered to be viral in nature.

    (D) This is felt to be a medical emergency.

    (E) Significant clinical findings include diplopia.

17. Which of the following is a cause of osteomyelitis?

    (A) *Moraxella catarrhalis*

    (B) *Pseudomonas aeruginosa*

    (C) *Streptococcus pneumoniae*

    (D) *Chlamydia trachomatis*

    (E) *Haemophilus influenzae*

18. What's the primary cause of acromegaly?

    (A) Adrenal gland tumor

    (B) Pancreatic hyperplasia

    (C) Paraneoplastic phenomenon

    (D) Pituitary adenoma

    (E) Medication adverse effect

19. What's the primary difference between gigantism and acromegaly?

    (A) Only acromegaly is associated with increased secretion of growth hormone.

    (B) Only those affected with gigantism are at risk for hypertension and left ventricular hypertrophy (LVH).

    (C) Only acromegaly has increased secretion of insulin-like growth factor (IGF-1).

    (D) Gigantism refers to tremendous growth before the growth plates fuse together; acromegaly is tremendous growth after fusion occurs.

    (E) Acromegaly refers to tremendous growth before the growth plates fuse together; gigantism is tremendous growth after fusion occurs.

Go on to next page

20. You are evaluating a 33-year-old woman who presents with complete delirium, including not knowing where she is. Her roommate states that the patient hasn't been acting right for days. She has been vomiting and has had multiple bouts of diarrhea. She has been unable to sleep, and the roommate reports that the patient couldn't stand being in a hot room and has had the air conditioner on full tilt in their apartment. On physical examination she has a temp of 40°C (104°F); her heart rate is 120 beats per minute. She appears agitated, and her reflexes are hyperactive. A urine drug screen is negative. This patient is likely experiencing which of the following conditions?

    (A) Myxedema

    (B) Thyroid storm

    (C) Addisonian crisis

    (D) Cocaine overdose

    (E) Pheochromocytoma

21. Which of the following would you prescribe for treating the symptoms of hyperthyroidism?

    (A) Beta blockers

    (B) Intravenous (IV) hydrocortisone

    (C) Phenoxybenzamine

    (D) Levothyroxine (Synthroid)

    (E) IV hydralazine

22. You're evaluating a 55-year-old man for anemia. He has a history of diabetes and a chronic osteomyelitis of his left foot. He has been in the hospital twice in the last year for transmetatarsal amputations. His hemoglobin is 8.5 mg/dL, his mean corpuscular volume (MCV) is 75, his ferritin is 1,200, and his iron saturation is 55%. What's the most likely cause of the anemia?

    (A) Lead poisoning

    (B) Iron-deficiency anemia

    (C) Thalassemia

    (D) Liver disease

    (E) Anemia of chronic disease

23. You're evaluating a 25-year-old woman who bruises easily. She states she has been noticing bleeding from her gums when she brushes her teeth as well as nose bleeding. She states her menses are heavier than before. She has a normal complete blood count (CBC). Her platelet count is normal. She has a normal Protime but a prolonged partial thromboplastin time (PTT). Her bleeding time is prolonged. Which of the following tests would you order next?

    (A) Factor VIII level

    (B) Liver function test (LFT)

    (C) Creatinine level

    (D) vWF assay and Factor VIII level

    (E) Fibrinogen level

24. The presence of Whipple's triad would be strongly suggestive of which condition?

    (A) Glucagonoma

    (B) Insulinoma

    (C) Diabetes mellitus

    (D) Diabetes insipidus

    (E) Hepatic failure

25. Which of the following is the most common histology of bladder cancer?

    (A) Transitional cell cancer

    (B) Squamous cell cancer

    (C) Adenocarcinoma

    (D) Small cell carcinona

    (E) Large cell carcinoma

26. A 35-year-old man was recently started on hydrochlorothiazide, or HCTZ, for high blood pressure. Which of the following abnormalities would you expect to find?

    (A) Hyperkalemia and metabolic acidosis

    (B) Hypokalemia and metabolic acidosis

    (C) Hypokalemia and metabolic alkalosis

    (D) Hyperkalemia and metabolic alkalosis

    (E) Hypokalemia only

Go on to next page

27. A 20-year-old man with type I diabetes mellitus presents to the hospital with a blood sugar of 800, a CO_2 of 10, and a pH of 7.28. His serum creatinine is 1.2 mg/dL, and his anion gap is 25. What's the initial step in treatment?

    (A) Normal saline followed by insulin infusion

    (B) Subcutaneous Lispro

    (C) Intravenous (IV) insulin infusion followed by normal saline

    (D) IV bicarbonate

    (E) Subcutaneous Lantus

28. What urinary microscopic finding is consistent with acute tubular necrosis (ATN)?

    (A) Dysmorphic red cells

    (B) Pyuria and white cell casts

    (C) Squamous epithelial cells

    (D) Muddy brown granular casts

    (E) Urine eosinophils

29. Which of the following is a side effect of sildenafil (Viagra)?

    (A) Hypertension

    (B) Pulmonary vasodilation

    (C) Ototoxicity

    (D) Hypokalemia

    (E) Neuropathy

30. Which of the following is associated with lung cancer?

    (A) Low calcium levels

    (B) Polycythemia

    (C) Ectopic ACTH production

    (D) Hematuria

    (E) High blood pressure

31. You're evaluating a patient who has a nasogastric (NG) tube. The NG tube has been on continuous suction for the last several hours. What acid-base abnormality would you expect to see?

    (A) Respiratory alkalosis

    (B) Metabolic acidosis

    (C) Metabolic alkalosis

    (D) Respiratory acidosis

    (E) Mixed acid-base disorder

32. What's the basic hemodynamic change in septic shock?

    (A) Decreased cardiac output

    (B) Decreased systemic vascular resistance

    (C) Increased afterload

    (D) Decreased preload

    (E) Changes in osmotic pressure

33. Which of the following is the primary side effect of indinavir (Crixivan)?

    (A) Nephrolithiasis

    (B) Proteinuria

    (C) Hypertension

    (D) Edema

    (E) Acute renal failure (ARF)

34. You are evaluating a 32-year-old man who presents with a sudden onset of pleuritic chest pain and shortness of breath. You're concerned about the possibility of a pulmonary embolism (PE). Which of the following tests, if negative, virtually excludes the possibility of a PE being present?

    (A) Fibrinogen

    (B) Fibrin degradation products

    (C) D-dimer

    (D) Erythrocyte sedimentation rate (ESR)

    (E) C-reactive protein

Go on to next page

35. You're seeing a 54-year-old man with worsening shortness of breath. You obtain a high-resolution CT scan that demonstrates a reticular pattern and honeycombing. What's the most likely diagnosis?

    (A) Sarcoidosis

    (B) Lymphoma

    (C) Interstitial pulmonary fibrosis (IPF)

    (D) Bronchogenic carcinoma

    (E) Aspergillosis

36. Those affected with phenylketonuria (PKU) lack the enzyme necessary to convert phenylalanine to which amino acid?

    (A) Tyrosine

    (B) Cystine

    (C) Methionine

    (D) Taurine

    (E) Arginine

37. You're evaluating a 65-year-old man admitted to the hospital for pulmonary edema. He's allergic to sulfa medications, but he also states he has had allergic reactions to furosemide (Lasix) and bumetanide (Bumex) as well. What could you give to this patient instead?

    (A) Torsemide (Demadex)

    (B) Ethacrynic acid (Edecrin)

    (C) Hydrochlorothiazide, or HCTZ (Microzide)

    (D) Acetazolamide (Diamox)

    (E) Metolazone (Zaroxolyn)

38. A 40-year-old healthcare worker asks you to read his purified protein derivative (PPD) that was administered two days ago. It shows an area of induration of 14 mm. What would you tell this individual?

    (A) This result is not considered to be positive.

    (B) He needs a repeat chest radiograph in six months.

    (C) He needs aggressive treatment because he has tested positive.

    (D) This may be a false positive, so he needs to be retested in three months.

    (E) He should take isoniazid (Tubizid) for one month only.

39. Which of the following statements concerning *Helicobacter pylori* is true?

    (A) It's a Gram-negative microaerophilic rod.

    (B) It's linked to the development of intestinal cancer.

    (C) It's a leading cause of Crohn's disease.

    (D) It can be detected via saliva.

    (E) The treatment includes the use of sucralfate (Carafate).

40. You are seeing an older man who presents with hemoptysis and acute renal failure (ARF). His blood pressure is 136/80 mmHg. A lung exam is clear to auscultation, and he has mild edema. Urinalysis demonstrates 3+ protein and 2+ blood. His serum creatinine is 2.6 mg/dL. Which of the following is the cause of his symptoms?

    (A) Goodpasture's syndrome

    (B) Lung cancer

    (C) Pulmonary embolism (PE)

    (D) Acute coronary syndrome (ACS)

    (E) Congestive heart failure (CHF)

41. Which of the following is used in the treatment of otitis media?

    (A) Trimethoprim/sulfamethoxazole (Bactrim)

    (B) Clindamycin (Cleocin)

    (C) Amoxicillin (Trimox)

    (D) Ceftriaxone (Rocephin)

    (E) Fluconazole (Diflucan)

42. What is the recommended treatment for erythema migrans?

    (A) Hydrocortisone (Cortaid) cream

    (B) Amoxicillin/clavulanic acid (Augmentin)

    (C) Clotirmiazole (Lotrimin)

    (D) Doxycycline (Vibramycin)

    (E) Metronidazole (Flagyl)

Go on to next page

43. What is the treatment for *trichomonas vaginalis* (vaginitis)?

    (A) Amoxicillin (Trimox)

    (B) Metronidazole (Flagyl)

    (C) Azithromycin (Zithromax)

    (D) Acyclovir (Cyclovir)

    (E) Doxycycline (Vibramycin)

44. You're evaluating a 25-year-old man who was involved in a motor vehicle accident. On exam, the person is complaining of double vision in his right eye. When evaluating his extraocular muscles, you note that he has difficulty with lateral gaze. What are you most likely dealing with?

    (A) Entropion

    (B) Optic neuritis

    (C) Amaurosis fugax

    (D) Blowout fracture

    (E) Myasthenia gravis

45. Which of the following is a common complication of a *Staphylococcus aureus* infection?

    (A) Splenic rupture

    (B) Hemolysis

    (C) Hepatitis

    (D) Acute kidney injury

    (E) Endocarditis

46. What's the treatment for Rocky Mountain spotted fever?

    (A) Amoxicillin (Trimox)

    (B) Azithromycin (Zithromax)

    (C) Doxycycline (Vibramycin)

    (D) Cefuroxime axetil (Ceftin)

    (E) Metronidazole (Flagyl)

47. Which of the following is a diagnostic criterion for tardive dyskinesia?

    (A) Inability to sustain a conversation with peers

    (B) Lack of interest in being socially interactive

    (C) Repeating the same word over and over

    (D) Lip smacking or repetitive facial movements

    (E) Being inflexible to changes in routine

48. Which of the following is a side effect of venlafaxine (Effexor)?

    (A) Hypertension

    (B) Hyperglycemia

    (C) Hypothyroidism

    (D) Hyperlipidemia

    (E) Weight gain

49. You're evaluating a 56-year-old obese man who can barely stay awake. He drives a truck and is afraid he's going to fall asleep on the road. He states that when he awakens in the morning, he feels as if he hasn't slept at all. What's your next step in management?

    (A) Obtain an MRI of the head.

    (B) Obtain a polysomnography.

    (C) Order an electroencephalogram (EEG).

    (D) Prescribe an antidepressant.

    (E) Check his thyroid-stimulating hormone (TSH) level.

50. You're evaluating a 60-year-old man who presents with difficulty speaking and left-sided weakness. What is the time frame in which tissue plasminogen activator (tPA) can be given in this setting?

    (A) Six hours from onset of symptoms

    (B) Three hours from onset of symptoms

    (C) One hour from onset of symptoms

    (D) Never

    (E) Within a 12-hour time frame

51. You're treating a pregnant woman who was recently diagnosed with hyperthyroidism. Which of the following is safe for her to use?

    (A) Methimazole (Tapazole)

    (B) Levothyroxine (Synthroid)

    (C) Propylthiouracil, or PTU

    (D) Iodine 131-I

    (E) Prednisone (Deltasone)

Go on to next page

52. Which of the following would not be an indication for the use of antibiotics for endocarditis prophylaxis?

   (A) Presence of congenital heart disease

   (B) Presence of a pacemaker

   (C) Presence of mechanical heart valves

   (D) Mitral valve prolapse (MVP)

   (E) Presence of a vascular graft

53. For a person who's undergoing dental surgery and is allergic to penicillin, which of the following antibiotics can be given prior to surgery for antibiotic prophylaxis?

   (A) Ciprofloxacin (Cipro)

   (B) Metronidazole (Flagyl)

   (C) Doxycycline (Doryx)

   (D) Cefuroxime axetil (Ceftin)

   (E) Clindamycin (Cleocin)

54. You're evaluating a pregnant woman in her third trimester who presents with painless vaginal bleeding. An ultrasound shows that the placenta is blocking the opening to her cervix. What is this condition called?

   (A) Abruptio placentae

   (B) Placenta previa

   (C) Ectopic pregnancy

   (D) Preeclampsia

   (E) Antiphospholipid antibody syndrome

55. What is the most common hypercoagulable state?

   (A) Prothrombin G mutation

   (B) Factor V Leiden mutation

   (C) Antithrombin III deficiency

   (D) Antiphospholipid antibody syndrome

   (E) Protein C deficiency

56. Which of the following supplements is recommended to women who are planning to become pregnant for the prevention of neural tube defects in babies?

   (A) Vitamin B_{12}

   (B) Vitamin C

   (C) Vitamin D

   (D) Folic acid

   (E) Niacin

57. What does this photo show?

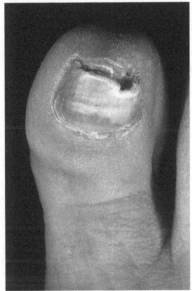

   (A) Paronychia

   (B) Herpetic whitlow

   (C) Koilonychia

   (D) Clubbing

   (E) Onychomycosis

Go on to next page

58. You're evaluating an 85-year-old woman with a history of chronic obstructive pulmonary disease (COPD) and diabetes who complains of belly pain. She states that she remembers having some kind of skin rash across her belly to her back that is slowly going away. She has developed an intense pain along the same area. She says it hurts constantly and nothing makes it better. A CT scan of the abdomen and blood work, including liver function tests (LFTs), report as normal. What is the likely cause of her abdominal and back pain?

    (A) Biliary colic

    (B) Irritable bowel syndrome (IBS)

    (C) Mesenteric angina

    (D) Postherpetic neuralgia

    (E) Pyelonephritis

59. Which of the following would you order to diagnose Cushing's syndrome?

    (A) MRI of the brain

    (B) 24-hour urinary free cortisol

    (C) Serum and urine β-human chorionic gonadotropin (β-hCG) levels

    (D) Ultrasound of the ovaries and measurement of follicle-stimulating hormone (FSH)/luteinizing hormone (LH) levels

    (E) Thyroid-stimulating hormone (TSH) level

60. Which of the following is a component of the antiphospholipid antibody syndrome?

    (A) Thrombocytosis

    (B) Anemia

    (C) Polycythemia

    (D) Hematuria

    (E) Second trimester spontaneous abortions

STOP DO NOT TURN THE PAGE UNTIL TOLD TO DO SO.
DO NOT RETURN TO A PREVIOUS TEST.

Block 5

> **Time:** 60 minutes for 60 questions
>
> **Directions:** Choose the *best* answer to each question. Mark the corresponding oval on the answer sheet.

1. You're evaluating a 40-year-old man during a routine physical. You notice a blood pressure of 182/40 mmHg. On cardiac auscultation you hear an early diastolic murmur. What cardiac abnormality does this person have?

   (A) Aortic stenosis

   (B) Aortic insufficiency

   (C) Mitral regurgitation

   (D) Mitral stenosis

   (E) Tricuspid regurgitation

2. What is the pulse pressure in someone whose blood pressure is 176/94 mmHg?

   (A) 220

   (B) 176

   (C) 132

   (D) 94

   (E) 82

3. You're evaluating a 26-year-old man who presents with fevers, chills, and rigors. He has a history of intravenous drug abuse (IVDA). His blood cultures are positive. On examination you hear a murmur. Which area of the heart is likely affected?

   (A) Mitral valve

   (B) Aortic valve

   (C) Tricuspid valve

   (D) Pulmonic valve

   (E) Sinoatrial node

4. Which of the following is a manifestation of infectious endocarditis (IE)?

   (A) Osler's nodes

   (B) Paronychia

   (C) Trousseau's sign

   (D) Cyanosis

   (E) Grey-Turner's sign

5. You obtain a chest radiograph for a 60-year-old man who presents with a cough, and the results demonstrate a lung nodule. Which of the following characteristics would portend a more benign prognosis?

   (A) Greater than 3 cm in size

   (B) Smooth, round borders

   (C) Spiculated borders

   (D) Lack of calcification within the nodule

   (E) Lack of fat noted within the nodule

6. Which of the following medications used for tuberculosis has color blindness as a possible side effect?

   (A) Ethambutol

   (B) Isoniazid

   (C) Rifampin

   (D) Pyrazinamide

   (E) Streptomycin

7. Which of the following is strongly associated with ulcerative colitis?

   (A) Cholecystitis

   (B) Primary biliary cirrhosis (PBC)

   (C) Cholangiocarcinoma

   (D) Sclerosing cholangitis

   (E) Biliary colic

Go on to next page

8. You're evaluating a 55-year-old woman who presents with an acute productive cough lasting five days. She states that the sputum is yellow colored. She has no smoking history and no other lung disease or chronic medical conditions. On examination you hear expiratory wheezing in both lung fields. A chest radiograph doesn't show any infiltrate or abnormal lung markings. What is the likely etiology of her cough?

    (A) Chronic bronchitis

    (B) Emphysema

    (C) Acute bronchitis

    (D) Sarcoidosis

    (E) Acute sinusitis

9. You're evaluating a 25-year-old house painter who presents with fatigue. On examination his conjunctivas are pale. He also complains of numbness and tingling in his legs. His labs demonstrate a hemoglobin of 8.5 mg/dL and a mean corpuscular volume (MCV) of 75. The smear shows basophilic stippling. What is the most likely cause of this person's anemia?

    (A) Iron deficiency

    (B) Thalassemia

    (C) Lead poisoning

    (D) Chronic disease

    (E) Glucose 6-phosphatase (G6PD) deficiency

10. Which of the following would you recommend for the treatment of a urinary tract infection (UTI)?

    (A) Azithromycin (Zithromax)

    (B) Trimethoprim/sulfamethoxazole (Bactrim)

    (C) Fluconazole (Diflucan)

    (D) Cephalexin (Keflex)

    (E) Acyclovir (Cyclovir)

11. You're evaluating a 64-year-old man who presents with dizziness. Approximately one week ago, he started on a new medication for hypertension. His blood pressure while sitting is 136/70 mmHg with a heart rate of 76 beats per minute. After standing up for 2 minutes, his blood pressure is 110/56 mmHg with a heart rate of 92 beats per minute, and he feels lightheaded. Does this scenario fit the criteria for symptomatic orthostatic hypotension?

    (A) Yes, it does meet the criteria.

    (B) No, it doesn't meet the criteria.

    (C) It fits the systolic blood pressure criteria but not the diastolic.

    (D) It fits the diastolic blood pressure criteria but not the systolic.

    (E) This is not symptomatic orthostatic hypotension because the patient has no symptoms.

12. You're evaluating a person who complains of dizziness when standing up. He has a history of diabetes, but he isn't on blood pressure medications. While sitting, his blood pressure is 118/80 mmHg with a heart rate of 70 beats per minute. When he stands up, his blood pressure is 90/66 mmHg with a heart rate of 60 beats per minute, and he needs to sit down because he's feeling dizzy. What is the underlying reason for this person's postural hypotension?

    (A) Volume depletion

    (B) Medication side effect

    (C) Infection

    (D) Autonomic neuropathy

    (E) Adrenal insufficiency

13. Which of the following medications can cause diabetes insipidus?

    (A) Lithium carbonate (Lithobid)

    (B) Carbamazepine (Tegretol)

    (C) Clofibrate (Atromid-S)

    (D) Furosemide (Lasix)

    (E) Amiloride (Midamor)

Go on to next page

14. Which of the following physical examination findings is consistent with anemia?

    (A) Dry mucous membranes

    (B) Dry buccal mucosa

    (C) Tachycardia

    (D) Diminished skin turgor

    (E) Pale conjunctivas

15. You're evaluating a person who presents with acute hematemesis. He has a history of cirrhosis and is actively drinking. You suspect that he has esophageal varices. Which of the following would be appropriate to administer to manage his acute variceal bleeding?

    (A) Warfarin (Coumadin)

    (B) Vitamin K

    (C) Intravenous (IV) hydrocortisone (Solu-Cortef)

    (D) IV octreotide (Sandostatin)

    (E) Vitamin B_{12}

16. You're evaluating a 55-year-old woman who presents with a lump on her right wrist. She states that it began a few weeks ago and has grown to the point of causing pain in her right hand, and the pain is made worse when she moves her right hand. On physical examination, you identify a lump about ½ inch in size on the dorsal aspect of the right wrist that is soft but not freely movable. What are you likely dealing with?

    (A) Carpal tunnel syndrome

    (B) Morton's neuroma

    (C) Lipoma

    (D) Ganglion cyst

    (E) Tenosynovitis

17. Which of the following side effects is associated with amiodarone (Cordarone)?

    (A) Leukopenia

    (B) Kidney failure

    (C) Pulmonary hemorrhage

    (D) Ototoxicity

    (E) Elevated liver function tests (LFTs)

18. You're seeing a 70-year-old man who complains of numbness when he sits down. He has a history of prostate cancer with bone metastasis. He states that over the last few days he has worsening numbness in his buttocks when he sits down. You probe further, and he states that it has been more difficult to "make it to the bathroom" and that he has been "wetting his pants more" over the last 24 hours. On physical examination, you note loss of tone in the anal sphincter as well as decreased ankle reflexes. What are you likely dealing with?

    (A) Spinal stenosis

    (B) Spondylolisthesis

    (C) Herniated disc

    (D) Muscle spasm

    (E) Cauda equina syndrome

19. You're seeing a 25-year-old man with low back pain. He denies any trauma or fall but states that it's painful to bend down. He's also complaining of his eye hurting. You order an HLA-B27, and it is positive. What would you expect to see on a back radiograph?

    (A) Degeneration of the nucleus pulposus

    (B) Curvature of his lumbar spine

    (C) Narrowing of the spinal canal

    (D) Inflammation of the sacroiliac joint

    (E) Vertebral fracture

20. Which of the following is an effect rather than a cause of pancreatitis?

    (A) Gallstones

    (B) Excessive alcohol use

    (C) Hyperglycemia

    (D) Hypertriglyceridemia

    (E) Medication adverse effects

Go on to next page

21. You're evaluating a 57-year-old man with a history of cirrhosis, admitted for evaluation of abdominal pain. He states that he has belly pain and that he has noticed increased swelling in his belly as well as his legs. His shirt, pants, and shoes are a little tighter than they were a few weeks ago. He denies any nausea, vomiting, or diarrhea. He denies any productive cough. On exam, his temperature is 38.1°C (100.5°F). His sclera are icteric, and his lungs are clear to auscultation. On abdominal examination, the patient has a distended abdomen. His examination is positive for shifting dullness, and bulging flanks are evident. He has diffuse abdominal tenderness to palpation. His white cell count is 18,000/uL, and his creatinine is 0.5 mg/dL. What is the likely cause of this person's abdominal pain?

    (A) Infectious colitis

    (B) Acute hepatitis

    (C) Spontaneous bacteria peritonitis

    (D) Hepatocellular cancer

    (E) Pneumonia

22. Which of the following labs is a true measure of the liver's synthetic function?

    (A) Protime (PT/INR)

    (B) Serum albumin level

    (C) Serum alanine aminotransferase (ALT) level

    (D) Blood glucose level

    (E) Fibrinogen level

23. You're examining a person who has had a change in mental status. During his evaluation, you notice that his blood sugar is low. He's experiencing palpitations and irritability. His symptoms improve after the administration of dextrose. You follow his fasting glucose levels, and again he is symptomatic until given intravenous (IV) dextrose. What is this constellation of symptoms called?

    (A) Beck's triad

    (B) Charcot's triad

    (C) Adrenal insufficiency

    (D) Whipple's triad

    (E) Thiamine deficiency

24. You're in the hospital on call and are asked to evaluate a patient who is bradycardic with a heart rate of 44 beats per minute. An electrocardiogram (ECG) is obtained and demonstrates a junctional rhythm. A stat potassium is obtained, and it is 7.5 mEq/L. What's the first treatment for the hyperkalemia in this patient?

    (A) Sodium polystyrene sulfate (Kayexalate)

    (B) Albuterol nebulizer treatment

    (C) Intravenous (IV) insulin followed by glucose

    (D) IV calcium gluconate

    (E) IV sodium bicarbonate

25. Which of the following would you order in the work-up for malabsorption syndrome?

    (A) Thyroid function test

    (B) Liver function test (LFT)

    (C) AM cortisol

    (D) Hemoglobin A1c

    (E) Anti-gliadin antibody

26. Which of the following is a cause of unconjugated hyperbilirubinemia?

    (A) Gilbert's syndrome

    (B) Cholestatic jaundice

    (C) Viral hepatitis

    (D) Cholecystitis

    (E) Pancreatic malignancy

27. You're examining a 27-week-old infant who is clearly in respiratory distress. You notice flaring of the nostrils as well as tachypnea. The chest radiograph shows atelectasis and a ground glass appearance. In addition to ventilation management, which of the following would you recommend to try to improve his respiratory function?

    (A) Nebulized albuterol

    (B) Intravenous (IV) steroids

    (C) Surfactant

    (D) Aggressive suctioning

    (E) Inhaled nitrous oxide

Go on to next page

28. Which area of the adrenal gland is responsible for cortisol production?

    (A) Zona fasciculata

    (B) Zona reticularis

    (C) Zona glomerulosa

    (D) All of the zones are responsible for cortisol production.

    (E) Marginal zone

29. You're evaluating a 65-year-old man with no history of lung disease. He asks you how often he should obtain a Pneumovax 23 vaccination. How often would you advise that he receive it?

    (A) Every ten years

    (B) Every five years

    (C) This is a lifetime vaccination, so only one dose is needed.

    (D) On an annual basis

    (E) Every three years

30. You're seeing an 18-year-old man who is preparing to go to college. He had a splenectomy as a result of a skiing accident while in high school. Which of the following vaccinations does he need to be given at this time?

    (A) Shingles vaccination

    (B) Tetanus vaccination

    (C) *Haemophilus influenzae* type B vaccination

    (D) Hepatitis B vaccination

    (E) Influenza vaccination

31. Which of the following patients is considered to be at risk for the development of breast cancer?

    (A) A woman with a late menarche

    (B) A woman whose sister was diagnosed with hypothyroidism

    (C) A woman who had her first pregnancy at 20 years of age

    (D) A woman with many children

    (E) A woman with a history of radiation treatments for thyroid cancer

32. Which of the following would be a cause of respiratory acidosis?

    (A) Pregnancy

    (B) Hypoxemia

    (C) Early sepsis

    (D) Kyphosis

    (E) Liver disease

33. You're evaluating a 63-year-old man who has been complaining of persistent heartburn-like symptoms. They have persisted despite lifestyle modification. He has a history of a recent myocardial infarction (MI). You note that he is currently on clopidogrel (Plavix). Which of the following medications may interact with the Plavix?

    (A) Ranitidine (Zantac)

    (B) Pantoprazole (Protonix)

    (C) Misoprostol (Cytotec)

    (D) Sucralfate (Carafate)

    (E) Metoclopramide (Reglan)

34. You're evaluating a 55-year-old man in the ER who presents with pain behind his right eye. He states that several times a year he gets a really bad pain in this location. Nothing over the counter seems to help. The pain is so bad that he says he "wants to stick a fork in his eyeball." On examination, you notice that the eye is tearing, the right pupil is constricted, and the eye is very red. Which of the following would you do next?

    (A) Obtain a sedimentation rate and start oral prednisone.

    (B) Obtain a lumbar puncture (LP).

    (C) Obtain an intraocular pressure.

    (D) Start the patient on a beta blocker.

    (E) Administer oxygen.

35. Which of the following would you order to evaluate for a possible subdural hematoma?

    (A) Radiograph of the skull

    (B) Lumbar puncture (LP)

    (C) Beck Depression Inventory questionnaire

    (D) CT scan of the head

    (E) Empiric trial of donepezil (Aricept)

Go on to next page

36. Which of the following would cause a cholestatic pattern of liver injury?

    (A) Hepatitis C

    (B) Erythromycin (E-Mycin)

    (C) Autoimmune hepatitis

    (D) Atorvastatin (Lipitor)

    (E) Hepatitis A

37. You're evaluating a 35-year-old woman who has just been diagnosed with Lyme disease. She is unable to tolerate doxycycline (Vibramycin) because it gives her severe stomach upset. Which of the following would you recommend to this patient?

    (A) Amoxicillin/clavulanic acid (Augmentin)

    (B) Benadryl 30 minutes prior to administration of doxycycline (Vibramycin)

    (C) Metoclopramide (Reglan) 30 minutes prior to the administration of doxycycline (Vibramycin)

    (D) Chloramphenicol

    (E) Ciprofloxacin (Cipro)

38. Which of the following would you order to diagnose a suspected retroperitoneal bleed?

    (A) Order a noncontrast CT scan of his abdomen and pelvis.

    (B) Check a peripheral smear for schistocytes.

    (C) Check an anti-gliadin antibody.

    (D) Order a chest radiograph.

    (E) Order a colonoscopy.

39. You're evaluating the blood work of a 40-year-old man for a follow-up office visit. When he comes in to visit you, you tell him that his fasting blood glucose level is elevated at 145 mg/dL and that he may have diabetes. You tell him he needs more testing to be sure, however. He nods and then asks you, "Why is my skin dark?" On exam, you notice the skin around his chest area and arms are a bronze color. On examination, you also note some testicular atrophy. Which of the following would you test for next?

    (A) Testosterone level

    (B) AM cortisol

    (C) Age-related cancer screening

    (D) Iron studies and ferritin level

    (E) Anti-nuclear antibody (ANA)

40. You're evaluating a 75-year-old man who presents to the hospital with worsening shortness of breath. He's an ornithologist and has lived in the Midwest for several years. On a chest radiograph you see what looks like small bullet holes across both lungs. He has no history of human immunodeficiency virus (HIV). What would you prescribe for this individual?

    (A) Diflucan (Fluconazole)

    (B) Amphotericin B (Amphotec)

    (C) Isoniazid

    (D) Isoniazid and ceftriaxone (Rifampin)

    (E) Ceftriaxone (Rifampin) and azithromycin (Zithromax)

41. For which group of people do you recommend screening for hypothyroidism?

    (A) Men greater than 21 years of age

    (B) Women greater than 25 years of age

    (C) Men greater than 65 years of age

    (D) Women greater than 30 years of age

    (E) Women and men greater than 35 years of age

Go on to next page

42. On fundoscopic examination of a patient, you notice the presence of whitish exudates and hemorrhages on retinal exam. What does this person most likely have?

    (A) Hypertension

    (B) Diabetes

    (C) Systemic lupus erythematosus (SLE)

    (D) Hyperthyroidism

    (E) Macular degeneration

43. You're evaluating a 64-year-old man who watches television continuously. He states that he doesn't like the TV shows themselves but that he is transfixed by the commercials. He receives "messages" from the television on an almost daily basis. Which of the following is most correct concerning his behavior?

    (A) He is suffering from a visual hallucination.

    (B) He is suffering from an auditory hallucination.

    (C) He is exhibiting manic behavior.

    (D) His behavior is likely a manifestation of schizophrenia.

    (E) He is suffering from a delusion.

44. You are evaluating a 30-year-old man who's complaining of dry, chapped hands. He's concerned about keeping his hands clean and washes them a minimum of 20 times a day. In addition to behavioral therapy, which of the following would you recommend?

    (A) Nortriptyline (Pamelor)

    (B) Sertraline (Zoloft)

    (C) Venlafaxine (Effexor)

    (D) Haloperidol (Haldol)

    (E) Bupropion (Wellbutrin)

45. Which of the following would be characteristic of the cerebral spinal fluid (CSF) in someone who has viral meningitis?

    (A) High protein, low glucose, and elevated white cell count with a neutrophilic predominance

    (B) Low protein, high glucose, and normal white cell count

    (C) Higher than normal protein, high glucose, and lymphocytic pleocytosis

    (D) Higher than normal protein, normal glucose, and lymphocytic pleocytosis

    (E) Low protein, low glucose, and elevated white cell count with a neutrophilic predominance

46. You're evaluating a male patient with chronic obstructive pulmonary disease (COPD) and notice that on a spirometry his FEV1/FVC is less than 50% of the predicted value. What would you classify the person's COPD as?

    (A) Mild

    (B) Moderate

    (C) Severe

    (D) Indeterminate, based on data given

    (E) Does not meet criteria for COPD

47. In addition to committing to a quit date and to smoking cessation classes, which of the following medications would you recommend to help someone stop smoking?

    (A) Paroxetine (Paxil)

    (B) Amitriptyline (Elavil)

    (C) Bupropion (Zyban)

    (D) Venlafaxine (Effexor)

    (E) Aripiprazole (Abilify)

Go on to next page

48. You're evaluating a 36-year-old man with human immunodeficiency virus (HIV) who has a persistently elevated lactic acid level. His serum lactic acid level is 3.5 mEq/L. He denies any sickness, he says he feels well, and he claims he has had no recent gastro-intestinal (GI) symptoms. His blood pressure is normal. Which of the following would you do next?

    (A) Review his HIV medication regimen.

    (B) Obtain a CT scan of his abdomen and pelvis, with both oral and intravenous (IV) contrast.

    (C) Check a D-lactate level.

    (D) Check liver function tests (LFTs).

    (E) Check a kidney function panel.

49. You're evaluating a 65-year-old man with a history of hypertension and diabetes. He has a creatinine of 1.4 mg/dL, giving him a glomerular filtration rate (GFR) of 55 mL/min. Which stage of chronic kidney disease (CKD) is he at?

    (A) Stage 1

    (B) Stage 2

    (C) Stage 3

    (D) Stage 4

    (E) Stage 5

50. A 45-year-old man presents with recurrent fevers. On physical examination you note a significant heart murmur and the presence of small macular lesions on the palmer aspect of the hand and the soles of the feet. What are these specific physical examination findings indicative of?

    (A) Rocky Mountain spotted fever

    (B) Infectious endocarditis (IE)

    (C) Lyme disease

    (D) Seronegative spondyloarthropathy

    (E) Rheumatoid arthritis (RA)

51. You are in the intensive care unit and plan to place an arterial line in a patient's radial artery in order to more closely monitor his blood pressure. What should you do before placing the arterial line?

    (A) Perform an ankle-brachial index (ABI).

    (B) Check radial pulses in both arms.

    (C) Obtain a Doppler evaluation of the carotid and axillary arteries.

    (D) Perform capillary refill testing on his fingers.

    (E) Perform an Allen's test.

52. Which of the following medications would be the best choice to treat a hypertensive crisis?

    (A) Sodium nitroprusside (Nipride)

    (B) Furosemide (Lasix)

    (C) Digoxin (Lanoxin)

    (D) Methyldopa (Aldomet)

    (E) Hydroxyurea (Hydrea)

53. You're evaluating an 80-year-old man who has a history of NYHA Class III heart failure. He's extremely short of breath. On exam, he is tachypneic, cyanotic, and his blood pressure is 99/60 mmHg. He has a signifi-cant jugular venous distention (JVD), an S3 gallop, rales in both lung fields, and 2+ lower extremity pitting edema. Which of the following would be an appropriate med-ication choice in this situation?

    (A) Dobutamine (Dobutrex)

    (B) Lactated Ringers

    (C) Octreotide (Somatostatin)

    (D) Vasopressin (Pitressin)

    (E) Neo-Synephrine

54. You're evaluating a 34-year-old man who comes to your office for a routine follow-up visit. He has a blood pressure of 120/88 mmHg. Which of the following would you classify him as having?

    (A) Normal blood pressure

    (B) Prehypertension

    (C) Stage I hypertension

    (D) Stage II hypertension

    (E) Stage III hypertension

Go on to next page

55. You're evaluating a 75-year-old man who passed out at home. The episode was witnessed, and he was out for less than a minute when he came to. He denies any shaking or loss of bowel or bladder function. On exam you see no bite marks on the tongue, and he is alert and oriented times three. What is the likely cause of his loss of consciousness?

    (A) Syncope

    (B) Seizure

    (C) Vestibular dysfunction

    (D) Hypertrophic cardiomyopathy

    (E) Adrenal insufficiency

56. You're evaluating a 75-year-old obese woman with shortness of breath. She has a significant smoking history and is still smoking about a half pack per day. She also has a history of diastolic dysfunction as seen on a recent cardiac echocardiogram (ECG). On physical examination, her body habitus makes it difficult to discern whether jugular venous distention (JVD) is present. She has decreased breath sounds at the bases and 1+ lower extremity edema, which the patient states is chronic. Which of the following tests would help you formulate a better treatment plan for this patient?

    (A) Obtain a CT scan of the thorax to help evaluate the lung parenchyma.

    (B) Obtain an arterial blood gas (ABG).

    (C) Obtain a lactic acid level.

    (D) Check a B-type natriuretic peptide (BNP) level.

    (E) Obtain a cardiac echo.

57. Which of the following human papillomavirus (HPV) serotypes is linked to the development of cervical cancer?

    (A) 14

    (B) 18

    (C) 25

    (D) 30

    (E) 37

58. You're evaluating a 30-year-old woman for the development of hypertension. In the office, she tells you that a lot of things "just aren't right." She hasn't had her period over the past several months. She's distraught because she has been trying (unsuccessfully) to become pregnant and is actually seeing a fertility specialist. On physical examination, she is obese with a BMI of 32. Her blood pressure is 160/94 mmHg. You note abnormal hair growth on her face, her chest, and her abdominal area. Concerning labs, you note that she has a blood glucose level of 140 mg/dL. What is this patient is suffering from?

    (A) Cushing's syndrome

    (B) Delayed pregnancy

    (C) Hypothyroidism

    (D) Pituitary adenoma

    (E) Polycystic ovarian syndrome (PCOS)

59. Which of the following would you prescribe for the treatment of postherpetic neuralgia?

    (A) Upper gastrointestinal (GI) series

    (B) Psychiatric consultation

    (C) Gabapentin (Neurontin)

    (D) Ibuprofen

    (E) Percocet

60. Which of the following statements concerning menopause is true?

    (A) Menopause is not a risk factor for the development of osteoporosis.

    (B) It is associated with an undetectable follicle-stimulating hormone (FSH) level.

    (C) It occurs most of the time to women in their early 30s.

    (D) The use of estrogen cream does not help with genitourinary symptoms.

    (E) Late menopause is a risk factor for endometrial cancer.

STOP DO NOT TURN THE PAGE UNTIL TOLD TO DO SO. DO NOT RETURN TO A PREVIOUS TEST.

Chapter 21

PANCE Practice Test Answers and Explanations

*U*se this answer key to score the practice test in Chapter 20. As you're going through the answer explanations, these techniques may be useful:

✔ **Look for trends in incorrect answers.** You may find that you need to study a particular body organ system more in order to do well on the test.

✔ **Count the number of correct answers.** While this check of correct answers won't correlate directly with the NCCPA "weighted scoring," you can be assured that the more questions you get right on the practice test, the more questions you'll get right on the PANCE.

✔ **Take a moment to review how you felt during the practice test.** While panic and frustration are normal parts of the test-taking process, you'll do better on the PANCE if you work on these feelings now. The idea is to let nothing break your cadence when you take the PANCE.

Block 1

1. **E.** Nephrotic syndrome includes edema, low blood albumin levels, hyperlipidemia, and a proteinuria of greater than 3.5 grams. Concerning Choice (E), hyperlipidemia is part of the nephrotic syndrome (the liver wants to "pump out" more protein to compensate for the protein that is being lost in the urine). Cholesterol is, after all, a lipoprotein, with emphasis on the word "protein." Hematuria, Choice (A), is not part of nephrotic syndrome. While hypertension and obstructive uropathy, Choice (C), can cause kidney disease, they would not be typical causes for nephrotic syndrome. Anemia, Choice (D), does not need to present for nephrotic syndrome to occur. Anemia is usually seen in advanced kidney disease, predominantly due to a lack of erythropoietin production by the kidneys.

2. **D.** Intravenous (IV) magnesium, Choice (D), is the recommended treatment for Torsades de Pointes. IV steroids, IV metoprolol (Lopressor), and IV digoxin (Lanoxin) — Choices (A), (B), and (E), respectively — are given to patients with rapid atrial fibrillation or supraventricular tachycardia, but not to patients with Torsades de Pointes.

3. **C.** Angiotensin-converting-enzyme (ACE) inhibitors, such as lisinopril (Zestril), Choice (C), are the only class of medications proven to reduce mortality in patients with systolic congestive heart failure (CHF). Digoxin (Lanoxin), Choice (A), helps improve symptoms of CHF and reduces duration of hospitalization; it improves morbidity but does not impact survival. Hydrochlorothiazide, or HCTZ, Choice (E), is used in the treatment of hypertension. Diltiazem (Cardizem), Choice (D), actually has a negative ionotropic effect on the heart and isn't used in the treatment of systolic CHF. It is used in the treatment of rate control for atrial fibrillation as well as diastolic dysfunction. Terazosin (Hytrin), Choice (B), is used in the treatment of hypertension as well as benign prostatic hypertrophy (BPH).

ACE inhibitors and angiotensin receptor blockers (ARBs) are both thought of as first-line modalities; however, it's unlikely that you would be asked a question where you would have to choose between ACE inhibitors and ARBs.

4. **D.** Angiotensin-converting-enzyme (ACE) inhibitors, not calcium channel blockers, can cause a cough, Choice (E), that requires discontinuing the medication. Angioedema is an uncommon but serious side effect that you need to be aware of with ACE inhibitors as well. The cough is thought to be bradykinin mediated. Constipation and edema, Choice (D), are side effects of calcium channel blockers. Diuretics can cause electrolyte abnormalities, including hypokalemia and hypomagnesemia, Choices (A) and (B).

5. **D.** A history of bleeding or falling is considered a contraindication to any type of anticoagulation. Because the gentleman from the question has a history of both, you have two important clues. You would want to have an inferior vena cava (IVC) filter placed in this patient. This solution is the only safe one you can use in someone with a pulmonary embolism (PE) in whom you can't anticoagulate.

6. **D.** This patient has Rocky Mountain spotted fever. A classic finding related to this disease is a petechial rash on the palms of the hands, wrists, and ankles. This disease is fatal if not treated. You treat Rocky Mountain spotted fever with doxycycline (Doxy-Caps), Choice (D), and by getting rid of the tick, if present. Intravenous (IV) ceftriaxone (Rocephin), Choice (B), is only given if Lyme disease with neurological manifestations is present. Azithromycin (Zithromax), Choice (C), is used to treat pulmonary infections, such as acute bronchitis or community-acquired pneumonia (CAP), not Rocky Mountain spotted fever. This patient's situation is more than a viral exanthema, so Choice (A) is inappropriate. The key in this question is recognizing the characteristic rash of Rocky Mountain spotted fever and the clue about a possible tick bite.

7. **C.** Polycythemia, Choice (E), is a paraneoplastic phenomenon most often related to renal cell cancer. Hypercalcemia, hyponatremia, and hypokalemia are paraneoplastic phenomenon with lung cancer. Ectopic ACTH secretion, Choice (C), is correct here; it's often seen with small-cell lung cancer.

8. **D.** If you see a question concerning the diagnosis of aortic dissection, you should be thinking about two tests: a transesophageal echocardiogram (TEE) or a CT scan of the chest (for thoracic aorta dissection), Choice (D), and a CT scan of the abdomen (for abdominal aortic dissection). Both scans require use of contrast. In an emergent situation, a CT scan with contrast is easier to get. A transthoracic echocardiogram (TTE), Choice (B), isn't as reliable as a TEE or CT scan. An MRI, Choice (C), takes time to obtain. A PET, Choice (E), scan is used in the staging of many malignancies, but it isn't used in the diagnosis of an acute aortic dissection.

9. **D.** While all the choices in this question can cause a macrocytic anemia, vitamin B_{12} deficiency (along with folic acid deficiency) can cause hypersegmented neutrophils on a peripheral smear.

10. **D.** The Dix-Hallpike maneuver, Choice (D), is a test used in the evaluation of vertigo. The Epley maneuver, Choice (C), is used in the treatment of vertigo (not in the evaluation of it). A Tensilon test, Choice (B), is used in the evaluation of myasthenia gravis. The Phalen's maneuver, Choice (A), is associated with carpal tunnel syndrome. Tilt table testing, Choice (E), can be used to evaluate orthostatic hypotension and syncope.

11. **A.** This person has a pleural fluid/serum LDH ratio of greater than 1.0. By Light's criteria, a pleural fluid/serum LDH ratio of greater than 0.6 is a criterion for a pleural effusion to be an exudative effusion. In this question, only pneumonia, Choice (A), is a cause of an exudative effusion. The rest of the choices are causes of a transudative effusion. In any question concerning pleural effusions, you need to be familiar with Light's criteria for evaluating the difference between transudative and exudative pleural effusions.

12. **D.** One of the treatments for a *Staphylococcus aureus* bacteremia is intravenous (IV) vancomycin (Vancocin)(MRSA is initially presumed), Choice (D). You aren't going to give steroids,

Choice (B), to someone who's actively bacteremic and infected. The patient doesn't have gout, so colchicine, Choice (C), isn't needed. The treatment for Lyme disease and Rocky Mountain spotted fever, both tick-borne illnesses, is oral doxycycline (Vibramycin), Choice (E).

13. **C.** You would treat autonomic neuropathy with an agent like midodrine (ProAmatine), which can help raise the blood pressure when standing. Nothing in the question suggests that the patient is volume depleted, infected, or suffering from adrenal insufficiency, thus requiring the other medications.

14. **D.** Lisinopril (Zestril) is an example of an angiotensin-converting-enzyme (ACE) inhibitor. These medications can't be given during pregnancy because they're teratogenic. All the other medications can be given during pregnancy. They also can be used if a patient chooses to breastfeed, because these other medications won't pass through to the breast milk.

15. **C.** Nonalcoholic steatohepatitis (NASH) is inflammation to the liver caused by fat deposition (also known as fatty liver). With the epidemic of obesity and diabetes, more and more people are diagnosed with a fatty liver. All the other choices can cause hepatitis but aren't as common.

16. **C.** Rovsing's sign, Choice (C), is one of several signs associated with acute appendicitis. With Rovsing's sign, palpation of the left lower quadrant (LLQ) causes pain at McBurney's point. Psoas and obturator signs, Choices (A) and (B), are two other signs associated with acute appendicitis. Murphy's sign, Choice (D), is associated with acute cholecystitis. Blumberg's sign, Choice (E), is associated with rebound tenderness caused by peritonitis.

17. **D.** This question requires you to pay attention to common causes of an acute change in mental status. The presentation of a waxing and waning mental status can be consistent with a subdural hematoma. The lack of a fever and neck rigidity should dissuade you from thinking about an infection or meningitis. Thiamine, Choice (A), would work only if Wernicke's encephalopathy was present secondary to thiamine deficiency. This gentleman may have fallen and hit his head. He needs a CT scan of his head, Choice (D), to look for a possible subdural bleed. The wording in the question should make you think that an infection is not present here, so a lumbar puncture (LP), blood and urine cultures, and a chest radiograph — Choices (B), (C), and (E), respectively — aren't necessary.

18. **C.** The preferred pharmacologic treatment for bacterial vaginosis (BV) is metronidazole (Flagyl). This fact is just something you need to memorize.

19. **A.** The following tests are or can be positive with systemic lupus erythematosus (SLE): anti-Smith antibody, Choice (A), anti-nuclear antibody (ANA), and anti-double-stranded antibody (anti-ds antibody). The anti-ribonucleoprotein (anti-RNP) antibody, Choice (C), is associated with mixed connective tissue disease (MCTD). The anti-SSA antibody, Choice (B), is associated with Sjögren's syndrome. HLA-B27, Choice (D), is associated with ankylosing spondylitis, inflammatory bowel disease (IBD), and psoriatic arthritis. Anti-mitochondrial antibody (AMA), Choice (E), is associated with primary biliary cirrhosis. For PANCE, you should be familiar with the rheumatologic conditions discussed in Chapter 6 along with their respective antibodies.

20. **C.** Lyme disease can cause a characteristic skin rash and be a cause of an acute arthritis as well as a cause of carditis and meningitis.

21. **A.** Hyponatremia is a common electrolyte abnormality associated with tricyclic antidepressants and selective serotonin reuptake inhibitors (SSRIs).

22. **D.** After ordering an AM cortisol and differentiating between primary and secondary adrenal insufficiency, you would order a cosyntropin stimulation test to confirm that adrenal insufficiency is present. The other tests listed in the answer choices are associated with Cushing's syndrome.

23. **E.** The patient has now developed an Addisonian crisis, which is an endocrine emergency. In this situation, which can be a cause of shock, you need to administer intravenous (IV) hydrocortisone. Nothing else will work unless you give the hydrocortisone.

24. **C.** Hyperthyroidism, not hypothyroidism, Choice (B), causes high-output heart failure. Anemia, not polycythemia, Choice (A), is a cause of high-output heart failure, as is thiamine deficiency, not a vitamin B_{12} deficiency, Choice (E). A vitamin D deficiency, Choice (D), is not associated with high-output heart failure. Severe vitamin D deficiency is associated with osteomalacia and rickets. Paget's disease of bone, Choice (C), is a cause of high-output heart failure.

25. **D.** Sclerosing cholangitis is a possible complication of ulcerative colitis but not of Crohn's disease. All the other choices are potential complications of both Crohn's and ulcerative colitis. This topic is a big one on the test, so make sure you're familiar with it.

26. **C.** This question tests your ability to recognize the cause of nephrotic syndrome in different age groups. In a young child with nephrotic syndrome, the cause is usually minimal change disease, Choice (C). IgA nephropathy, Choice (E), would show hematuria and proteinuria. Membranous nephropathy and focal segmental glomerulosclerosis, Choices (A) and (B), are causes of nephrotic syndrome in adults. Benign orthostatic proteinuria, Choice (D), would cause tubular range proteinuria (less than 3 grams of protein in a 24-hour urine collection).

27. **D.** This question is about pure memorization. A cause of osteomyelitis in someone with sickle cell anemia is *Salmonella enteritidis.*

28. **D.** The patient has anemia, thrombocytopenia, and schistocytes. The combination of these features along with a change in mental status should make you think about thrombotic thrombocytopenic purpura (TTP). The treatment for TTP is plasmapheresis, Choice (D). You wouldn't give platelets, Choice (A), because this would only "add fuel to the fire." Intravenous (IV) steroids, emergent splenectomy, and intravenous gamma globulin (IVIG) — Choices (B), (C), and (E), respectively — would be used in the treatment of idiopathic thrombocytopenic purpura (ITP).

29. **C.** The symptoms the patient is having are characteristic of Kawasaki disease. While some of the symptoms may overlap with a viral exanthem, the characteristic findings of a red or strawberry tongue and a truncal rash are associated primarily with Kawasaki disease. This condition is commonly asked about on tests.

30. **E.** All of the organs except the lung produce alkaline phosphatase.

31. **D.** The S1 is the closing of the tricuspid and mitral valves. S1 may be accentuated in mild to moderate mitral stenosis, Choice (D). So in the case of an absent S1, the mitral valve isn't closing and is indicative of severe mitral stenosis. On an electrocardiogram (ECG), you'll also see a short PR interval. The physical exam findings of the patient presented in the question match this condition. *Tip:* Review the link between rheumatic heart disease and mitral stenosis.

32. **B.** For any nursing home resident, healthcare-associated pneumonia is often caused by Gram-negative organisms like *Pseudomonas aeruginosa,* Choice (B), so the clue is in the first part of the question. *Legionella pneumophilia* and *Candida albicans,* Choices (A) and (E), are causes of a community-acquired pneumonia (CAP). *Streptococcus viridans,* Choice (C), is a cause of subacute bacterial endocarditis.

33. **A.** Acanthosis nigricans is a medical condition characterized by the presence of pigmented areas in the neck, inguinal, axillary, and abdominal areas of the body. It can be familial or associated with many medical conditions, including diabetes and malignancy.

34. **B.** The most common causes of amenorrhea are pregnancy, hypothyroidism, and hyperprolactinemia. So in a woman whose β-hCG is negative, the next step is to check the thyroid-stimulating hormone (TSH), Choice (B), and prolactin levels. Anemia in and of itself isn't a known cause of amenorrhea. Repeating the serum β-hCG level, Choice (D), would not make any sense.

35. **C.** Hyperparathyroidism is the most common cause of hypercalcemia, followed by malignancy. The other answer choices are also causes of hypercalcemia, but they aren't as prevalent.

36. **A.** This person has all the findings of cystic fibrosis (CF), including lung involvement, pancreatic insufficiency causing malabsorptive diarrhea, and small testes. You would order an alpha-1 antitrypsin level to test for alpha-a antitrypsin deficiency, which would present with shortness of breath, emphysema, and elevated liver function. The patient with sarcoid would have a chronic nonproductive cough and hypercalcemia. The length of time the young man has experienced his symptoms is too long to indicate a pneumonia, and tuberculosis (TB), whether primary or extrapulmonary, wouldn't typically present this way.

37. **D.** If you see a decrease in the hemoglobin level of a patient on warfarin (Coumadin), especially if he has no evidence of any gastrointestinal (GI) bleeding, think of a retroperitoneal bleed, Choice (D). The patient may have pain in the back or flank with an acute bleed, and skin ecchymosis may or may not be present. A retroperitoneal bleed can occur spontaneously in the absence of a fall or trauma. A hemothorax, Choice (E), would cause bleeding in the pleural space and would cause the person to have shortness of breath or a cough productive of blood.

38. **C.** This patient is having uremic symptoms. The metallic taste is actually one of the primary symptoms of uremia. To diagnose, you would check a serum blood urea nitrogen (BUN) and creatinine level. Note that some of the patient's fatigue may be due to anemia, which often coexists with kidney disease.

39. **E.** The triad of miosis, ptosis, and anhidrosis is seen with a Pancoast tumor, which is a lung malignancy. You'll see variations of this question on the test.

40. **A.** The gist of this question is evaluating for dementia. Vitamin B_{12} deficiency, Choice (A), is a reversible cause of dementia that needs to be evaluated for. A 24-hour urinary free cortisol, Choice (D), is the evaluation for Cushing's syndrome. Phosphorous levels, potassium levels, and vitamin D levels, — Choices (B), (C), and (E), respectively — if low, would not account for any confusion.

41. **B.** Lamotrigine (Lamictal), Choice (B), is a medication used in the treatment of seizure disorders that can cause a characteristic skin rash. It's maculopapular in nature and usually goes away with the discontinuation of the medication. You may have chosen phenytoin (Dilantin), Choice (A), because it's also used to treat seizures, and it, too, can cause a rash. However, the clues are in the question. The rash associated with Dilantin, such as Stevens-Johnson syndrome, is a major desquamating rash. This rash is potentially fatal — much different than your typical drug rash. The patient in the question is nontoxic, afebrile, and otherwise healthy. The presentation would be the complete opposite in a patient presenting with Stevens-Johnson syndrome.

42. **A.** This gentleman is having an acute coronary syndrome (ACS). He his having unstable angina. The initial treatment of this patient would include oxygen, aspirin, morphine, and a beta blocker as well as nitroglycerin and intravenous (IV) heparin, Choice (A). If this person were experiencing a ST elevation myocardial infarction (STEMI), the patient would be taken directly to a catheterization lab, Choice (B), which is a standard of care. You would never do a stress test, Choice (C), on someone with active chest pain or active ischemic symptoms. Because the gentleman has no symptoms to suggest congestive heart failure (CHF), a chest radiograph, Choice (E), wouldn't be warranted. A stat echocardiogram, Choice (D), wouldn't need to be done urgently either.

43. **E.** The goal Protime (PT-INR) for someone with atrial fibrillation is 2.0–3.0.

44. **C.** This patient has signs and symptoms consistent with celiac sprue. The combination of anemia, low iron, and low vitamin B_{12} levels should make you think about a malabsorption issue. So you should order a tissue transglutaminase antibody test, Choice (C). It is

unusual to find a colonic malignancy in someone his age with no family history of colon cancer. The stools being negative and his lack of family history are tip-offs that no cancer is present. You wouldn't need a bone marrow biopsy, Choice (A), in this situation. The person needs both vitamin B_{12} replacement and intravenous (IV) iron, Choices (D) and (E), but a definitive diagnosis must be made first with Choice (C).

45. **C.** An MRI of the hips is the test of choice to evaluate for avascular necrosis. The MRI can catch changes of early avascular necrosis better than other imaging modalities. You'll likely see this popular topic area on the test.

46. **C.** To ace the test, you need to be familiar with the various orthopedic physical exam signs. The orthopedic test for the issue in this question is Finkelstein's test. When this test is positive, it indicates that the patient may have a Dupuytren's tenosynovitis. This test question is a classic one, so remember the association.

47. **B.** Common causes of a chronic cough include cough variant asthma, allergic rhinitis, and gastroesophageal reflux disease (GERD). You'll encounter variations of this question on the test. So if you read a question concerning a cough that occurs primarily at night, think of GERD. The first step is to advise the patient not to eat before bedtime and to keep the head of his bed elevated to minimize the gastric reflux.

48. **C.** Ménière's disease involves the ear. It is a cause of vertigo, Choice (C), hearing loss, nausea, and tinnitus. Visual symptoms, such as decreased vision, Choice (E), aren't associated with Ménière's disease. The other choices also aren't associated with Ménière's disease.

49. **A.** The esophagus is lined by squamous epithelium, except near the GE junction where you have columnar epithelium.

50. **D.** In a patient with rhabdomyolysis, the standard is the use of intravenous (IV) normal saline, Choice (D), to keep the kidneys flushed. The use of bicarbonate, Choice (E), is still controversial.

51. **D.** In a young woman without a smoking history who presents with a lung mass, the answer is bronchoalveolar carcinoma until proven otherwise. This cancer has a favorable prognosis compared to the other lung malignancies.

52. **B.** Quetiapine (Seroquel) and the other atypical antipsychotics can cause weight gain, Choice (B). Other potential side effects include hyperglycemia — not hypoglycemia, Choice (A) — hyperlipidemia, and dry mouth. Agranulocytosis, Choice (D), is a side effect of clozapine (Clozaril). Hypothyroidism, Choice (C), can be seen with lithium as a side effect. Hyponatremia, Choice (E), is a side effect of the selective serotonin reuptake inhibitors (SSRIs).

53. **B.** In a young child with rectal bleeding and right lower quadrant (RLQ) pain, you need to think about Meckel's diverticulum, Choice (B). Acute appendicitis, Choice (A), can also present with RLQ pain, but it wouldn't typically present with rectal bleeding. It's classically associated with mid-epigastric pain that migrates to McBurney's point. Diverticulitis, Choice (C), presents with left lower quadrant (LLQ) tenderness and is usually seen in older adults. Regional enteritis, Choice (D), is a fancy name for Crohn's disease, and, again, this condition is usually seen in young adults. Pyloric stenosis, Choice (E), presents with projectile vomiting and abdominal pain.

54. **A.** Diltiazem (Cardizem), Choice (E), is used in the treatment of diastolic heart failure and atrial fibrillation. Because it's a negative ionotrope, this drug isn't used in the treatment of systolic heart failure. Hydrochlorothiazide, or HCTZ (Microzide), Choice (B), is used in the treatment of hypertension. Terazosin (Hytrin), Choice (C), is used in the treatment of hypertension and benign prostatic hyperplasia (BPH). Clonidine (Catapres), Choice (D), is used in the treatment of refractory hypertension. Angiotensin-converting-enzyme (ACE) inhibitors like lisinopril (Zestril), Choice (A), are a great choice for someone with systolic heart failure.

55. **D.** The treatment for prehypertension is lifestyle modification and dietary changes, Choice (D). An angiotensin-converting-enzyme (ACE) inhibitor, Choice (A), or calcium channel blocker, Choice (B), is often considered first line for the treatment of Stage I hypertension. Sometimes two medications need to be started simultaneously for Stage II hypertension. This person has prehypertension. Having the patient start on hydrochlorothiazide, or HCTZ (Microzide), Choice (E), is put in as a distractor; the take-home message is that the treatment of prehypertension doesn't involve the use of antihypertensive medications.

56. **D.** Rheumatoid arthritis (RA) can be a cause of subcutaneous nodules, Choice (D). Recall that other common clinical manifestations of RA can include morning stiffness lasting more than one hour and a symmetric polyarthritis. Scleroderma can be a cause of elevated pulmonary pressures, Choice (B). It can also be a cause of high blood pressure and heartburn, Choices (A) and (E). Sclerodactyly, Choice (C), can be seen with CREST syndrome.

57. **B.** This young man's symptoms indicate a typical presentation of Osgood-Schlatter disease, Choice (B), which is common in adolescent male athletes. The pain in this condition is below the kneecap at the tibial tubercle. Chondromalacia, Choice (A), is pain under the kneecap. A stress fracture, Choice (C), in a runner typically occurs in the ankle or foot rather than the knee. A quadriceps tear, Choice (D), causes pain and swelling around the thigh area, depending on which muscle of the quadriceps is torn. Sciatica, Choice (E), typically presents in the gluteal region and has more of a posterior distribution, following the anatomy of the sciatic nerve.

58. **B.** All the choices concerning iron therapy are false, except Choice (B): The reticulocyte count can be used to assess the bone marrow response to iron therapy. The addition of vitamin C, or ascorbic acid, not vitamin D, Choice (C), enhances the absorption of oral iron. Iron can be replaced either orally or intravenously, not subcutaneously as suggested in Choice (E). The most common complaint with iron is constipation, not diarrhea, Choice (A). Iron should be given separately from other medications because it can interfere in their absorption, making Choice (D) incorrect.

59. **A.** Hearing loss can be conductive or sensorineural in etiology. Any process that affects sound conduction from the outer ear to the inner ear is a cause of conductive hearing loss. Examples of conductive hearing loss include all of the choices except Choice (A), Ménière's disease, which causes sensorineural deafness. This type of deafness concerns sound transmission from the inner ear to the nerves in the ear and to the brain.

60. **B.** *Clostridium difficile* colitis is an epidemic cause of hospital-acquired infections. You'll encounter questions about this type of colitis on the PANCE. The key to this question is simply memorizing the treatments for this colitis. Oral metronidazole (Flagyl) and oral vancomycin, Choice (B), can be given to treat this condition. Intravenous (IV) vancomycin, Choice (E), however, isn't used to treat *C. difficile*. The most common use of IV vancomycin is in treating methicillin-resistant *Staphylococcus aureus* (MRSA) bloodstream infection. Clindamycin (Cleocin), Choice (A), is a significant cause of *C. difficile* colitis. Amoxicillin (Amoxil) and doxycycline (Doryx), Choices (C) and (D), can be causes of this type colitis as well (as can any antibiotic class).

Block 2

1. **C.** An S2 is a physiologic heart sound that represents closing of the aortic and pulmonic valves.

2. **B.** Intermittent asthma is defined as less than two exacerbations per week with no more than two nocturnal exacerbations per month. Peak flow meter readings should be at baseline in between exacerbations. Mild persistent asthma, Choice (A), is defined as having more than two asthma exacerbations per week but not occurring on a daily basis. This distinction is subtle, but it's important to be aware of.

3. **E.** Metformin (Glucophage), Choice (D), is indicated for the treatment of type II diabetes. Type I diabetes is caused by insulin deficiency, not insulin resistance, as suggested in Choice (A). Concerning Choice (B), type I diabetes is seen at a younger age compared to type II diabetes. C-peptide levels can only be measured in type II diabetes, not type I, as noted in Choice (C). Hypertriglyceridemia and low HDL levels can be found in uncontrolled diabetes mellitus, as discussed in Choice (E).

4. **C.** The apple-core deformity is a radiologic sign that signals significant concern for a colonic malignancy.

5. **C.** Hypertrophic cardiomyopathy is characterized by a murmur that increases in intensity in response to the Valsalva maneuver and softens as you increase resistance (with the handgrip, for example).

6. **A.** This patient has *Pneumocystis jiroveci* pneumonia. The initial treatment is intravenous (IV) trimethoprim/sulfamethoxazole (Bactrim). This question is popular on tests, so commit it to memory. Note that this type of pneumonia used to be called *Pneumocystis carinii* and is still known by the abbreviation PCP.

7. **D.** Histoplasmosis is a fungal pulmonary process, so the recommended treatment is itraconazole (Sporanox).

8. **B.** The child is suffering from fifth disease, or erythema infectiosum, caused by parvovirus B19, Choice (B). A common description of this condition is the slapped-cheek appearance. Rhinovirus, Choice (E), is the cause of the common cold, which wouldn't present this way. Respiratory syncytial virus (RSV), Choice (D), is a usual cause of bronchiolitis. If the child is up to date on his vaccinations, it's unlikely that he would contract measles, Choice (A).

9. **B.** The most common causes of acute bronchitis are actually viral, not bacterial. However, if the person has underlying lung disease, you need to think of bacterial etiologies, including *Haemophilus influenzae* and *Moraxella catarrhalis.*

10. **C.** In someone diagnosed with aortic stenosis, dyspnea has the worst prognosis, with an average survival of only two years.

11. **A.** In a person you suspect may have carcinoid syndrome, the confirmatory biochemical diagnosis is a 24-hour urinary 5-hydroxyindoleacetic acid (5-HIAA) level.

12. **E.** The fundoscopic findings represent papilledema. Any process that increases intracranial pressure (ICP) can cause papilledema. A negative CT scan argues against an intracranial bleed, Choice (C). Her blood pressure isn't elevated enough to cause papilledema, as suggested in Choice (B). In a young woman with increased body mass index (BMI), a common cause of papilledema is pseudotumor cerebri, Choice (E), or benign intracranial hypertension.

13. **E.** Acetazolamide (Diamox) is a diuretic that's used in the treatment of glaucoma.

14. **B.** The patient has symptoms of hypothyroidism. The most common cause of hypothyroidism is Hashimoto's thyroiditis, Choice (B). Grave's disease and toxic adenoma, Choices (A) and (D), are causes of hyperthyroidism, not hypothyroidism. Usually in questions concerning a pituitary microadenoma, Choice (E), you read something about peripheral vision loss. No evidence in this question exists to suggest that a tumor is present, as suggested in Choice (C).

15. **C.** A Mallory-Weiss tear, Choice (C), is a tear in the esophagus that's brought on by repeat vomiting. None of the other choices fit here. Esophageal varices, Choice (A), is caused by long-term alcohol use, which isn't mentioned in the question. Barrett's esophagus, Choice (E), is caused by a history of long-standing gastroesophageal reflux disease (GERD), which isn't mentioned. Nor is there any mention of any GERD symptoms, Choice (D). Duodenal ulcer, Choice (B), presents with abdominal pain that is relieved with food. You wouldn't see a tear in the esophagus on endoscopy with this condition either. You'd instead see an ulceration in the duodenal area.

16. **C.** In someone with bulimia, you normally see parotid gland enlargement, Choice (C), not parotid gland atrophy. You would expect to see dry mucous membranes, not moist mucous membranes, Choice (A), because the person is likely volume depleted. Skin hyperpigmentation, Choice (B), can be seen in adrenal insufficiency. Macular rash, Choice (D), is seen with systemic lupus erythematosus (SLE), and buffalo hump, Choice (E), is seen with Cushing's syndrome.

17. **C.** Fludrocortisone (Florinef), Choice (C), can be used in treating adrenal insufficiency, hyperkalemia, and orthostatic hypotension. Side effects of this medication include edema and hypokalemia. Furosemide (Lasix), Choice (D), causes hypokalemia, and it's used in treating edema. Spironolactone (Aldactone), Choice (E), causes hyperkalemia, and it's used in treating hypertension. Terazosin (Hytrin), Choice (B), can cause orthostatic hypotension. Midodrine (ProAmatine), Choice (A), is also used in treating hypotension. This question is a tricky one, so keep your causes and side effects straight!

18. **D.** Pancreatitis, Choice (D), can be a cause of adult respiratory distress syndrome (ARDS). Congestive heart failure (CHF), Choice (A), isn't a common etiology of this condition, and neither are any of the other choices.

19. **B.** This 16-year-old boy has a urinalysis positive for both protein and blood, so you're likely dealing with IgA nephropathy, Choice (B). Henoch-Schonlein purpura, Choice (C), presents with abdominal pain, arthralgias, purpura, and kidney disease — none of which are present in this patient's case. Minimal change disease, Choice (D), presents with proteinuria and no hematuria. The patient has no history of diabetes to suggest diabetic nephropathy, Choice (E). And you wouldn't expect to see the blood and protein in the urinalysis in some who has hypertension, Choice (A).

20. **D.** The key in this question is recognizing the risk factors and the synovial fluid analysis concerning gout. High purine intake and alcohol use can precipitate a gout attack. With a gout attack, you'd see needle-shaped crystals with negative birefringence under polarized light, Choice (D). Positively birefringent, rhomboid-shaped crystals, Choice (C), are what you would expect to find with pseudogout. A synovial fluid white cell count greater than 100,000, Choice (A), is the typical synovial fluid analysis you would see with septic arthritis. Eosinophils in the synovial fluid, Choice (E), isn't something coauthor Rich has ever seen clinically.

21. **B.** Huntington's disease, Choice (B), is autosomal dominant, and one can see chorea-like movements with this condition. Sydenham chorea, Choice (A), is associated with streptococcal infection and rheumatic fever. Parkinson's disease, Choice (C), is associated with bradykinesia and a shuffling gait, and it usually affects older people. Multiple sclerosis (MS), Choice (E), can present with ocular problems, including optic neuropathy as well as tremors, muscle weakness, and spasticity. While cerebral palsy, Choice (D), can have choreiform-type movements, it can cause many other symptoms that aren't present in this individual.

22. **A.** The rhythm strip shows atrial fibrillation. Note the irregularly irregular rhythm and the lack of P waves.

23. **C.** In anyone with atrial fibrillation, evaluating for a hyperthyroid state, Choice (C), is important because it can predispose the person to atrial fibrillation. Be aware that a strong association exists between chronic obstructive pulmonary disease (COPD), Choice (B), and another type of arrhythmia, multifocal atrial tachycardia (MAT).

24. **E.** Of the conditions listed, hyperparathyroidism can be a cause of pseudogout.

25. **B.** With *Clostridium difficile* colitis being a leading hospital-acquired infection, you may see several questions on this topic on the PANCE. The patient in this question has a toxic megacolon, which is a dreaded complication of *Clostridium difficile* colitis. It can be a surgical emergency and often results in high morbidity and mortality.

26. **E.** Intravenous (IV) steroids, Choice (E), are used in the treatment of an acute asthma exacerbation. Urine eosinophils, Choice (A), are ordered if you're looking for acute interstitial nephritis. Asthma can have a mild serum eosinophilia, but you wouldn't expect to see any eosinophils in the urine. A methacholine challenge test, Choice (C), is actually a test that's used in diagnosing someone with asthma, not treating it acutely. IV antibiotics, Choice (D), aren't indicated for an acute asthma attack unless you note evidence of an underlying bacterial infection.

27. **C.** This is a tension pneumothorax, and a medical emergency. The key is in the physical findings. In someone with this condition, you would hear no breath sounds on the affected side as well as a tracheal deviation and mediastinal shift to the side opposite the pneumothorax. Venous return can be affected and cause the subsequent low blood pressure.

28. **E.** The emergent treatment for a tension pneumothorax is a needle decompression, Choice (E), to allow reexpansion of the lung. A chest tube, Choice (C), is often used in the treatment of a pneumothorax, but it isn't the first action you would perform in this emergent situation.

29. **E.** In acute prostatitis, which is likely what the gentleman in the question is suffering from, you avoid invasive procedures, Choice (E), because you can make things worse. The treatment for this condition is intravenous (IV) antibiotics. Usually the fluoroquinolones or cephalosporins can be used. Don't use a Foley catheter, Choice (B), and don't do a digital rectal exam, Choice (D). A prostate ultrasound isn't a routine test for the evaluation of benign prostatic hyperplasia (BPH), as suggested in Choice (C), nor would it help in acute prostatitis.

30. **B.** You'll likely encounter test questions that ask you to differentiate polymyalgia rheumatica (PMR), fibromyalgia, and polymyositis. The main difference between fibromyalgia, Choice (C), and PMR, Choice (B), is the erythrocyte sedimentation rate (ESR). In fibromyalgia, it will be normal; in PMR, it will be elevated. In polymyositis, Choice (A), you'd expect an elevated creatine phosphokinase (CPK).

31. **A.** Conjunctivitis related to swimming is usually associated with a viral etiology, not a bacterial or fungal cause.

32. **A.** Atrial septal defect, Choice (A), is associated with a fixed split S2. Ventricular septal defect, Choice (B), usually demonstrates a holosystolic murmur. The intensity of the murmur associated with the hypertrophic cardiomyopathy, Choice (C), increases in response to the Valsalva maneuver. Remember that the test makers like to ask questions about congenital heart disease.

33. **B.** If you encounter a question where a patient has a "black mouth" or "bad dentition," consider aspiration of anaerobes as a cause of pneumonia. One of the most common places in the lung to find an anaerobic infection is the right lower lobe.

34. **D.** *Pseudomonas aeruginosa* is one of the most common causes of external otitis, which can be seen in diabetes. *Pseudomonas aeruginosa* is also one of the causes of osteomyelitis.

35. **D.** Of all the thyroid cancers, anaplastic cancer of the thyroid, Choice (D), has the worst prognosis. Papillary, follicular, and medullary — Choices (A) through (C), respectively — represent the different types of thyroid cancer. Squamous-cell cancer of the thyroid, Choice (E), doesn't exist.

36. **D.** The treatment of an essential tremor is a beta blocker, especially propanolol (Inderal). Because it's lipophilic, it can penetrate the blood-brain barrier (BBB) better than the other classes of beta blockers. None of the other medications here are indicated in the treatment of essential tremor.

37. **B.** Trimethoprim/sulfamethoxazole (Bactrim) is a sulfa antibiotic that can precipitate anemia in a patient with glucose 6-phosphatase deficiency, or G6PD. The scenario in the question is a classic presentation for G6PD.

38. **C.** This person has hepatocellular carcinoma secondary to hepatitis C. Risk factors for hepatitis C include intravenous (IV) drug use and blood transfusions.

39. **C.** The patient in question has scabies. The treatment is Permethrin cream. The information in this question is typical of a scabies outbreak, especially the fact that multiple nursing home residents are affected.

40. **E.** The treatment for uric acid stones is a low-purine diet and alkalinization of the urine, Choice (E). Loop diuretics, Choice (D), should never be used in the treatment of kidney stones because they can increase urine calcium and sodium excretion, which is a huge no-no. Calcium-based stones, Choice (B), are the most common type of stone, and they can be seen on radiography. Uric acid stones are radiolucent, however, and can't be seen on radiography. Struvite stones aren't hereditary, as suggested in Choice (C); they're caused by urease-producing organisms. Usually you see a history of recurrent urinary infections with struvite stones.

41. **B.** This question has a lot of erythema in it, but erythema chronicum migrans, Choice (B), is the one you're looking for. It's associated with Lyme disease, which is often asked about on the test (so know it well!). Erythema marginatum, Choice (C), is associated with rheumatic fever. Erythema nodosum, Choice (E), is associated with many conditions, including sarcoidosis (Lofgren's syndrome). Erythema multiforme, Choice (A), is a skin hypersensitivity reaction that has many causes, including medications, such as antibiotics and anti-seizure medications. Erythema infectiosum, Choice (D), is another name for fifth disease, a common childhood viral exanthem that often presents with a "slapped-cheek appearance."

42. **E.** The patient has a positive Chvostek's sign, which can be seen with hypocalcemia. This patient with neck surgery likely had thyroid surgery, and the surgeon may have removed a parathyroid gland, which is causing the hypocalcemia.

43. **C.** The child has significant scoliosis. Scoliotic curves greater than 40° as diagnosed by radiograph require orthopedic referral.

44. **A.** Most of the time, a person with pellagra, which is a deficiency of niacin (vitamin B_3), presents with diarrhea, not obstipation (severe constipation in which nothing in the bowel is moving). All the other choices are manifestations of pellagra.

45. **C.** You're seeing manifestations of Still's disease, which is also known as juvenile rheumatoid arthritis (JRA). For both JRA and RA, remember that a patient's rheumatoid factor (RF) doesn't need to be positive for these arthritic conditions to be present.

46. **E.** This person has Guillain-Barré syndrome, which typically presents as an ascending neurologic weakness. If you see a presentation like the woman's in this question, which first affects the legs and arms and then causes difficulty speaking, you should think of this syndrome. None of the other choices present this way.

47. **D.** Carbidopa/Levodopa (Sinemet), Choice (D), is used to treat Parkinson's disease. The treatment for Guillain-Barré syndrome is plasmapheresis, Choice (C), which can remove circulating antibodies responsible for the syndrome. Intravenous (IV) steroids, Choice (A), are used for an acute exacerbation of multiple sclerosis (MS), and interferon, Choice (B), is often used as maintenance therapy for MS. Cyclophosphamide (Cytoxan), Choice (E), is used for vasculitis.

48. **B.** Mania, Choice (B), is an example of a mood disorder. Paranoia and catatonia, Choices (A) and (C), are types of schizophrenia. Note that paranoia can be a type of personality disorder as well. Agoraphobia, Choice (D), is an example of a phobia. Anhedonia, Choice (E), is an inability to experience joy or pleasure. This can be seen with a variety of conditions, including mood disorders and schizophrenia and isn't specific for a mood disorder.

49. **A.** Patients with paranoid schizophrenia, Choice (A), believe that someone is always out to get them. A person affected by catatonic schizophrenia, Choice (C), is either in a coma-like state or is bizarre and hyperactive — two opposite ends of the spectrum. With disorganized schizophrenia, Choice (E), everything about the person is disorganized — his or her thought patterns, word choices, and writing. Nothing makes sense. Undifferentiated schizophrenia, Choice (D), has many of the symptoms of the other three types. Mania, Choice (B), isn't a type of schizophrenia.

50. **A.** Pelvic inflammatory disease (PID) is a risk factor for endometriosis. Other factors include early menarche, menorrhagia, nulliparity, and having a first-degree relative with endometriosis. Endometrial cancer is not a risk factor for endometriosis.

51. **D.** Endometritis, Choice (D), can be very painful. Common risk factors for this condition include a recent surgical or invasive procedure, such as the placement of an intrauterine device (IUD) or a D&C. The lack of back pain and urinary symptoms would argue against pyelonephritis, Choice (C), or cystitis, Choice (A). Vaginitis, Choice (B), which is often painless, would present with a discharge and maybe a history of sexual intercourse. Colitis, Choice (E), would present with abdominal pain and diarrhea.

52. **B.** A transesophageal echocardiogram (TEE), Choice (B), is the gold standard to evaluate the heart valves to make sure no vegetation is present. A transthoracic echocardiogram (TTE), Choice (A), isn't as accurate. And a CT scan, Choice (C), or MRI, Choice (D), won't give you a good look at the heart valves. Blood culture positivity, Choice (E), in and of itself, doesn't give a diagnosis of endocarditis; you need to see that vegetation is present.

53. **D.** This question literally fits the definition of chronic bronchitis, Choice (D), which is a type of chronic obstructive pulmonary disease (COPD) where the patient has a productive cough three months out of a year for two consecutive years. The short, stocky build (also known as "the blue bloater") is also stereotypical of chronic bronchitis. Emphysema, Choice (A), is more consistent with a thin, asthenic type of build. Acute epiglottitis, Choice (B), is usually an emergency seen in children; they present with drooling and an inability to maintain a patent airway. Alpha-1 antitrypsin deficiency, Choice (E), is usually seen in a younger age group.

54. **C.** This person has all the characteristics of borderline personality disorder. The self-mutilation (for example, the razor marks on his skin) is a less common characteristic of this personality disorder, however.

55. **C.** This person is cirrhotic and has end-stage liver disease. He likely has a coagulopathy secondary to liver disease. Vitamin K, oral or subcutaneous, Choices (A) and (B), wouldn't work because the liver may not be able to metabolize it. In addition, this patient is acutely bleeding. Vitamin K, even if it were to work, isn't indicated for an acute bleeding problem, because it can take a few hours to work. The answer is to administer fresh frozen plasma (FFP), Choice (C), to replace the low levels of clotting factors. Because this person doesn't have hemophilia A, factor VIII concentrate, Choice (E), isn't needed.

56. **B.** One big test topic is being able to differentiate delirium from dementia. An acute change in mental status is usually due to delirium, Choice (B), and this commonly can be seen in hospitalized settings. Dementia, Choice (A), is more of a chronic diagnosis — the change in mental status and confusion has been occurring for months. Dysthymia and mania, Choices (C) and (E), are both mood disorders. Pseudodementia, Choice (D), which is seen more in the older population, exists when symptoms of depression get mistaken for dementia.

57. **A.** This is one of those congenital heart disease questions that you just need to memorize. Be aware of the four components of tetralogy of Fallot, which are present in the patient in this question.

58. **E.** A great mnemonic for remembering reactive arthritis is DUCA: D is dermatitis, U is urethritis, C is conjunctivitis, and A is arthritis. Alopecia is a criterion seen in systemic lupus erythematosus (SLE), but not reactive arthritis.

59. **E.** This patient has a significant salicylate intoxication and metabolic acidosis. Because his salicylate level is 100 and his pH is below 7.35, you need to call the nephrologist for dialysis, Choice (E). The medication 4-methylpyrazole (Fomepizole), Choice (C), is used in treating ethylene glycol and methanol overdose. Flumazenil (Romazicon), Choice (D), is used in treating a benzodiazepine overdose. Intravenous (IV) N-acetylcysteine (Mucomyst), Choice (B), is used in treating an acetaminophen (Tylenol) overdose.

60. **B.** The picture in this question shows acne rosacea, a common skin condition. The main treatments for this condition include topical metronidazole (Flagyl), Choice (B), and oral doxycycline (Vibramycin). Vitamin A derivatives, not Vitamin D derivatives, Choice (D), can also be prescribed. Topical clotrimazole and betamethasone (Lotrisone), Choice (A), is a combination topical steroid and antifungal that wouldn't be used to treat this condition. Oral cephalexin (Keflex), Choice (C), would be used to treat a superficial skin infection, cellulitis, or impetigo.

Block 3

1. **B.** This rhythm strip is classic for torsades de pointes (also known as R on T phenomenon). A good way of thinking about this strip is by picturing a wire wrapping itself around a stick. This rhythm indicates a medical emergency as it is a type of ventricular tachycardia.

2. **D.** The presence of accelerated blood pressure and hypokalemia should make you think about renal artery stenosis (RAS), Choice (C), and/or hypokalemia. A key phrase in the question, however, is "no abdominal or femoral bruit." This is a significant clue that RAS isn't present. The other real cause of hypertension and profound hypokalemia such as this is hyperaldosteronism, Choice (D). The other choices would not cause this degree of hypokalemia. A pheochromocytoma, Choice (A), can present with flushing, palpitations, and an elevated urinary metanephrines and vanillylmandelic acid (VMA) level. Carcinoid syndrome, Choice (B), can also cause hypertension, flushing, and palpitations, and the test of choice would be a urinary 5-HIAA level. Hyperthyroidism, Choice (E), can present with labile blood pressure, tachycardia, and heat intolerance.

3. **E.** A key to answering pulmonary questions is recognizing patterns of presentation. When you see restrictive disease, one of the pulmonary conditions that should enter your mind is interstitial pulmonary fibrosis (IPF). The reticular nodular pattern is classic for IPF. Often the lung sounds (dry rales, for example) can be mistaken for congestive heart failure (CHF). The other choices here relate to obstructive airway disease, not restrictive disease.

4. **D.** This person likely has irritable bowel syndrome. One clue is the pattern of her stool habits — diarrhea during the day and normal at night. She doesn't need a colonoscopy, Choice (A), just yet, and she shows no indication for a proton pump inhibitor (PPI), Choice (C). None of her symptoms suggest lactose intolerance, Choice (E). And because the stool is already negative for blood, you have no reason to recheck, Choice (B). So begin with lifestyle management, including stress management and relaxation techniques, Choice (D).

5. **B.** Rheumatoid arthritis (RA) is a symmetric polyarthritis that commonly affects women more than men. RA can be present even in the setting of a negative rheumatoid factor (RF). The RF can be negative more than 50% of the time with RA. Sulfasalazine (Azulfidine) is used in the treatment of ulcerative colitis, but not as much in RA. Chondrocalcinosis can be a radiographic feature of pseudogout; you would expect joint space narrowing and erosive arthritis with this condition.

6. **D.** The patient in this question suffers from labrynthitis, Choice (D). She isn't dizzy when she stands up, so you know her symptoms aren't from orthostatic hypotension, Choice (A). She has no other symptoms, including hearing loss or tinnitus, to suggest Ménière's disease, Choice (B), or an acoustic neuroma, Choice (C). A cholesteatoma, Choice (E), refers to scarring and the remnants of a bad middle ear infection.

7. **C.** Galactorrhea is caused by an elevation in prolactin levels. Common causes of elevated prolactin levels include prolactinomas and medications, including antipsychotics, which raise prolactin levels by inhibiting dopamine.

8. **A.** This question relies on the fact that you know the definition of a somatoform disorder. An older term associated with this syndrome is *conversion disorder.*

9. **B.** This person has polyuria, polyphagia, and polydipsia, which are hallmarks of diabetes. In someone this young, you would suspect a new onset type I diabetes, so her serum blood glucose level should be checked, Choice (B). Nausea and vomiting associated with pregnancy wouldn't cause these other symptoms, so no need for a beta-hCG level, Choice (A). Hyperthyroidism would cause weight loss but none of the "three P's" mentioned here, so, again, you don't need to check her thyroid-stimulating (TSH) level, Choice (C). Sometimes people on drugs or alcohol don't eat and are cachectic as a result, and that doesn't appear to be the case here. So you can skip the urine drug screen, Choice (E).

10. **D.** Oseltamivir (Tamiflu), Choice (D), is indicated for both influenza A and B. Amantidine (Symmetrel), Choice (A), is only used for treating influenza B. Acyclovir (Cyclovir), Choice (B), is used to treat herpes simplex. Amoxicillin-clavulanic acid (Augmentin), Choice (C), and doxycycline (Doryx), Choice (E), are antibiotics and aren't used to treat viral infections.

11. **D.** Given this person's work-up, which noted microcytic anemia, normal iron levels, and no evidence of any chronic conditions, you need to look for thalassemia with a hemoglobin electrophoresis.

12. **D.** Seminomas are germ cell tumors in the testes of younger men. They have a good prognosis and are very radiosensitive. Radiation is the predominant therapy. Seminomas won't show an elevated alpha-fetoprotein level.

13. **A.** The photo in this question is a classic appearance of lower-extremity cellulitis, which is commonly seen in those with diabetes and venous insufficiency and those who are obese. It causes an infection of the skin's subcutaneous and dermis layers. The treatment usually consists of a first-generation cephalosporin, such as cephalexin (Keflex).

14. **B.** This question encourages you to think about microvascular disease or vascular dementia. The patient is loaded with risk factors, including atrial fibrillation (which puts him at risk for small embolic strokes) and significant cardiovascular and peripheral vascular disease that both increase the risk of developing vascular dementia.

15. **B.** The classic electrocardiogram (ECG) findings in acute pericarditis are diffuse ST segment elevation and PR segment depression.

16. **D.** The one physical examination sign associated with cirrhosis is shifting dullness, Choice (D), which is found with ascites. Jugular venous distension (JVD), Choice (A), can be found with congestive heart failure (CHF). The other choices are physical exam signs you would see with cardiac tamponade.

17. **E.** Metronidazole (Flagyl) is more often used to treat anaerobic infections, and it's also the treatment of choice for pseudomembranous colitis. The other choices are used in the treatment of community-acquired pneumonia (CAP).

18. **D.** The usual treatment for diverticulitis in a hospital setting involves using antibiotics that cover Gram-negatives and anaerobes. The usual prescribed cocktail is Choice (D), ciprofloxacin (Cipro) and metronidazole (Flagyl). Ceftriaxone (Rocephin) and azithromycin (Zithromax), Choice (A), represents the treatment for community-acquired pneumonia (CAP). Choices (B), (E), and (C) are random combinations of antibiotics and antifungals that have no place in this situation.

19. **A.** Cauda equina is an emergency and requires that you call the neurosurgeon. If, on a test, this choice weren't available, and you could ask for an emergent CT scan with contrast or an MRI of the lumbar spine that would be the next best answer. The other choices concern back pain that you have more time to evaluate and treat.

20. **C.** Niacin, Choice (C), is prescribed for raising HDL levels. Atorvastatin (Lipitor), cholestyramine (colestipol), and ezetemibe (Zetia) — Choices (A), (D), and (E), respectively — are used to lower LDL levels. Fenofibrate (Tricor), Choice (B), is used to lower triglyceride levels.

21. **D.** In a young person who has difficulty controlling blood pressure, especially with claudication symptoms, you need to think about coarctation of the aorta. Those affected have upper-extremity high blood pressure and barely palpable pulses in their lower extremities. They also may complain of claudication-like symptoms, as in this question.

22. **B.** The chest radiograph shows pulmonary edema. You use intravenous (IV) nitroglycerin, Choice (B), to treat pulmonary edema. It is a vasodilator. IV steroids, Choice (E), are used in an acute exacerbation of asthma or chronic obstructive pulmonary disease (COPD), but not in pulmonary edema. IV ceftriaxone (Rocephin), Choice (D), is given to someone with pneumonia. IV heparin, Choice (C), is given to someone with an acute coronary syndrome (ACS), pulmonary embolism (PE), or atrial fibrillation. This gentleman does have pulmonary edema, but you aren't given any information that leads you to believe that he has an ACS. You wouldn't give IV saline, Choice (A), to someone with pulmonary edema.

23. **A.** Diarrhea caused by *Giardia lamblia,* Choice (A), can result from drinking lake water polluted by animal fecal material. Some PANCE questions may also cite drinking from a well. In diarrhea questions, the key is in the setting of what someone ate and where someone was before the onset of the diarrheal symptoms. *Cryptosporidium,* Choice (D), would be found in someone who was immunosuppressed, such as a person with human immunodeficiency virus (HIV). *Shigella, Salmonella,* and *Campylobacter jejuni* — Choices (B), (C), and (E), respectively — are related to food contamination as a cause of diarrhea.

24. **D.** The Lachman test is the definitive test for evaluating an injury to the anterior cruciate ligament. Another diagnostic maneuver for examining the anterior cruciate ligament is the anterior drawer test.

25. **B.** This patient shows a typical presentation for epiglottitis, Choice (B). You will see questions on the test where you must differentiate between the choices in this question. While both epiglottitis and croup, Choice (A), can present with stridor, the drooling and sitting forward in order to breathe are synonymous with epiglottitis. Pertussis or whooping cough, Choice (E), present with a barking type of cough.

26. **E.** The patient in this question likely has group A beta hemolytic strep (GABHS). The treatment for GABHS is a penicillin derivative first line, such as amoxicillin (Trimox), Choice (E). One of the differences between the clinical presentation of mononuclelosis and GABHS is the location of the adenopathy. Expect to see posterior cervical adenopathy with GABHS. The lack of splenomegaly argues against this being mononucleosis, which is caused by the Epstein-Barr virus. If you see a question regarding adenopathy, exudative pharyngitis, and splenomegaly on the test, think mono. Hand-foot-and-mouth disease, a common pediatric viral illness, is caused by the coxsackievirus, Choice (D). Coxsackievirus is also thought to be a cause of viral pericarditis. Concerning Choice (C), parainfluenza is a cause of croup.

27. **D.** This person likely has a vitamin D deficiency. If a young man suffers a femur fracture, you know something weird is going on. He doesn't spend any time outdoors (no vitamin D from the sun), and he doesn't consume any dairy products, which are fortified with vitamin D. So he needs vitamin D supplementation.

28. **B.** Primary hyperparathyroidism can be a cause of hypophosphatemia as it causes increased phosphate excretion in the kidney.

29. **C.** The woman in this question has all the clinical findings of preeclampsia, Choice (C). She has proteinuria and hypertension that began after her 20th gestational week. Eclampsia, Choice (E), refers to seizure activity that can occur as a result of preeclampsia. Gestational hypertension, Choice (A), also presents with an elevated blood pressure after 20 weeks gestation, but proteinuria isn't present. Gestational diabetes, Choice (B), refers to elevated blood glucose levels discovered during pregnancy.

30. **B.** Fibrocystic breast disease isn't a pre-malignant condition, as suggested in Choice (D). It's a benign condition of the breast. It can be a painful condition that can make both breasts painful, Choice (A), but it's usually temporally related to the menstrual cycle, not unrelated. Patients can complain of breasts feeling swollen or full, Choice (B). A nipple discharge may be present, which is the opposite of what's discussed in Choice (C). Because it is a benign condition, mastectomy and/or lumpectomy with radiation, Choice (E), is not needed. The treatment involves the use of analgesics and warm compresses.

31. **B.** An anterior wall myocardial infarction (MI), Choice (B), is characterized by ST elevation in the anterior leads, namely V1–V4. The leads for an inferior wall MI, Choice (A), are ST elevation in leads II and III and aVF. The lateral wall, Choice (C), is leads V5 and V6. The posterior wall, Choice (D), is tricky in that you can see ST depression in the anterior leads, with a prominent R wave in leads V1 and V2.

32. **D.** The standard of care for an ST elevation myocardial infarction (STEMI) is a catheterization, Choice (D). The morbidity and mortality of STEMI patients are improved when they're taken directly to the catheterization lab. You should only use a medication like tissue plasminogen activator (tPA), Choice (B), when access to a cardiac catheterization lab isn't available. Intravenous (IV) heparin and nitroglycerin, clopidogrel (Plavix), and IV beta blockers — Choices (A), (C), and (E), respectively — are used in the treatment of an acute coronary syndrome (ACS).

33. **E.** A little anatomy never hurt anyone. The arterial supply to the left ventricle is the left anterior descending artery.

34. **B.** The patient's waxing and waning mental status indicates a subdural hematoma. The key to answering this question correctly is recognizing the history of the fall.

35. **B.** The patient has an essential tremor, Choice (B), which can be worsened in times of stress or anxiety. She has no symptoms present to suggest Parkinson's disease, Choice (C), and she isn't suffering from myoclonic jerks, Choice (E), which are more spastic movements. Post-traumatic stress disorder, Choice (A), is an anxiety disorder, but it isn't associated with tremor. Tardive dyskinesia, Choice (D), is choreiform facial movements (for example, lip-smacking), which usually appear as a side effect of certain antipsychotic medications that inhibit dopamine.

36. **C.** The triad of eye pain, loss of vision, and loss of papillary response is consistent with closed-angle glaucoma, Choice (C), which is an ocular emergency. Another key in the question is the high intraocular pressure. Macular degeneration, Choice (D), usually presents in both eyes and causes a gradual loss of vision. Amaurosis fugax, Choice (B), is a loss or partial loss of vision in one eye, usually painless, that's secondary to carotid disease or occlusion of the retinal artery. Temporal arteritis, Choice (A), is associated with loss of vision and pain in one eye as well as tenderness over the temporal area and an elevated sedimentation rate. Jaw claudication can also be present with temporal arteritis.

37. **A.** Optic neuritis is associated with multiple sclerosis (MS) and, in fact, can be the presenting symptom.

38. **C.** Murphy's sign is associated with acute cholecystitis, Choice (C). Hepatitis, Choice (A), can be painless or associated with right upper quadrant (RUQ) tenderness to palpation, if hepatomegaly is present. Diverticulitis, Choice (D), presents with left lower quadrant (LLQ) pains, and regional enteritis (Crohn's disease), Choice (E), presents with right lower quadrant (RLQ) tenderness. The hallmark of ischemic colitis, Choice (B), is pain out of proportion to physical findings, which can include LLQ pain and blood in the stool.

39. **C.** Pyelonephritis can be a cause of costovertebral tenderness. This physical examination finding can be seen with many types of kidney problems, including pyelonephritis and kidney stones. You can see this sign by gently tapping on the left and right flank area (and hoping the patient doesn't jump off the table in pain).

40. **B.** This question shows a classic incidence of otitis media, Choice (B), an infection frequently seen in childhood. External otitis, Choice (C), occurs on the outer ear and outer part of the canal, usually in those with recent water exposure or with diabetes. Mastoiditis, Choice (D), is a complication of otitis media. This complication, which can be determined on exam by finding tenderness of the mastoid processes, isn't suggested by the physical exam findings in the question. No physical findings suggest acute sinusitis, Choice (E), either. You would see a perforated tympanic membrane, Choice (A), with an otoscopic examination.

41. **D.** The motor vehicle accident is the most common cause of mortality among teenagers.

42. **C.** This question is pure memorization. Obesity is defined as a body mass index (BMI) greater than 30.

43. **B.** Hypocalcemia causes a prolonged QT interval, Choice (B). Hypercalcemia causes a shortened QT interval, Choice (A). Hypokalemia causes a QT prolongation or a U wave, Choice (C). Neither a diffuse PR interval prolongation, Choice (D), nor a widened QRS complex, Choice (E), is applicable here.

44. **D.** This person has *vaginal candidiasis* (often referred to as a yeast infection). The treatment of choice for *vaginal candidiasis* is fluconazole (Diflucan), usually given one time.

45. **B.** You'll see several questions on the PANCE concerning tuberculosis (TB); several of them related to medications and medication side effects. One pronounced effect of rifampin is that it can turn body secretions (including tears and urine) a reddish-orange color.

46. **A.** A common cause of bacterial meningitis in the elderly is *Streptococcus pneumoniae,* Choice (A). *Pneumocystis jiroveci,* Choice (B), isn't a cause of meningitis but of pneumonia in an immunocompromised adult, such as one who has human immunodeficiency virus (HIV). *Cryptococcus neoformans,* Choice (E), is a cause of meningitis, but it's more often seen in those who are immunosuppressed, such as those with HIV. *Staphylococcus aureus,* Choice (D), isn't considered a common cause of meningitis. Even though *Hemophilus influenzae,* Choice (C), is a cause of bacterial meningitis in the older population, *Streptococcus pneumonia* is more predominant.

47. **C.** Hydroxychloroquine (Plaquenil), which is used to treat systemic lupus erythematosus (SLE) and other autoimmune diseases, has the potential to cause macular degeneration. So anyone using this medication should have annual follow-ups with an ophthalmologist.

48. **B.** Morning stiffness lasting more than one hour is commonly seen in rheumatoid arthritis (RA). The remaining choices are all associated with fibromyalgia.

49. **C.** This person likely has rhabdomyolysis, Choice (C). One clue to the answer is the statement that the person was down on the ground for several hours, which can cause muscle damage. This scenario is common after an alcohol or drug binge when the individual passes out and doesn't move from one spot for several hours. The lack of red blood cells on microscopic examination argues against Wegener's granulomatosis, acute glomerulonephritis, and nephrolithiasis — Choices (A), (B), and (E), respectively. The question provides no evidence to suggest any type of hemolysis, Choice (D).

50. **B.** Vitamin B_6 deficiency is associated with a peripheral neuropathy, Choice (B). Brittle bones, Choice (E), are associated with a vitamin D deficiency. Easy bruising, Choice (D), occurs with a vitamin K deficiency. Any B vitamin deficiency can be associated with weakness. A decrease in nighttime vision, Choice (A), would be associated with a vitamin A deficiency.

51. **B.** Common causes of polyuria include diabetes, diuretics, and diabetes insipidus. In this gentleman, who had brain trauma and bleeding after a motor vehicle accident, the most likely cause is diabetes insipidus. His blood sugar is normal, and he's not on any diuretics. His kidney function is normal. No medications would be given in this situation.

52. **B.** Digoxin (Lanoxin) is used to treat systolic congestive heart failure (CHF), not diastolic CHF. It is also used in the treatment of atrial fibrillation as it works as an AV nodal blocker not as an SA nodal blocker. It can't be removed by dialysis, and it decreases morbidity but not mortality.

53. **A.** If you see a question with eggshell calcifications on chest radiograph, you have a clue that you're dealing with silicosis, Choice (A). Another clue is the patient's occupation, because glass or sand workers are at an increased risk of developing silicosis. Asbestosis, Choice (B), has different lung findings, including fibrosis, pleural thickening, and plaques. Interstitial pulmonary fibrosis, Choice (E), isn't associated with eggshell calcifications.

54. **D.** *Escherichia coli* 0175:H7 is the most common cause of hemolytic uremic syndrome (HUS).

55. **B.** The cell type most commonly seen with Hodgkin's lymphoma is the Reed-Sternberg cell, Choice (B). The Auer rod, Choice (A), is associated with acute myelogenous leukemia. Atypical lymphocytes, Choice (C), can be seen with mononucleosis. Schistocytes or "helmet cells," Choice (E), are seen in many hemolytic states, including thrombotic thrombocytopenic purpura (TTP). Target cells, Choice (D), are associated with liver disease.

56. **B.** Vegans are often deficient in a few key nutrients, vitamin B_{12}, Choice (B), being one of them, because it's only found in animal products. So addressing this deficiency should be your first line of action in this situation. Signs of vitamin B_{12} deficiency can include a red, swollen tongue; diarrhea; peripheral neuropathy; fatigue; and weakness. The person, as a vegan, won't likely be deficient in folic acid, Choice (A), which is readily available in vegetables and legumes. The other choices aren't applicable in this question.

57. **C.** Metformin (Glucophage) is commonly used in treating diabetes. It increases peripheral utilization of insulin into the tissues, Choice (C), as its main mechanism of action. Metformin is associated with weight loss, not weight gain, as suggested in Choice (A). It can cause diarrhea more so than constipation, Choice (D). Its use needs to be watched in someone with kidney disease, not liver disease, Choice (E). Metformin can inhibit the liver's production of glucose rather than inhibit carbohydrate absorption in the intestine, Choice (B).

58. **A.** Tophi, Choice (A), are the uric acid crystals that are deposited on multiple joints of the body. Podagra, Choice (B), is gout that involves the first metatarsal. Pellagra, Choice (C), refers to a deficiency of niacin (vitamin B_3). Tender points and trigger points, Choices (D) and (E), are usually talked about in relation to rheumatologic diseases and fibromyalgia.

59. **B.** This gentleman's thoughts are an example of a delusion, Choice (B), or a belief in something that isn't true. A hallucination, Choice (A), is actively seeing or hearing something that isn't present. Those who are paranoid, Choice (E), often have delusions of persecution; however, other symptoms are present as well. Mania, Choice (D), is a mood disorder, usually part of the bipolar syndrome. Somatoform disorder, Choice (C), refers to a physical ailment without an identifiable organic cause.

60. **A.** In a young man who presents with uncontrolled hypertension and tachycardia, you first need to think about drug use and obtain a urine drug screen, Choice (A). Looking at the person's electrolytes, including blood glucose, Choice (C), wouldn't be the first test you would order here. He has no evidence of any focal neurologic symptoms that would require brain imaging, Choice (D). Salicylate intoxication would cause a metabolic acidosis and respiratory alkalosis, not uncontrolled hypertension as in this patient. So you don't need to check a salicylate level, Choice (E).

Block 4

1. **A.** An S3 refers to ventricular volume overload. It can often be heard as an "S3 gallop."

2. **A.** You need to start this gentleman on intravenous (IV) fluids, Choice (A). You wouldn't give a beta blocker like metoprolol (Lopressor), Choice (C), to this patient. Sinus tachycardia occurs for many reasons. Pain, volume depletion, fever, and anemia are just a few. The key in this situation isn't to simply give a beta blocker to slow down the heart rate; instead, you need to find out the cause of the sinus tachycardia. This person doesn't need a stress test, Choice (E). He also shows no indication that he's adrenally insufficient requiring IV steroids, including IV hydrocortisone (Solu Medrol), Choice (D). This gentleman is volume depleted, so you wouldn't give him a diuretic, Choice (B).

3. **D.** In anyone who's volume depleted, you first use isotonic saline, Choice (D), to fill the vascular space and volume resuscitate. You would only give fresh frozen plasma (FFP), Choice (E), in this situation if the person had a coagulopathy and was actively bleeding. More hypotonic fluids can be given if the person is hypernatremic and you need to give a more dilute intravenous (IV) solution. The most important point here, however, is to give isotonic saline to raise the blood pressure.

4. **C.** You're dealing with diabetic gastroparesis secondary to diabetic neuropathy. One effective medication is metoclopramide (Reglan), Choice (C). It has been used to treat this condition as a prokinetic agent because it can decrease gastric emptying. Ranitidine (Zantac), sucralfate (Carafate), and pantoprazole (Protonix) — Choices (A), (B), and (D), respectively — are used to treat ulcer disease and gastritis. Cisapride (Propulsid), Choice (E), is a prokinetic agent like Reglan, but it was taken off the market because it produced cardiac side effects.

5. **D.** Ipratropium bromide (Atrovent) works synergistically with albuterol to promote better bronchodilatory effects. It is used in the treatment of asthma as well as chronic obstructive pulmonary disorder (COPD). It isn't used in the treatment of bronchiectasis. It has anticholinergic side effects and works as a muscarinic receptor antagonist.

6. **E.** The person is presenting with histoplasmosis, Choice (E). The key to this question concerns where the person lives. If you see a question where a person lives in the Ohio River Valley, near the Mississippi River, you should consider histoplasmosis. If you encounter a question where the person lives in the San Joaquin area in California, you should think about coccidiomycosis, Choice (D). The chest radiograph appearances of all the choices can be similar in nature.

7. **B.** The patient likely has either a renal cell cancer or a bladder cancer. He needs to go for a CT scan and cystoscopy, Choice (B). The patient has hematuria, and the microscopic sediment is positive for red blood cells. He has no proteinuria, which argues against a nephritis being present. He doesn't need a kidney biopsy, Choice (A), nor does a 24-hour urine protein need to be repeated, Choice (E). If the patient had rhabdomyolysis, no red blood cells would be present on the microscopic sediment. So you don't need to obtain a creatine phosphokinase (CPK) level, Choice (D). Risk factors for bladder cancer include smoking and certain occupational exposures, including working in the dye industry. The patient shows no evidence that he has a urinary tract infection (UTI). For instance, he shows no pyuria and his urinalysis isn't positive for leukocyte esterase or nitrites. So he doesn't need a urine culture and trimethoprim/sulfamethoxazole (Bactrim), Choice (C).

8. **A.** This person has Barrett's esophagus that has transformed into an adenocarcinoma, Choice (A). One significant risk is gastroesophageal reflux disease (GERD), and the person has had heartburn for years. Barrett's esophagus is actually a metaplasia and is associated with an increased risk of adenocarcinoma. Squamous cell carcinoma, Choice (B), is another type of esophageal cancer, but it's less common. Transitional cell cancer, Choice (C), is usually seen with bladder cancer. The esophagus isn't a common site for lymphoma, Choice (E).

9. **D.** The risks of cholesterol-based gallstones are female gender, obesity, and older age. Those who have had gastric bypass surgery are at an increased risk of cholesterol-based gallstones as well. The risk factors for pigment gallstones are hematologic conditions that cause intravascular hemolysis. Sickle cell disease and hepatic cirrhosis are additional risk factors for pigment stones. Actually, any process that can cause the release of bilirubin is responsible for the formation of pigment stones.

10. **B.** We include this question because you're likely to encounter some basic science on the PANCE. The propensity for heartburn and popularity of Barrett's also make this topic important. Here are two basic things to know about Barrett's esophagus: You see goblet cells, Choice (B), and you see columnar metaplasia of the normal squamous cells located there. Peyer's patches, Choice (A), are seen on the small intestine. Howell-Jolly bodies, Choice (C), can be seen on a peripheral smear either as a result of a splenectomy or in sickle cell disease. Epithelial cell hyperplasia and keratinized epithelium, Choices (D) and (E), are made up.

11. **E.** This person has positive blood cultures and vegetation located on a heart valve. His condition is likely an endocarditis caused by *Staphylococcus aureus*. The patient likely has seeding of the shoulder joint, for example, a septic arthritis of the shoulder joint caused by *Staph aureus,* Choice (E). If he had pain in his back, you would worry about an osteomyelitis caused by *Staph aureus*. Nothing in the question suggests gout or pseudogout, Choice (A) or (B). Osteoarthritis, Choice (C), of the right shoulder can certainly occur, but this gentleman is 36 years old, so he's likely too young for it unless he has been an athlete with repetitive motion injuries. While Lyme disease, Choice (D), can cause a monoarticular arthritis, he shows no indication of exposure: no tick bite, no living near the woods, no deer, and so on.

12. **D.** An S4 represents atrial contraction in a noncompliant ventricle. It's heard before an S1 and never in atrial fibrillation (in a fibrillating atria, the atria isn't contracting, so you should not hear an S4). An S3 represents ventricular volume overload. You can hear an "S3 gallop" on cardiac auscultation in someone with systolic congestive heart failure (CHF). An S2 is a closure of the aortic and pulmonic valves. This is a physiologic heart sound (as is S1).

13. **B.** All the choices in the question have been implicated in causing osteoporosis except hydrochlorothiazide, or HCTZ, Choice (B). Hydrochlorothiazide may actually have a beneficial effect on bone density by promoting calcium retention in the kidney, and by directly stimulating osteoblast differentiation and bone mineral formation. Long-term use of heparin, Choice (D), has been linked to osteoporosis. Phenytoin (Dilantin), Choice (E), has been linked to low vitamin D levels, which is a risk factor for osteoporosis. In men, testosterone deficiency, Choice (C), has been linked to osteoporosis. This question is one of those where you would eliminate the answers that couldn't be correct (those that can cause osteoporosis and have a negative effect on bone density).

14. **C.** This person has temporomandibular joint, or TMJ, syndrome, Choice (C). Risk factors include grinding of the teeth at night. Any significant movement of the jaw can elicit pain. The finding of tenderness to palpation of the jaw suggests TMJ may be present. Although temporal arteritis (TA), Choice (A), can present with jaw claudication, the patient has no visual symptoms to suggest TA. The dentist didn't suggest cavities, Choice (B). She also has no neurologic signs to suggest disc disease, Choice (D). Bell's palsy, Choice (E), is facial nerve paralysis, which isn't present here.

15. **A.** This gentleman shows a classic presentation of adhesive capsulitis, Choice (A), which is also known as "frozen shoulder." This condition is usually seen after a fall affecting the shoulder, and because of the pain, the person doesn't move the shoulder much. As a result, the shoulder is limited in range of motion. An acute gout flare, Choice (E), doesn't usually hit the shoulder. You would be able to see a shoulder dislocation, Choice (B), on physical examination. Certainly osteoarthritis, Choice (C), can affect the shoulder, but that condition is more of a gradual phenomenon occurring over time.

16. **B.** Dacryocystitis is a bacterial infection of the lacrimal sac, Choice (B), not a viral infection of the conjunctiva, as noted in Choices (A) and (C). Treatment consists of the use of antibiotics. It is not a medical emergency, Choice (D). Clinical findings include erythema and edema around the lacrimal duct, not diplopia, Choice (E).

17. **B.** *Pseudomonas aeruginosa* is a common cause of osteomyelitis, especially in someone with diabetes mellitus. *Moraxella catarrhalis* and *Streptococcus pneumoniae,* Choices (A) and (C), are common causes of bacterial sinusitis and otitis media. *Chlamydia trachomatis,* Choice (D), is a common cause of a sexually transmitted infection.

18. **D.** Acromegaly is caused by an oversecretion of growth hormone. The most common reason a patient will have too much growth hormone is a pituitary adenoma. None of the other choices are applicable.

19. **D.** Gigantism and acromegaly are part of the same continuum; both conditions occur as a result of growth hormone excess. The difference is that gigantism occurs before the growth plates fuse, and acromegaly occurs after. Choices (A), (B), and (C) are all applicable to both syndromes.

20. **B.** This patient is suffering from thyroid storm, Choice (B). All the symptoms are present, including the delirium, confusion, high fever, and tachycardia. A myxedema coma, Choice (A), is the opposite of a thyroid storm; the person with this condition is lethargic and comatose, not agitated and delirious. With an Addisonian crisis, Choice (C), the presenting symptoms are hypotension and weakness. A cocaine overdose, Choice (D), could cause similar symptoms to thyroid storm, but you're told that her urine drug screen is clean. Pheochromocytoma, Choice (E), certainly could present with an acute change in blood pressure (either hypertensive crisis or profound hypotension), but the person wouldn't be delirious nor would she experience the other symptoms mentioned in the clinical scenario.

21. **A.** Beta blockers (usually propanolol), Choice (A), are used in the treatment of hyperthyroidism. An intravenous (IV) steroid like hydrocortisone, Choice (B), is used in the treatment of an Addisonian crisis. Levothyroxine (Synthroid), Choice (D), is given for the treatment of myxedema. Phenoxybenzamine, Choice (C), is used in treating a pheochromocytoma. IV hydralazine, Choice (E), isn't applicable.

22. **E.** This person has a history of diabetes and osteomyelitis, a long-standing chronic infection, which corresponds with Choice (E). The iron studies show an elevated ferritin level, which is elevated in inflammatory states. With a iron saturation of 55%, this person isn't iron deficient, Choice (B). Liver disease, Choice (D), is a cause of a macrocytic anemia. Nothing in the history suggests lead poisoning, Choice (A).

23. **D.** This patient has Von Willebrand disease, which is usually seen in young people. The key is in the lab values. The platelets are normal. The ProTime is normal, which rules out liver disease as a cause. Fibrinogen levels are low in liver disease and are also low in disseminated intravascular coagulation (DIC). If DIC were present, however, you would expect to see thrombocytopenia, which isn't the case here. You have no reason to suspect uremia as a cause; no uremic symptoms are present. You would order a vWF assay and Factor VIII level, because vWF is bound to Factor VIII. In other words, you wouldn't just order Factor VIII alone.

24. **B.** Whipple's triad is suggestive of an insulinoma, Choice (B). A glucagonoma, Choice (A), is actually the opposite problem, one of persistent hyperglycemia. Diabetes mellitus, Choice (C), is diagnosed by an average fasting blood glucose greater than 126 mg/dL on two separate occasions. Diabetes insipidus, Choice (D), refers to polyuria caused by a problem with antidiuretic hormone (ADH) deficiency or resistance.

25. **A.** The most common histology of bladder cancer is transitional cell cancer, Choice (A). Squamous cell carcinoma, Choice (B), is the second most common type. Adenocarcinoma, Choice (C), isn't a histologic cell type of bladder cancer; it's usually associated with other organs, such as the lung and pancreas. Small cell carcinoma, Choice (D), refers to a type of lung cancer, and large cell carcinoma, Choice (E), is an invented term. A histologic cell type of lymphoma, called large cell lymphoma, does exist, however.

26. **C.** You'd expect to find hypokalemia and metabolic alkalosis with hydrochlorothiazide, or HCTZ. Potassium-sparing diuretics like spironolactone (Aldactone) can cause high potassium and metabolic acidosis, Choice (A). Acetazolamide (Diamox) causes a hypokalemic metabolic acidosis, Choice (B).

27. **C.** The key to this question is noting that the patient has all the characteristics of diabetic ketoacidosis (DKA). The initial treatment is intravenous (IV) insulin infusion followed by normal saline (because the patient has a significant component of volume depletion), Choice (C). Lispro and Lantus, Choices (B) and (E), aren't used in the initial treatment of DKA.

28. **D.** Muddy brown granular casts, Choice (D), are seen with acute tubular necrosis (ATN). Dysmorphic red cells, Choice (A), are often seen with glomerulonephritis. Urine eosinophils, Choice (E), are seen with acute interstitial nephritis. Pyuria and white cell casts, Choice (B), can be seen with pyelonephritis. Squamous epithelial cells, Choice (C), have no pathologic significance; if they're present, you know the person didn't give a midstream urine sample.

29. **B.** Sildenafil (Viagra) is a vasodilator that's used in treating erectile dysfunction (ED) by increasing blood supply to the area. This medication is also used to treat other conditions, including pulmonary hypertension, because it dilates the pulmonary vasculature, Choice (B). It can be a cause of hypotension, not hypertension, Choice (A). It can cause blindness in rare instances, not ototoxicity, Choice (C). It isn't a cause of hypokalemia or other electrolyte abnormalities, Choice (D). It isn't a cause of neuropathy, Choice (E).

30. **C.** Ectopic ACTH production is a paraneoplastic response usually seen in small cell lung cancer (SCLC). The other choices are findings associated with the setting of renal cell carcinoma (RCC).

31. **C.** Nasogastric suction and vomiting are common gastrointestinal (GI) causes of metabolic alkalosis due to losses of hydrogen ions and potassium.

32. **B.** Septic shock is characterized by a reduction in systemic vascular resistance, Choice (B). Cardiogenic shock is characterized by a decreased cardiac output, Choice (A), in addition to an increased systemic vascular resistance (for example, afterload), Choice (C). Changes in osmotic pressure gradient, Choice (E), can often be seen in shock associated with liver failure. Decreased preload, Choice (D), can be seen in multiple types of shock, including hypovolemic shock and septic shock.

33. **A.** Indinavir (Crixivan) is used in treating human immunodeficiency virus (HIV). A main side effect is the development of renal calculi, or kidney stones. None of the other choices apply in this situation.

34. **C.** The D-dimer is useful for its negative predictive value. A negative D-dimer nearly eliminates the possibility that a pulmonary embolism (PE) is present. Note that a positive D-dimer is sensitive but not specific, however. Many conditions can cause a positive D-dimer, including malignancy, infection, and inflammation. Thus, a positive D-dimer test doesn't confirm that a PE is present.

35. **C.** A high-resolution CT scan can be used in evaluating interstitial pulmonary fibrosis (IPF). The description in the question is classic for IPF. You would also see a restrictive defect in pulmonary function tests (PFTs).

36. **A.** Phenylketonuria (PKU) is an inherited metabolic disorder caused by an inability to convert phenylalanine to tyrosine.

37. **B.** Ethacrynic acid (Edecrin) is a loop diuretic that isn't sulfa related. It can be used in the treatment of pulmonary edema.

38. **C.** For any healthcare worker, an induration above 10 mm is considered positive. The person needs to be treated aggressively.

39. **A.** *Helicobacter pylori* is a Gram-negative microaerophilic rod, Choice (A). It can't be detected via saliva, as suggested in Choice (D). Instead, it can be detected on an endoscopic biopsy, a blood test, and a fecal assay. It's linked to the development of gastric cancer, not intestinal cancer, Choice (B). It's a leading cause of peptic ulcer disease, not Crohn's disease, Choice (C). The treatment includes the proton pump inhibitor with a macrolide and a penicillin, not sucralfate (Carafate), as noted in Choice (E).

40. **A.** This gentleman has a lung-kidney vasculitis. The only choice that matches this is Goodpasture's syndrome, Choice (A). Lung cancer and pulmonary embolism (PE), Choices (B) and (C), can present with hemoptysis, but you wouldn't expect renal failure with either of these. Acute coronary syndrome (ACS), Choice (D), doesn't present with hemoptysis. Congestive heart failure (CHF), Choice (E), can present with hemoptysis, but the question said that the patient's lungs were clear, which would argue against this condition.

41. **C.** The usual first-line treatment for otitis media is a first-generation penicillin, such as amoxicillin (Trimox), Choice (C). Trimethoprim/sulfamethoxazole (Bactrim), Choice (A), wouldn't be indicated here first line. Ceftriaxone (Rocephin), Choice (D), is an intravenous (IV) or intramuscular antibiotic that isn't required, because the patient only needs an oral antibiotic. The patient also shows no need for an antifungal medication such as fluconazole (Diflucan), Choice (E), or a potent antibiotic like clindamycin (Cleocin), Choice (B).

42. **D.** The recognized treatment for Lyme disease is doxycycline. This is one of those facts you just have to memorize; know the rash and know the treatment. You'll also encounter other questions concerning complications of Lyme disease.

43. **B.** The treatment of *Trichomonas vaginalis* is metronidazole (Flagyl). This is a fact you just have to commit to memory.

44. **D.** In any motor vehicle accident case where a patient experiences double vision and a cranial nerve palsy, you need to evaluate for a blowout fracture, Choice (D). Optic neuritis, Choice (B), can present with pain and vision disturbances, but you wouldn't expect a history of trauma. Myasthenia gravis, Choice (E), affects both eyes. Amaurosis fugax, Choice (C), presents as a lampshade covering the eye; this condition can be seen with carotid stenosis. Entropion, Choice (A), is a retraction of the eyelid.

45. **E.** Endocarditis is a common complication of a *Staphylococcus aureus* infection. The other choices are actually complications of a malaria infection.

46. **C.** Doxycycline (Vibramycin) is the treatment of choice for Rocky Mountain spotted fever.

47. **D.** Lip smacking and repetitive facial movements are criteria for diagnosing tardive dyskinesia. All the other choices are features of autism.

48. **A.** A significant side of effect of venlafaxine (Effexor) is hypertension, Choice (A). Hyperglycemia, hyperlipidemia, and weight gain — Choices (B), (D), and (E), respectively — are side effects of many of the atypical antipsychotics and some of the mood stabilizers.

49. **B.** This gentleman likely has obstructive sleep apnea and needs to be evaluated with a sleep study, or polysomnography. The lack of a restorative sleep pattern and excessive daytime somnolence are two important clues to this medical condition.

50. **B.** For a cerebrovascular accident (CVA), tissue plasminogen activator (tPA) can be given within three to four-and-a-half hours from the onset of symptoms.

51. **C.** For hyperthyroidism in a pregnant woman, you usually use propylthiouracil, or PTU, Choice (C). Methimazole, Choice (A), and iodine 131-I, Choice (D), can't be given in pregnancy. You'd use prednisone (Deltasone), Choice (E), only in treating a thyroid storm and if the patient presents with a significant ophthalmopathy secondary to thyroid disease.

52. **D.** Be aware of indications for endocarditis prophylaxis. Mitral valve prolapse (MVP) in and of itself isn't an indication for endocarditis prophylaxis. The patient needs to have a significant prolapse with valvular dysfunction in order to require prophylaxis. The other answer choices are criteria for endocarditis prophylaxis.

53. **E.** The usual medication prescribed before a dental procedure for antibiotic prophylaxis is a penicillin derivative, most often amoxicillin. If a patient is allergic to penicillin, the oral surgeon can prescribe either erythromycin (E-Mycin) or clindamycin (Cleocin).

54. **B.** This woman shows the classic presentation of placenta previa, Choice (B). It's diagnosed by ultrasound and presents with painless bleeding. Abruptio placentae, Choice (A), presents with bleeding and abdominal pain. Ectopic pregnancy, Choice (C), presents with abdominal or perineal pain and a positive β-hCG. Preeclampsia, Choice (D), is the presence of hypertension and proteinuria after the 20th week of pregnancy. Antiphospholipid antibody syndrome, Choice (E), is associated with second trimester abortions.

55. **B.** Factor V Leiden mutation is the most common hypercoagulable state. Those affected can be heterozygous or homozygous for this condition.

56. **D.** Folic acid replacement reduces the risk of fetal neural tube defects, especially spina bifida. The other choices aren't applicable.

57. **E.** The photo in question shows onychomycosis, or nail fungus. Treat this condition with an antifungal regimen, such as Lamisil or Sporanox. Risk factors include a suppressed immune system and diabetes. Liver function tests (LFTs) need to be monitored with the use of either of these two medications.

58. **D.** The evaluation of abdominal pain, especially in an older person can sometimes be puzzling. If you encounter a question that states that a rash had been present before (particularly a unilateral linear rash), think varicella zoster and postherpetic neuralgia, Choice (D), as the cause of pain. The pain pattern for the woman in the question follows a dermatomal distribution. All the other causes of pain, except for pyelonephritis, Choice (E), are usually more episodic. Mesenteric angina, Choice (C), is pain that occurs after eating, usually related to blood flow issues. Irritable bowel syndrome (IBS), Choice (B), is usually more a diagnosis of exclusion, but the patient didn't report altered bowel habits. Pyelonephritis could present with fever and abnormal urinalysis with pyuria. A CT scan could be benign or show perinephric stranding.

59. **B.** The initial diagnosis for Cushing's syndrome is either a 24-hour urinary free cortisol, Choice (B), or a low-dose dexamethasone suppression test. For the diagnosis of polycystic ovarian syndrome (PCOS), you would order an ultrasound of the ovaries as well as follicle-stimulating hormone (FSH)/luteinizing hormone (LH) blood levels, Choice (D). An MRI of the brain, Choice (A), would be used to confirm the diagnosis of a pituitary adenoma. Serum and urine β-human chorionic gonadotropin (β-hCG) levels, Choice (C), are used to confirm the diagnosis of pregnancy; note that the β-hCG is also used in the diagnosis of a hydatidiform mole. A thyroid-stimulating hormone (TSH) level, Choice (E), would be used to evaluate for hypothyroidism.

60. **E.** The antiphospholipid antibody syndrome consists of second trimester abortions, thrombocytopenia, and deep venous thrombosis (DVT). It isn't associated with thrombocytosis, anemia, polycythemia, or hematuria — Choices (A), (B), (C), or (D).

Block 5

1. **B.** Aortic insufficiency is characterized by a widened pulse pressure and diastolic murmur. You should know these key components of the murmur for the test.

2. **E.** The pulse pressure is the difference between the systolic and diastolic blood pressures.

3. **C.** This patient likely has infectious endocarditis (IE). In someone with a history of intravenous drug abuse (IVDA), the usual causative organism is *Staphylococcus aureus*. With IVDA, the most common valve affected is the tricuspid valve. ***Remember:*** For testing purposes,

the mitral valve is associated with rheumatic fever. Realize clinically, however, that the mitral valve is also commonly affected by IE.

4. **A.** Clinical manifestations of infectious endocarditis (IE) include Osler's nodes, Choice (A), Janeway lesions, and Roth spots. Paronychia, Choice (B), is a bacterial infection of the nail bed. Trousseau's sign, Choice (C), is associated with the migratory thrombophlebitis associated with pancreatic cancer. The other Trousseau's sign can actually be associated with hypocalcemia. Cyanosis, Choice (D), isn't a recognized manifestation of infective endocarditis. Grey-Turner's sign, Choice (E), is associated with hemorrhagic pancreatitis.

5. **B.** When evaluating a pulmonary nodule, you need to figure out whether you're dealing with a benign or malignant problem. Bigger nodules with spiculated edges, lack of calcium, and lack of fat — Choices (C), (D), and (E), respectively — increase the risk that you're dealing with a malignant process. Smooth, round borders, Choice (B), confer a more benign risk. Fat and calcification within the nodule also confer a more benign risk. The pattern of calcification is also important in determining whether it's benign or malignant. Refer to Chapter 4 to review the evaluation of lung nodules.

6. **A.** Ethambutol, Choice (A), is the one medication used in the treatment of tuberculosis (TB) that can affect the eyes and cause color blindness or an optic neuritis. Isoniazid, Choice (B), is associated mainly with increased liver function tests (LFTs) and a peripheral neuropathy. Isoniazid is noted to deplete the body of vitamin B_6, so the patient should be supplemented with that vitamin.

7. **D.** Sclerosing cholangitis, Choice (D), is strongly associated with ulcerative colitis. Make sure you're aware of this important association for the test. Cholangiocarcinoma, Choice (C), is a cancer of the biliary tract that's not associated with ulcerative colitis or any other inflammatory bowel disease (IBD). Primary biliary cirrhosis (PBC), Choice (B), is an autoimmune disease that affects younger to middle-aged women. The laboratory marker for PBC is antimitochondrial antibodies.

8. **C.** The person has acute bronchitis, Choice (C). She has no prior history of lung disease to suggest chronic bronchitis (productive cough three months a year for two consecutive years), emphysema, or sarcoidosis — Choices (A), (B), and (D), respectively. She also shows no symptoms to suggest a diagnosis of acute sinusitis, Choice (E). For example, she has no sinus pressure, frontal headache, and so on.

9. **C.** The person likely has lead poisoning, Choice (C). He works as a house painter, which is one clue in the question. It's unlikely that a 25-year-old man with no other medical conditions would have an anemia of chronic disease, Choice (D). In addition, a young man would be unlikely to have iron losses, Choice (A).

10. **B.** Trimethoprim-sulfamethoxazole (Bactrim), Choice (B), is used for the treatment of a urinary tract infection (UTI). Azithromycin (Zithromax), Choice (A), is used in the treatment of a community-acquired pneumonia (CAP). Fluconazole (Diflucan), Choice (C), is used to treat fungal infections. Cephalexin (Keflex), Choice (D), is used to treat skin infections, such as cellulitis. Acyclovir (Cyclovir), Choice (E), is used in the treatment of herpes and varicella zoster infections.

11. **A.** Orthostatic hypotension is commonly seen in clinical practice, especially after beginning an antihypertensive medication. The accepted definition of this type of hypotension is a decrease of more than 20 mmHg in the systolic blood pressure or more than 10 mmHg in the diastolic blood pressure after standing. At this point, the patient is usually symptomatic. The patient in the question fits all these criteria comparing the sitting to the standing blood pressures.

12. **D.** If a patient's blood pressure is low when he stands up, you should see a compensatory tachycardia, an increase in heart rate. The patient in the question has no increase in heart rate. In all the choices except Choice (D), you would expect to see a compensatory tachycardia. The most common reason for the heart rate not to increase when standing is an autonomic neuropathy. Those patients with diabetes can have an autonomic neuropathy as well as a peripheral neuropathy. Often the two coexist.

13. **A.** Lithium carbonate (Lithobid), Choice (A), is a commonly prescribed medication used for the treatment of bipolar disorder and can cause diabetes insipidus. Carbamazepine (Tegretol), Choice (B), causes the opposite symptoms of lithium and can cause a syndrome of inappropriate diuretic hormone (SIADH). Clofibrate (Atromid-S), Choice (C), also causes a SIADH-like phenomenon. Furosemide (Lasix), Choice (D), causes a diuresis but not a diabetes insipidus. Amiloride (Midamor), Choice (E), is used for diabetes insipidus second to lithium. It's also a potassium-sparing diuretic that can be used for the treatment of hypertension.

14. **E.** The physical examination sign of pale conjunctivas often suggests that anemia may be present.

15. **D.** The use of intravenous (IV) octreotide (Sandostatin), Choice (D), is used in the treatment of esophageal varices. You wouldn't give warfarin (Coumadin), Choice (A), to someone who is actively bleeding. IV hydrocortisone (Solu-Cortef), Choice (C), is used in the treatment of adrenal insufficiency. Vitamin B_{12}, Choice (E), is used to help someone with B_{12} deficiency; it doesn't have a place in the treatment of acute esophageal varices. A person with advanced liver disease can't effectively metabolize vitamin K, Choice (B). Note also that vitamin K takes several hours to correct hypoprothrombinemia.

16. **D.** This patient likely has a ganglion cyst, Choice (D), which usually presents on the extremities, such as on the elbows or the wrists. The affected person may be asymptomatic, or she may experience pain with movement. Morton's neuroma, Choice (B), affects the foot, not the hand. Carpal tunnel syndrome, Choice (A), affects the median nerve and isn't associated with any palpable lump. A lipoma, Choice (C), is a freely movable lump that's painless and can be found in various places on the body, including the extensor surfaces of many extremities. Tenosynovitis, Choice (E), presents with pain in the thumb, especially on flexion, but it doesn't present with a palpable lump.

17. **E.** Amiodarone (Cordarone) is a popular antiarrhythmic used in treating various atrial and ventricular arrhythmias, including atrial fibrillation. This medication has a lot of side effects, including hypothyroidism and hyperthyroidism, corneal eye deposits, and elevated liver function tests (LFTs), Choice (E). Amiodarone is associated with pulmonary fibrosis, not pulmonary hemorrhage, Choice (C). The other choices listed do not pertain to amiodarone.

18. **E.** The patient has cauda equina syndrome, Choice (E), which can cause saddle anesthesia and loss of bowel and bladder function. While all the other choices are causes of pain, the symptoms are specific to cauda equina syndrome. Spinal stenosis, Choice (A), can be debilitating and painful, usually causing pseudoclaudication, but it's not in itself a neurologic emergency. Spondylolisthesis, Choice (B), is an anterior slipping of the vertebrae.

19. **D.** This person has ankylosing spondylitis. On a lumbar spine radiograph, you may see the classic bamboo spine as well as inflammation of his sacroiliac joint, or sacroiliitis.

20. **C.** All the choices except hyperglycemia, Choice (C), are common causes of pancreatitis. Hyperglycemia can be a consequence of pancreatitis rather than a cause.

21. **C.** The patient likely has spontaneous bacteria peritonitis, Choice (C). He has ascites, shown by physical examination, including the presence of shifting dullness and bulging flanks. You don't have enough information in the question to make an informed decision as to whether the patient has acute hepatitis or cancer, Choices (B) or (D). The lack of diarrhea and cough in the patient's symptoms make the presence of colitis or pneumonia, Choices (A) or (E), highly unlikely.

22. **A.** The Protime (PT/INR), Choice (A), is a measure of the liver's synthetic function. The liver is the body's metabolizer as well as a part in the clotting process. So the loss of this clotting ability is the first sign that the liver is losing its metabolic integrity. Liver enzymes, Choice (C), aren't a true measure of the synthetic function of the liver. In fact, they may not even be elevated if chronic cirrhosis is present. Even though the liver is involved in gluconeogenesis, the blood glucose level, Choice (D), isn't a reliable enough marker for liver disease. However, if hypoglycemia is present, you can certainly consider liver disease in your differential diagnosis. Serum albumin levels and fibrinogen levels, Choices (B) and (E), are acute phase reactants and in advanced cirrhosis may be low, just secondary to end-stage liver disease.

23. **D.** This patient has the constellation of symptoms referred to as Whipple's triad. The other triad choices aren't applicable to this condition. Thiamine deficiency is characterized by Wernicke's encephalopathy.

24. **D.** The patient has electrocardiogram (ECG) changes and is exhibiting bradycardia secondary to hyperkalemia. Intravenous (IV) calcium gluconate, Choice (D), is indicated to be given first to stabilize the heart. After the calcium is administered, regular IV insulin and glucose is administered, Choice (C). These medications shift the potassium from the extracellular compartment into the intracellular compartment. The albuterol nebulizer, Choice (B), works by a similar mechanism to force potassium into the cell (via the beta-2 receptor activation); however, it's not as effective as insulin and glucose.

    Sodium polystyrene sulfate (Kayexelate), Choice (A), is an osmotic diarrheal agent used to rid the body of excess potassium via the gastrointestinal (GI) tract. It can take three to four hours to work (not to mention it tastes terrible), which isn't quickly enough in this situation to lower the potassium. You need to make quick work of lowering the potassium because the ECG changes are due to the high potassium levels.

25. **E.** Celiac disease can cause malabsorption of vitamins and nutrients; you would order an anti-gliadin antibody to work up this condition. The other choices don't have a place here.

26. **A.** Gilbert's syndrome is a hereditary cause of unconjugated hyperbilirubinemia. This condition occurs because of a deficiency of the enzyme responsible for conjugating bilirubin. No acute treatment exists for this condition.

27. **C.** Hyaline membrane disease (HMD) causes significant respiratory distress in newborn infants, usually before the age of 28 weeks. The chest radiograph can show hazy infiltrates and ground glass appearance. A deficiency of surfactant is thought to be the cause of HMD. In addition to ventilation, the treatment is the administration of surfactant through nebulized aerosol.

28. **A.** Cortisol is made in the zona fasciculata, Choice (A). The zona glomerulosa, Choice (C), makes aldosterone, which is the outermost layer of the adrenal gland. The zona reticularis, Choice (B), is responsible for the production of androgens. The adrenal gland doesn't have a marginal zone, Choice (E).

29. **C.** The Pneumovax 23 vaccination recommendation is once for those older than 65. If a person has significant lung disease, some question whether revaccination is appropriate. The official recommendation is that Pneumovax 23 is a "once and done" vaccination, but some medical professionals may choose to vaccinate again after five years. However, this revaccination is somewhat controversial. For the purposes of test taking, stick with official recommendations.

30. **C.** When a person has lost the spleen, he or she is at risk for bacterial infections, especially from the encapsulated organisms. A *Haemophilus influenzae* type B vaccination, Choice (C), should be administered to prevent this potentially fatal complication. It's also recommended that the person receive an influenza vaccine, Choice (E), annually. Hepatitis B, Choice (D), is a vaccination usually given to newborns, and immunity isn't affected by asplenia.

31. **E.** History of radiation treatments for another type of cancer, Choice (E), increase one's risk for the development of breast cancer. Early menarche, not late menarche, Choice (A), is associated with an increased risk of breast cancer. In addition, nulliparity, not multiparity, Choice (D), is a risk factor for breast cancer. Being pregnant later in life compared to earlier, Choice (C), is also a risk factor. A family history of a first-degree relative with breast cancer and/or endometrial cancer, not hypothyroidism, Choice (B), would be a risk factor for breast cancer.

32. **D.** Kyphosis, especially when severe, can interfere with a normal breathing pattern. It's associated with a restrictive defect shown on pulmonary function testing and is a cause of respiratory acidosis. All the other choices are causes of respiratory alkalosis.

33. **B.** Being aware of medication interactions is important, especially concerning cardiac medications. A significant interaction is possible between clopidogrel (Plavix) and some of the proton pump inhibitors (PPIs), including pantoprazole (Protonix).

34. **E.** The person in the question is suffering from a cluster headache. It's classic, occurring more often in men and unilateral in presentation. Treatment can include medications that abort the headache, but the most important treatment to consider is oxygen. You know this gentleman isn't suffering from temporal arteritis or glaucoma, because he has no loss of vision. He also has no other symptoms of temporal arteritis (for example, jaw claudication). Plus, temporal arteritis is seen more commonly in women. Narrow-angle glaucoma would present with a fixed, dilated pupil versus the pupillary constriction that you see with a cluster headache. Beta blockers are used for prophylaxis for migraine headaches, so they wouldn't have a role here.

35. **D.** A noncontrast CT scan of the head is the test of choice for evaluating a possible subdural hematoma.

36. **B.** Two different types of liver injury exist: a transaminitis and a cholestatic pattern of liver injury. The macrolide antibiotics, particularly erythromycin (E-Mycin), Choice (B), can cause a cholestatic pattern of liver injury. The other choices would cause a hepatitis, or transaminitis type of liver injury.

37. **A.** In someone who's unable to tolerate doxycycline (Vibramycin), an appropriate alternative is amoxicillin/clavulanic acid (Augmentin), Choice (A). Benadryl 30 minutes prior to administration of doxycycline and metoclopramide (Reglan) 30 minutes prior to the administration of doxycycline, Choices (B) and (C), don't make any sense. Chloramphenicol and ciprofloxacin (Cipro), Choices (D) and (E), aren't indicated for the treatment of Lyme disease.

38. **A.** A noncontrast CT scan of the abdomen and pelvis will evaluate for a retroperitoneal bleed. None of the other answers are applicable.

39. **D.** This person has all the features of hemochromatosis, including diabetes, bronze pigmentation of the skin, and testicular atrophy. The screening test for this syndrome is an iron saturation and ferritin level, which can determine whether the patient has elevated transferrin saturation.

40. **B.** This person has histoplasmosis. The key in this question is his occupation — he loves birds as an ornithologist. It's likely that he's been exposed to bird droppings, which causes the disease. The location (the Midwest) is important as well given the higher incidence of histoplasmosis in that region. He likely was on oral itraconazole as an outpatient, and when this therapy didn't work, he came into the hospital. (Note that itraconazole sounds like Miconazole, an imidazole antifungal agent, which is an over-the-counter treatment for tinea pedis.) In the hospital, the treatment for worsening histoplasmosis is amphotericin B (Amphotec). His chest radiograph shows a pattern that can be seen with histoplasmosis as well as military tuberculosis (TB), but the patient shows no signs of having TB.

41. **E.** The answer for this question isn't without controversy. Different medical groups have different recommendations regarding the screening for hypothyroidism. The most recommended practice is screening for both men and women older than 35 years of age by checking a thyroid-stimulating hormone (TSH) level.

42. **B.** This patient likely has diabetes affecting his eyes, which is referred to as diabetic retinopathy. This condition is characterized by cotton-wool exudates and retinal hemorrhages, which is a classic presentation.

43. **D.** Schizophrenia is a psychotic disorder where both delusions and hallucinations are present. The scenario presented in the question would at least suggest that a medical professional look beyond diagnosing a hallucination or delusion and think about the possibility that schizophrenia may indeed be present. This gentleman shows no indications that he's manic.

44. **B.** The person likely has obsessive-compulsive disorder (OCD). Selective serotonin reuptake inhibitors (SSRIs), such as sertraline (Zoloft), have been used for the treatment of OCD. The other medications in this question aren't as efficacious as SSRIs.

45. **D.** One biggie on the test is being able to tell from a cerebral spinal fluid (CSF) analysis the difference between bacterial and viral (aseptic) meningitis. Basically, the CSF protein will be higher, and the CSF glucose will be normal or low normal. The white blood count (WBC) will show more lymphocytes and/or monocytes.

46. **C.** Different stages of chronic obstructive pulmonary disease (COPD) exist depending on the ratio of FEV1/FVC. Someone whose FEV1 is less than 50% of the predicted value has severe COPD. It's important to do spirometry/pulmonary function tests (PFTs) early because many people can have a decline in pulmonary function before they even have symptoms.

47. **C.** Quitting smoking is difficult. The combination of committing to a quit date and to smoking cessation classes as well as the use of the medication bupropion (Zyban) seems to have the best results. This medication is approved for smoking cessation.

48. **A.** You need to review this gentleman's human immunodeficiency virus (HIV) medications. When it comes to HIV medications, you need to be aware of some things. You'll be asked about these meds in the many practice tests you'll no doubt take. Some of the medications used to treat HIV can cause an elevated lactic acid level because they can interfere with mitochondrial function. One example is stavudine.

    Many times a patient's lactic acid will be elevated but presents no lactic acidosis (though the patient is still at risk of developing lactic acidosis with a severe infection, shock-like state, or other immune-compromising condition). Remember that two different types of lactic acid exist, an L-type and a D-type. The L-type is the most common type you deal with. The D-type is specific to bowel problems, such as bacterial overgrowth syndrome.

49. **C.** With a glomerular filtration rate (GFR) of 55 mL/min, this person has Stage 3 chronic kidney disease (CKD), which is defined as an estimated GFR of between 30–59 mL/min.

50. **B.** These macular lesions on the patient's palms and soles are Janeway lesions, which are a cutaneous manifestation of infectious endocarditis (IE), Choice (B). Certainly other conditions can also cause skin lesions on the palms and soles. The clinical scenario points to IE versus Rocky Mountain spotted fever, Choice (A). Lyme disease, Choice (C), causes the characteristic erythema chronicum migrans, or bull's-eye lesion, which can occur anywhere on the body. Seronegative spondyloarthropathy and rheumatoid arthritis (RA), Choices (D) and (E), don't usually cause a skin rash with this kind of distribution.

51. **E.** Before putting in an arterial line, you want to be sure the patient has decent circulation, so performing an Allen's test, Choice (E), is crucial. If, for some unseen reason, the patient has damage to his radial artery, you still have a collateral blood supply to the hand. The ankle-brachial index (ABI), Choice (A), is used to assess the arterial blood flow to the lower extremities. The capillary refill, Choice (D), doesn't give you enough information in this circumstance; although, in general, it's a good indicator of digital perfusion. Dopplers of the carotid arteries, Choice (C), can be used to evaluate for carotid stenosis, especially if someone has transient ischemic attack (TIA) symptoms or an audible carotid bruit. Coauthor Rich has never ordered an axillary Doppler, but it sounds like an awesome test with which to confuse people.

52. **A.** Ah, the wonderful world of pharmacology! Sodium nitroprusside (Nipride), Choice (A), is a potent arterial and venous vasodilator and is commonly prescribed for the treatment of a hypertensive crisis. Furosemide (Lasix), Choice (B), is used in the treatment of congestive heart failure (CHF). Digoxin (Lanoxin), Choice (C), is used in the treatment of CHF and atrial fibrillation. Methyldopa (Aldomet), Choice (D), is an oral antihypertensive but is not the best choice to use in the setting of a hypertensive crisis because it isn't as potent as Choice (A). Choice (D) is commonly prescribed for the treatment of hypertension in pregnant women. Hydroxyurea (Hydrea), Choice (E), is used in the treatment of polycythemia vera.

53. **A.** This person has decompensated heart failure. Dobutamine (Dobutrex), Choice (A), is a positive ionotrope, which is indicated. Lactated Ringers, Choice (B), is a type of intravenous (IV) fluid that is contraindicated in the setting of heart failure. Octreotide (Somatostatin) and vasopressin (Pitressin), Choices (C) and (D), are used in the management of esophageal varices. Neo-Synephrine, Choice (E), is used in treating septic shock because it's a potent vasoconstrictor. As a result, you wouldn't want to use it for the man in the question.

54. **B.** If you missed this question, you should review the JNC 7 criteria for hypertension in Chapter 3. This person by definition has prehypertension, Choice (B) — the systolic blood pressure is less than 130 mmHg, and the diastolic is less than 90 mmHg. Normal blood pressure, Stage I hypertension, and Stage II hypertension — Choices (A), (C), and (D), respectively — represent the different categories of blood pressure. However, Stage III, Choice (E), isn't a valid category.

55. **A.** For test questions concerning loss of consciousness, many times you're asked to differentiate between syncope and seizure. The historical elements in the question are important: The lack of a postictal state and tongue biting and the patient's continued control of his bowel or bladder function during the episode argue against seizure, Choice (B) and point toward syncope, Choice (A). Vestibular dysfunction, Choice (C), would present with vertigo-like symptoms. Hypertrophic cardiomyopathy, Choice (D), can be a cause of syncope and sudden death characteristically in a younger individual. Adrenal insufficiency, Choice (E), is an uncommon cause of syncope.

56. **D.** Here you encounter that age-old question, "Is the patient wet or dry?" This question was formulated because you're trying to figure out whether the person is experiencing a congestive heart failure (CHF) exacerbation or a chronic obstructive pulmonary disease (COPD) exacerbation. A B-type natriuretic peptide (BNP) level should help you, because it's expected to be elevated in states of CHF and lower in COPD. The other choices, while helpful, wouldn't be as specific in this situation as a BNP level. (***Note:*** You'd choose Choice (D) for the PANCE; clinically, it's not as clear cut, however.)

57. **B.** Certain serotypes of human papillomavirus (HPV) are linked to the development of cervical cancer. Choice (B), 18, is one of them.

58. **E.** This woman almost certainly has polycystic ovarian syndrome (PCOS), Choice (E). She has all the symptoms, including amenorrhea, infertility (which is a biggie with PCOS), hypertension, metabolic syndrome, and hirsutism.

    You may be reading this answer explanation and thinking, what about Cushing's syndrome, Choice (A)? Certainly some features can overlap, including the hypertension and metabolic syndrome, but if this woman were experiencing Cushing's you'd notice some description consistent with the syndrome, including buffalo hump and so forth. Delayed pregnancy, Choice (B), makes no sense, and hypothyroidism, Choice (C) (while it is a cause of amenorrhea), usually isn't associated with hirsutism and some of the other features of PCOS. With a pituitary adenoma, Choice (D), one could have bitemporal hemianopsia. Pituitary adenoma is also a cause of Cushing's disease.

59. **C.** Nerve pain responds to a neuralgesic medication such as gabapentin (Neurontin), Choice (C). This patient doesn't need an upper gastrointestinal (GI) series or psychiatric consultation, Choices (A) and (B). Neuralgia pain can be debilitating, so an opioid analgesic would likely be prescribed after starting with a medication like gabapentin. Ibuprofen, Choice (D), isn't considered first-line for neuropathic pain.

60. **E.** As noted in Choice (E), late menopause is a risk factor for the development of endometrial cancer. Menopause is associated with an elevated follicle-stimulating hormone (FSH) level, not an undetectable one, as suggested in Choice (B). It commonly affects women in their early 50s, not those in their 30s, Choice (C). Menopause is a risk factor for the development of osteoporosis, which is the opposite of what's noted in Choice (A). Regarding Choice (D), estrogen cream does help with genitourinary symptoms.

Answer Key

Block 1

1. E	13. C	25. D	37. D	49. A
2. D	14. D	26. C	38. C	50. D
3. C	15. C	27. D	39. E	51. D
4. D	16. C	28. D	40. A	52. B
5. D	17. D	29. C	41. B	53. B
6. D	18. C	30. E	42. A	54. A
7. C	19. A	31. D	43. E	55. D
8. D	20. C	32. B	44. C	56. D
9. D	21. A	33. A	45. C	57. B
10. D	22. D	34. B	46. C	58. B
11. A	23. E	35. C	47. B	59. A
12. D	24. C	36. A	48. C	60. B

Block 2

1. C	13. E	25. B	37. B	49. A
2. B	14. B	26. E	38. C	50. A
3. E	15. C	27. C	39. C	51. D
4. C	16. C	28. E	40. E	52. B
5. C	17. C	29. E	41. B	53. D
6. A	18. D	30. B	42. E	54. C
7. D	19. B	31. A	43. C	55. C
8. B	20. D	32. A	44. A	56. B
9. B	21. B	33. B	45. C	57. A
10. C	22. A	34. D	46. E	58. E
11. A	23. C	35. D	47. D	59. E
12. E	24. E	36. D	48. B	60. B

Block 3

1. B	13. A	25. B	37. A	49. C
2. D	14. B	26. E	38. C	50. B
3. E	15. B	27. D	39. C	51. B
4. D	16. D	28. B	40. B	52. B
5. B	17. E	29. C	41. D	53. A
6. D	18. D	30. B	42. C	54. D
7. C	19. A	31. B	43. B	55. B
8. A	20. C	32. D	44. D	56. B
9. B	21. D	33. E	45. B	57. C
10. D	22. B	34. B	46. A	58. A
11. D	23. A	35. B	47. C	59. B
12. D	24. D	36. C	48. B	60. A

Block 4

1. A	13. B	25. A	37. B	49. B
2. A	14. C	26. C	38. C	50. B
3. D	15. A	27. C	39. A	51. C
4. C	16. B	28. D	40. A	52. D
5. D	17. B	29. B	41. C	53. E
6. E	18. D	30. C	42. D	54. B
7. B	19. D	31. C	43. B	55. B
8. A	20. B	32. B	44. D	56. D
9. D	21. A	33. A	45. E	57. E
10. B	22. E	34. C	46. C	58. D
11. E	23. D	35. C	47. D	59. B
12. D	24. B	36. A	48. A	60. E

Block 5

1. B	13. A	25. E	37. A	49. C
2. E	14. E	26. A	38. A	50. B
3. C	15. D	27. C	39. D	51. E
4. A	16. D	28. A	40. B	52. A
5. B	17. E	29. C	41. E	53. A
6. A	18. E	30. C	42. B	54. B
7. D	19. D	31. E	43. D	55. A
8. C	20. C	32. D	44. B	56. D
9. C	21. C	33. B	45. D	57. B
10. B	22. A	34. E	46. C	58. E
11. A	23. D	35. D	47. C	59. C
12. D	24. D	36. B	48. A	60. E

Part VII
The Part of Tens

The 5th Wave   By Rich Tennant

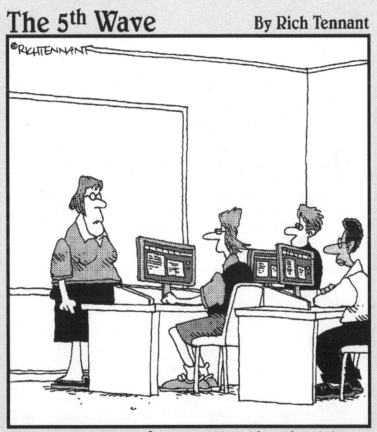

"In celebration of completing the Physician Assistant Exam, I'd like you all to stick out your tongues and say 'Ahhhhh.'"

In this part . . .

The three chapters in Part VII are filled with useful information in compact form. Chapter 22 gives you a brief rundown of 11 big-payoff medical triads, Chapter 23 contains common medical abbreviations, and Chapter 24 describes what we think are the top ten mistakes that test-takers make.

Chapter 22

The Top Ten (Plus a Bonus) Medical Triads

In This Chapter

▶ Looking at associated signs and symptoms

▶ Knowing common triads for the PANCE

*P*ANCE/PANRE question-makers love clinical triads because they're a great resource for test questions. When you understand common triads, you're one step ahead of everyone else. It's important not only to recognize the components of the triads themselves but also to see how they can apply to other clinically related test problems. Here are the top 11 triads (we give you both Charcot's triads) you should be aware of as you prepare for the test.

Virchow's Triad: Thrombosis

Virchow's triad of *stasis, hypercoagulable state,* and *endothelial dysfunction* are thought to be components of or causes of thrombosis. When you're reading questions concerning a *deep venous thrombosis (DVT)* or hypercoagulable state, you may well be dealing with some abnormality of this triad.

Scenarios you encounter on an exam typically include a person who's been on a long plane trip or car ride who develops a lower extremity DVT. In other scenarios, the person may have had a prolonged surgery or have been immobilized for a long period of time. You may need to determine the duration of anticoagulation. All these scenarios concern issues of stasis predisposing to a DVT.

Concerning the hypercoagulable states, you need to recognize their common causes. For details, see Chapter 18.

Charcot's Two Triads: Ascending Cholangitis or Multiple Sclerosis

Jean-Martin Charcot actually came up with two different triads. The first Charcot's triad concerns the triad of *ascending cholangitis,* and the second is related to the triad of *multiple sclerosis (MS).*

Ascending cholangitis is an infection of the biliary tract and is a medical emergency. Charcot's triad concerning the biliary tract is *right upper-quadrant (RUQ) pain, fever,* and *jaundice.* Here's a high-yield fact: The most common medical condition associated with ascending cholangitis is *inflammatory bowel disease (IBD).*

If you see a test question about someone with ulcerative colitis who develops right upper-quadrant pain, fever, and jaundice, it's ascending cholangitis until proven otherwise.

Charcot's triad concerning MS is *nystagmus, intention tremor,* and *dysarthria.* These symptoms can clue you in that MS may be present. Another big symptom for MS is optic neuritis.

Don't confuse Charcot's triad as it pertains to MS with the triad of Wernicke's encephalopathy. Wernicke's is caused by a thiamine deficiency, usually secondary to alcoholism and poor nutritional status. The triad associated with Wernicke's consists of *ataxia, ophthalmoplegia,* and *confusion.* The immediate treatment is thiamine; the longer term treatment is to stop drinking.

Beck's Triad: Cardiac Tamponade

You don't want to miss Beck's triad, either clinically or on the test. The triad consists of three important signs of *cardiac tamponade.* The signs are *jugular venous distention (JVD), shock,* and *distant or muffled heart sounds.* Cardiac tamponade is a surgical emergency requiring emergent pericardiocentesis.

On the PANCE, you'll be given a patient scenario and asked about managing a patient in shock. From a cardiac perspective, your main differentials will be cardiogenic shock due to a failing left ventricle and cardiac tamponade. With cardiogenic shock, you may hear rales on lung exam and see pulmonary edema on CXR; JVD may also be present. See Chapter 3 for more details.

Saint's Triad: Gallstones, Hiatal Hernia, Diverticular Disease

Saint's triad consists of *gallstones, hiatal hernia,* and *diverticular disease.* This triad teaches an important lesson, both in test-taking and in clinical medicine. Although many people have all three of these separate conditions, there isn't one unifying diagnosis that explains them.

Many of us in medicine are conditioned to look for one syndrome or disease process that explains everything. This concept is called *Occam's razor:* The practitioner should look for the fewest possible causes that will account for all the symptoms. For the most part, the PANCE asks you to identify one medical condition that can explain all the findings together. Sometimes, however, the test-makers throw you a curveball and present things that are seemingly unrelated.

Whipple's Triad: Insulinoma

Whipple's triad consists of three criteria that alert the clinician that a person's *diaphoresis, tremulousness,* and *shakiness* may be due to hypoglycemia. If symptoms are present and the following happens, insulinoma may be present. The procedure goes like this:

1. The patient demonstrates diaphoresis, tremulousness, and shakiness.

2. While the person is having the symptoms, the clinician checks the blood glucose level to be certain that hypoglycemia is present *at the same time* as the symptoms.

Normalizing the blood glucose normalizes the person's symptoms.

Don't confuse Whipple's triad with *Whipple's disease,* which is a malabsorption syndrome caused by the *Tropheryma whipplei* bacterium. Whipple's disease, which is also referred to as tropical sprue, involves two big-ticket points:

- ✔ Recognition of the disease by means of a positive periodic acid-Schiff stain as found on intestinal biopsy

- ✔ Treatment for 1 year with trimethoprim/sulfamethoxazole (Bactrim)

Dieulafoy's Triad: Acute Appendicitis

Dieulafoy's triad deals with acute appendicitis. This is a big-payoff surgical test question, and it's easy to grasp.

Dieulafoy's triad consists of *abdominal tenderness, skin hypersensitivity,* and *contraction of the muscle* at McBurney's point. *McBurney's point* is a point on the right side of the abdomen, one-third the distance from the anterior superior iliac spine (ASIS) to the umbilical area.

Other common clinical signs of acute appendicitis you may be tested on include *Rovsing's sign,* the *psoas sign,* the *obturator sign,* and *Blumberg's sign.* See Chapter 7 for details.

Sampter's Triad: Aspirin Sensitivity

Sampter's triad, also known as the *aspirin triad,* is a medical condition consisting of *asthma, sensitivity to aspirin,* and *nasal polyps.* This is one of those medical syndromes where you either recognize the clinical presentation or you don't. It usually occurs in young people in their late twenties and early thirties. They have significant sensitivity to acetylsalicylic acid; however, people with this syndrome are able to tolerate acetaminophen.

The treatment is to desensitize the person to aspirin. Steroids and leukotriene agonists may be needed.

Waddell's Triad: High-Impact Childhood Trauma

Waddell's triad is a recurrent topic in test questions. The triad is associated with childhood trauma, specifically in a child hit by a motor vehicle. With this triad, we're talking about high impact trauma. The triad consists of *femur fracture, traumatic injuries to the chest or abdomen,* and *injuries to the opposite side of the head.* Waddell's triad isn't a very common childhood injury (we're glad to report), but it is something to be aware of for test-taking purposes.

Another useful pediatric-injury topic is causes of injury based on the pediatric age group. Falls are a leading cause of injury overall. For children under 1 year of age, airway obstruction is among the leading causes of injury. For children ages 1 to 14, bicycle-related accidents are among the most common, followed by drowning.

Cushing's Triad: Head Trauma

If you see test questions about any type of head trauma, remember Cushing's triad. This triad consists of a *decreased heart rate, altered respiratory pattern,* and *increased systolic blood pressure.* These three changes are a consequence of increased intracranial pressure associated with head trauma.

Don't confuse Cushing's triad with *Cushing's syndrome* or *Cushing's disease.* Any medical condition that causes the adrenal gland to secrete excess cortisol is called *Cushing's syndrome.* If the cause of the excess cortisol is a tumor in the pituitary gland (making excess ACTH), then the condition is called *Cushing's disease.* In other words, Cushing's disease is one of myriad causes of Cushing's syndrome. Go figure — neither of these have anything to do with Cushing's triad.

Bergmann's Triad: Fat Embolism

Bergmann's triad is often seen in the context of a fat embolism. This triad consists of abrupt onset of *shortness of breath, change in mental status,* and *petechial lesions along the chest and axillary area.* Fat embolism is an emergent medical condition.

Fat embolism is a common occurrence after many orthopedic procedures. It's also described after a trauma, usually if there are fractures of the long bones. In addition to the triad, note that fat embolism can cause bilateral pulmonary infiltrates consistent with acute respiratory distress syndrome (ARDS).

If you read a test question with the words "acute shortness of breath," get ready. These buzzwords should prompt you to consider putting *pulmonary embolism* at the top of your diagnosis. Fat embolism is also in the differential as well. The keys are in the question. If the person was the victim of a trauma or has had an orthopedic procedure, think fat embolus.

Chapter 23

Ten Important Medical Abbreviations

*W*hen some abbreviations appear on a test, in study materials, and in textbooks, they seem to cause great angst. This needn't happen to you! In this chapter, we review those medical abbreviations that you're most likely to see when studying for the PANCE/PANRE. Our hope is to ease any fear or consternation as you approach these abbreviations (even though medicine has thousands of them). We start by reviewing the many abbreviations associated with thrombocytopenia, and from there things only get better!

Delineating DIC from TTP in Thrombocytopenia

When you're evaluating someone with thrombocytopenia, you need to sift through several abbreviations, including ITP, HIT, DIC, HUS, and TTP (flip back to Chapter 18 for details on thrombocytopenia). One of the biggest hurdles seems to be differentiating disseminated intravascular coagulation (DIC) from thrombotic thrombocytopenic purpura (TTP).

We bring this up here because the PANCE always includes a question or two on this topic, either about identifying the platelet problem or picking the most appropriate management step. Here's the story in a nutshell:

▶ **DIC:** Low platelets, elevated INR, low fibrinogen; treatment is usually fresh frozen plasma (FFP) if the patient is bleeding and heparin if the patient is clotting

▶ **TTP:** Low platelets, schistocytes (helmet cells) on peripheral smear, and elevated LDH level; treatment is either plasmapheresis or, if unavailable, giving fresh frozen plasma

Figuring Out Fever of Unknown Origin (FUO)

When it comes to fevers, nothing is more frustrating for a clinician than trying to figure out where a fever is coming from, especially if it has persisted for a long time. *Fever of unknown origin* (FUO for short) isn't *UFO* misspelled, but it's just as mysterious. Here are the two requirements for calling a fever an FUO:

▶ The temperature has to be > 38.3°C (101°F) documented several times for more than 3 weeks.

▶ After 1 week of intensive investigation in the hospital, the cause of the fever remains elusive.

Common causes of FUO are infection and inflammation. Concerning inflammatory processes that cause FUO, the two broad etiologies you should think about are malignancy and connective tissue disease states. Also, when nothing else makes sense, think about drug fever as a cause of refractory fevers.

Treating Sexually Transmitted Infections (STIs)

Not only are sexually transmitted infections (STIs) painful to have, but STI questions can also be painful to answer on a test — that is, if you aren't familiar with your bugs and drugs. The questions concerning STIs usually deal with identification and management, with a strong focus on management. Here are some key points:

✔ **Chlamydia and gonorrhea:** People with *Chlamydia trachomatis* can often be co-infected with *Neisseria gonorrhoeae,* and the recommended treatment is azithromycin (Zithromax) 1 g PO for one dose only. Alternately, give doxycycline 100 mg PO BID for 1 week for chlamydia along with Ceftriaxone 125 mg IM × 1 for gonorrhea.

✔ **Bacterial vaginosis:** Recall that *bacterial vaginosis* (BV) is treated only if symptoms are present. The recommended treatment is metronidazole (Flagyl) 500 mg PO BID for 1 week.

✔ **Syphilis:** If the person has primary *syphilis,* the recommended treatment is one intramuscular injection of benzathine penicillin, 2.4 million units, in the buttocks. That's a real pain in the you-know-what.

Be aware and beware of the *Jarisch-Herxheimer reaction,* in which antibiotics cause zillions of bacteria to die, releasing large quantities of toxins into the body. This clinical syndrome is characterized by a fever and muscle aches that occur within 24 to 48 hours after initiating treatment for syphilis.

Understanding the Differential Diagnosis (DDx) of Really High Blood Pressure (HBP)

The PANCE usually includes several questions about identifying and managing really high blood pressure (HBP). Usually, the gist of the question is recognizing either a pattern of symptoms or abnormal laboratory values — that's a tipoff to the answer. Here are some general patterns of questions that can lead you to the right answer about renal artery stenosis, primary hyperaldosteronism, and pheochromocytoma, which are all typical causes of resistant HBP:

✔ If you're asked the cause of refractory HBP in someone with carotid disease, CAD, and/ or PAD, think about renal artery stenosis (RAS). The question usually gives you a clue that vascular disease exists elsewhere in the body. Here are other tipoffs in the question that point to RAS: the presence of an abdominal or femoral bruit, worsening renal failure and hyperkalemia after being given an ACE inhibitor, and recurrent CHF (and the heart isn't to blame).

✔ If you're asked about the cause of refractory HBP in someone with problems of low potassium, you should first think about *primary hyperaldosteronism.* Your next step is to obtain serum aldosterone and renin levels in order to evaluate for this.

✔ The PANCE often asks a question or two about evaluating pheochromocytoma. Classically, there can be flushing, palpitations, and labile blood pressure. The diagnosis is confirmed biochemically with a positive 24-hour urine metanephrines and a vanillyl mandelic acid (VMA) test.

Minding Mean Corpuscular Volume (MCV)

When evaluating anemia, a good way to think about the differential diagnosis is based on the mean corpuscular volume (MCV), which you read about in Chapter 18. Here's how the MCV levels compare:

- ✔ **Low MCV:** Anemias associated with a low MCV are the microcytic anemias. They include iron deficiency anemia, thalassemia, lead poisoning, anemia of chronic disease, and sideroblastic anemia.

- ✔ **High MCV:** Anemias with a high MCV are the macrocytic anemias. They include B_{12} and folate deficiencies (the megaloblastic anemias), hypothyroidism, hemolysis, and liver disease.

- ✔ **Normal MCV:** Anemias associated with a normal MCV include anemia secondary to kidney disease, myelophthisic anemia, acute GI bleeding, and certain forms of bone marrow failure.

Learning the Lumbar Puncture (LP)

Test questions about lumbar puncture (LP, informally called a *spinal tap*) often concern interpreting lab results in the setting of acute meningitis. Understanding the results is a popular topic on tests, given the prevalence of meningitis and the high mortality if the condition is left undiagnosed. On the PANCE, the key to acing these types of questions is to know the cerebrospinal fluid (CSF) results for the different types of meningitis.

- ✔ **Bacterial meningitis:** The pattern for bacterial meningitis includes a high CSF protein, a low CSF glucose, and a CSF glucose level that's less than two-thirds of the value of the serum glucose. Often, a significant number of white cells are in the CSF, usually with a neutrophilic predominance.

- ✔ **Aseptic meningitis:** For aseptic meningitis, the protein levels can be slightly high, but the CSF glucose levels are normal. In the first 24 hours, a large number of leukocytes are in the CSF with a neutrophilic predominance, only to later show a more lymphocyte-predominant pattern.

Treating Tuberculosis (TB)

Getting through the test without being asked a question about tuberculosis (TB) is pretty much impossible. We cover TB in detail in Chapter 4, but here, we want to provide some high-yield points about the side effects of medications used in treating TB:

- ✔ **Isoniazid (INH):** INH, which is usually the first-line treatment, can cause a peripheral neuropathy. It may also cause low levels of vitamin B_6 (pyridoxine), so supplementation with vitamin B_6 is recommended. Because INH also carries a risk of hepatitis, liver function needs to be monitored while the person is on the medication.

- ✔ **Rifampin (RIF):** RIF can turn the urine and secretions a funky orange color. Rifampin is a potent enzyme inducer that can affect the metabolism of many drug classes (as we explain in Chapter 14). It has GI effects, can cause thrombocytopenia, and can be toxic to the liver.

✔ **Pyrazinamide (PZA):** PZA can cause some minor joint pains, but the main effect is liver toxicity. It can also raise serum uric acid levels.

✔ **Ethambutol (EMB):** EMB's significant side effect involves the eye. EMB can cause color blindness, and in some studies it has caused optic neuropathy.

Controlling Congestive Heart Failure (CHF)

CHF is a very popular abbreviation, as it represents *congestive heart failure,* the most common reason that someone is admitted to the hospital. Recall that CHF is a symptom of an underlying problem. Conditions that can cause CHF include systolic dysfunction, diastolic dysfunction, valvular abnormalities, and metabolic problems, such as anemia, hyperthyroidism, and some nutritional deficiencies causing a heart failure state. (See Chapter 3 for more on CHF.)

The treatment of acute CHF includes using an intravenous diuretic such as furosemide (Lasix), oxygen, and nitroglycerin (given orally, intravenously, or via a transdermal patch). Other medications, including an ACE inhibitor and digoxin, may be added, especially if there's reduced systolic function.

Identifying Inflammatory Bowel Disease (IBD)

You can read about inflammatory bowel disease (IBD) in Chapter 5. IBD includes two separate but overlapping conditions, Crohn's disease and ulcerative colitis (UC). Having IBD puts the patient at increased risk for colorectal cancer.

Remember FOAPS, the acronym concerning the potential complications of IBD:

F: Fistula

O: Obstruction

A: Abscess

P: Perforation

S: Stricture

Confronting Chronic Obstructive Pulmonary Disease (COPD)

Chronic obstructive pulmonary disease (COPD) is a very common cause of admission to the hospital. So is advanced lung disease. Success points for the PANCE concerning COPD include recalling the inpatient management of COPD: intravenous steroids, nebulizer treatments, and supportive care.

The best treatment for COPD is for the patient to stop smoking. Oxygen should be administered as needed.

Chapter 24

Ten Mistakes that Test-Takers Make

In This Chapter

▶ Managing your time

▶ Reading for understanding

▶ Understanding the tricks in questions

▶ Trusting your instincts

▶ Preparing for the exam

Assume for a moment that everything has gone according to plan. You've studied for the PANCE. You registered for the exam and have arrived at the test center in one piece. All that remains is for you to take the test and pass with a high score.

The PANCE is 5 hours long and contains 300 multiple-choice questions. You have 60 minutes to answer each block of 60 questions with breaks between blocks. That's plenty of time to finish if you avoid getting caught in any test-taker traps.

The PANRE is 4 hours long and contains 240 multiple-choice questions. Again, you have 60 minutes to answer each block of 60 questions with breaks between blocks. Remember that you have a choice for the PANRE; you can choose the adult medicine option, the surgical option, or the primary care option. This allows you to pick an area that you may have more expertise in and that reflects more of your daily practice.

This chapter contains ten cautions about test taking. Be smart! A big part of being smart is not to do the dumb things we discuss here.

Taking Too Much Time on One Question

At the start of a block of questions, time is your friend. Toward the end of the hour, time — the lack of it — can become a deadly enemy.

Don't linger too long on tough questions. Enter your best answer and move on. Later questions in the block may even give you insight into a question that's causing you grief. If so, you can go back and change your answer.

On the other hand, don't rush. You *do* have time to read and understand the questions thoroughly. If you rush, you may fall prey to the trick in the question. See the later section "Not Knowing Common Traps in Questions" for details.

Passing on an Answer

You can skip a question, but it's risky. If you skip questions, you run the risk of leaving questions unanswered as time runs out. Each unanswered question is scored as a 0, the same as a wrong answer, so what's the point?

If all else fails, choose what you feel is the most likely answer. Guessing is better than not answering the question at all (on a test, not in clinical practice). You have a 1-in-5 chance of being right, and your odds improve if you can eliminate obviously wrong answer choices first.

While you're taking the test, you can go back and change an answer during the allotted time. After you exit a test block, however, what's there is permanent. You can keep track of the questions you want to go back to on the white board that the testing center provides.

Approaching Questions Randomly

Bouncing all over the questions in a block is a bad idea. Remember, many questions are relatively lengthy, and figuring out the right answer requires some time to sort the facts and think. That doesn't change, so it won't serve you to say to yourself, "Oh, I'll save time by answering the easy ones first." Naw, there aren't any easy questions. When you have to go back to a question and reread it, especially a lengthy, complex question, you waste time. You want to use your time as efficiently as possible.

Answer the questions in an orderly way. Otherwise, you run the risk of failing to answer a question (with a guaranteed score of 0). You don't want to be dashing through unanswered questions in the last 2 minutes of the block. Start at the beginning and end at the end.

Reading the Part and Not the Whole

Marriages and business partnerships can fail because the parties don't practice active listening. Your test-taking can fail if you don't practice active reading. *Active reading* means trying to drill past the extraneous information being presented to get to the meat of the question. When Rich first took his medical boards, he often would look at the answer choices first to try to get a sense of where the question was heading. If you're the type of person who needs to list key points and take notes, then by all means, use the white board provided by the testing center to do just that.

Don't be careless! Read the whole question *and the possible answers* carefully. Read the text twice if you have trouble the first time.

Don't skip a key word or phrase, because the correct answer often hinges on it. For example, if a question says a person presents with a painless condition, you can eliminate diagnoses where you'd expect pain to be present. Similarly, any question in which the person presents with a persistent fever should immediately help you eliminate some possible diagnoses and consider others.

Reading carefully means reading slowly. This may sound silly, but you can read a word incorrectly (Barry does this all the time). For example, if you misread "patient is *now* in pain" as "patient is *not* in pain," you'll likely discard the correct diagnosis and pick an incorrect one.

Not Eliminating the Question's Excess

Test-makers love to throw test-takers a few curveballs, which come in the form of TMI — too much information. The smart test-taker eliminates elements in both the question and the answers that don't fit:

- For questions, look out for "too many symptoms." One symptom may be interesting but not germane to the diagnosis.

- For answers, watch for (and eliminate) nonsensical choices. For example, if you see no evidence of deep venous thrombosis in a what-to-prescribe question, then an anticoagulant like warfarin (Coumadin) wouldn't make any sense.

Your goal is to ignore any underbrush in the questions and to narrow the answer choices so the best answer is easier to find.

Not Knowing Common Traps in Questions

Test-makers are resourceful, but they're not infinitely resourceful. You're generally going to be asked two types of questions. The first type is the one-liner question that tests your knowledge base and probably has short answer choices. The second type of question concerns clinical scenarios in which you may be asked to name a diagnosis, interpret a patient's symptoms or abnormal lab values, and/or manage the patient's condition. Knowing the structure types can help you, and not knowing them can hurt you.

Within these question types lie a number of logical traps. Beware the following:

- **Qualifying words in the question:** A correct reading of the question can point you to the correct answer — or at least help you eliminate some answer choices. For example, look for words and phrases such as "physical examination" (that's not a history), "painless" (eliminate conditions associated with pain), "unconscious" (you won't be asking the patient questions), "in utero" (the baby isn't born yet), and "alcoholism" (a factor in many conditions).

- **Patently false answer choices:** If you see a word you've never encountered in your studies, it probably doesn't exist. Eliminate it. By our count, there are at least 210 syndromes, but we assure you that there's no Lennon-McCartney syndrome.

- **Oversimplification:** If an answer choice seems too simple, it probably is. Test-makers love this sort of easy answer choice. Once in a while it's correct, but don't bet your certification/registration/license on it.

- **Overcomplication:** If one of the answer choices seems way too elaborate, it's likely wrong. You can probably eliminate it.

- **Funky ranges:** Some questions present you with ranges of values — time since onset, duration of condition, typical patient age at onset, and so on. Usually, but not always, the correct answer isn't the smallest or the largest value. For example, with fever of unknown origin (FUO), the temperature has to be > 38.3°C (101°F) documented several times for more than 3 weeks. So a temperature of 37.0°C (98.6°F) or a duration of 3 days wouldn't indicate FUO.

Misunderstanding the Question's Essence

What does a question really say? Which answer do the test-makers really want? The idea is to study the question for its essence. How do you learn how to get to the essence of a question? By practice. Lucky for you, there are more than 1,500 practice questions in this book and on its accompanying DVD, not counting those in the chapters.

Some questions are straightforward, and that's good news. You know the answer, or you don't. For example, is *Streptococcus pneumoniae* a cause of community-acquired pneumonia? You can bet your sweet antibiotic it is! For this type of "you know it or you don't" question, build your vocabulary of terms. Also, take a look at the next section on key relationships.

Unfortunately, the good news ends here. Most questions are not straightforward. For example, consider this question from Chapter 4:

What is the treatment of choice for mild persistent asthma?

(A) Inhaled steroids

(B) Daily albuterol

(C) Methacholine (Provocholine)

(D) Daily ipratropium bromide (Atrovent)

(E) Nebulized albuterol and daily ipratropium bromide (Atrovent)

The correct answer is Choice (A). For *mild persistent* asthma, use inhaled steroids. For *intermittent* asthma, using a short-acting inhaler like albuterol is okay. Notice that the essence of this question is "mild persistent" asthma. If the question asked about "intermittent" asthma, the best answer would be Choice (B).

So read the question for its essence. Remember, this is only a test, and passing isn't that hard. Real life is much tougher.

Not Knowing Key Relationships

One of the tools you have in studying for the PANCE are the 300 or so digital flashcards that came with this book. These flashcards enable you to remember the key relationships concerning the many medical conditions that you learned. Especially for the one-liner type of questions that test your medical knowledge base, knowing relationships is the key to answering those questions correctly.

For example, if you're asked a question about Rocky Mountain spotted fever, three quick but important related points should come into your head immediately: it's fatal if not treated, the rash can be on the palms and soles, and the treatment is doxycycline (Vibramycin). We've organized the material in this book so you can review key associations, not just random medical facts.

One way you can make associations is by knowing the key words. The big value in this is on the "you know it or you don't" questions. Look at the following example:

Which one of the following bacteria is associated with a community-acquired pneumonia?

(A) *Streptococcus pneumoniae*

(B) *Pneumocystis jeruvecii*

(C) *Pseudomonas aeruginosa*

(D) *Escherichia coli*

(E) *Klebsiella pneumoniae*

You read this question, and your brain should open its "community-acquired pneumonia" file. You remember that there are the "typicals" and "atypicals." Choice (A) is a common cause of community-acquired pneumonia. How do you eliminate the other choices? By remembering the key associations you made when studying. Choice (B) is associated with HIV. Choice (C) is a cause of external otitis and osteomyelitis in those with diabetes mellitus. If *Pseudomonas aeruginosa* is a cause of any pneumonia, it would be a healthcare-associated pneumonia (it's Gram-negative). Choice (D) is associated with a UTI. Choice (E) can be associated with a healthcare pneumonia, but a big association is a pneumonia in someone with a history of alcoholism.

In general, you can branch out from key words to related groups of key words. Aside from increasing your PANCE score, knowing the relationship among etiologies, conditions, lab values, and treatments is essential in clinical practice. Here are a few sample groups:

- ✔ **Causative organisms:** Know major bacteria, fungi, and viruses and the diseases they relate to. Or consider the converse — know major diseases and the bacteria, fungi, and viruses that can cause them.

- ✔ **Triads:** Know your triads by name, know the three elements of each triad, and of course, be able to equate the presentation of the triad to the condition it suggests. For example, although knowing how Dieulfoy's triad presents is important, knowing that it suggests acute appendicitis is equally important. That suggests a close encounter with a surgeon, because you don't want to risk peritonitis. We list some need-to-know triads in Chapter 22.

- ✔ **Related conditions:** Know which conditions "may also be present." This can influence your answer to a test question. For example, consider the meaning when hypernatremia, hyponatremia, hypercalcemia, or hypocalcemia is present. Recall some of the top two or three differential diagnoses for each medical condition.

- ✔ **Labs:** Granted, there are hundreds of labs, each one with a reference range. Just the same, if you know the biggies, you'll be in better shape. For example, among ions, sodium, calcium, and potassium are the most important. Among the arterial blood gases, think pO_2 and pCO_2. Don't forget about pH and glomerular filtration rate (GFR), either. During the exam, you have access to a list of laboratory reference ranges for the most common tests.

- ✔ **Disease vectors:** How is a disease spread? It may be handy to know that West Nile virus, dengue fever, malaria, epidemic polyarthritis, Rift Valley fever, Ross River fever, St. Louis encephalitis, Japanese encephalitis, yellow fever, and La Crosse encephalitis are all carried by several different mosquitoes.

Not Going with Your Gut

You completed a comprehensive set of courses to acquire your medical knowledge. You used this fine book to hone your awareness of key test topics. Why, then, wouldn't you trust yourself? When your lower GI says an answer is right, follow the instinct. This process puts an answer in place and moves you along to the next question.

If you go blank at some point, man up (or woman up) to overcome this. Let your gut be the basis for action here. Believe us, in the ER you have *less* time to make critical decisions than you'll ever have on the PANCE or PANRE. If you're a working PA or if you've done a clinical rotation in the ER, you know this already. Whenever Rich answered a test question with an answer that went against his initial gut reaction, the majority of the time it was wrong. Don't ignore your intuition.

Not Memorizing Key Points

This is a test. Like any other exam you've taken, you need to memorize key facts. To make the associations that you read about in the prior section, you need to commit some basic information to memory.

If you look at the cardiology chapter (Chapter 3), for example, you need to know the physical exam findings of the various cardiac conditions. You may be familiar with some of these conditions, like aortic stenosis, because you've seen them on your clinical rotations or in your clinical practice, but you need to know the hard facts. Fortunately for you, with the flashcards and the many practice questions in this book, the repetition will breed a sense of familiarity.

Take asthma as another example where memorization is useful. Not only do you need to know the various stages of asthma, but you also need to know the treatments for them. This requires some degree of memorization.

Here are some suggestions on what to focus on as you're memorizing:

✔ Pay attention to our predictions about the likelihood that certain topics will appear on the test. In the various body organ system chapters, we usually declare that a certain subject is virtually guaranteed to appear on the test.

✔ Be familiar with the proportions of questions from different subject areas. The topics of the four chapters in Part II of this book, which deal with four organ systems, historically account for 50 percent of the PANCE questions. See Chapter 2 for more info on the category breakdown.

Don't worry, though. Your knowledge and memorization will all come together with the proper preparation.

Appendix A

About the CD

*Y*ou take many standardized tests using a computer, and the PANCE/PANRE is no exception. This book contains one complete practice exam in Chapter 20 and the answers in Chapter 21. The companion CD gives you four additional practices exams: three for the PANCE and one for the PANRE. All the tests, except one, can be taken timed or untimed. One of the PANCE practice tests can be taken only with the timer ticking away, just like the real test.

As a bonus, the CD contains a set of more than 300 flashcards and a slideshow of dermatologic pictures.

This appendix explains how to use the CD, what it contains, and what to do if you run into problems. *Note:* If you are using a digital version of this book, this appendix does not apply. Please go to http://booksupport.wiley.com for access to the additional content.

System Requirements

Make sure your computer meets the minimum system requirements in the following list. If your computer doesn't match up to most of these requirements, you may have problems using the software and files on the CD.

- ✔ A PC with a Pentium or faster processor or a Mac OS computer with a 68040 or faster processor.
- ✔ Microsoft Windows 98 or later; or a Macintosh running Apple OS X or later.
- ✔ At least 32MB of total RAM installed on your computer.
- ✔ A CD-ROM drive.
- ✔ A monitor capable of displaying at least 256 colors or grayscale.
- ✔ Adobe Reader for viewing the PDFs. If you need a copy, go to http://get.adobe.com/reader/.

If you need more information on the basics, check out these books published by John Wiley & Sons, Inc.: *PCs For Dummies* by Dan Gookin; *Macs For Dummies* by Edward C. Baig; *iMacs For Dummies* by Mark L. Chambers; and *Windows XP For Dummies* and *Windows Vista For Dummies,* both by Andy Rathbone.

Using the CD

To use the CD, follow these steps.

1. **Insert the CD into your computer's CD-ROM drive.**

   The license agreement appears.

   Note to Windows users: The interface won't launch if you have autorun disabled. In that case, choose Start⇨Run. (For Windows Vista, choose Start⇨All Programs⇨ Accessories⇨Run.) In the dialog box that appears, type ***D:\Start.exe***. (Replace *D* with the proper letter if your CD drive uses a different letter. If you don't know the letter, see how your CD drive is listed under My Computer or Computer.) Click OK.

   Notes for Mac Users: When the CD icon appears on your desktop, double-click the icon to open the CD and double-click the Start icon. Also, note that the content menus may not function as expected in newer versions of Safari and Firefox; however, the documents are available by navigating to the Contents folder.

2. **Read through the license agreement and then click the Accept button if you want to use the CD.**

   The CD interface appears. The interface allows you to browse the contents with just a click of a button or two.

What You'll Find on the CD

This section provides a summary of the goodies you can find on the CD.

Practice tests

To help you prepare for the PANCE/PANRE, the CD includes three full-length PANCE practice exams and one full-length PANRE to supplement the practice PANCE from the book. Like the real test, each practice PANCE on the CD has five sections (or blocks) consisting of 60 questions. For two of the practice tests, you can take each block with or without a timer; for the third PANCE, you can take only a timed version, which can give you an idea of how it feels to answer 60 questions in an hour without stopping. The PANRE practice test consists of four sections (blocks) containing 60 questions each. You can take each block with or without a timer.

Of course, the CD contains the answers as well as explanations that tell you why each answer is correct.

Test results can't be saved. We recommend that after you complete a block of questions, you write down the topics of the questions you missed so you can go back and review those areas.

Flashcards

We've included more than 300 flashcards on the CD to test your medical knowledge. We've weighted the number of flashcards to correspond to the proportions of questions from different subject areas on the test.

You'll find the flashcards useful in two ways: First, when you know the answer, just flip the card over to confirm your choice. Second, when a question gives you trouble, you can flip the card over and study the answer.

For your convenience, we categorize the flashcards according to organ system, and we also present all 300+ cards together so you can really test your knowledge. In any category, you can work through the cards in order or choose a random selection.

Slideshow

When you're a PA, you'll be examining and diagnosing patients' conditions first-hand. Because we can't send dozens of diseased patients to you so you can examine their ailments, we've included a slideshow with a few dozen color photos showing you rashes and skin lesions and other bumps and lumps that you'll encounter in your practice. Study these color photos and descriptions to increase your chances of recognizing the conditions on sight.

PDFs

You can find the following PDF (portable document format) files on this CD:

- A summary of general information about the test
- An explanation of how the test is scored

To view a file saved as a PDF, you need a PDF-viewer program. Not to worry — it's probably already installed on your computer, so all you have to do is double-click on the document filename to launch the viewer and see the file. However, if you get an error message, you can go to `get.adobe.com/reader` to download the free Adobe Reader.

Troubleshooting and Customer Care

We tried our best to compile programs that work on most computers with the minimum system requirements. Alas, your computer may differ, and some programs may not work properly for some reason.

The two likeliest problems are that you don't have enough memory (RAM) for the programs you want to use, or you have other programs running that are affecting installation or running of a program. If you get an error message such as `Not enough memory` or `Setup cannot continue`, try one or more of the following suggestions and then try using the software again:

- ✔ **Turn off any antivirus software running on your computer.** Installation programs sometimes mimic virus activity and may make your computer incorrectly believe that it's being infected by a virus.

- ✔ **Close all running programs.** The more programs you have running, the less memory is available to other programs. If you have several other programs running, try closing a couple and then starting the CD again.

- ✔ **Add more RAM to your computer.** This is, admittedly, a somewhat expensive step. However, adding more memory can really help the speed of your computer and allow more programs to run at the same time.

If you have trouble with the CD-ROM, please call Wiley Product Technical Support at 877-762-2974. Outside the United States, call 317-572-3993. You can also contact Wiley Product Technical Support at `http://support.wiley.com`. Wiley will provide technical support only for installation and other general quality control items. For technical support on the applications themselves, consult the program's vendor or author.

To place additional orders or to request information about other Wiley products, please call 877-762-2974.

Index

John Wiley & Sons, Inc.
End-User License Agreement

READ THIS. You should carefully read these terms and conditions before downloading any media from this CD/DVD or website (the "Media"). This is a license agreement "Agreement" between you and John Wiley & Sons, Inc. "Wiley". By downloading Media from this CD/DVD or website, you agree that you have read and accept the following terms and conditions.

1. **License Grant.** Wiley grants to you (either an individual or entity) a nonexclusive license to use one copy of the Media solely for your own personal or business purposes on a single computer (whether a standard computer or a workstation component of a multi-user network). The Media is in use on a computer when it is loaded into temporary memory (RAM) or installed into permanent memory (hard disk, CD-ROM, or other storage device). Wiley reserves all rights not expressly granted herein.

2. **Ownership.** Wiley is the owner of all right, title, and interest, including copyright, in and to the compilation of the Media. Copyright to the individual programs of the Media is owned by the author or other authorized copyright owner of each program. Ownership of the Media and all proprietary rights relating thereto remain with Wiley and its licensers.

3. **Restrictions On Use and Transfer.**

    (a) You may not (i) rent or lease the Media, (ii) copy or reproduce the Media through a LAN or other network system or through any computer subscriber system or bulletin-board system, or (iii) modify, adapt, or create derivative works based on the Media.

    (b) You may not reverse engineer, decompile, or disassemble the Media. You may transfer the Media and user documentation on a permanent basis, provided that the transferee agrees to accept the terms and conditions of this Agreement and you retain no copies. If the Media is an update or has been updated, any transfer must include the most recent update and all prior versions.

    (c) You may not remove or destroy any copyright notices or other proprietary markings on the Media.

    (d) You may not use the Media in any unlawful manner, for any unlawful purpose, or in any manner inconsistent with this EULA.

4. **Restrictions on Use of Individual Programs.** You must follow the individual requirements and restrictions detailed for each individual program on the Media. These limitations are also contained in the individual license agreements contained in the Media. These limitations may include a requirement that after using the program for a specified period of time, the user must pay a registration fee or discontinue use. By downloading the Media, you will be agreeing to abide by the licenses and restrictions for these individual programs that are detailed in the Media. None of the material on this Media may ever be licensed, reproduced, or redistributed by you, in original or modified form, for commercial purposes.

5. **Limited Warranty.**

    (a) WILEY AND THE AUTHOR(S) DISCLAIM ALL WARRANTIES, EXPRESS OR IMPLIED, INCLUDING WITHOUT LIMITATION IMPLIED WARRANTIES OF MERCHANTABILITY AND FITNESS FOR A PARTICULAR PURPOSE, WITH RESPECT TO THE MEDIA, THE PROGRAMS, AND/OR THE SOURCE CODE CONTAINED THEREIN. WILEY DOES NOT WARRANT THAT THE FUNCTIONS CONTAINED IN THE MEDIA WILL MEET YOUR REQUIREMENTS OR THAT THE OPERATION OF THE MEDIA WILL BE ERROR FREE.

    (b) This limited warranty gives you specific legal rights, and you may have other rights that vary from jurisdiction to jurisdiction.

6. **Remedies.**

    (a) In no event shall Wiley or the author be liable for any damages whatsoever (including without limitation damages for loss of business profits, business interruption, loss of business information, or any other pecuniary loss) arising from the use of or inability to use the Media, even if Wiley has been advised of the possibility of such damages.

    (b) Because some jurisdictions do not allow the exclusion or limitation of liability for consequential or incidental damages, the above limitation or exclusion may not apply to you.

7. **U.S. Government Restricted Rights.** Use, duplication, or disclosure of the Media for or on behalf of the United States of America, its agencies and/or instrumentalities "U.S. Government" is subject to restrictions as stated in paragraph (c)(1)(ii) of the Rights in Technical Data and Computer Software clause of DFARS 252.227-7013, or subparagraphs (c) (1) and (2) of the Commercial Computer Software - Restricted Rights clause at FAR 52.227-19, and in similar clauses in the NASA FAR supplement, as applicable.

8. **General.** This Agreement constitutes the entire understanding of the parties and revokes and supersedes all prior agreements, oral or written, between them and may not be modified or amended except in a writing signed by both parties hereto that specifically refers to this Agreement. This Agreement shall take precedence over any other documents that may be in conflict herewith. If any one or more provisions contained in this Agreement are held by any court or tribunal to be invalid, illegal, or otherwise unenforceable, each and every other provision shall remain in full force and effect.